Medical Pharmacology

Principles and Concepts

Medical Pharmacology

Principles and Concepts

Andres Goth, M.D.

Professor
Department of Pharmacology
The University of Texas Health Science Center at Dallas
Southwestern Medical School
Dallas, Texas

Consulting Editor
Elliot S. Vesell, M.D.

Evan Pugh Professor and Chairman
Department of Pharmacology
Pennsylvania State University College of Medicine
Hershey, Pennsylvania

Eleventh edition
With 124 illustrations

The C. V. Mosby Company

ST. LOUIS   TORONTO   1984

MOSBY

A TRADITION OF PUBLISHING EXCELLENCE

Editor: Samuel E. Harshberger
Assistant editor: Anne Gunter
Editing supervisor: Judi Wolken
Manuscript editors: April Nauman, Rebecca A. Reece
Design: Nancy Steinmeyer
Production: Judith A. England, Susan Trail

Eleventh edition

Printed in the United States of America

The C.V. Mosby Company
11830 Westline Industrial Drive, St. Louis, Missouri 63146

Library of Congress Cataloging in Publication Data

Goth, Andres.
    Medical pharmacology.

    "About 20 chapters have been either completely
rewritten or significantly revised by contributors who
are experts in their field."—Pref.
    Includes bibiliographies and index.
    1. Pharmacology.   I.   Vesell, Elliot S., 1933-   .
II. Title. [DNLM: 1.   Pharmacology.   QV 4 G684m]
RM300.G65   1984   615'.7   83-17398
ISBN 0-8016-1962-9

GW/VH/VH   9   8   7   6   5   4   3   2   1   01/B/087

Contributors

CHESTON M. BERLIN, M.D.
Professor of Pediatrics and Pharmacology, Pennsylvania State University College of Medicine, Hershey, Pennsylvania

KARL H. BEYER, Jr., M.D., Ph.D.
Visiting Professor of Pharmacology, Pennsylvania State University College of Medicine, Hershey, Pennsylvania

BURNELL R. BROWN, Jr., M.D., Ph.D.
Professor and Head, Department of Anesthesiology, University of Arizona School of Medicine, Tucson, Arizona

JOHN D. CONNOR, Ph.D.
Professor of Pharmacology, The Pennsylvania State University College of Medicine, Hershey, Pennsylvania

GREGORY G. DIMIJIAN, M.D.
Clinical Assistant Professor of Psychiatry, The University of Texas Health Science Center at Dallas, Southwestern Medical School, Dallas, Texas

SAMSON T. JACOB, Ph.D.
Professor of Pharmacology, Pennsylvania State University College of Medicine, Hershey, Pennsylvania

ANTHONY KALES, M.D.
Professor and Chairman, Department of Psychiatry; Director, Sleep Research and Treatment Center, Pennsylvania State University College of Medicine, Hershey, Pennsylvania

JOAN Y. SUMMY-LONG, Ph.D.
Associate Professor of Pharmacology, Pennsylvania State University College of Medicine, Hershey, Pennsylvania

JOHN R. LUDERER, M.D.
Assistant Professor of Medicine and Pharmacology, Pennsylvania State University College of Medicine, Hershey, Pennsylvania

G. THOMAS PASSANANTI, Ph.D.
Assistant Professor of Pharmacology, Pennsylvania State University College of Medicine, Hershey, Pennsylvania

KATHLEEN M. ROSE, Ph.D.
Associate Professor of Pharmacology, University of Texas Medical School at Houston, Houston, Texas

WALTER B. SEVERS, Ph.D.
Professor of Pharmacology, Pennsylvania State University College of Medicine, Hershey, Pennsylvania

CONSTANTIN R. SOLDATOS, M.D.
Clinical Professor, Department of Psychiatry, Pennsylvania State University College of Medicine, Hershey, Pennsylvania; Chief, Sleep Research Unit, University of Athens School of Medicine, Athens, Greece

ELLIOT S. VESELL, M.D.
Evan Pugh Professor and Chairman, Department of Pharmacology, Pennsylvania State University College of Medicine, Hershey, Pennsylvania

Preface

The eleventh edition of *Medical Pharmacology* is essentially a new book. About 20 chapters have been either completely rewritten or significantly revised by contributors who are experts in their fields. All other chapters have also been brought up to date. The most significant feature of this new edition is its presentation of the most modern pharmacological literature in a readable and easily understood manner.

I am very grateful to the various contributors for their chapters and to Dr. Elliot Vesell for selecting them and coordinating this team effort. The contributors maintained the basic organization and philosophy of the book, which is based on the presentation of the medically relevant aspects of modern pharmacology in a readable manner.

I would like to give special thanks to Dr. Wesley G. Clark and Dr. George W. Read for their help in the completion of the manuscript.

With the tremendous expansion of the discipline, it seemed impractical to include an extensive bibliography, so only a few recent, key references are mentioned at the end of each chapter.

Essentially all new drugs and new pharmacological concepts are discussed in the text. The reader may feel confident that the information presented is based on the most recent pharmacological literature. Furthermore, the importance of this information to medicine and therapeutics is stressed.

Andres Goth

Contents

section three — Psychopharmacology

section four — Depressants and stimulants of the central nervous system

section five — Anesthetics

section six — Drugs used in cardiovascular disease

section seven Drug effects on the respiratory and gastrointestinal tracts

section eight Drugs that influence metabolic and endocrine functions

section nine Chemotherapy

Chapter 1

Introduction

Chemical agents not only provide the structural basis and energy supply of living organisms but also regulate their functional activities. The interactions between potent chemicals and living systems contribute to the understanding of life processes and provide effective methods for the treatment, prevention, and diagnosis of many diseases. Chemical compounds used for these purposes are *drugs*, and their actions on living systems are referred to as *drug effects*.

Pharmacology deals with the properties and effects of drugs or, in a more general sense, with the interactions of chemical compounds and living systems. It is a discipline of biology and is closely related to other disciplines, particularly physiology and biochemistry.

Despite the considerable overlap among the various disciplines of biology, pharmacology is unique in that it deals primarily with the mechanism of action of biologically active substances.

Although its specific aim is to define the biological activity of chemical compounds, pharmacology also contributes greatly to knowledge of living systems. This contribution to the understanding of life processes is valuable to biological sciences in general and to medicine in particular. An understanding of drugs is necessary for the diagnosis, prevention, and treatment of disease. Some aspects of pharmacology are of remote relevance to the study of medicine. To emphasize this distinction, the title *Medical Pharmacology* was chosen for this book.

There are several fields of study that may be considered subdivisions of pharmacology or disciplines related to it.

Pharmacodynamics is the study of drug effects and the handling of drugs by the body. This aspect of pharmacology is perhaps nearest to a basic science of medicine.

Emphasis on mode of action of chemical compounds distinguishes pharmacology from some of the other basic sciences of medicine. As used in medicine, the term *pharmacology* is essentially synonymous with pharmacodynamics.

Chemotherapy is that subdivision of pharmacology which, according to the definition first proposed by Paul Ehrlich, deals with drugs that are capable of destroying invading organisms without destroying the host.

Pharmacy is concerned with the preparation and dispensing of drugs. Today the physician seldom has the need to prepare or dispense drugs. Even the pharmacist has very little to do with the preparation of drugs; most of them are manufactured by large companies. The pharmacist may provide useful services, however, as a member of the health team having special knowledge about drug preparations.

Therapeutics is the art of treatment of disease. *Pharmacotherapeutics* is the application of drugs in the treatment of disease.

Toxicology is the science of poisons and poisonings. Although toxicology may be viewed as a special aspect of pharmacology, it developed into a separate discipline for a variety of reasons. Forensic and environmental medicine requires the services and knowledge of toxicologists with special training in drug identification and poison control.

| HISTORICAL DEVELOPMENT OF PHARMACOLOGY | Although no detailed discussion will be attempted, it should be pointed out that the history of pharmacology can be divided into two periods. The early period goes back to antiquity and is characterized by empirical observations in the use of crude drugs. It is interesting that even primitive people could discover relationships between drugs and disease. The use of drugs has been so prevalent throughout history that Sir William Osler stated (1894) with some justification that "man has an inborn craving for medicine." |

In contrast to this ancient period, modern pharmacology is based on experimental investigations concerning the site and mode of action of drugs. The application of the scientific method to studies on drugs was initiated in France by François Magendie and was expanded by Claude Bernard (1813-1878). The name of Oswald Schmiedeberg (1838-1921) is commonly associated with the development of experimental pharmacology in Germany, and John Jacob Abel (1857-1938) played a similar role in the United States.

The growth of pharmacology was greatly stimulated by the rise of synthetic organic chemistry, which provided new tools and new therapeutic agents. More recently, pharmacology has benefited from developments of other basic sciences and in turn has contributed to their growth.

One of the most dynamic areas of pharmacological research is that which deals increasingly with drug receptors and important new developments; for example, the discovery of the endorphins was made possible by the existence of drug receptors being recognized. There are those who feel that one of the basic functions of pharmacology is to map out drug receptors in the body.

Some of the greatest changes in medicine that have occurred during the last few decades are directly attributable to the discovery of new drugs. Progress in this field has not been without its problems, however. Success in the search for new therapeutic agents has not been matched by equal expertise in the evaluation of their clinical safety and efficacy. Furthermore, the practicing physician has not always been prepared for some of the new drugs whose clinical use requires considerable understanding of basic principles. Nevertheless, in the recent history of pharmacology the main successes more than make up for the problems created by drugs.

There are several reasons for considering pharmacology one of the increasingly important basic sciences of medicine. Some of these are obvious; others are not yet generally recognized.

PLACE OF PHARMACOLOGY IN MEDICINE

Large numbers of drugs are used in the practice of medicine. They cannot be applied intelligently or even safely without some understanding of their mode of action, side effects, toxicity, and metabolism. As powerful new drugs are introduced, adequate pharmacological knowledge on the part of the physician becomes mandatory. Pharmacological terms and concepts are used so commonly in the clinical journals that a physician without a good grounding in the subject would find it difficult to read and understand the current medical literature.

Pharmacology is taught in medical schools for other reasons. As a basic science it contributes important concepts to the understanding of various functions in health and disease. In research, drugs are used increasingly as chemical tools for elucidating basic mechanisms. Also, drugs are being used more frequently for diagnostic purposes.

Pharmacology is also important in medicine because of the commercial influences that are exerted on the physician in the selection of drugs. A good understanding of the principles of pharmacology should provide the physician with a critical attitude and the ability to evaluate rationally the claims made for various new drug preparations.

Finally, it is increasingly recognized that numerous functions in the body are regulated by endogenous compounds, which interact with specific receptors. Many commonly used drugs mimic or oppose the action of these endogenous compounds or alter their metabolism. When viewed in this light, pharmacology is not only the scientific basis of drug therapy but also is a basic science of medicine, which contributes to our understanding of how the body functions in health and disease.

PROBLEM 1-1. In view of the importance of pharmacology in the practice of medicine and the current preoccupation with adverse drug reactions, why is there so little time devoted to it in the medical curriculum? The answer seems to lie in the interdisciplinary nature of the subject and in tradition. Because of its interdisciplinary nature, many areas of pharmacology could be taught in other courses. On the other hand, as has been pointed out by the Nobel Laureate Carl Cori,[1] information on drugs can be taught by experts in various disciplines, but an organized course outside a medical school pharmacology department is difficult.

Tradition is an obstacle to the adequate teaching of pharmacology. It is believed by many medical educators that students will learn about drugs "later," perhaps in residency training or as they pick up information when they need it in their practice. Many critical physicians will admit, however, that what they pick up "later" is some practical information essential for therapeutics but not much basic knowledge of pharmacology, which is often badly needed.

CLINICAL
PHARMACOLOGY

Although pharmacology is concerned with drug effects in all species of animals, in medicine there is increasing interest in clinical pharmacology, which concerns itself with pharmacological effects in human beings.

There are many reasons for this increasing interest. Results of pharmacological studies on animals sometimes cannot be applied to human beings because of species variations in the response to the drug or in its metabolism. Clinical pharmacology also provides scientific methods for the determination of usefulness, potency, and toxicity of new drugs in humans.

Pharmacological knowledge essential for good medical practice includes not only the findings of clinical pharmacology but also those principles and concepts generally derived from animal experiments, which are necessary for thorough understanding of drug effects. Without these principles and concepts, rational therapeutics is impossible.

REFERENCE   1. Cori, C.C.: The call of science, Annu. Rev.
                 Biochem. **38**:1, 1969.

section one

General aspects of pharmacology

Chapter 2

Drug-receptor interactions

Most drugs exert their potent and specific effects in the body by forming a bond, generally reversible, with some cellular constituent. This cellular constituent is the *receptor*. Drugs that interact with a receptor and elicit a response are termed *agonists;* compounds that interact with receptors preventing the action of agonists are referred to as *specific antagonists*.

The existence of receptors for a drug in cells can be deduced from (1) relationships between structure and activity in a homologous or congeneric series, (2) quantitative studies on agonist-antagonist pairs, and (3) selective binding of radioactive drugs to isolated cells or membranes.

The role of a receptor is to recognize a chemical signal and to discriminate between such a signal and other molecules. The drug-receptor interaction is then coupled to an effector mechanism to provide an appropriate cellular response. The presence of receptors at an anatomical site determines the selective nature of many drug effects. For example, acetylcholine applied directly to a motor end-plate produces an action potential. When the same drug is applied a short distance from the end-plate, it has no effect.

Not all drug actions are mediated by receptors. Volatile anesthetics, metal chelating agents, or osmotic diuretics exert effects that are not mediated by specific receptors. On the other hand, drugs of the autonomic nervous system, the opiate narcotics, and most antipsychotic drugs act on specific receptors.

The *receptor concept* was first proposed by Langley in 1878 and was used extensively by Paul Ehrlich in his studies on chemotherapy. Investigating the opposing actions of pilocarpine and atropine on salivary section, Langley hypothesized the presence of some substance in the nerve endings or glands with which the drugs may combine. To Ehrlich, receptors were groups of protoplasmic macromolecules with which drugs could combine *reversibly* or *irreversibly*.

According to current concepts,[3] there are several types of drug receptors. Type I receptors are on the external surface of the plasma membrane of target cells. They interact with drugs that mimic or block the actions of autonomic mediators, such as

RECEPTOR THEORY

7

catecholamines and some peptide hormones and releasing factors. Type II receptors are located in the cytoplasm of target cells and combine with drugs that mimic or block the actions of steroid hormones. The drug-receptor combination may be modified and translocated to the nucleus where it may regulate the concentration of a specific messenger ribonucleic acid (RNA) and, ultimately, the synthesis of proteins. Type III receptors are in the cell nucleus. The thyroid hormone is the best example of a drug that interacts with nuclear receptors.

The binding forces in the drug-receptor interaction are represented by covalent bonds, ionic and hydrogen bonds, and van der Waals bonds. Covalent bonds, because of their high binding energy, provide essentially irreversible effects. If the drug is an antagonist such as phenoxybenzamine, the covalent bond formation results in noncompetitive antagonism. Ionic bonds are important because most drugs contain cationic and anionic groups. Consequently the pH may influence their interaction with receptors. The van der Waals bond is a weak interaction between dipoles. Although the bond energy is only about 0.5 kcal per mole—compared with 100 kcal per mole for the covalent bond—van der Waals bonds are very important in drug-receptor interactions for several reasons. First, the binding forces are summed over a large number of interacting atoms. Second, since drugs and receptors "fit" in three-dimensional space, the critical role of interatomic distances allows the receptor to discriminate between the specific drug and a related compound having a different conformation. Finally, the relatively weak van der Waals bond allows for reversible interactions and drug effects of short duration.

DRUG-RECEPTOR INTERACTIONS

The basic requirement for a receptor is the ability to discriminate signal from noise.[3] To receive the signal the receptor must have an affinity for the drug. At the same time, receptors must have specificity, in other words, an appropriately low affinity for less active drugs.

Affinity is quantitated by studying the dose-response relationship between a drug and a receptor, using one of several methods. In systems in which only dose and response can be determined, the log dose is plotted against the response (Fig. 2-1). In such studies, the dose of a drug that produces a response which is 50% of the maximum is referred to as ED_{50}.

With newer methods usually requiring radioactive drugs, the relationships between free and specifically bound drugs can be quantitated, and much additional useful information can be obtained.

The binding of a drug (D) and a receptor (R) can be represented as follows:

$$[D] + [R] \overset{k_1}{\rightarrow} [DR]$$

The rate at which they combine is described by the rate constant k_1. Since most drug-receptor interactions are reversible, it is also true that

$$[DR] \overset{k_2}{\rightarrow} [D] + [R]$$

Log dose-response curves illustrating difference between potency and efficacy. **A,** *Drug* **FIG. 2-1**
A is much more potent than drug B, but both have the same maximum effect. **B,** *Drug* A
is not only more potent but also has a greater efficacy. It produces a higher peak effect
than drug B.

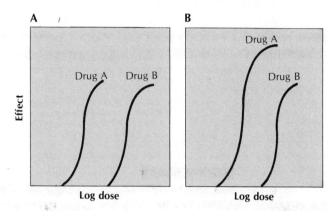

At equilibrium the rates of the forward and backward reactions are equal, and

$$k_1[D][R] = k_2[DR]$$

The concept of K_d emerges if the above equation is rewritten:

$$\frac{[D][R]}{[DR]} = \frac{k_2}{k_1} = K_d$$

K_d is the equilibrium dissociation constant, and it is related to affinity. In the
above equation, if half of the receptors are combined with a drug, the concentrations
of R and DR are equal and will be canceled. It follows then that under those conditions
K_d = D. This means that the free concentration of drug necessary to saturate 50%
of the receptors equals the K_d. If this concentration is low, affinity is high.

In the model described before, the magnitude of a response is a function of the *Affinity and intrinsic*
number of receptors occupied. *Affinity* is the tendency of a drug to form a combination *activity*
with the receptor.

It is known, however, that there are *partial agonists,* which act on the same
receptor as a full agonist but which cannot produce the same maximum effect regardless of concentration. Also, a drug may not only have a higher affinity than
another compound but also may produce a higher maximum effect (Fig. 2-1). Therefore the response is not only a function of the concentration of the drug-receptor
complex but also depends on what is termed *intrinsic activity* or efficacy. This concept
may be defined as the capacity to stimulate for a given receptor occupancy.

An agonist is a drug that has affinity for a receptor and that has intrinsic activity.
A competitive antagonist has affinity for the receptor but lacks significant intrinsic
activity.

Rate models of
drug action

In the foregoing discussion it has been implied that response to a drug is proportional to the concentration of the drug-receptor complex. There are some observations that are difficult to explain by this receptor occupation theory. For example, some drugs stimulate first and then act as antagonists. Nicotine does this in ganglionic transmission.

It is conceivable that the response to a drug is not dependent on the *concentration* of the drug receptor complex but on the *rate* of drug-receptor combinations. Furthermore, the receptor and the rate constants may be altered by the initial drug action. Initial stimulation followed by block as in the case of nicotine would be explained by such alterations of the receptor and the rate constants for association and dissociation.

Drugs that do not
act on specific
receptors

The biological activity of anesthetics, hypnotics, and alcohol depends not on drug-receptor interactions but on the *relative saturation* at some cellular phase (Ferguson's principle).[5] Whenever chemically unrelated drugs give the same effect at the same relative saturation, they are unlikely to act on specific receptors. It is more probable that by reaching a certain level of saturation at some cellular site (the so-called biophase) they hinder some metabolic function.[5]

Receptor regulation

The response to drugs depends on the number of the receptors. This number may be affected by the continued presence of the drug. Generally, receptors that activate adenyl cyclase, α receptors for catecholamines, and insulin receptors tend to decrease in number or undergo down regulation with continued administration of the drugs. This phenomenon is sometimes referred to as *desensitization* or *tachyphylaxis*. Although there is great interest in this form of down regulation, it should be pointed out that most drugs can be administered repeatedly or continuously over periods of hours without much desensitization occurring. Furthermore, only agonists produce homologous down regulation.

There are a few examples of increased receptor numbers produced by certain hormones. For example, the thyroid hormone increases the number of β receptors in the myocardium, which fits with the clinical impression of an increased sensitivity of hyperthyroid individuals to catecholamines.

Receptor-related
diseases

There is great interest in the role of receptor changes in certain diseases. Practically all patients with myasthenia gravis have antibodies to acetylcholine receptors present in the motor end-plate. In some forms of insulin-resistant diabetes, there are antibodies to insulin receptors. Other interesting examples of receptor-related diseases are testicular feminization (androgen insensitivity), familial hypercholesterolemia (decrease in "receptors" for low density lipoproteins), and a number of endocrine diseases that may depend on receptor insensitivity rather than on hormonal deficiencies.

A drug is said to be potent when it has great biological activity per unit weight. When the dose of a drug is plotted on a logarithmic scale against a measured effect, a sigmoid curve is obtained, usually referred to as a log *dose-response* curve. Any point on such a curve could indicate the potency of a drug, but for comparative purposes the dose that gives 50% of the total or maximal effect is most often selected. This dose is the ED_{50}, or effective dose$_{50}$. In Fig. 2-1 drugs A and B produced parallel dose-response curves. The ED_{50} of drug B may be 10 times greater than that of drug A. As a consequence, it may be said that drug A is 10 times as potent as drug B. *It is essential to remember that potencies are compared on the basis of doses that produce the same effect and not by comparing the magnitudes of effects elicited by the same dose.*

A clinically important example of a potency relationship very similar to that given in Fig. 2-1, *A*, is given by the diuretic drugs chlorothiazide and hydrochlorothiazide. One hundred milligrams of hydrochlorothiazide given orally to a patient promotes a significant increase in the urinary output of sodium chloride. It takes about 1 g of chlorothiazide to achieve the same effect. As a consequence, one may say that hydrochlorothiazide is 10 times as potent as chlorothiazide.

Fig. 2-1, *B*, illustrates another property of a drug that should not be confused with potency. Drug A is not only 10 times as potent as drug B, but it also has a higher maximum or "ceiling" of activity. The maximum effect is commonly referred to as *efficacy,* or *power,* and is illustrated by the following example.

Chlorothiazide as well as hydrochlorothiazide has a definite "ceiling" of activity. Two grams of chlorothiazide will exert the maximum effect. Furosemide, however, has not only greater potency than chlorothiazide but also a higher ceiling. It can cause the excretion of a larger percentage of the total amount of sodium chloride filtered by the glomeruli. Consequently, furosemide is not only more *potent* than chlorothiazide but also has greater *efficacy,* or power.

Potency and efficacy are often confused in medical terminology. Potency alone is an overrated advantage in therapeutics. If drug A is 10 times as potent as drug B but has no other virtues, this means only that the patient will take smaller tablets. Pharmaceutical companies often emphasize that a drug is more potent than some other drug. This in itself has little importance to the physician. On the other hand, if the drug has a greater efficacy, it may accomplish things that are unattainable with a less efficacious compound.

QUANTITATIVE ASPECTS OF DRUG POTENCY AND EFFICACY

Parallel shifts in the log dose-response curve may be attributed to varying affinities, whereas variations in the maximum height of the curves are expressions of varying intrinsic activities, or efficacies. In Fig. 2-1, *B*, drug B is less potent than drug A and has less affinity for the receptor. The relative actions of chlorothiazide, hydrochlorothiazide and furosemide discussed previously are examples of the differences between potency and efficacy.

GRAPHIC PRESENTATION OF AFFINITY, INTRINSIC ACTIVITY, AND EFFICACY

FIG. 2-2   *Effect of acetylcholine on tension development of guinea pig ileum. Atropine, a competitive antagonist, causes a parallel shift to the log dose-response curve.*

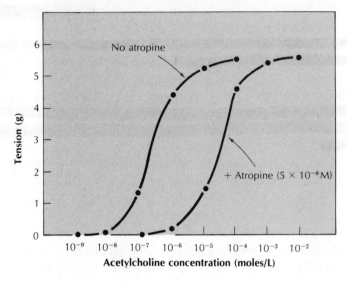

Acetylcholine concentration (moles/L)

AGONIST,
ANTAGONIST,
AND PARTIAL
AGONIST

An agonist is a drug that has affinity and efficacy. It interacts with receptors and elicits a response. Acetylcholine is a good example of an agonist. However, if a log dose-response curve to acetylcholine is obtained in the presence of atropine (an antagonist), it will be found that atropine has no effects of its own but that it shifts the log dose-response curve of acetylcholine to the right.

Atropine is viewed as competing with acetylcholine for the same receptors; in other words, the antagonist has affinity but lacks efficacy. This is an example of *competitive* or *surmountable* antagonism. The key feature of this kind of antagonism is *parallel displacement of the log dose-response curve to the right without a shift in the maximum* (Fig. 2-2).

Somewhere between pure agonists and pure antagonists are the drugs termed partial agonists. They have affinity and some efficacy but may antagonize the action of other drugs that have a higher efficacy.

NONCOMPETITIVE
ANTAGONISM

In the case of atropine and acetylcholine the antagonist and agonist were competing for the same receptor, as evidenced by the parallel shift in the log dose-response curve without a shift in the maximum. In some instances the antagonist may combine irreversibly with the receptor or a portion of the receptor, in which case increasing the concentration of the agonist will never fully overcome the inhibition. The net effect will be a decrease in the maximum height of the log dose-response curve, which is interpreted to reflect a decrease in the number of drug-receptor complexes.

The potency of an antagonist may be measured by several methods. One of the earliest, the measurement of pA2, was introduced by Schild.[14] The value of pA2 is the negative logarithm of the concentration of an antagonist, which necessitates doubling the concentration of the agonist to obtain the same response as in the absence of the antagonist. For example, the pA2 for diphenhydramine as determined on histamine contractions of the guinea pig ileum is approximately 8. This means that a concentration of 10^{-8} M diphenhydramine necessitates the doubling of the concentration of histamine to obtain the same concentration.

PROBLEM 2-1. How is the potency of an antagonist related to its pA2 value? Clearly, the higher the pA2, the more potent the antagonist. If, instead of measuring pA2, the value of pA10 is measured, would it be greater or smaller than the pA2?

For other methods of expressing drug antagonism, the reader should consult the review of Gaddum.[7]

PROBLEM 2-2. What is the role of receptors in causing the opposite effects of the same drug in different organs? For example, acetylcholine relaxes vascular smooth muscle but causes contraction of intestinal or bronchial smooth muscle. Are the receptors different? This is not likely since the same antagonist, atropine, blocks all of these effects. It seems that the drug-receptor interaction only initiates or triggers a series of events, the final outcome of which is built into the system beyond the receptor.

REFERENCES

1. Albert, A.: Relations between molecular structure and biological activity: stages in the evolution of current concepts, Annu. Rev. Pharmacol. 11:13, 1971.
2. Ariëns, E.J., and Beld, A.J.: The receptor concept in evolution, Biochem. Pharmacol. 26:913, 1977.
3. Baxter, J.D., and Funder, J.W.: Hormone receptors, N. Engl. J. Med. 301:1149, 1979.
4. Burgen, A.S.V.: Receptor mechanisms, Annu. Rev. Pharmacol. 10:7, 1970.
5. Ferguson, J.: Use of chemical potentials as indices of toxicity, Proc. R. Soc. Biol. 127:387, 1939.
6. Flier, J.S., Kahn, R., and Roth, J.: Receptors, antireceptor antibodies and mechanisms of insulin resistance, N. Engl. J. Med. 300:413, 1979.
7. Gaddum, J.H.: Drug antagonism, Pharmacol. Rev. 9:211, 1957.
8. Hurwitz, L., and Suria, A.: The link between agonist action and the response in smooth muscle, Annu. Rev. Pharmacol. 11:303, 1971.
9. Jacobs, S., and Cuatrecasas, P.: Cell receptors in disease, N. Engl. J. Med. 297:1383, 1977.
10. King, A.C., and cuatrecasas, P.: Peptide hormone-induced receptor mobility, aggregation and internalization, N. Engl. J. Med. 305:77, 1981.
11. Lefkowitz, R.J.: Direct binding of adrenergic receptors: biochemical, physiologic, and clinical implications, Ann. Intern. Med. 91:450, 1979.
12. Overstreet, D.H., and Yamamura, H.I.: Receptor alterations and drug tolerance, Life Sci. 25:1865, 1979.
13. Porter, R., and O'Connor, M., editors: Molecular properties of drug receptors, Ciba Foundation Symposium, London, 1970, J & A Churchill.
14. Schild, H.O.: pA, a new scale for the measurement of drug antagonism, Br. J. Pharmacol. Chemother. 2:189, 1947.
15. Snyder, S.H.: Receptors, neurotransmitters and drug responses, N. Engl. J. Med. 300:465, 1979.

Chapter 3

Pharmacokinetic principles in the use of drugs

Pharmacokinetics is the study of the time course of absorption, distribution, metabolism, and excretion of drugs and their metabolites in the intact organism. A schematic representation of pharmacokinetics is shown below:

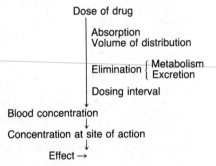

Dose of drug

Absorption
Volume of distribution

Elimination { Metabolism
Excretion

Dosing interval

Blood concentration

Concentration at site of action

Effect →

PASSAGE OF DRUGS ACROSS BODY MEMBRANES

For a drug to reach its site of action it must pass across various body membranes. This can be seen in Fig. 3-1, which depicts the general course of a drug in the body. Absorption, capillary transfer, penetration into cells, and excretion are basic examples of the passage of drugs across body membranes.

Because of its lipoid nature, the cell membrane is highly permeable to lipid-soluble substances. Since the cell is also easily penetrated by water and other small lipid-insoluble substances such as urea, it is postulated that the lipid membrane has pores or channels that allow passage of lipid-insoluble molecules of small dimensions.

In addition to the passive movement of many substances across body membranes, it is necessary to postulate more complex processes for the passage of glucose, amino acids, and some inorganic ions and drug substances. A simplified summary of the various types of passage across body membranes follows:

1. Passive transfer
   a. Simple diffusion
   b. Filtration

2. Specialized transport
   a. Active transport
   b. Facilitated diffusion
   c. Pinocytosis

The essential features of these transfer mechanisms will be described briefly.

Absorption and fate of a drug.

FIG. 3-1

Modified from Brodie, B.B.: Clin. Pharmacol. Ther. 3:374, 1962.

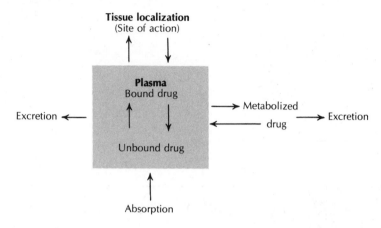

Simple diffusion is characterized by the rate of transfer of a substance across a membrane being directly proportional to the concentration gradient on both sides of the membrane. Both lipid-soluble substances and lipid-insoluble molecules of small size may cross body membranes by simple diffusion. *Filtration* is spoken of when a porous membrane allows the bulk flow of a solvent and the substances dissolved in it except for those that are large. The glomerular membrane of the kidney is a good example of a filtering membrane.

Passive transfer

A special situation exists in the case of partly ionized drugs, since cell membranes are more permeable to the nonionized form of a given drug than to its ionized form because of the greater lipid solubility of the nonionized form. As a consequence, the passage of many drugs into cells and across other membranes becomes a function of the pH of the internal environment and the pK_a of the drug.

The concept of pK_a is derived from the Henderson-Hasselbalch equation. For an acid:

$$pK_a = pH + Log \frac{Molecular\ concentration\ of\ nonionized\ acid}{Molecular\ concentration\ of\ ionized\ acid}$$

For a base:

$$pK_a = pH + Log \frac{Molecular\ concentration\ of\ ionized\ base}{Molecular\ concentration\ of\ nonionized\ base}$$

It follows from these equations that, when a substance is half-ionized and half-nonionized at a certain pH, its pK_a is equal to this pH. In other words, a substance is half-ionized at a pH value that is equal to its pK_a.

Although these concepts may seem academic, they have become of great importance in explaining a number of clinically important facts. For example, weak acids such as salicylic acid (pK_a = 3) are well absorbed from the stomach, whereas

TABLE 3-1   pK$_a$ values for some weak acids and bases (at 25° C)

Weak acids	pK$_a$	Weak bases	pK$_a$
Salicylic acid	3.00	Reserpine	6.6
Aspirin	3.49	Codeine	7.9
Sulfadiazine	6.48	Quinine	8.4
Barbital	7.91	Procaine	8.8
Boric acid	9.24	Ephedrine	9.36
		Atropine	9.65

TABLE 3-2   Effect of pH on the ionization of salicylic acid (pK$_a$ 3)

pH	Percent nonionized
1	99.0
2	90.0
3	50.0
4	9.09
5	1.00
6	0.10

weak bases such as quinine (pK$_a$ = 8.4) are not absorbed until they reach the less acidic intestine. The influence of urinary pH on the excretion of salicylic acid and phenobarbital represents another example of the dependence of diffusion on the pK$_a$ of drugs.

The pK$_a$ values for a number of acidic and basic drugs are listed in Table 3-1. It should be remembered that for acidic drugs the lower the pK$_a$, the stronger the acid, whereas for basic drugs the higher the pK$_a$, the stronger the base.

The relationships between pH, pK$_a$, and ionization of an acidic drug are illustrated in Table 3-2, with salicylic acid as an example.

Specialized transport   The passage of many substances into cells and across body membranes cannot be explained simply on the basis of diffusion of filtration. For example, compounds may be taken up against a concentration gradient, great selectivity can be shown for compounds of the same size, competitive inhibition can occur among substances handled by the same mechanisms, and in some instances metabolic inhibitors can block the transport processes.

To explain these phenomena the existence of specific *carriers* in membranes has been postulated. *Active transport* is spoken of when, in addition to many other criteria, substances are moving against a concentration or electrochemical gradient. *Facilitated diffusion* is a special form of carrier transport that has many of the characteristics of active transport, but the substrate does not move against a concentration gradient. The uptake of glucose by cells is an example of facilitated diffusion. *Pinocytosis* refers to the ability of cells to engulf small droplets. This process may be of some importance in the uptake of large molecules.

PRINCIPLES OF PHARMACO-KINETICS

Studies on drug distribution, absorption, and excretion led to the concept that the body may be treated as if it consisted of different compartments. A drug is transferred from one compartment to another in conformance with first-order kinetics. The simplest model, the "one-compartment model," assumes that after administration drugs are homogeneously distributed throughout the tissues and fluids of the body (Fig. 3-1). In this model the *apparent volume of distribution* (V_d) is determined using the following equation:

$$V_d = \frac{\text{Amount of drug in the body}}{\text{Concentration of drug in plasma}}$$

In determining the apparent volume of distribution, it is not implied that the concentration of the drug in various tissues is the *same* as in plasma. It is assumed, however, that changes in plasma concentrations reflect changes in tissue concentrations. If a drug is concentrated in some tissues, its apparent volume of distribution may be very large, even greater than total body water.

In most instances both the absorption and elimination of drugs take place according to an exponential decay curve (Fig. 3-2). This exponential process follows first-order kinetics; in other words, a constant fraction of the drug is absorbed or eliminated per unit time. The time required for 50% completion of the process is known as the *half-time* or $t_{1/2}$, which is independent of the concentration of the drug. Measurement of the half-time may be understood by examining Fig. 3-2. It can be calculated that it requires four half-times for the exponential processes to become 94% complete. Thus, it takes more than four half-times for the drug to be completely eliminated.

In a few instances elimination is a zero-order process; that is, the same quantity of drug is eliminated per unit time. The best example is alcohol. It is assumed that the saturation of the metabolizing enzymes is responsible for the deviation from first-order kinetics. In other cases, the rate of elimination may be dose related so that small doses are handled by first-order kinetics, but as the dose is increased half-times become prolonged. Examples of drugs that show dose-related elimination are aspirin and phenytoin.

Two-compartment open model

The single-compartment model just discussed assumes an instantaneous and homogeneous distribution of drugs throughout the body. This is obviously an oversimplification. A *two-compartment open model* describes more adequately the observed changes in the concentration of drugs in the body (Fig. 3-3).

The two-compartment model envisions the existence of a small central compartment and a larger peripheral compartment. Although no specific anatomical spaces are implied, the central compartment usually corresponds to the blood volume and the extracellular fluid volume of highly perfused organs. The peripheral compartment consists of more poorly perfused tissues such as skin, fat, and muscle.

It is assumed further that drugs enter the central compartment and are eliminated from that compartment, although some reversible transfer occurs to the peripheral compartment that acts as a reservoir.[6]

FIG. 3-2   *Schematic representation of drug disappearance curves and biological half-life. The y axis is on the arithmetic scale in* **A** *and on the logarithmic scale in* **B**. *Drug* A *has a biological half-life of 1 hour. The biological half-life of drug* B *is 2 hours.*

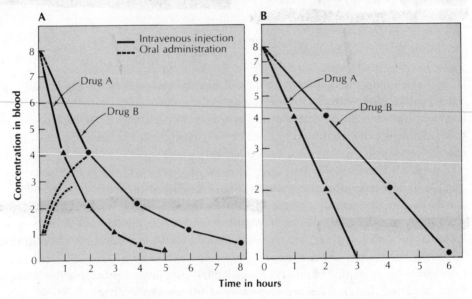

FIG. 3-3   *Diagram of two-compartment open model.*

Modified from Greenblatt, D.J., and KochWeser, J. Reprinted, by permission. From the New England Journal of Medicine 293:702, 1975.

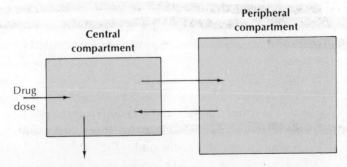

The process whereby a drug is made available to the fluids of distribution is referred to as *absorption*. The rate of this process depends on the method of administration, solubility, and other physical properties of the drug.

ABSORPTION

Drugs are administered by the oral route in many different forms—solutions, suspensions, capsules, and tablets with various coatings. When the drug is not in solution, its rate of absorption will be the net result of the two processes: the process of solution and the absorption process itself. The solution process can be altered by pharmaceutical manipulations, thus influencing the absorption rate, but the absorption process is a basic characteristic of the membranes of the gastrointestinal tract.

Absorption from the gastrointestinal tract

In general, the absorption of drugs from the gastrointestinal tract can be explained by simple diffusion across a membrane having the characteristics of a lipoid structure with water-filled pores. Simple diffusion does not account for the uptake of sugars and other nutrients, in which case absorption can only be explained in terms of active mechanisms. A useful principle, derived from experimental data, is that the limiting membrane is permeable to nonionized lipid-soluble forms of drugs and less permeable to the ionized form. This principle has considerable predictive value. Weak acids such as salicylates and barbiturates are largely nonionized in the acidic gastric contents and are therefore well absorbed from the stomach. Such weak bases as quinine or ephedrine and highly ionized quaternary amines such as tetraethylammonium are not significantly absorbed from the stomach. Alkalinization of gastric contents would be expected to decrease absorption of weak acids from the stomach and increase that of weak bases.

Absorption from the small intestine is similar in principle to that from the stomach, except that the pH of intestinal contents is usually 6.6. Interestingly, drug distribution studies between plasma and small intestinal fluid would indicate a possible pH value of 5.3 for the area just adjacent to the intestinal absorbing membrane. Weakly acidic and weakly basic drugs are well absorbed from the small intestine, but highly ionized acids and bases are not well absorbed. Special mechanisms exist for the absorption of sugars, amino acids, and compounds related to normal nutrients. Some inorganic ions such as sodium and chloride are well absorbed despite the fact that they are in the ionic form.

In the oral cavity the oral mucosa also appears to behave as a lipid pore membrane, and drugs may be absorbed in sublingual administration. Nitroglycerin is usually administered in this manner.

Drug effects on gastric emptying may greatly affect absorption. For example, chloroquine has a much higher LD_{50} when given by mouth to rats than after its direct administration into the intestine. This difference is a consequence of inhibition of gastric emptying by chloroquine.

When injected intravenously, a drug is rapidly distributed in the various compartments of the body.

The rate of absorption following subcutaneous or intramuscular injection depends

Absorption with parenteral administration

largely on two factors: solubility of the preparation and blood flow through the area. Suspensions or colloidal preparations are absorbed more slowly than aqueous solutions. Advantage is taken of this fact in many instances when prolonged absorption is desirable. For example, protamine is added to insulin to form a suspension and thereby decrease the rate of absorption from the subcutaneous depot site. The various injectable penicillin suspensions are good examples of prolonging the action of a therapeutic agent by slowing its absorption.

The blood flow through a tissue has much to do with the speed of absorption of a drug from its site of injection. Absorption from a subcutaneous site may be very slow in the presence of peripheral circulatory failure. This has been observed in the subcutaneous administration of morphine to patients in shock. Similarly, the greater blood flow per unit weight of muscle is responsible for the more rapid absorption of drugs from this tissue than from subcutaneous fat.

Certain practical consequences of these facts may be of real clinical importance. Cooling an area of injection will slow absorption, a desirable effect if an excessive dose has been inadvertently injected or if untoward reactions begin to develop in an unusually susceptible patient. On the other hand, massage of the site of injection will speed up absorption.

Rate-controlled drug delivery	There is increasing interest in methods of administration of drugs that maintain a fairly uniform concentration of the active agent at its site of action. Examples of these methods are pumps, local delivery systems, and transdermal devices. Pumps can be worn externally or can be implanted under the skin. The insulin infusion pump is finding application in correcting the metabolic abnormalities of patients with diabetes. Pilocarpine is ordinarily used as eyedrops. Frequent administration is necessary because of rapid clearance. A device can be placed under the lower eyelid that releases the drug uniformly without systemic side effects. Transdermal devices are used increasingly for the administration of scopolamine and nitroglycerin.
Clinical pharmacology of absorption: bioavailability	Drugs used in medicine seem to fall into three categories of absorption. Some are completely absorbed, some are not significantly absorbed, and still others are partially absorbed. Examples of well-absorbed drugs are most sulfonamides, digitoxin, aspirin, and barbiturates. Drugs not absorbed significantly include streptomycin, neomycin, and kanamycin. Examples of partially or variably absorbed drugs are penicillin G, certain digitalis glycosides, and dicumarol.

Drugs that are incompletely and variably absorbed present a problem to the physician, since dosage cannot be used as a guide to adequate treatment. In this situation it is helpful to monitor the concentration of the drug in the blood or to carefully follow a characteristic effect of the drug.

The dosage form of the drug has a great influence on absorption. Solutions are absorbed most rapidly and coated tablets most slowly. Enteric-coated tablets are commonly used to provide a sustained level of the drug in the body, but despite the popularity of this dosage form, it cannot be considered a predictable method of administering drugs. There are great individual variations in gastric emptying and rate of dissolution of such preparations. They may even be eliminated unchanged in the feces.

There is much current interest in observations indicating that various preparations of the same drug administered orally may give different serum concentrations. The term *bioavailability* has been defined as the relative absorption efficiency of a test dosage form relative to a standard oral or intravenous preparation.

The most popular mode of drug administration is the oral route. After oral administration, the area under blood drug concentration–time curve (AUC) reflects the amount of drug that reaches the systemic sampling site. The ratio of $AUC_{oral}/AUC_{intravenous}$ is a measure of the bioavailability of the drug after oral administration.[3]

BIOAVAILABILITY

When administered orally, drugs must pass through the intestinal wall and ordinarily must traverse the liver before reaching the systemic sampling site. Even with complete gastrointestinal absorption a fraction of the dose may not reach the sampling site because of metabolism within gut or liver. This concept is referred to as "first-pass" effect and is important for drugs such as imipramine, lidocaine, meperidine, nortriptyline, phenacetin, propranolol, and others.[3]

"FIRST-PASS" EFFECT

Once a drug reaches the plasma, its main fluid of distribution, it must pass across various barriers to reach its final site of action. The first of these barriers is the capillary wall. Through processes of diffusion filtration, most drugs rapidly cross the capillary wall, which has the characteristics of a lipid membrane with water-filled pores. Lipid-soluble substances diffuse through the entire capillary endothelium, whereas lipid-insoluble drugs pass through pores, which represent a fraction of the total capillary surface. The capillary transfer of lipid-insoluble substances is inversely related to molecular size. Large molecules such as dextran are transferred so slowly that they can be used as plasma substitutes.

DISTRIBUTION OF DRUGS IN THE BODY

There are several factors that contribute to the unequal distribution of drugs in the body. Some of these are (1) binding to plasma proteins, (2) cellular binding, (3) concentration in body fat, and (4) the blood-brain barrier.

The *binding of drugs to plasma proteins* creates a higher concentration of the drug in the blood than in the extracellular fluid. It also provides a depot, since the bound portion of the drug is in equilibrium with the free form. As the unbound fraction is excreted or metabolized, additional amounts are eluted from the protein. Protein binding prolongs the half-life of a drug in the body, since the bound fraction is not filtered through the renal glomeruli and is not exposed to processes of biotransformation until freed.

The protein-bound fraction of a drug is generally inactive until it becomes free. Thus the protein-bound fractions of sulfonamides and penicillins exert no chemotherapeutic effect. The protein responsible for binding is usually albumin, although

Factors contributing to the unequal distribution of drugs

globulins may be very important in relation to the binding of some hormonal agents and drugs.

The binding capacity of proteins is not unlimited. Once it becomes saturated, a sudden increase in toxicity may occur with further administration of some drugs. In hypoalbuminemia, toxic manifestations to drugs may appear as a consequence of deficiency in the binding protein.

Drugs may influence the protein binding of other substances or drugs. Thus salicylates decrease the binding of thyroxine to proteins. The binding of bilirubin to albumin may be inhibited by a variety of drugs such as sulfisoxazole or salicylates, the free bilirubin thereby becoming ultrafiltrable.

Binding to plasma protein influences not only the biological activity of drugs but also their distribution. A highly protein-bound drug could displace another and increase its pharmacological activity and toxicity, which changes its distribution.[1] Fatal kernicterus has occurred in premature infants who were given sulfisoxazole. The sulfonamide displaced bilirubin from plasma protein and thereby promoted the penetration of the bile pigment into the brains of the infants. Sulfinpyrazone can increase the concentration of sulfonamides in the fetus by a similar mechanism of displacement on plasma proteins of the mother. Other examples of drug interactions based on displacement in protein binding will be discussed in Chapter 63.

The *cellular binding* of drugs is usually a result of an affinity for some cellular constituent. The high concentration of the antimalarial drug quinacrine (Atabrine) in the liver or muscle is probably caused by the affinity of this drug for nucleoproteins.

The short duration of action of certain drugs such as the thiobarbiturate intravenous anesthetics has been explained on the basis of the rapid uptake by the brain, followed by a rapid decrease as the concentration of the drug in the blood falls.

The *blood-brain barrier* represents a unique example of unequal distribution of drugs. Even if injected intravenously, many drugs fail to penetrate the central nervous system, the cerebrospinal fluid, or the aqueous humor as rapidly as they do other tissues. Known exceptions to this principle are the neurohypophysis and the area postrema.

The capillaries in the central nervous system (CNS) are enveloped by glial cells, which represent a barrier to many water-soluble compounds, although they are permeable to lipid-soluble substances. Thus quaternary amines penetrate the CNS poorly, but the general anesthetics do so with ease.

A fact of great importance in medicine is the change in the permeability of various barriers produced by inflammation. In the early days of penicillin therapy it was known that the administration of large doses to normal persons failed to produce detectable levels of the antibiotic in the cerebrospinal fluid. It was found, however, that penicillin would penetrate into the spinal fluid of patients with meningitis.

Although many drugs do not penetrate the cerebrospinal fluid well, they can move efficiently in the reverse direction when administered by intracisternal injection. Perhaps they are removed from the cerebrospinal fluid by filtration across the arachnoid villi. In addition, the choroid plexus is capable of pumping out certain substances from the cerebrospinal fluid—for example, penicillin.[8]

The passage of drugs into *milk* may be explained by diffusion of the nonionized, nonprotein-bound fraction. Since most drugs are weak electrolytes, they will appear in varying amounts in milk and may exert adverse effects on the breast-fed infant. When taken in larger than average doses by the mother, atropine, bromides, anthraquinones, metronidazole, and ergot alkaloids may cause intoxication in the breast-fed infant. On the other hand, the following drugs appear in milk only in small quantities and are generally of no clinical significance for the infant: morphine, codeine, phenolphthalein, tolbutamide, quinine, and salicylates. Large doses of drugs in general should not be administered to the mother who is breast-feeding her child without considering the possible danger to the infant.

The most important route of excretion for most drugs is the kidney. Many drugs are also excreted into bile, but they are then usually recycled through the intestine, making this route quantitatively unimportant. Excretion of drugs into milk may have some significance for the breast-fed child but is not an important avenue of excretion for the mother. Elimination of drugs through the lungs, salivary and sweat glands, and feces is important only in special cases to be discussed under individual drugs.

EXCRETION OF DRUGS

Two major mechanisms are involved in the renal handling of drugs: glomerular filtration with variable tubular reabsorption and tubular secretion. The half-life of a drug in the body will be influenced also by such extrarenal factors as plasma protein binding, the existence of tissue depots and, most important, by the rate of drug metabolism.

The usual course of the drug is filtration through the glomeruli and partial resorption by the tubules. Since water is reabsorbed to a much greater extent than are most drugs, the concentration of drugs in the urine is most frequently greater than in plasma.

A study of the excretion of weak electrolytes has revealed an interesting connection between the pH of urine and renal handling of these drugs. Generally, drugs that are bases are excreted to a greater extent if the urine is acidic, whereas acidic compounds are excreted more favorably if the urine is alkaline. The magnitude of this pH dependence is influenced also by the dissociation constant of a given drug. To explain these results it has been postulated that the undissociated fraction is reabsorbed more readily than the ionic form of a drug. This thesis is favored by the known lipid solubility of undissociated electrolytes.

A practical application of this knowledge has been proposed in the treatment of phenobarbital poisoning. Since phenobarbital is a weak acid having a pK_a of 7.3, its dissociation is greatly influenced by changes in pH at levels obtainable in mammalian urine. Alkalinization of the urine by the administration of sodium bicarbonate causes a significant increase in the excretion of phenobarbital.

Since urine is normally acidic, the excretion of weakly acidic drugs by renal handling alone would require a very long time. Fortunately, drug metabolism tends to transform these into stronger acids, thereby increasing the percentage of the ionic forms and hindering their tubular resorption.

In addition to glomerular filtration with passive tubular resorption, the renal tubule can actively secrete organic anions and cations. Examples of organic anions are aminohippurate sodium, iodopyracet (Diodrast), phenol red, and penicillin; examples of organic cations are tetraethylammonium, mepiperphenidol (Darstine), and N-methylnicotinamide. These active secretory processes may also handle other anions and cations such as salicylic acid, quinine, and tolazoline (Priscoline). Competition for active tubular secretion exists among the various anions and cations.

Drugs that, in addition to undergoing glomerular filtration, are also secreted by the tubules (such as penicillins) have a very short half-life. Efforts have been made to inhibit the process of tubular secretion by drugs such as probenecid, which was specifically developed for this purpose. Usually, however, it is simpler to prolong the half-life of drugs by slowing their absorption. This is the reason for the development of many penicillin preparations that are absorbed slowly following intramuscular injection.

DRUG DISAPPEARANCE CURVES　　The final net effect of absorption, excretion, distribution, and drug metabolism can be described in the form of drug disappearance curves, using blood or tissue concentration data.

A careful examination of Fig. 3-2 and most other drug disappearance studies indicates that they follow an *exponential decay* curve.

Nonlinear pharmacokinetics and interindividual variations　　Many drug disappearance curves are not as smooth as the hypothetical ones shown in Fig. 3-2. There are several reasons for nonlinearity. The limited capacity of drug-metabolizing enzymes may lead to increased half-times with increasing doses of plasma concentrations. For example, increasing the dose of aspirin from 0.5 to 1.0 g every 8 hours may delay the steady state from 2 days to 1 week.

Interindividual variations may also be considerable.[4] Drugs such as desipramine, dicumarol, and phenylbutazone may vary greatly in regard to half-life or steady state plasma concentrations, although the patients are receiving the same dosage regimen.[4]

Implications of exponential drug disappearance curve　　The frequency of drug administration to patients is often dependent on the biological half-life of the drug. This is always the case when a sustained blood level of the drug is desirable. For example, the sulfonamides should be used in such a manner that a sustained blood level is achieved. The frequency with which various members of the sulfonamide group of drugs is administered depends then on the biological half-life. The $t_{1/2}$ of sulfisoxazole in humans is 8 hours, whereas that of sulfamethoxypyridazine is 34 hours. It is not surprising, then, that the former is administered orally every 4 hours and the latter every 24 hours. The delay in ab-

Logarithm of drug concentration in blood plotted against time (solid line) after intravenous   **FIG. 3-4**
administration of a drug whose disposition can be described by a two-compartment model.
Broken line (----) represents extrapolation of terminal (B) phase. The ·-·-··-·- line was
obtained by method of residuals.

From Dvorchik, B.H., and Vesell, E.S.: Clin. Chem. 22:868, 1976.

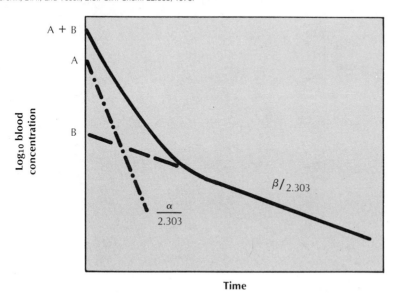

sorption after oral administration is the main reason why these drugs are administered more frequently than could be predicted by their half-lives.

Occasionally the physician wishes to obtain a steadily rising blood or tissue level of a drug until a certain effect is achieved. Quinidine is sometimes given orally every hour for several doses until atrial fibrillation stops. In this case the physician deliberately creates drug cumulation by giving quinidine more frequently than would be justified on the basis of its $t_{1/2}$.

Failure to appreciate the exponential nature of drug disappearance can lead to erroneous ideas in therapeutics. For example, if a drug has a short duration of action, doubling the dose will not double the duration of its effect.

Drugs may be administered in a single dose or in a repetitive fashion. Fig. 3-4   ***DOSAGE***
shows a drug concentration curve following a single intravenous administration. From   ***SCHEDULES AND***
such a curve it is possible to calculate the apparent volume of distribution, since the   ***PHARMACO-***
total amount of drug is known and blood concentration can be extrapolated to zero   ***KINETICS***
time. The ratio of these figures gives the apparent volume of distribution.

If the drug is administered orally in a single dose, the curve will have an ascending limb, a peak, and a descending limb. Variations in absorption and elimination may

FIG. 3-5 *Plot of concentration of a drug in blood after repetitive oral administration of equal doses at equal time intervals.*

From Dvorchik, B.H., and Vesell, E.S.: Clin. Chem. *22:*868, 1976.

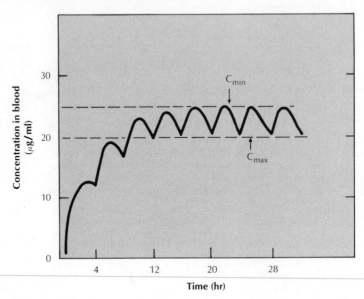

greatly influence the concentration curve reflecting changes in the peak effect, the time required for achieving the peak effect, and the duration of action of the drug.

Repetitive dosing If a drug is given repetitively at intervals shorter than the time necessary for its complete elimination, it will accumulate in the body. As stated before, more than four half-times are required for complete clearance. A typical plot of the concentration of a drug in blood after repetitive oral administration of equal doses at equal time intervals is depicted in Fig. 3-5. It may be seen that the drug concentration rises until it reaches a *plateau*. The curve also shows *fluctuations*.

The plateau concentration is reached in little more than four half-times. More precisely, in four half-times a concentration equal to 94% of the maximum is reached. The time required to reach the plateau depends *only* on the elimination half-time. The maximum concentration of the drug at the plateau level depends on the maintenance dose and the elimination half-time. The maintenance dose is the amount of drug administered at each dosage interval.

It is useful to compare the maximum drug concentration reached after a single dose with that obtained after repetitive dosage. If a drug is administered at intervals equal to its elimination half-time, its concentration at the plateau will be about 1.5 times that reached after a single dose. Many drugs are administered at intervals shorter than their elimination half-time. If a drug has a half-time of 7 days and it is administered once a day, it will take more than 28 days (four half-times) to reach a plateau concentration.

The fluctuations in drug concentration depend on the maintenance dose, the dose interval, and the elimination half-time. Frequent administration of a drug tends to minimize fluctuations in the drug concentration, since the ratio of dosage interval per half-time is decreased.

As shown in Fig. 3-5, repetitive administration of equal doses of a drug will produce a desired plateau concentration, which may require many hours or days, depending on the elimination half-time. In many clinical situations, the physician does not consider such a long wait desirable and administers an *initial loading dose,* followed by a maintenance dose. This is usually done with digitalis glycosides, which have a long half-time of elimination. In this case, the initial loading dose is larger than the maintenance doses.

The importance of fluctuations depends on the drug and on the clinical situation. With some drugs, such as penicillin, large fluctuations are quite acceptable, whereas with the sulfonamides sustained blood levels are necessary to achieve a therapeutic objective. Impaired renal function has an important effect on dosage of drugs that are cleared by the kidney. In this situation, either the dose must be decreased or the dose interval must be increased with corresponding changes in drug concentrations.

Total body clearance of a drug, which results from all processes of elimination, may be determined by the following equation:

Total body clearance

$$\text{Clearance} = (V_c)(k_e) = \text{Dose}/\text{AUC}$$

(where V_c is the apparent volume of distribution, k_e is the rate constant for the overall elimination of drug from the body, and AUC is the area under the blood concentration curve)

PROBLEM 3-1. *A sleeping medication has a half-life of 1 hour. It is administered in a dose of 100 mg, and the patient wakes up when only 12.5 mg remain in the body. How many hours will the patient sleep? If 200 mg of the same drug is administered, how much longer will the patient sleep? The answer can be found by examining Fig. 3-2. Doubling the dose simply adds one half-life to the duration of sleep.*

In general, if a drug has a short duration of action, the following methods are available for prolonging its action:

1. Frequent administration. Most sulfonamides are administered every 4 hours.
2. Slowing absorption. Enteric coating and other pharmaceutical maneuvers can accomplish this.
3. Interfering with renal excretion. Probenecid blocks the excretion of penicillin.
4. Inhibiting drug metabolism. Allopurinol was originally developed for blocking the metabolic degradation of mercaptopurine.

REFERENCES

1. Anton, A.H., and Rodriguez, R.E.: Drug induced change in the distribution of sulfonamides in the mother rat and its fetus, Science **180**:974, 1973.
2. Bennett, W.M., Singer, I., and Coggins, C.H.: A practical guide to drug usage in adult patients with impaired renal function, JAMA **214**:1468, 1970.
3. Dvorchik, B.H., and Vesell, E.S.: Pharmacokinetic interpretation of data gathered during therapeutic drug monitoring, Clin. Chem. **22**:868, 1976.
4. Gibaldi, M., and Levy, G.: Pharmacokinetics in clinical practice, JAMA **235**:1864, 1976.
5. Goldman, P.: Rate-controlled drug delivery, N. Engl. J. Med. **307**:286, 1982.
6. Greenblatt, D.J., and Koch-Weser, J.: Clinical pharmacokinetics, N. Engl. J. Med. **293**:702, 1975.
7. LaDu, B.N., Mandel, H.G., and Way, E.L.: Fundamentals of drug metabolism and drug disposition, Baltimore, 1971, The Williams & Wilkins Co.
8. Levine, R.R.: Pharmacology: drug actions and reactions, Boston, 1973, Little Brown & Co.
9. Ther, L., and Winne, D.: Drug absorption, Annu. Rev. Pharmacol. **11**:57, 1971.

Chapter 4

Drug metabolism and enzyme induction

If the body depended solely on excretory mechanisms for ridding itself of drugs, lipid-soluble compounds would be retained almost indefinitely (p. 23). Drug metabolism generally results in the formation of more water-soluble metabolites that are not well reabsorbed by the renal tubules and are efficiently excreted (Fig. 4-1).

Drug metabolism varies greatly in different species and in individuals of the same species. For example, in humans the effect of a single therapeutic dose of meperidine lasts 3 to 4 hours, but the drug has very transient effects in dogs. This is understandable, since meperidine is metabolized in humans at a rate of 20% per hour, in contrast with 90% per hour in dogs.

Elimination of drugs.   *FIG. 4-1*

From Remmer, H.: Am. J. Med. **49**:617, 1970.

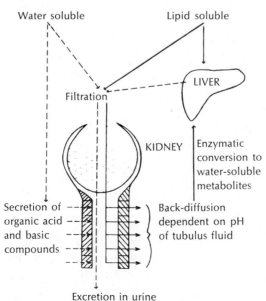

TABLE 4-1	Drug metabolism and enzymes of the endoplasmic reticulum	
Drug metabolism		Enzyme
Oxidations of aliphatic and aromatic groups		Cytochrome P-450
Barbiturates		
Diazepoxides		
Phenothiazines		
Meprobamate		
Phenytoin		
Antihistaminics		
Acetophenetidin		
Aminopyrine		
Some synthetic steroids		
Reductions of azo and nitro groups		Flavin enzymes
Hydrolyses of esters and amides		Esterases
Conjugations with glucuronic acid		Transferases
Alcohols		
Phenols		

Modified from Remmer, H.: Am. J. Med. **49**:617, 1970.

DRUG METABOLISM

Chemical reactions in drug metabolism

The chemical reactions involved in drug metabolism or *biotransformation* are classified as microsomal oxidations, nonmicrosomal oxidations, reductions, hydrolyses, and conjugations.[6] The various pathways of drug metabolism will be discussed, with specific examples given. Since microsomal enzymes play a predominant role in biotransformation (Table 4-1), their functions will be summarized first.

MICROSOMAL ENZYMES

The microsomal enzymes of the liver, which are part of the smooth endoplasmic reticulum, convert many lipid-soluble drugs and foreign compounds into more water-soluble metabolites. Early studies on this system were performed by several investigators.[6]

The microsomal drug-metabolizing enzymes represent a mixed-function oxidase system. In the presence of nicotinamide adenine dinucleotide phosphate (NADPH) and oxygen the enzyme system transfers one atom of oxygen to the drug while another atom of oxygen is reduced to form water. The general scheme is as follows:

$$NADPH + A + H_2 \rightarrow AH_2 + NADP^+$$

$$AH_2 + O_2 \rightarrow \text{``Active oxygen''}$$

$$\text{``Active oxygen''} + Drug \rightarrow \text{Oxidized drug} + A + H_2O$$

$$NADPH + O_2 + Drug = NADP^+ + H_2O + \text{Oxidized drug}$$

In this general scheme A is cytochrome P-450, which is the terminal oxidase for a variety of drug oxidative reactions. Cytochrome P-450 is so named because this hemoprotein in its reduced form can combine with carbon monoxide, the product having an absorption peak at 450 nm. Other essential enzymes in the reaction include NADPH cytochrome P-450 reductase, which reduces the oxidized P-450.

The reactions catalyzed by the microsomal drug-metabolizing enzymes include hydroxylation of aromatic rings, aliphatic hydroxylations, *N*-dealkylations, *O*-dealkylations, deaminations, sulfoxidations, and *N*-oxidations.

Induction and inhibition of microsomal hydroxylase. Phenobarbital and many other lipid-soluble drugs may cause hypertrophy of the smooth endoplasmic reticulum and an increase in the amount of microsomal hydroxylase.

Premature infants and persons with liver disease may have a deficiency of the microsomal enzymes. Some drugs may also inhibit the drug-metabolizing enzymes.

Hydroxylation of aromatic rings. Acetanilid is changed to *p*-hydroxyacetanilid, more commonly known as *N*-acetyl-*p*-aminophenol. Phenobarbital is changed to the inactive *p*-hydroxyphenobarbital.

Phenobarbital   [o]   *p*-Hydroxyphenobarbital

Side chain oxidation (aliphatic hydroxylation). Pentobarbital is changed to pentobarbital alcohol. Meprobamate is changed to hydroxymeprobamate.

Pentobarbital   [o]   Pentobarbital alcohol

N-dealkylation. Mephobarbital is demethylated to phenobarbital.

Mephobarbital   [o]   Phenobarbital

N-oxidation. Trimenthylamine is changed to trimethylamine oxide.

$$(CH_3)_3N \xrightarrow{[o]} (CH_3)_3N = O$$

Trimethylamine   Trimethylamine oxide

Sulfoxidation. Chlorpromazine is changed to chlorpromazine sulfoxide.

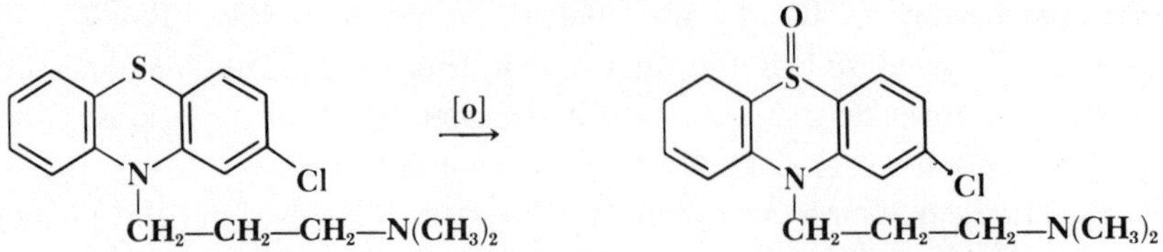

Chlorpromazine   Chlorpromazine sulfoxide

O-dealkylation. Acetophenetidin is changed to *N*-acetyl-*p*-aminophenol.

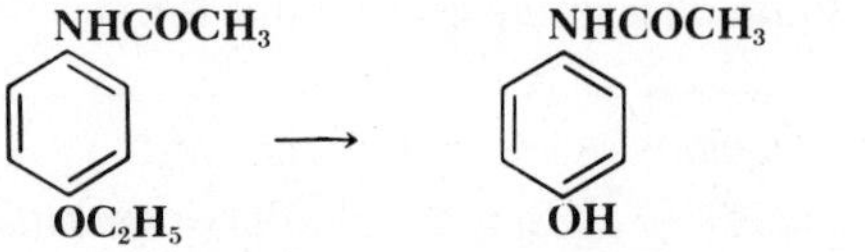

Acetophenetidin   *N*-Acetyl-*p*-aminophenol

S-dealkylation. 6-Methyl thiopurine is changed to 6-mercaptopurine.

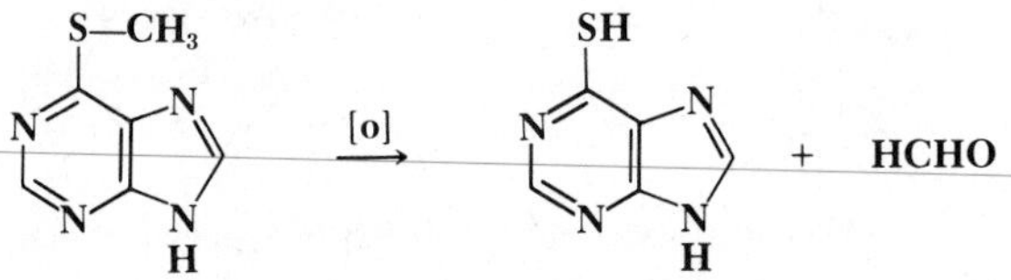

6-Methyl thiopurine   6-Mercaptopurine

Deamination. Amphetamine is oxidized to phenylacetone.

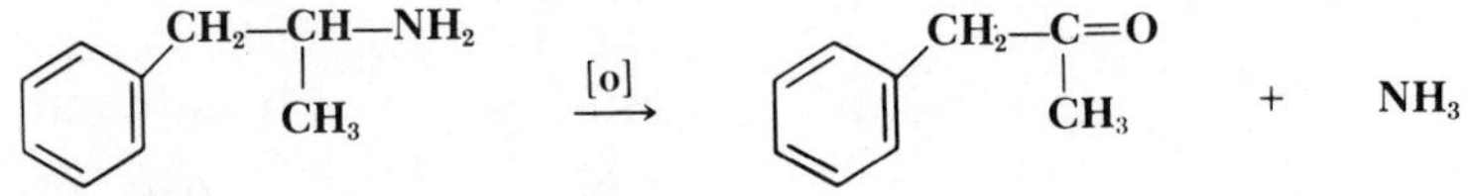

Amphetamine   Phenylacetone

Desulfuration. Parathion is oxidized to paraoxon.

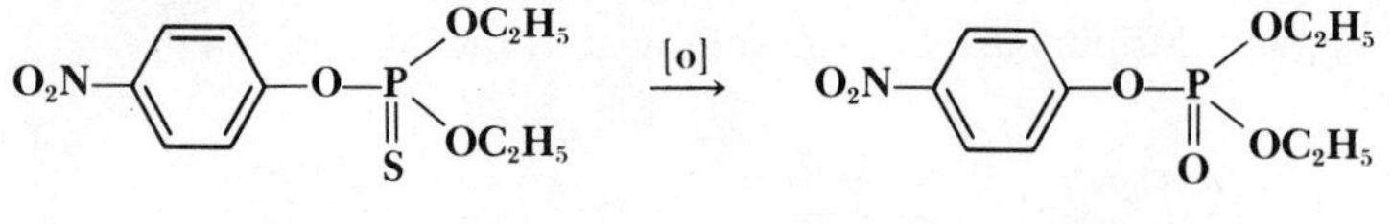

Parathion   Paraoxon

NONMICROSOMAL (ALCOHOL) OXIDATION   *p*-Nitrobenzyl alcohol is changed to *p*-nitrobenzaldehyde.

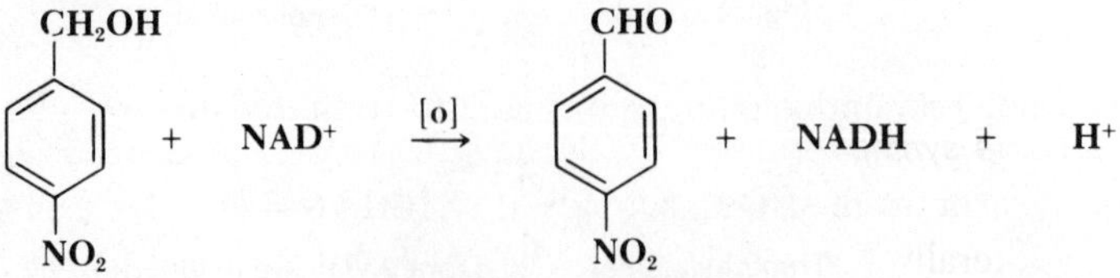

p-Nitrobenzyl alcohol   *p*-Nitrobenzaldehyde

Nitroreduction. Chloramphenicol is reduced to the arylamine.

Chloramphenicol   "Arylamine"

Azoreduction. Prontosil is reduced to sulfanilamide.

Prontosil   Sulfanilamide

Alcohol dehydrogenation. Chloral hydrate is changed to trichloroethanol.

Chloral hydrate   Trichloroethanol

Procaine is hydrolyzed to *p*-aminobenzoic acid and diethylaminoethanol.

Procaine   *p*-Aminobenzoic   Diethylaminoethanol
acid

The most important conjugation reactions are glucuronide synthesis, glycine con-

jugation, sulfate conjugation, acetylation, mercapturic acid synthesis, and methylation.

Glucuronide synthesis. Phenols, alcohols, carboxylic acids, and compounds containing amino or sulfhydryl groups may undergo glucuronide conjugation. Since glucose is generally available in the body, glucuronide formation is a common route of drug metabolism. The mechanism of the reaction is as follows:

$$\text{Uridine diphosphoglucuronate} + \text{ROH} \xrightarrow[\text{transferase}]{\text{Glucuronyl}} \text{RO glucuronide} + \text{Uridine diphosphate}$$

An example of a drug excreted almost entirely as the glucuronide is salicylamide.

Salicylamide   Salicylamide glucuronide

Glycine conjugation. Glycine conjugation is characteristic for certain aromatic acids. It depends on the availability of coenzyme A, glycine, and glycine-*N*-acylase. A typical reaction is as follows:

$$\text{Benzoic acid} \xrightarrow{\text{ATP + CoA}} \text{Benzoyl-CoA} \xrightarrow{\text{Glycine}} \text{Hippuric acid}$$

Some of the drugs conjugated with glycine in humans are salicylic acid, isonicotinic acid, and *p*-aminosalicylic acid. These drugs are metabolized by other pathways also, which may be more important quantitatively than glycine conjugation.

Sulfate conjugation. Phenols, alcohols, or aromatic amines may undergo sulfate conjugation. The sulfate donor is 3′-phospho-adenosine-5-phospho-sulfate (PAPS).

Acetylation. Derivatives of aniline are acetylated in the body. In addition to sulfanilamide and related compounds, widely used drugs such as *p*-aminosalicylic acid, isoniazid, and aminopyrine are transformed by this mechanism. The general reaction involving an amine, acetyl coenzyme A, and a specific acetylating enzyme may be depicted in the following manner:

$$\text{RNH}_2 + \text{CoASCOCH}_3 \xrightarrow{\text{Acetylase}} \text{RNHCOCH}_3 + \text{CoASH}$$

The acetylating ability of different patients may vary considerably. In the case of isoniazid, a low degree of acetylation shows some correlation with incidence of toxic reactions such as peripheral neuritis.

Isoniazid   Acetylated isoniazid

Mercapturic acid synthesis. This is not a common pathway in humans, although it may occur. Some drugs containing an active halogen or a nitro group may be changed to mercapturates.

Methylation. Norepinephrine and epinephrine are metabolized in part to normetanephrine and metanephrine by a process of *O*-methylation, whereas nicotinic acid is metabolized to *N*-methylnicotinic acid, an example of *N*-methylation. The source of methyl groups for drug methylations is *S*-adenosylmethionine.

Norepinephrine → Normetanephrine

Drug metabolism generally changes a drug to more water-soluble metabolites. The term *detoxication* is not accurate, since the body can form a toxic metabolite from a less toxic drug. Drug metabolism generally produces inactive metabolites from active drugs. It may, however, produce an active metabolite from an inactive drug or from an initially active drug.

Drug metabolism and detoxication

The toxicity of some compounds may be caused by a metabolite. The insecticide parathion is changed in the body to the more toxic paraoxon.

An even more remarkable example of the possible deleterious effects of the so-called detoxication process is given by the example of liver damage caused by carbon tetrachloride and probably some other drugs. Carbon tetrachloride is a well-known hepatotoxic agent. The curious finding that newborn rats are more resistant to the toxic effect of carbon tetrachloride[1] along with the observation that phenobarbital increases not only the metabolism of the halogenated hydrocarbon but also its toxicity, suggests that drug metabolism is involved in the hepatotoxicity of the compound. It is believed that free radicals are formed as a result of the interaction of some drugs and the drug-metabolizing enzymes. The free radicals may be directly toxic, perhaps through an interaction with membrane phospholipids. They may also make endogenous proteins antigenic, thus accounting for some forms of drug allergy.

Details of metabolism must be considered in connection with the individual drugs, but one very interesting generalization has been made concerning the evolutionary importance of certain detoxication mechanisms.

As we have seen in the previous section, the clearance of weakly acidic or basic drugs is hindered by the tubular resorption of the undissociated molecule. But for terrestrial animals there is no alternate route of excretion. In contrast, aquatic animals have no difficulty with such foreign compounds because the lipid membranes of the gills offer a ready avenue for their excretion. In the course of evolution, terrestrial organisms seem to have solved this problem by utilizing such mechanisms as side chain oxidation and conjugation, which make these foreign compounds more acidic and hence more easily rejected by the renal tubules.

The development of detoxication mechanisms appears to have been an evolutionary necessity, since terrestrial animals ingest many foreign compounds with their food. The mechanisms of detoxication, perhaps developed for the handling of such compounds, serve also at the present time for the biotransformation of a large variety of drugs.

Factors that delay
the metabolism
of drugs

It has been pointed out that drugs are usually metabolized at rates proportional to their plasma levels because at therapeutic levels their concentration is not high enough to saturate the drug-metabolizing enzymes. Any conditions that lower the concentration of drugs at the level of the metabolizing enzymes or decrease the amount or activity of the enzymes would be expected to prolong the biological half-life of the drug. Several of these factors are of great importance, whereas others may become significant only in particular diseases or in the presence of certain drug combinations. The following are some examples:

1. The reversible protein binding limits drug metabolism. Phenylbutazone, for example, is highly protein bound—up to 98% after therapeutic doses. If the dose is increased so that only 88% of the drug is protein bound, the free portion is metabolized much more rapidly. As a consequence, not much is gained by increasing the dose.

2. Localization of the drug in the adipose tissue (thiopental) or in the liver (quinacrine) protects it against metabolic degradation and prolongs its half-life. Precipitation of the drug in the gastrointestinal tract may similarly prolong its half-life (zoxazolamine).

3. Diseases of the liver and immaturity of drug-metabolizing enzymes during the neonatal period may interfere with the biotransformation of some drugs.

4. A drug may inhibit the metabolism of another drug and thus may prolong and intensify its action. This is why monoamine oxidase (MAO) inhibitors may cause alarming reactions when tyramine-containing food or beverages are ingested. The very interesting experimental drug SKF-525A (β-diethylaminoethyl diphenylpropylacetate) inhibits the microsomal enzymes that metabolize a large variety of drugs. Iproniazid is another inhibitor of drug-metabolizing enzymes.

ENZYME
INDUCTION

When several drugs are used simultaneously in a patient, it is difficult enough to keep in mind their various pharmacological interactions. An additional difficulty comes from observations indicating that some drugs can induce the formation of microsomal drug-metabolizing enzymes. Some cases of tolerance to a drug may be caused by microsomal enzyme induction. There are well-authenticated cases in both the experimental and the clinical literature of such drug interactions.

Stimulation of
drug-metabolizing
enzymes by drugs
and foreign
compounds

It was first shown in 1954[2] that mice fed the carcinogen 3-methylcholanthrene developed an increased capacity for demethylating 3-methyl-4-dimethylaminoazobenzene by liver microsomal enzymes. Several other examples of increased drug metabolism induced by various preparations followed. The long-acting barbiturate phenobarbital was found to stimulate the metabolism of such short-acting barbiturates as hexobarbital.

Effect of phenobarbital on plasma levels of dicumarol and on prothrombin time in a human   *FIG. 4-2*
subject treated chronically with 75 mg/day of dicumarol.

From Cucinell, S.A., Conney, A.H., Sansur, M., and Burns, J.J.: Clin. Pharmacol. Ther. 6:420, 1965.

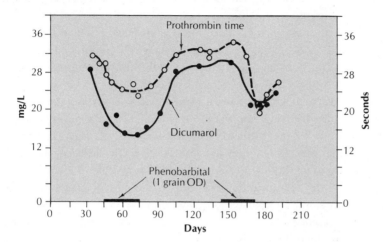

The following examples of stimulated drug metabolism have been demonstrated   *Stimulation of drug*
in humans.   *metabolism in*

Phenobarbital stimulates the metabolism of phenytoin (Dilantin), griseofulvin,   *humans*
and dicumarol (Fig. 4-2). Barbiturates stimulate the glucuronide conjugation of bilirubin in mice; this finding suggested the use of phenobarbital in the treatment of
congenital nonhemolytic jaundice in infants. The administration of 15 mg of phenobarbital two or three times daily lowered the free serum bilirubin concentration
in these infants. Additionally, it improved the conjugation of salicylamide in the same
infants, another example of glucuronide formation.

Phenylbutazone speeds the metabolism of aminopyrine. **Meprobamate** and **glutethimide** may induce tolerance to their action by enzyme induction.

Phenytoin interferes with the effect of dexamethasone, probably by promoting
microsomal enzyme activity.

The inducers may promote the metabolism of certain hormones as well as that
of various drugs and foreign compounds. Oxidative drug-metabolizing enzymes hy-
droxylate such endogenous compounds as testosterone, estradiol, progesterone, and
cortisol.

Although several examples of abnormal drug reactions in inherited diseases are   *PHARMACO-*
well known, the systematic study of pharmacogenetics is recent.[5] Among the well-   *GENETICS*
known examples of adverse drug reactions occurring in certain inherited diseases
are the following: barbiturates may produce severe attacks in congenital porphyria;
salicylates are dangerous in individuals in whom glucuronyl transferase is congenitally

absent (Crigler-Najjar syndrome); hypersensitivity to atropine occurs in patients suffering from Down's syndrome; and epinephrine or glucagon fails to produce hyperglycemia in individuals who are deficient in the enzyme glucose-6-phosphatase (von Gierke's disease).

A broad classification of pharmacogenetic abnormalities[5] would attribute most genetically conditioned anomalous drug responses to (1) receptor site abnormalities, (2) drug metabolism disorders, (3) tissue metabolism disorders, and (4) anatomical abnormalities.

Although there are not many well-known examples of *receptor site abnormalities*, they must undoubtedly contribute to the variation in drug responses. The resistance of some individuals to the coumarin anticoagulants is probably an example of a receptor site abnormality. The best known examples of pharmacogenetics are provided by *drug metabolism* disorders, in which abnormal blood levels of a drug can be measured after the administration of a normal dose. In *tissue metabolism* disorders an individual may show an adverse reaction to a normal blood level of a drug because of a special vulnerability caused by an abnormality in tissue metabolism. For example, in glucose-6-phosphate dehydrogenase deficiency a usual dose of primaquine may cause hemolytic anemia. Finally, an *anatomical abnormality* may cause adverse drug reactions. For example, in a patient with an inherited subaortic stenosis, digitalis may cause fatal reactions.[5]

Continuous and discontinuous variation	It is generally recognized that the response to a drug in a population shows *continuous variation*. Drug effects such as the LD_{50} or ED_{50} (pp. 40-42) and rate of destruction of a drug in the body generally show a normal distribution in a population, as shown in Fig. 4-3, *A*. Some of the great discoveries in pharmacogenetics occur when the response to some drug or the metabolism of a drug indicates a *discontinuous variation*, as shown in Fig. 4-3, *B*. Follow-up of such a bimodal distribution often reveals a genetic basis and provides the explanation for unusual responses to drugs, which is more satisfying than simply calling them idiosyncrasies.

Hemolytic anemia caused by the ingestion of the bean *Vicia fava* and reactions to several other drugs have similarly been traced to a deficiency of glucose-6-phosphate dehydrogenase. The following drugs have been suspected: acetophenetidin, acetanilid, probenecid, and others.

As discussed on pp. 60-61, the enzyme glucose-6-phosphate dehydrogenase in the red cell is responsible for the formation of NADPH (reduced form of nicotinamide adenine dinucleotide phosphate, or reduced triphosphopyridine nucleotide). NADPH is a cofactor for gluthathione reductase, which converts glutathione to the reduced form. When there is a genetically determined deficiency of glucose-6-phosphate in the red cell, severe hemolytic episodes may be caused by the administration of oxidant drugs.

Schematic illustration of continuous *and* discontinuous *variation. When a standard dose*   *FIG. 4-3*
of a drug is given to a large number of persons and a drug effect or metabolism is measured,
the usual finding is a normal frequency distribution as in **A.** *On the other hand, a discon-*
tinuous variation, as exemplified by the bimodal distribution shown in **B,** *may indicate a*
genetically determined abnormality in drug action or metabolism.

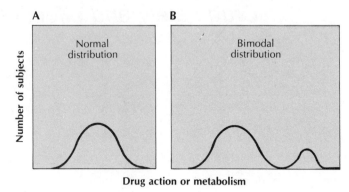

REFERENCES

1. Anders, M.W.: Enhancement and inhibition of drug metabolism, Annu. Rev. Pharmacol. **11:**37, 1971.
2. Brown, R.R., Miller, J.A., and Miller, E.C.: The metabolism of methylated aminoazo dyes, J. Biol. chem. **209:**211, 1954.
3. Conney, A.H., and Burns, J.J.: Metabolic interactions among environmental chemicals and drugs, Science **178:**576, 1972.
4. Gelehrter, T.D.: Enzyme induction, N. Engl. J. Med. **294:**589, 1976.
5. La Du, B.N.: The genetics of drug reactions, Hosp. Pract., p. 97, June, 1971.
6. La Du, B.N., Mandel, H.G., and Way, E.L.: Fundamentals of drug metabolism and drug disposition, Baltimore, 1971, The Williams & Wilkins Co.
7. Remmer, H.: The role of the liver in drug metabolism, Am. J. Med. **49:**617, 1970.
8. Schreiber, E.C.: The metabolic alteration of drugs, Annu. Rev. Pharmacol. **10:**77, 1970.
9. Vesell, E.S.: Pharmacogenetics, N. Engl. J. Med. **287:**904, 1972.

Chapter 5

Drug safety and effectiveness

With the expansion of drug therapy and with the introduction of potent agents that have complex effects and even more complex interactions with each other, it is increasingly necessary for the physician to have a scientific attitude and considerable knowledge of drug evaluation.

Since the most extensive studies on drug evaluation are carried out in connection with the development of *new* drugs, this subject will be discussed in some detail along with factors that modify drug safety and effectiveness.

DEVELOPMENT OF A NEW DRUG

New drugs originate from many different sources. Accidental observations of natural products, unexpected clinical findings of known compounds, basic physiological or biochemical investigations, and even test tube experiments have provided leads for great therapeutic discoveries. Most new drugs are discovered today by screening. Large numbers of natural products or synthetic compounds are tested for a variety of possible biological activities. A highly effective drug that seems safe enough on preliminary testing is then carried through a series of steps:

1. Animal studies
   a. Acute, subacute, and chronic toxicity
   b. Therapeutic index
   c. Absorption, excretion, distribution, and metabolism
2. Human studies
   a. Phase 1: preliminary pharmacological evaluation
   b. Phase 2: basic controlled clinical evaluation
   c. Phase 3: extended clinical evaluation

Animal studies
ACUTE, SUBACUTE, AND CHRONIC TOXICITY

The most common measure of acute toxicity is the median lethal dose (LD_{50}). The LD_{50} is determined by giving various doses of the drugs to groups of animals. Ordinarily only a single dose is given to each animal. The percentage of animals dying in each group within a selected period (for example, 24 hours) is plotted against the dose. From this curve the dose that kills 50% of the animals is estimated and is

Illustrating concept of therapeutic index (TI).

FIG. 5-1

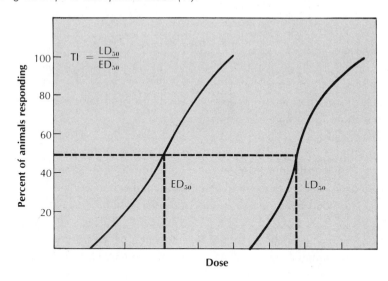

referred to as the LD_{50}. This particular dose-mortality figure is chosen because it can be determined more precisely; the curve approaches a straight line at the LD_{50}. It should be emphasized that the LD_{50} of any drug is of interest only to experimental pharmacologists, not to clinicians.

Customarily at least three different species are used for acute toxicity determinations, and observations are made not only on the LD_{50} but also on the type of toxic symptoms that the animals develop.

In subacute toxicity studies the mode of administration and the dosage depend on the proposed clinical trial. Usually the drug is administered orally. Several doses are used, some within the range of the estimated human dose and others that produce toxic manifestations. Careful observations are carried out on these animals, including a variety of laboratory studies such as hematological examinations, renal and hepatic function tests, and many others.

The chronic toxicity studies are of long duration. They may last many months and may be carried out through several generations to detect the possible teratogenic effect of a drug. Again several species are necessary because even in prolonged studies some species are much more suitable than others for the demonstration of adverse effects. The animals are killed periodically and thorough pathological studies are performed.

The LD_{50} of a drug is not nearly as important as its therapeutic index, or therapeutic ratio. This concept in *animal experiments* refers to the ratio of the LD_{50} to the median effective dose (ED_{50}), as illustrated in Fig. 5-1.

THERAPEUTIC INDEX

$$\text{Therapeutic index} = \frac{LD_{50}}{ED_{50}}$$

In clinical medicine the therapeutic index based on median lethal doses has no meaning. Instead, the ratio of a toxic dose over the effective dose is sometimes used. Even in animal experiments, the ratio of LD_1/ED_{100} would give a better idea of safety, but it has no particular application. The concept of effectiveness in relation to toxicity is more important than any special ratio.

The concept of toxicity in relation to effectiveness, the basis of the therapeutic index, is of interest to clinicians as well as to experimental pharmacologists. A physician may not be greatly interested in the exact number of milligrams of a drug that will produce toxic effects but is vitally interested in knowing how far the therapeutic dose can be exceeded before adverse effects are likely to be encountered.

ABSORPTION, EXCRETION, DISTRIBUTION, AND METABOLISM	The development of analytic methods for determining the absorption, excretion, distribution, and metabolism of a drug in animals adds much to the proper design of animal experiments on the toxicity and efficacy of the drug. In addition, these methods are desirable for the initiation and pursuit of clinical studies.

Human studies: clinical pharmacology	Animal studies provide a general profile of the toxicity, pharmacological activities, and pharmacokinetics of a new drug. Even with all this information available, the initiation of clinical studies is risky. There are numerous examples of drugs that pass all the preclinical criteria for safety but show serious adverse effects in humans. The clinical pharmacologist should consider not only the data obtained previously in animals but also the chemical nature of the drug and its possible similarity to hazardous drugs.

The lack of correlation between toxicity data in animals and adverse effects in humans is well known. Not only is there great species variation in toxicity, an example of comparative pharmacology, but many adverse effects simply cannot be ascertained in animals. Zbinden[4] claims that of the 45 most frequent drug-related symptoms observed in 11,000 patients treated with 77 different drugs or drug combinations, at least one half would probably not be recognized in animal experiments. Such symptoms include drowsiness, nausea, dizziness, nervousness, epigastric distress, headache, weakness, insomnia, fatigue, tinnitus, heartburn, skin rash, depression, dermatitis, increased energy, vertigo, lethargy, nocturia, abdominal distention, flatulence, stiffness, and urticaria.

Because of these discrepancies between animal data and human effects, the initial clinical studies on any drug should be undertaken with great care, with the methodology meticulously planned, and with special attention given to *relevance* (pertinence of data), *representativeness* (selection of material to eliminate bias), and *reliability* (repeatability of results). The new drug application must be filed before any clinical evaluation studies are initiated.

Very small doses of the drug are administered to human volunteers to obtain a preliminary idea of its safety in humans. With increasing doses, an attempt is made to extend the previously demonstrated effects in animals to humans. The ethical aspects of human experimentation have been the subject of much discussion in recent years and will not be taken up in detail. The important points are, however, that the volunteer must be truly a volunteer (that is, able to give an informed consent) and that the investigator must be competent. In some instances it is essential to have methods for the determination of blood levels of the new drug. Without such determinations the investigator cannot tell whether lack of effectiveness in humans is a consequence of lack of absorption or too rapid excretion and metabolism.

PHASE 1: PRELIMINARY PHARMACOLOGICAL EVALUATION

Whereas the phase 1 studies are usually performed by one or two clinical investigators, in phase 2 a somewhat larger number of clinical investigators attempt to find out in blind or double-blind studies as much information as possible about the safety and efficacy of the new drug. Adverse effects must be reported promptly to the sponsoring company and to the Food and Drug Administration (FDA), and specific studies are sometimes initiated to ascertain the significance of such unexpected findings.

PHASE 2: BASIC CONTROLLED CLINICAL EVALUATION

As many as 50 to 100 physicians participate in the large-scale clinical trial of a new drug. The investigators must not only be competent clinicians but must also have some experience and training in the field of drug evaluation.

Assuming that the phase 3 studies demonstrate to the satisfaction of the FDA that the drug is safe and effective, the investigational drug may be approved to be distributed and used when prescribed by a physician.

It would seem that with all these safeguards a drug approved by the FDA would be free of all hazard. Unfortunately there are many unusual side effects, idiosyncrasies, and drug allergies that show up only after extensive use in large numbers of patients.

PHASE 3: EXTENDED CLINICAL EVALUATION

Experimental studies in animals show that the dose of a drug that will give an all-or-nothing response (such as the death of the animal) varies considerably. Fig. 5-2 illustrates the gaussian distribution of susceptibility, which can be demonstrated easily in animals. The biological variation in drug effect is an important reason why dosages must be individualized and treatment adjusted to the requirements of a given patient.

FACTORS INFLUENCING THE SAFETY AND EFFECTIVENESS OF DRUGS
Biological variation

Because of biological variation, disease, or presence of another medication, some persons may show a much greater than normal response to the ordinary dose of a drug. For example, a thyrotoxic patient may have an exaggerated cardiovascular response to injected epinephrine. A patient with subclinical asthma may evidence symptoms of bronchial constriction from doses of acetyl-β-methylcholine or histamine that would be innocuous in normal persons. These patients are at the susceptible

Hypersusceptibility

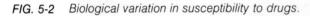

FIG. 5-2   *Biological variation in susceptibility to drugs.*

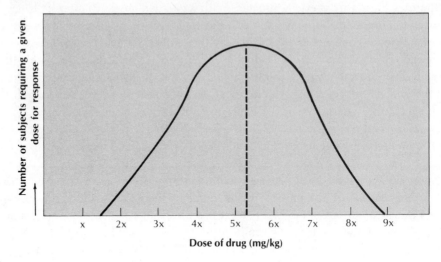

end of a normal frequency distribution curve and their responses are quantitatively different. Hypersusceptibility is sometimes referred to as *drug intolerance*.

Drug idiosyncrasy and drug allergy

The term *idiosyncrasy* has been used rather vaguely in medicine to cover drug reactions that are *qualitatively* different from the usual effects obtained in the majority of patients and cannot be attributed to drug allergy. Occasionally extreme susceptibility of an individual to the expected pharmacological effect of a drug has also been included in the drug idiosyncrasies.

With the increasing knowledge of pharmacogenetics (discussed on p. 50), many drug idiosyncrasies have been found to be genetically conditioned enzymatic deficiencies. Such deficiencies can interfere with the metabolic degradation of a drug, as in prolonged apnea caused by succinylcholine, or they may make certain cells more vulnerable to an adverse effect of a drug, as is the case in hemolytic anemia elicited by primaquine and other drugs in patients whose red cells are deficient in glucose-6-phosphate dehydrogenase.

It is quite likely that all drug idiosyncrasies will turn out to be genetically conditioned abnormalities of enzymes or receptors.

Drug allergy is an altered response to a drug resulting from a previous sensitizing exposure and an immunological mechanism. It differs from drug toxicity in a number of respects. (1) The altered reaction occurs in only a fraction of the population. (2) Its dose-response is unusual in that a minute amount of an otherwise safe drug elicits a severe reaction. (3) The manifestations of the reaction are different from the usual pharmacological effects of the drug. (4) There is a primary sensitizing period before the individual responds with an unusual reaction to a further exposure. (5) When the sensitizing drug is a protein or a compound that forms covalent bonds with proteins, circulating antibodies may be demonstrated in sensitized individuals, and skin tests, although hazardous, may show a positive reaction to the offending drug.

In most drug allergies, it is not known what the complete antigen is or in what form the drug acts as a haptene. A patient may react to the ingestion of a sulfonamide by developing a skin rash and still show no positive reaction to the same drug when injected intracutaneously. This is generally true for drugs of small molecular weight and the *immediate* type of allergies elicited by them. In *contact dermatitis*, on the other hand, positive patch tests are regularly obtained.

The terms *immediate* and *delayed reactions* originated from observations of the rapidity with which the positive skin test to allergens becomes manifest. Thus in anaphylactic hypersensitivity, skin test results are immediate, but in delayed states such as tuberculin hypersensitivity, it is many hours before there is a visible change in the skin where the antigen was injected. In addition, there are profound differences in the immunological basis of the two types of hypersensitivities. Circulating antibodies are believed to be important in immediate but not in delayed hypersensitivities. The latter can be transferred to normal individuals only by means of sensitized cells.

IMMEDIATE AND DELAYED DRUG ALLERGIES

Among the many types of drug allergies, some are considered immediate, others delayed, and still others are not classifiable at present. *Anaphylaxis, urticaria, angioneurotic edema, drug fever,* and *asthma* clearly belong in the category of immediate reactions. *Serum sickness* reactions are characterized by a delay in the appearance of manifestations following the initial sensitization to a drug; this same delay is observed after the first administration of a foreign serum. Once sensitized, however, an individual often reacts to the same drug rather rapidly. For example, methyldopa (Aldomet) may be taken daily by an individual for 1 to 2 weeks before fever and joint pain develop. The subsequent administration of a small dose of the drug will produce the same reaction in a matter of hours. *Contact dermatitis* is undoubtedly a delayed allergy. Many other cutaneous reactions and *some* severe hematological disturbances elicited by drugs probably also belong in the delayed category.

In experimental investigations, drugs are administered on the basis of a certain number of milligrams per kilogram of body weight, since the volume of distribution of a drug is roughly a function of body mass. For the same reason the weight of the patient should be taken into consideration when a dose is calculated. Certain formulas allow adjustment of dosage according to weight. For example, Clark's rule is as follows:

Age and weight of patient

$$\text{Dose for child} = \text{Adult dose} \times \frac{\text{Weight of child in pounds}}{150}$$

It is assumed in this formula that a child needs a smaller dose because the weight is less, but this is only an approximation. It has been pointed out that the child is not simply a "small adult" and that reactions to drugs in children may result from problems in growth and development rather than size.[2] Catastrophes have resulted from the routine adaptation of adult dosages for children. The gray baby syndrome caused by chloramphenicol, kernicterus by vitamin K, and blindness by the use of oxygen in premature infants are examples of the peculiar problems of drug use in pediatrics.

DOSE FOR CHILDREN BASED ON SURFACE AREA

The dose of a drug for children is proportional to weight to the 0.7 power.[1] Since body surface is similarly related to body weight, it has been suggested that pediatric dosages should be calculated on the basis of surface area of the body in square meters. Tables relating the weight of a child in pounds to surface area in square meters and approximate percentage of adult dose are available. According to such tables, a 22-pound child having a surface area of 0.46 sq m should receive 27% of the adult dose. A child weighing 121 pounds with a surface area of 1.58 sq m would receive 91% of the adult dose.

Disease processes influencing susceptibility and detoxication

Pathological processes influence susceptibility to drugs. In some instances this can be explained by altered detoxication processes induced by the disease, but in other cases the explanation may be obscure.

It is obvious that in severe renal disease one must use with caution those drugs such as phenobarbital that depend on renal clearance for excretion. In severe liver disease, similar care must be exercised in the use of drugs that are normally detoxified by hepatic processes.

Abnormal susceptibility to drugs in disease states may depend on other mechanisms. The asthmatic patient is said to be hypersusceptible to the bronchoconstrictor action of histamine or methacholine, whereas the thyrotoxic patient is hypersusceptible to epinephrine. Patients with subclinical glaucoma may respond with an acute attack to doses of a mydriatic that would be harmless in a normal person.

Presence of other drugs

When more than one drug is given to the same patient, their actions may be completely independent of one another. Often, however, the combined effect may be greater than that which could have been obtained with a single drug, or a drug may have even less effect than if it were given alone.

ADDITIVE EFFECT, SYNERGISM, AND POTENTIATION

When the combined effect of two drugs is the algebraic sum of the individual actions, it is referred to as *summation* or *additive effect*. Another way of stating the additive effect is in terms of doses rather than effects. If a certain dose of drug A and another dose of drug B produce the same effect quantitatively, the additive effect concept implies that one half the dose of each drug used simultaneously would elicit the same effect. *Synergism* is defined in various ways. To some it means an additive, or greater than additive, effect. Others reserve the term for cases in which one drug increases the action of another by interfering with its destruction or disposition, thus greatly increasing its action. *Potentiation* generally mens a greater than additive effect. The terms synergism and potentiation are commonly abused in pharmaceutical promotion.

Drug antagonism may be of several types: chemical antagonism, physiological antagonism, and pharmacological antagonism.

Chemical antagonism. A drug may actually combine with another in the body. This is the basis of the action of the chemical antidotes. For example, dimercaprol (British antilewisite; BAL) can combine with mercury or arsenic in the body. The diuretic effect of a mercurial can be blocked by the injection of BAL.

Physiological antagonism. Two drugs may influence a physiological system in opposite directions, one drug canceling the effect of another. The simultaneous injection of properly adjusted doses of vasodilator and vasoconstrictor drugs may cause no change in blood pressure. Stimulants and depressants of the CNS can antagonize each other by a similar mechanism.

Pharmacological antagonism. Two drugs may compete for the same receptor site, the inactive or weak member of the pair preventing the access of the potent drug. This is the phenomenon of pharmacological antagonism.

Examples of pharmacological antagonism are the histamine-antihistaminic drug relationships and also atropine-acetylcholine antagonism. It is quite likely that many examples of competitive antagonism in pharmacology are not competition for enzymes but rather for receptor surfaces.

The key point in pharmacological antagonism is parallel displacement of the dose-response curve of a drug by a second drug. If the two drugs compete for the same receptor, the curves should remain parallel and the maximum height of the curves should remain the same (p. 12).

ANTAGONISM

A drug may interact with another by many different mechanisms. Some of these are (1) absorption from the gastrointestinal tract, (2) binding to plasma proteins, (3) renal excretion, (4) inhibition of metabolic degradation, (5) promotion of metabolic degradation by enzyme induction, and (6) alteration of electrolyte patterns. These and other drug interactions have acquired such an importance in clinical pharmacology that the problem is discussed in detail in Chapter 63.

COMPLEX DRUG INTERACTIONS IN CLINICAL PHARMACOLOGY

Response to dosage can be greatly influenced by certain special features of drug metabolism such as cumulation, tolerance, and tachyphylaxis.

Cumulation, tolerance, and tachyphylaxis

Most drugs are eliminated from the body by a first-order reaction. This means that a constant fraction of the drug present in the body is eliminated per unit time. It also means that it takes four half-lives to eliminate 93% of the drug. If the drug is administered repeatedly and frequently in relation to its half-life, it will accumulate

CUMULATION

FIG. 5-3   *Illustrating concept of cumulation. Drug a is completely destroyed or excreted in less than 24 hours. Thus it does not accumulate when administered once a day. Drug b requires more than 24 hours for its metabolic degradation or excretion. It is a cumulative drug when it is administered once a day.*

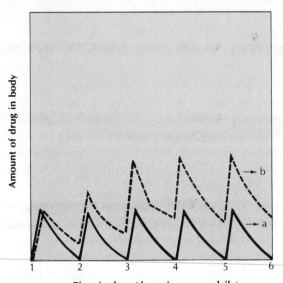

Time in days (drug given once daily)

in the body. Eventually, however, a *plateau* will be reached, since elimination is increasing as the amount of drug in the body increases. Digitoxin is a good example of a drug having a long half-life, leading to cumulation when administered daily.

Fig. 5-3 shows the resulting curve of the amount of drug in the body plotted schematically against the number of doses. The plateau in the case of drug *b* (Fig. 5-3) indicates that, in general, the amount of drug metabolized in a day is proportional to the amount in the body.

When dealing with cumulative drugs, the dosage will vary greatly, depending on whether loading or maintenance doses are administered. The former must be large enough to build up a therapeutically effective level in the body, whereas maintenance doses are adjusted to the daily metabolic and excretory rates.

TOLERANCE   Tolerance is an interesting phenomenon characterized by the need for increasing amounts of a drug to obtain the same therapeutic effect. Drugs vary greatly in their tendency to induce tolerance; perhaps the best-known examples are the opium alkaloids. The adult therapeutic dose of morphine is ordinarily 10 to 15 mg, but if the drug is administered repeatedly to a patient, increasing doses are necessary to obtain the same analgesic effect. Finally, enormous doses are sought by the addict who has gradually developed tolerance. Although it is a well-studied phenomenon, the actual mechanism of tolerance remains mysterious.

Drugs that produce significant tolerance are not numerous. Many are similar to the digitalis glycosides, which can be taken daily for years without tolerance developing.

Tachyphylaxis is the term reserved for rapidly developing tolerance. This is noted in laboratory experiments with certain drugs—for example, vasopressin or certain adrenergic compounds such as amphetamine. In these experiments the first injection of the drug produces a much greater elevation of blood pressure than subsequent injections given after only a brief interval.

The mechanism of tachyphylaxis is understood only in some cases. For example, indirectly acting sympathomimetic amines such as amphetamine release norepinephrine from adrenergic nerve endings. Tachyphylaxis probably is a consequence of depletion of available norepinephrine. The same mechanism plays a role in tachyphylaxis to histamine releasers. In other instances the action of a drug may persist at the receptor site, but its overt manifestations are concealed by compensatory reflexes or by desensitization of the receptor.

TACHYPHYLAXIS

Drug effects are greatly influenced by genetically determined variations in susceptibility. Idiosyncrasies in general are most commonly related to pharmacogenetic abnormalities. This subject is discussed in detail on p. 50.

Pharmacogenetics

---

1. Done, A.K.: Drugs for children. In Modell, W., editor: Drugs of choice 1978-1979, St. Louis, 1978, The C.V. Mosby Co.
2. Shirkey, H.C., and Ericson, A.S.: Adverse reactions to drugs—their relation to growth and development. In Shirkey, H.C., editor: Pediatric therapy, ed. 6, St. Louis, 1980, The C.V. Mosby Co.
3. Stewart, G.T.: Allergy to penicillin and related antibiotics: antigenic and immunochemical mechanisms, Annu. Rev. Pharmacol. 13:309, 1973.
4. Zbinden, G.: Animal toxicity studies: a critical evaluation, Appl. Ther. 8:128, 1966.

REFERENCES

Chapter 6

Pharmacogenetics: the individual response to drugs

VARIATIONS IN DRUG RESPONSE

A perplexing problem for both pharmacologists and physicians is the large variation that occurs among normal subjects as well as patients in response to a particular drug. Such interindividual variations have been demonstrated for many drugs. They signify correspondingly large variations in the dose of these drugs required by different patients. The clinical consequences of such differences among patients in dose requirement cannot be overemphasized.

The magnitude of interindividual variations in rate of elimination of a drug given to a group of subjects, all in the same dose and by the same route, can range from fourfold to fortyfold, depending on both the particular drug and the population.

Drug elimination rates and drug toxicity

Every physician learns to take into account variations among patients in rates of drug elimination by individualizing the dose of certain drugs, particularly drugs with low therapeutic indices. For clinical purposes, the therapeutic index of a drug may be defined as the ratio of the toxic dose of that drug to its effective dose. (For further discussion of this concept and its derivation see p. 42.) If the dose of a drug with a low therapeutic index is not individualized, the same dose administered by the same route can produce toxicity in some patients, the desired pharmacological effect in other patients, and therapeutic ineffectiveness in still others. By contrast, physicians have a greater margin of safety in administering a drug with a high therapeutic index because for such drugs the physician can select from a wider range of nontoxic doses.

In recent years numerous drugs with low therapeutic indices have been introduced, thereby increasing the risk of toxicity when these drugs are administered. Although the frequency of drug toxicity is high, its exact incidence is unknown and probably differs from one hospital to another and from one geographical region to another. On the medical wards of several university hospitals (such as Cornell and Johns Hopkins), the incidence of adverse drug reactions was reported to comprise 5% of all admissions.

The epidemiological data on adverse drug reactions emphasize the practical need to understand precise causes for extensive differences among patients in drug response. Understanding these mechanisms could lead to safer ways to use drugs. Probably many adverse drug reactions arise from a failure to tailor the dosage of drugs with low therapeutic indices closely enough to widely different individual needs.

Determining causes of variations in drug elimination rates

Pharmacogenetics deals with genetically caused variations in drug response. Some pharmacogenetic conditions in humans that affect either drug metabolism or the interaction of drugs at different sites (including receptor sites) are listed in Table 6-1. Pharmacogenetic conditions in humans transmitted by genes at a single locus are divided for convenience into those that affect drug absorption, distribution, metabolism, excretion, and receptor action.

In pharmacogenetics the screening of populations by a simple, rapid, safe test is necessary to ascertain how a particular trait is inherited, what its incidence is in a given group, and how the frequency of the genes controlling the trait varies from one group and geographical area to another.

Although in pharmacogenetic studies the plasma half-life or clearance of a drug has been conveniently employed as the principal test of gene structure and function, such measurements may not be sensitive enough to serve as an index of possible variations among subjects in genes that control proteins, which are directly involved in the disposition of certain drugs.

*PHARMACO-
GENETICS*

Several curves can be generated when the same dose of a drug is given by the same route to a large population of normal subjects and a specific quantitative response to the drug is measured and plotted. The three most common shapes of this distribution curve are *unimodal*, *bimodal*, and *trimodal*. Pharmacological responses of a normal population generally exhibit large interindividual variations, again indicating that the same dose of drug cannot be administered to all subjects with the expectation of an identical response and that the doses of many drugs must be individualized. Although the *shape* of the curve can provide *clues* to the mechanisms responsible for this large interindividual variation in drug response, the shapes by themselves must not be regarded as conclusive evidence. Thus it must be emphasized that genetic factors, environmental factors, or both may be responsible for producing any shaped curve. For many drugs, when a population is tested, it is customary to obtain a unimodal, normal gaussian distribution curve of drug response. This curve can arise from purely environmental differences among the subjects or, by contrast, from purely genetic differences in which genes at multiple loci contribute to the variation. This latter type of genetic control is called *polygenic*. Polygenic control is generally observed to be at least partially involved in the regulation of such metric traits as blood pressure, intelligence, and intensity of skin color. Similarly, bimodal or trimodal distribution curves of drug response are usually produced by monogen-

*DISTRIBUTION
CURVES OF DRUG
RESPONSE*

TABLE 6-1 Genetic conditions, probably transmitted as single factors, that alter drug response

Condition	Aberrant enzyme and location	Mode of inheritance*	Agent provoking response
Altering the way the body acts on drugs			
Acatalasia	Catalase in erythrocytes	AR	Hydrogen peroxide
Suxamethonium sensitivity or atypical cholinesterase	Cholinesterase in plasma	AR	Suxamethonium or succinylcholine
Slow inactivation of isoniazid	Isoniazid acetylase in liver	AR	Isoniazid, sulfamethazine, sulfamaprine, procainamide, phenelzine, dapsone, and hydralazine
Acetophenetidin-induced methemoglobinemia	? Mixed function oxidase in liver microsomes that deethylates acetophenetidin	AR	Acetophenetidin
Deficient N-glucosidation of amobarbital	? Mixed function oxidase in liver microsomes that N-glucosidates amobarbital	AR	Amobarbital
Polymorphic hydroxylation of debrisoquine in man	Mixed function oxidase in liver microsomes that 4-hydroxylates debrisoquine	AR	Debrisoquine
Altering the way drugs act on the body			
Warfarin resistance	? Altered receptor or enzyme in liver with increased affinity for vitamin K	AD	Warfarin
Inability to taste phenylthiourea or phenylthiocarbamide	Unknown	AR	Drugs containing N—C $=$ S group such as phenylthiourea, methyl, and propylthiouracil
Glucose-6-phosphate dehydrogenase deficiency, favism, or drug-induced hemolytic anemia	Glucose-6-phosphate dehydrogenase	XL incomplete codominant	Various analgesics (acetanilid, acetylsalicylic acid, acetophenetidin [phenacetin], antipyrine, aminopyrine [Pyramidon]); sulfonamides and sulfones (sulfanilamide, sulfapyridine, N²-acetylsulfanilamide, sulfacetamide, sulfisoxazole [Gantrisin], thiazosulfone, salicylazosulfapyridine [Azulfidine], sulfoxone, sulfamethoxypyridazine [Kynex]); antimalarials (primaquine, pamaquine, pentaquine, quinacrine [Atabrine]); nonsulfonamide antibacterial agents (furazolidone, nitrofurantoin [Furadantin], chloramphenicol, p-aminosalicylic acid); and miscellaneous drugs (naphthalene, vitamin K, probenecid, trinitrotoluene, methylene blue, dimercaprol [BAL], phenylhydrazine, quinine, and quinidine)

*AR, Autosomal recessive; AD, autosomal dominant; XL, X linked.

ically controlled conditions, such as those listed in Table 6-1, but can also arise from environmental differences among the subjects investigated.

The second, most critical step is to perform a family study on individuals located at the extremes of the distribution curve. Individuals at the extremes are most likely to exhibit a response to drugs sufficiently distinctive to permit clear-cut identification and tracing through several generations. By determining whether this particular type of drug response is in fact transmitted through several generations in conformity to mendelian laws for inheritance of dominant and recessive traits, investigators can tell whether a genetic mechanism controls the variation in drug response observed in the population. Furthermore, the specific kind of genetic control (autosomal dominant or recessive; X-linked dominant or recessive) can be discovered.

PHARMACO-
GENETIC
DIFFERENCES IN
ELIMINATION
RATES OF
COMMONLY USED
DRUGS

Before some of the pharmacogenetic conditions listed in Table 6-1 are discussed, the causes of genetic variation in drug response more common than any of those listed in Table 6-1 will be described. Evidence exists that in several populations large interindividual variations in the disposition of numerous drugs are controlled by genetic factors. Twin studies demonstrated that fivefold to tenfold interindividual variations in disposition of antipyrine, phenylbutazone, and bishydroxycoumarin were genetically controlled (Fig. 6-1). For this purpose, twins may be considered representative of partial family units, since monozygotic twins are identical with respect to all their genes, whereas dizygotic twins have approximately 50% of their genes in common, just as do any siblings. Genetic factors controlling interindividual variations in rates of drug elimination proved, unlike most conditions listed in Table 6-1, to occur commonly and to involve many rather than few drugs.

Although the precise genetic mechanisms responsible for large interindividual variations in the hepatic metabolism of these commonly used drugs have not yet been firmly established, techniques to measure the major metabolites of many of these drugs are now being used in family studies that should soon provide definitive answers to this important question.[4]

Genetic differences that exist among normal subjects in rates of drug elimination from the body help to explain the markedly different dosage requirements of many patients. These results constitute the scientific basis for the long-recognized need to individualize doses of many commonly used drugs.

GENETIC AND
ENVIRONMENTAL
CAUSES OF
VARIATIONS IN
DRUG RESPONSE

Because so many environmental factors can alter rates of drug elimination in patients and because the relative role that each of these factors plays in influencing rates of drug metabolism changes even in the same subject with time and with numerous other variables, it is difficult to identify, even at a particular time, which factors are operating and what contribution each factor actually makes to the total drug-metabolizing capacity of a person. For this reason, the role of each of these factors is generally investigated in normal, nonmedicated volunteer subjects in a near basal state with respect to most of the variables known to alter hepatic drug-metabolizing capacity.[11] Measurements with a test drug (such as antipyrine) are then performed to quantify this basal capacity in each volunteer subject; a single environmental alteration is introduced, during which the subject's drug-metabolizing activity is remeasured; and the change from basal values is taken to quantitate the effect exerted by the single environmental change (Table 6-2).[11] This approach, introduced in 1969 and now widely used to explore gene-environment interactions, clearly has limitations, since results cannot always be extrapolated with accuracy to other drugs or will certain environmental factors that alter the disposition of other drugs always alter antipyrine pharmacokinetics. Clearly other test drugs are therefore required.

FIG. 6-1 *Plasma half-lives of bishydroxycoumarin and antipyrine were measured separately at an interval of more than 6 months in healthy monozygotic (identical) and dizygotic (fraternal) twins. Values for each set of twins for each drug are joined by a solid line. Note that intratwin differences in plasma half-life of both bishydroxycoumarin and antipyrine are smaller (as indicated by a shorter line joining the circles) in monozygotic than in dizygotic twins.*

*Based on data from Vesell, E.S., and Page, J.G.: J. Clin. Invest. **47**:2657, 1968; and Vesell, E.S., and Page, J.G.: Science **161**:72, 1968.*

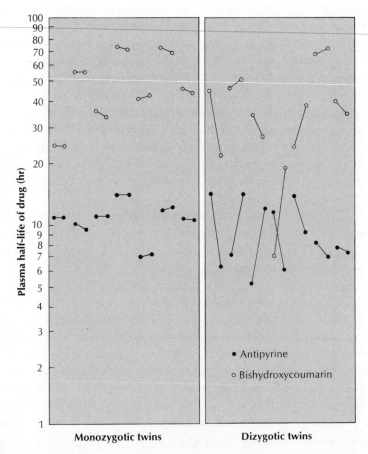

TABLE 6-2   Applications of the antipyrine test in humans where antipyrine was measured before and after a single environmental change

Environmental change	Effect of each factor on antipyrine half-life ($t_{1/2}$)
Drugs	
Adrenocorticotropic hormone (ACTH)	Unaltered $t_{1/2}$
Allopurinol	↑ $t_{1/2}$
Aminopyrine (administered simultaneously with anti-pyrine)	↑ $t_{1/2}$
Amobarbital	↓ $t_{1/2}$
Barbiturate overdose	↓ $t_{1/2}$
Chlorimipramine	↓ $t_{1/2}$
Delta-9-tetrahydrocannabinol	↑ $t_{1/2}$
Dexamethasone	Unaltered $t_{1/2}$
Disulfiram	↑ $t_{1/2}$
Ethanol (for 21 days)	↓ $t_{1/2}$
Ethinyl estradiol plus *dl*-norgestrel	↑ $t_{1/2}$
Fenfluramine	Unaltered $t_{1/2}$
Halofenate	↓ $t_{1/2}$
Hydrocortisone infusion	↓ $t_{1/2}$ ↑ $t_{1/2}$ Unaltered $t_{1/2}$
Levodopa	↑ $t_{1/2}$
Mandrax[R] (diphenhydramine-methaqualone)	↓ $t_{1/2}$
Norethynodrel plus mestranol	↑ $t_{1/2}$
Paracetamol overdose	↑ $t_{1/2}$
Phenobarbital	↓ $t_{1/2}$
Propranolol	↑ $t_{1/2}$
Quinine	↓ $t_{1/2}$
Rifampicin	Unaltered $t_{1/2}$
Spironolactone	↓ $t_{1/2}$
Spironolactone plus butobarbitone	↓ $t_{1/2}$

Tricyclic antidepressants
   Amitriptyline
   Chlorimipramine
   Desmethylimipramine
   Imipramine
   Nortriptyline
	↓ $t_{1/2}$ or unaltered
	 ↑ $t_{1/2}$

Vitamin C	↓ $t_{1/2}$
Disease states	
Etiocholanolone-induced fever	↑ $t_{1/2}$
Hyperthyroid	↓ $t_{1/2}$
Hypothyroid	↑ $t_{1/2}$
Lead poisoning	↑ $t_{1/2}$

Based on data from Vesell, E.S.: Clin. Pharmacol. Ther. **25**:675, 1979.   *Continued.*

TABLE 6-2   Applications of the antipyrine test in humans where antipyrine was measured before and after a single environmental change—cont'd

Environmental change	Effect of each factor on antipyrine half-life ($t_{1/2}$)
Environmental factors and chemicals	
Bed rest (for 3 days)	$\downarrow t_{1/2}$
Brussels sprouts and cabbage diet	Small $\downarrow t_{1/2}$
Charcoal-broiled beef diet	$\downarrow t_{1/2}$
Cigarette smoking	$\downarrow t_{1/2}$
Circadian variations	Circadian variations in antipyrine metabolism occur in some subjects
Cola nut chewing	Unaltered $t_{1/2}$
Obese subjects fasting for 10 days	Unaltered $t_{1/2}$
High carbohydrate–low protein isocaloric diet	$\uparrow t_{1/2}$
Low carbohydrate–high protein isocaloric diet	$\downarrow t_{1/2}$
Menstrual cycle	Small $\downarrow t_{1/2}$ at midcycle (single subject)
Metabolism in the neonate	Antipyrine $t_{1/2}$ 4 days after birth is shorter than 1 day after birth
Pharmacokinetics of oral and intravenous antipyrine administration	$t_{1/2}$ same after oral or intravenous administration
Piperonyl butoxide	Unaltered $t_{1/2}$
Relationship between D-glucaric acid excretion in urine and antipyrine metabolism	High correlation between antipyrine $t_{1/2}$ and D-glucaric acid excretion in urine
Stress of heat, exercise, and fluid deprivation	Small $\downarrow t_{1/2}$
Miscellaneous factors	
Reproducibility of antipyrine disposition in a subject up to 1 year	$t_{1/2}$ highly reproducible in individual subjects

PHARMACO-GENETIC CONDITIONS (SINGLE-LOCUS TRANSMISSION) THAT ALTER DRUG METABOLISM

A number of pharmacogenetic conditions result from changes in an enzyme controlling the metabolism of a drug. In these conditions, the mutations result in drug accumulation, which causes toxicity. Drug accumulation and toxicity arise from genetically transmitted defects in metabolism of the drug. These defects cause decreased conversion of pharmacologically active drug to pharmacologically inactive metabolite(s). It is of interest that the genetic abnormality long precedes administration of the drug. Thus if individuals possessing such genetic abnormalities can be identified *before* they receive the drug, toxicity can be avoided by either not giving the drug or by giving a much reduced dose. For these reasons, familiarity with pharmacogenetic conditions can help physicians administer drugs more safely and can reduce the high incidence of drug toxicity.

Acatalasia

The condition acatalasia was discovered in a patient on application of hydrogen peroxide to the gums to sterilize a wound after surgery. Instead of bubbles of oxygen evolving from the action of the enzyme catalase as occurs in normal individuals, the hydrogen peroxide remained unchanged and caused toxicity by denaturing tissue proteins. The patient lacked catalase in her oral mucosa and erythrocytes, as did three of her five siblings. The parents were second cousins—consanguinity is a hallmark of autosomal recessive inheritance, which proved to be the mode of transmission of acatalasia. The incidence of this condition reached 1% in certain regions of Japan and also occurred in slightly lower frequency in certain areas of Switzerland. Only a few sporadic cases have been reported in the United States. An impressive lesson from the discovery of acatalasia is that the clinician (in this case, the Japanese oral surgeon Takahara[7-10]) can make an important contribution if alert to the possibility that genetic differences can cause unusual reactions to drugs. Takahara postulated, after completing oral surgery on his patient who then exhibited a toxic response to the antiseptic hydrogen peroxide, that she responded inappropriately because she lacked the normal form of the enzyme required to eliminate the drug. He proved his theory to be correct by gathering similar cases from 27 Japanese families.

Atypical plasma cholinesterase

Another example of how a pharmacogenetic lesion can produce drug toxicity is that of atypical plasma cholinesterase. Individuals possessing a double dose of a mutant gene cannot adequately hydrolyze succinylcholine, a compound administered before surgical procedures to produce muscle relaxation. Normally succinylcholine is rapidly metabolized by a plasma esterase. However, in patients with two mutant genes that control the structure of the plasma enzyme cholinesterase, the drug is retained in the body for much longer periods than usual. Succinylcholine can produce respiratory failure for prolonged periods of time and potentially death if appropriate respiratory resuscitation is not available. When succinylcholine was introduced in 1952 and administered widely in England as a preanesthetic agent, several deaths caused by paralysis of the respiratory muscles did in fact occur in individuals who had inherited from each parent a mutant gene at the cholinesterase locus. Although 1 in 25 persons carries a single dose of the mutant gene, affected persons with two doses occur only once among 2500 individuals.

Studies on the plasma cholinesterase activity of affected individuals, their families, and normal individuals showed considerable overlap until a refinement in technique was introduced. This refinement consisted of a determination of the "dibucaine number," or percent inhibition of plasma cholinesterase by the drug dibucaine (Nupercaine). The dibucaine numbers of 135 individuals of seven unrelated families gave a trimodal curve with no overlap. It has been postulated that plasma cholinesterase activity is determined by two genes at a single locus (alleles), one responsible for the *usual*, the other for the *atypical* form of the enzyme. Most individuals, having a dibucaine number of about 80, are postulated to have two of the usual alleles, $E_1{}^u E_1{}^u$. Individuals of the atypical phenotype, having dibucaine numbers of about 22, have the genotype $E_1{}^a E_1{}^a$. Finally, a third or intermediate group, with dibucaine numbers of about 62, may have a genotype $E_1{}^u E_1{}^a$.[7]

Genetic differences in rates of acetylation of isoniazid, hydralazine, procainamide, and some sulfonamides

Isoniazid is used to treat tuberculosis. Individuals with the genetically transmitted trait of fast acetylation of isoniazid may not be adequately treated on a fixed low dose because of rapid biotransformation of the drug. By contrast, slow acetylators, when receiving the higher, normal dose, may develop toxic effects. Isoniazid-induced polyneuritis—pain and tingling and possibly muscular weakness in the upper and lower extremities—occurs more frequently in slow than in rapid acetylators of isoniazid.[1] Fortunately, the neuritis can be effectively treated with vitamin B$_6$ (pyridoxine).

Isoniazid is metabolized by a liver acetylase. Approximately 50% of the population in this country are acetylators by virtue of possessing a double dose of a recessive form of the gene at this locus. Fast acetylators are either heterozygous or homozygous for the dominant allele. Like several other genetically controlled variations in humans, this hereditary variation in acetylation exhibits marked geographical differences in gene frequency. For example, slow inactivation is uncommon in Eskimos, 95% of whom are rapid acetylators, and only slightly more common in Japanese, 90% of whom are rapid acetylators. In Latin America, approximately 67% of the population are rapid acetylators.

Genetically controlled fast and slow acetylation occurs for several other drugs, including certain sulfonamides; the antihypertensive drug hydralazine; procainamide, an antiarrhythmic drug; and phenelzine, an antidepressant drug. However, several drugs metabolized by acetylation, such as the antitubercular drug *p*-aminosalicylic acid, do not show this difference in rate. Therefore a different enzyme must acetylate these drugs. Continued administration of high doses of hydralazine in slow but not fast acetylators can lead to severe toxicity.

Toxicity can develop not only from drug accumulation resulting from genetically induced retardation in the normal rate of metabolism of a drug but also from the metabolites themselves. For example, rapid acetylators of isoniazid may be more liable than slow acetylators to develop hepatitis after chronic isoniazid administration; presumably a metabolite of the drug is the offending agent. Thus, compared to parent drugs, metabolites cannot all be considered innocuous. An exciting new branch of toxicology is devoted to exploration of how highly reactive, transient drug metabolites covalently bind to tissue components, thereby producing pathological lesions. In this manner, these metabolites are believed to cause some types of teratogenesis, cancer, drug toxicity, and hypersensitivity.

Acetophenetidin-induced methemoglobinemia

Severe methemoglobinemia and hemolysis occurred in a 17-year-old girl after ingestion of the analgesic phenacetin (acetophenetidin). Heritable erythrocytic disorders, including hemoglobinopathies, were excluded as a cause of her hemolysis by multiple laboratory studies. As much as one half of the patient's hemoglobin was occasionally in the form of methemoglobin. After administration of phenacetin, large amounts of the 2-hydroxyphenetidin metabolite and its conjugates appeared in her urine. In normal persons more than 70% of a single 2 g dose of phenacetin can be accounted for in the urine as *N*-acetyl-*p*-aminophenol (acetaminophen), with only minute amounts of the hydroxylated products that predominated in the patient's urine. One sister, a brother, and both parents of the patient had a normal response to phenacetin, but another sister responded abnormally.

These facts suggested an autosomal recessive mode of inheritance of a defect in which the patient's hepatic drug-metabolizing enzymes were deficient in deethylating capacity. Phenacetin, instead of being deethylated to form acetaminophen as in normal persons was hydroxylated in the patient and her 38-year-old sister.

In this patient and her sister, toxicity after phenacetin administration probably arose from these abnormal hydroxylated products, since induction by phenobarbital of hepatic phenacetin-hydroxylating enzymes before administration of phenacetin exacerbated the condition, producing severe neurological symptoms, including bilateral positive Babinski responses, and profound methemoglobinemia. By contrast, in a normal volunteer, phenacetin administration after the same pretreatment with phenobarbital failed to give rise to either methemoglobinemia or neurological changes.

A twin study suggested that large interindividual variations in elimination rates of amobarbital were under genetic control.[2] Pursuing their initial observations, Kalow and associates investigated the family of one set of twins with a deficiency in *N*-hydroxylation, but not *C*-hydroxylation, or amobarbital.[8] The family study of these twins disclosed that this deficiency probably arose from autosomal recessive transmission of a mutant gene.[8]

Deficient N-glucosidation of amobarbital

The antihypertensive drug debrisoquine is widely used in England but is not yet used in the United States. It was observed that patients receiving debrisoquine vary widely in the hypotensive response to the adrenergic-blocking action of the drug and that a close correlation exists between debrisoquine plasma concentrations and the resultant decline in blood pressure.[6] In 94 unrelated volunteers the urinary ratio of the parent drug to the primary metabolite, 4-hydroxydebrisoquine, was measured after a single oral dose of 10 mg debrisoquine.[5] In 3 of these 94 subjects the ratio was very high, suggesting a possible deficiency of the hepatic cytochrome P-450–dependent monooxygenase that 4-hydroxylates debrisoquine. Furthermore, family studies of these three volunteers with abnormally high ratios of debrisoquine to 4-hydroxydebrisoquine in the 8-hour urinary collection suggested transmission of the metabolic deficiency as an autosomal recessive trait.[5] Most side effects as well as most pronounced antihypertensive activity of debrisoquine occurred in the slow metabolizers—those individuals with the highest urinary ratio of parent drug to metabolite.

Polymorphic hydroxylation of debrisoquine

Another fundamental pharmacogenetic principle is underscored by the work of the British group on the genetic control of debrisoquine metabolism and by the previously described example of genetic differences in isoniazid metabolism. When a genetically controlled variation is discovered in the disposition of a particular drug, a search should be undertaken to determine whether the disposition of structurally related drugs is similarly affected by the same genes. The British group reported that the metabolism of 22 drugs in addition to debrisoquine is regulated by this same genetic locus; these other metabolic reactions include *O*-deethylation of phenacetin, hydroxylation of sparteine, nortriptyline, phenformin, metoprolol, alprenolol, timolol, propranolol, perhexiline, and encainide.[3]

PHARMACO-GENETIC CONDITIONS (SINGLE-LOCUS TRANSMISSION) THAT ALTER DRUG INTERACTIONS *Warfarin resistance*	Resistance to warfarin is one of several mutations in humans that modify the pharmacological response to a drug by altering the drug receptor (Table 6-1). One might envision the mutation changing the receptor shape so that it is unable to bind the drug as efficiently as the normal receptor does. In subjects with the mutant gene, the therapeutic effect is not achieved after normal doses of warfarin. Anticoagulation occurs only after the physician administers many times the normal dose of warfarin. Warfarin acts by inhibiting the production of several blood components necessary for clotting, probably by competing with vitamin K for the receptor. In cases of warfarin resistance the mutant receptor is an altered molecule that fails to bind warfarin as strongly as the normal one and therefore does not produce anticoagulation; this alteration results also in a stronger than normal binding of vitamin K. The first family discovered to exhibit this genetically transmitted resistance to warfarin is represented in Fig. 6-2; the index case was a 71-year-old man who came to the hospital with an acute myocardial infarction, the standard treatment of which includes anticoagulation with warfarin.
Genetic differences in capacity to taste phenyl-thiocarbamide	Most persons are able to taste dilute solutions of phenylthiocarbamide (PTC, phenylthiourea) and chemically related compounds containing the thiocyanate group, whereas others, called nontasters, cannot. These differences in ability to taste PTC, in addition to the fact that metabolism of some thiocyanate compounds appears to be no different in tasters and nontasters, suggest that a receptor mutation exists in nontasters. Enlargement of the thyroid gland, called goiter, can be produced in rats by PTC, and certain of these compounds are used in antithyroid drugs in cases of thyroid overactivity. A number of common vegetables including turnips, brussels sprouts, and kale contain a goiter-producing chemical, and nodular goiters are more common among nontasters than among tasters of PTC. These differences in taste threshold may influence food preferences and, thus, consumption of potential goitrogenic compounds.
Genetic control of glucose-6-phosphate dehydrogenase deficiency	A more complicated condition is glucose-6-phosphate dehydrogenase (G-6-PD) deficiency, which affects 100 million people in the world, primarily in areas where malaria is endemic. In the United States 1 in 10 black males is affected. Individuals with any one of 80 different mutations that occur at a specific site on the X chromosome develop hemolytic anemia after exposure to a large number of different drugs, some of which are listed in Table 6-1. Some dietary constituents, such as fava beans (of the plant *Vicia fava*), can cause hemolysis in susceptible subjects. The mechanism believed responsible for development of hemolysis is complex but prob-

Transmission of warfarin resistance through three generations of a family, indicating au-   *FIG. 6-2*
tosomal codominant inheritance of resistance to pharmacological effects of this drug.

From O'Reilly, R.A., Aggler, P.M., Hoag, M.S., Leong, L.S., and Kropatkin, M.L.: Reprinted by permission from The New England Journal of Medicine 271:809, 1964.

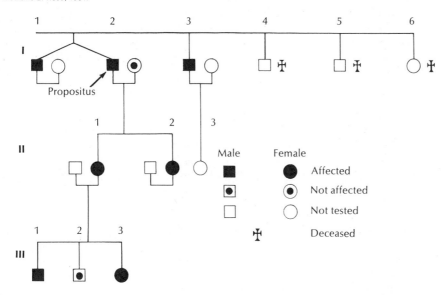

ably initially involves a shortage of NADPH, the reduced form of the cofactor nicotinamide adenine dinucleotide phosphate. NADPH is produced by the enzyme G-6-PD. NADPH itself then serves as a cofactor for glutathione reductase, an enzyme that converts glutathione to the reduced form. Thus G-6-PD deficiency ultimately leads to deficiency of reduced glutathione.

In normal individuals, the red cell membrane is maintained in a functional state by having an adequate supply of reduced glutathione available to keep membrane proteins in a reduced and operative condition. Highly reactive drug metabolites oxidize membrane proteins; if these oxidized proteins are not rapidly reduced by glutathione, hemolysis ensues. Thus a genetically induced enzyme deficiency results in decreased usable glutathione, thereby creating an altered receptor in the cell membrane. Reactive drug metabolites binding to this new receptor produce hemolysis.

It has recently become apparent that there is a high degree of genetically controlled variation among the total complement of enzymes in humans. As many as one third of all enzymes in humans exist in electrophoretically distinguishable forms that vary markedly within many white populations. These variant forms are determined by genes that, like the previously discussed traits affecting drug disposition, are located at a single genetic locus and transmitted from generation to generation according to mendelian law.

REFERENCES

1. Drayer, D.E., and Reidenberg, M.M.: Clinical consequences of polymorphic acetylation of basic drugs, Clin. Pharmacol. Ther. **22**:251, 1977.
2. Endrenyi, L., Inaba, T., and Kalow, W.: Genetic study of amobarbital elimination based on its kinetics in twins, Clin. Pharmacol. Ther. **20**:701, 1976.
3. Idle, J.R., Sloan, T.P., Smith, R.L., and Wakile, L.A.: Application of the phenotyped panel approach to the detection of polymorphism of drug oxidation in man, Br. J. Pharmacol. **66**:430P, 1979.
4. Kalow, W., Kadar, D., Inaba, T., and Tang, B.K.: A case of deficiency of N-hydroxylation of amobarbital, Clin. Pharmacol. Ther. **21**:530, 1977.
5. Mahgoub, A., Dring, L.G., Idle, J.R., Lancaster, R., and Smith, R.L.: Polymorphic hydroxylation of debrisoquen in man, Lancet **2**:584, 1977.
6. Silas, J.H., Lennard, M.S., Tucker, G.T., Smith, A.J., Malcolm, S.L., and Marten, T.R.: Why hypertensive patients vary in their response to oral debrisoquen, Br. Med. J. **1**:422, 1977.
7. Takahara, S.: Progressive oral gangrene probably due to lack of catalase in the blood (acatalasemia), Lancet **263**:1101, 1952.
8. Takahara, S., and Doi, K.: Statistical study of acatalasemia (a review of thirty-eight cases appearing in the literature), Acta Med. Okayama **13**:1, 1959.
9. Takahara, S., Hamilton, H.B., Neel, J.V., Kobara, T.Y., Ogura, Y., and Nishimura, E.T.: Hypocatalasemia: a new genetic carrier state, J. Clin. Invest. **39**:610, 1960.
10. Takahara, S., Sato, H., Doi, M., and Mihara, S.: Acatalasemia. III. On the heredity of acatalasemia, Proc. Japan Acad. **28**:585, 1952.
11. Vesell, E.S., and Page, J.G.: Genetic control of the phenobarbital-induced shortening of plasma antipyrine half-lives in man, J. Clin. Invest. **48**:2202, 1969.

Chapter 7

Effects of age on drug disposition

For many years physicians recognized that patients receiving drugs with low therapeutic indices had to have the usual adult doses reduced to avoid drug toxicity. Precise causes for increased drug sensitivity of geriatric patients have been difficult to identify. Accordingly, only in the last 6 years have some mechanisms responsible for reduced dosage requirements of elderly patients been firmly established. In the last 6 years multiple studies corrected this relative neglect, and the results revealed that for almost every drug investigated the values obtained for rates of drug absorption, distribution, metabolism, or excretion differed in geriatric subjects compared to young adults.

Geriatric subjects, compared to middle-aged subjects, present special problems to the pharmacologist and the clinician. To identify how drugs are handled in "normal" geriatric subjects, such subjects must be carefully examined to exclude pathological conditions. However, the very changes that occur in drug disposition in geriatric subjects occur largely because of degenerative alterations in the structure and function of the heart, liver, and kidney. These degenerative changes have as consequences decreased physiological function of each tissue. For example, cardiac output declines approximately 1% per year from age 19 to 86 years, and with age a decreased proportion of the remaining blood goes to the liver and kidneys. Age-induced changes in the structure and function of critical organs probably occur at different rates in different subjects. Accordingly, subjects of the same chronological age can exhibit different degrees of cardiovascular, hepatic, or renal degeneration and hence different degrees of impairment in the physiological function of each organ.

Although complete data concerning effects of age on gastrointestinal absorption of drugs are presently unavailable, certain changes that occur with age should, from a purely theoretical point of view, alter rates of drug absorption from the gastrointestinal tract. For example, with age gastric emptying time decreases, probably as a result of increased stomach pH. Shortened retention of drugs in the stomach would be anticipated to accelerate their absorption, since drug absorption in the gut occurs mainly in the small intestine because of the large absorbing surface available there.

PROBLEMS OF INVESTIGATING

DRUG ABSORPTION FROM SITES OF ADMINISTRATION

However, drug absorption is complex and involves several distinct steps, including disintegration of tablets or capsules and dissolution of active ingredients.

Another critical factor that affects gastrointestinal drug absorption is intestinal blood perfusion, which has been demonstrated to decrease by 40% to 50% from rates measured in young adults.[1] This reduction would be expected to slow drug absorption in the gut because of decreased transfer of some drugs by active transport across the serosal membrane. Reduction with age in the rate of phosphorylation in the intestinal mucosa retards active absorption of galactose, whereas passive absorption of xylose in the gut declines by 40% from ages 18 to 40 years to ages 70 to 80 years.[9]

Despite these theoretical considerations suggesting reduced rates of gastrointestinal drug absorption with age, Castleden and George[2] reported that age exerted no significant effect on either the rate or amount of gastrointestinal absorption of aspirin, an acidic drug, or the β-adrenergic blocker practolol, a basic drug excreted unchanged by the kidney after absorption from the small intestine.

DRUG DISTRIBUTION	

DRUG DISTRIBUTION

The paucity of studies quantitating age-associated effects on drug distribution may be due in part to the formidable difficulty of distinguishing between the normal aging process on one hand and physiological dysfunction resulting from degenerative diseases of the heart, liver, and kidney that commonly afflict the elderly on the other hand. These degenerative diseases can change the composition of fluid compartments of the body such as total body water, extracellular water, and intracellular water. Therefore selection of appropriate geriatric subjects for pharmacokinetic investigations influences the results; some conflicting reports can probably be attributed to failure of some studies to employ sufficiently rigorous criteria of "normality" in selecting geriatric subjects.

Albumin concentrations decline with age (Fig. 7-1).[7] Whether this decrease occurs as a consequence of reduced albumin synthesis, increased albumin catabolism, or a combination of these is uncertain. From the theoretical viewpoint of what effect reduced albumin concentration would exert on rates of drug elimination from the body, one would predict that for drugs not highly bound to albumin, no change in elimination rate would occur. By contrast, one would predict that for highly bound drugs elimination rates would be accelerated. This anticipated acceleration in the elimination rate of highly bound drugs in the elderly would arise from having more of the drug present in its active unbound form, with consequently greater opportunity for metabolism and excretion. In practice, the opposite of this theoretical expectation occurs. In geriatric patients elimination rates of several highly bound drugs either decrease or remain unchanged, but they do not increase.

When the percent binding of specific drugs to albumin is compared in geriatric subjects and normal middle-aged adults, a variety of results are obtained; only a few drugs exhibit reduced binding in older individuals. No changes with age were observed for plasma binding of phenobarbital, penicillin G, or phenytoin, although mean albumin concentrations declined in the subjects investigated from 4.0 g/ml in those under 50 years old to 3.4 g/ml in those over 50 years old.[1] Also in other studies

Change in mean (±SE) serum albumin concentrations according to age in 11,090 hos-   *FIG. 7-1*
pitalized medical patients.

From Greenblatt, D.J.: J. Am. Geriatr. Soc. **27**:20, 1979.

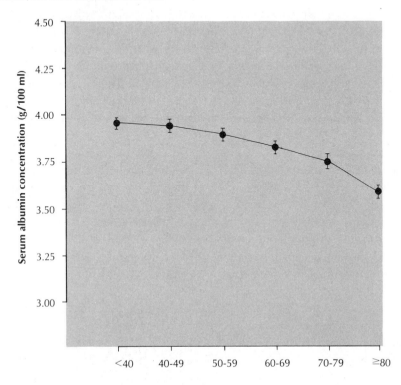

the percent binding of warfarin or diazepam did not change with age. However, another report showed reduced plasma binding of phenylbutazone occurring with age but no change in plasma binding of sulfadiazine or salicylate. In still another study, phenytoin binding declined with age when subjects less than 45 years old who had a mean serum albumin concentration of 4.1 mg/ml were compared with subjects over 65 years old whose mean serum albumin concentrations were 2.9 g/ml.[14] In this and a confirmatory paper on phenytoin from a different laboratory,[8,9] the decrease in percent drug binding with age paralleled the decline in plasma albumin concentrations.

Practical consequences of decreased albumin concentrations in geriatric subjects are noteworthy. Wallace, Whiting, and Runcie showed that the magnitude of interactions affecting displacement from albumin of one drug by another was greater in older than in younger subjects.[14] Binding to plasma proteins of three drugs—phenylbutazone, salicylate, and sulfadiazine—was measured in young and geriatric subjects. In subjects receiving one or more other drugs, geriatric subjects exhibited markedly higher concentrations of the free form of phenylbutazone, salicylate, or sulfadiazine than concentrations found in geriatric subjects not taking other drugs or in younger subjects taking other drugs.[14] The increase in free drug concentration in plasma of geriatric subjects correlated with the number of drugs taken. Wallace, Whiting, and Runcie suggested that geriatric subjects are more susceptible than younger subjects to displacement of one drug from albumin by another because geriatric subjects have lower plasma albumin concentrations.[14]

With respect to other age-related alterations in drug distribution, it was mentioned before that total body weight declines with age but that the proportion of total body weight occupied by fat increases with age. Thus it would be expected that, compared to young adults, geriatric subjects should exhibit increased apparent volumes of distribution (aVd) of very lipid-soluble drugs and environmental compounds (such as DDT). Data on this subject are sparse.

DRUG METABOLISM

Table 7-1 summarizes studies that show the influence of age on drug disposition in human subjects. Effects of age on drug metabolism had previously been demonstrated in rodents.[6] With increasing age rats exhibited reduced activity of several hepatic cytochrome P-450–dependent monooxygenases, the system responsible for biotransformation of most drugs in mammals. Cytochrome P-450 exists in distinct molecular forms, or isozymes, each molecular form probably having different affinity for the same as well as for different drug substrates. These multiple molecular forms have different genetic control and different responses to inducing agents. Heterogeneity of cytochrome P-450 complicates attempts to understand how the drug-metabolizing enzyme system changes under diverse conditions. For example, heterogeneity of cytochrome P-450 may be responsible in part for the complex, age-associated changes observed in both rodents and humans in which, in general, the hepatic drug-metabolizing capacity is very low during the fetal and neonatal periods, reaches a peak in the pediatric age range, and declines thereafter. Possibly different forms of cytochrome P-450 display different developmental patterns.

Studies of two drugs, antipyrine and propranolol, illustrate the complexities of reaching valid interpretations of such pharmacokinetic values obtained in apparently normal subjects of different ages. One of the earliest papers comparing the pharmacokinetics of a drug in young and geriatric subjects revealed that in subjects whose average age was 78 years, antipyrine plasma half-life was 17.4 hours compared to 12.0 hours in subjects of an average age of 26 years.[10] Less marked differences between young and geriatric subjects occurred in antipyrine aVd. Subjects of the same age of different sexes also had different rates of antipyrine elimination. This paper concluded that older subjects exhibited reduced capacity to eliminate the test drug antipyrine because of age-associated reductions in hepatic drug-metabolizing capacity. Subsequently, cigarette smoking was claimed to be mainly responsible for the smaller age-associated reduction in antipyrine elimination observed.[12]

Not adequately recognized is the complexity of "cigarette smoking" as a habit involving subtle psychological, social, and genetic aspects. To consider cigarette smoking as only an environmental factor consisting of exposing the subject to inducing chemicals is to ignore many contributing but discrete individual factors associated

TABLE 7-1   Effects of age on drug disposition

Drug	Elimination rate		aVd	Apparent mechanism for age-related change
	Young adult	Geriatric		
Acetanilid	$t_{1/2}$ = 1.45 hr	$t_{1/2}$ = 2.07 hr	—	Decreased metabolism
Aminopyrine	$t_{1/2}$ = 3.0 hr	$t_{1/2}$ = 10.0 hr	—	—
Ampicillin	$t_{1/2}$ = 1.0 hr	$t_{1/2}$ = 1.2 hr	—	Decreased metabolism
Amylobarbitone (amobarbital)	Urinary metabolite excretion = 14.2% Plasma drug level = 1.3 µg/ml	Urinary metabolite excretion = 4.3% Plasma drug level = 1.0 µg/ml	—	—
Antipyrine	First study: $t_{1/2}$ = 12 hr Second study: No change in MCR* of nonsmokers; MCR* decreased with age in smokers	First study: $t_{1/2}$ = 17.4 hr	—	—
Chlordiazepoxide	Clearance = 26.6 ml/min	Clearance = 46.3 ml/min	↑ in geriatric subjects	—
Diazepam	$t_{1/2}$ = 20 hr	$t_{1/2}$ = 80 hr	↑ ×3 in geriatric subjects	—
Digoxin	$t_{1/2}$ = 51 hr	$t_{1/2}$ = 73 hr	—	Decreased renal function
Dihydrostreptomycin	$t_{1/2}$ = 5.2 hr	$t_{1/2}$ = 8.4 hr	—	Decreased renal function
Doxycycline	$t_{1/2}$ = 11.95 hr	$t_{1/2}$ = 17.74 hr	—	Decreased renal function
Flurazepam	Incidence of flurazepam toxicity increased with age		—	—
Indocyanine green	MCR* decreased with age		—	Decreased liver blood flow
Isoniazid	$t_{1/2}$ = 2.5 hr	$t_{1/2}$ = 2.9 hr	—	—
Kanamycin	$t_{1/2}$ = 107 min	$t_{1/2}$ = 282 min	—	Decreased renal function
Lithium	Clearance = 41.5 ml/min	Clearance = 7.7 ml/min	—	—
Lorazepam	Clearance = 0.99 ml/min/kg	Clearance = 0.77 ml/min/kg	↑ ×2.5 in geriatric subjects	—
Nitrazepam	Clearance = 4.1/1 hr	Clearance = 4.7/1 hr	↑ ×2.0 in geriatric subjects	—
Penicillin	$t_{1/2}$ = 0.55 hr (penicillin G) $t_{1/2}$ = 10 hr (procaine penicillin)	$t_{1/2}$ = 1.0 hr (penicillin G) $t_{1/2}$ = 18 hr (procaine penicillin)	—	—
Pethidine/meperidine	Plasma levels twice as high in geriatric subjects		—	—
Phenobarbital	$t_{1/2}$ = 71 hr	$t_{1/2}$ = 107 hr	—	Decreased metabolism
Phenylbutazone	First study: $t_{1/2}$ = 81 hr Second study: $t_{1/2}$ = 87 hr	$t_{1/2}$ = 105 hr $t_{1/2}$ = 110 hr	—	—
Phenytoin	Clearance = 26 ml/kg/hr	Clearance = 42 ml/kg/hr	—	—
Practolol	$t_{1/2}$ = 7.1 hr	$t_{1/2}$ = 8.6 hr	—	Decreased renal function
Propicillin	Serum levels are twice as high in geriatric subjects		↓ in geriatric subjects	Decreased distribution volume
Propranolol	Clearance decreases with age only in smokers		—	—
Quinidine	Clearance = 4.04 hr	Clearance = 2.64 hr	No change	Decreased metabolism and renal function
Tetracycline	$t_{1/2}$ = 3.5 hr	$t_{1/2}$ = 4.5 hr	—	—

*MCR, Metabolic clearance rate.

with the habit. These individual factors ultimately determine whether a subject makes the decision to smoke cigarettes in a sufficiently high dose to alter hepatic drug-metabolizing capacity.

Propranolol illustrates again the complexities inherent in assessing age-associated effects on pharmacokinetics. Two studies published in 1979 reached different conclusions concerning reasons for prolonged propranolol elimination rates and higher plasma concentrations with age.[2,13] Higher propranolol concentrations in the elderly were attributed both to increased propranolol bioavailability in the elderly, assessed by comparing concentration-time curves after intravenous and oral dosing, and to slowed propranolol distribution to tissues.[2] Increased bioavailability of propranolol after its oral administration in the elderly suggested to the authors that hepatic metabolism of the drug declined with age.

DRUG EXCRETION

Many drugs and their metabolites are eliminated from the body by renal excretion. The extent to which renal mechanisms control drug elimination from the body can vary from 0% to 100%, depending on the drug. For drugs whose elimination depends mainly on renal function, such as barbital, digoxin, gentamicin, and penicillin, impairment of renal function can greatly prolong their sojourn in the body by reducing real clearance. Estimates of the degree of renal dysfunction as judged by reductions in creatinine clearance form the basis for published nomograms that permit selection of appropriately lowered doses of drugs with relatively small therapeutic indices such as digoxin and gentamicin. Since, on the basis of age-associated reductions in renal perfusion, endogenous creatinine clearance declines in the elderly, even without overt renal disease, to approximately one half the values observed in normal young adults,[5] these nomograms show, once endogenous creatinine clearance has been measured, what dose of a drug such as digoxin or gentamicin should be administered to a geriatric patient.[3,4]

CONCLUSIONS

Effects of age on drug absorption, distribution, metabolism, elimination, and various combinations of these have been reviewed.[11] The magnitude of such age-related changes depends on both the pharmacological profile of the particular drug and certain critical environmental and genetic characteristics of each geriatric subject. Because so many diverse environmental factors that can influence drug disposition change concomitantly in elderly subjects, it is often difficult to determine what specific factors are responsible for the pharmacokinetic characteristics of a given drug in a particular geriatric patient. Detailed investigations disclosed that the mechanisms involved are more complex than initially suspected and more pharmacokinetic measurements were required for resolution than were actually obtained in the experiments. For these reasons and because of the incompleteness of our present knowledge, physicians need to exercise special care to avoid toxicity when drugs are administered singly or in combination to geriatric patients. Thus special care is necessary to individualize the dose of many drugs according to the particular requirement of each geriatric patient.

1. Bender, D.A., Post, A., Meier, J.P., Higson, J.E., and Reichard, G.: Plasma protein binding of drugs as a function of age in adult human subjects, J. Pharm. Sci. **64**:1711, 1975.

2. Castleden, C.M., and George, C.F.: The effect of aging on the hepatic clearance of propranolol, Br. J. Clin. Pharmacol. **7**:49, 1979.

3. Christiansen, N.J.B., Kolendorf, K., Siersback-Nielsen, K., and Hansen, J.M.: Serum digoxin values following a dosage regimen based on body weight, sex, age and renal function, Acta Med. Scand. **194**:257, 1973.

4. Dettli, L.C.: Drug dosage in renal disease, Clin. Pharmacokinet. **1**:126, 1976.

5. Friedman, S.A., Raizner, A.E., Rosen, H., Solomon, N.A., and Sy, W.: Functional defects in the aging kidney, Ann. Intern. Med. **76**:41, 1972.

6. Gorrod, J.W.: Absorption, metabolism and excretion of drugs in geriatric subjects, Gerontol. Clin. **16**:30, 1974.

7. Greenblatt, D.J.: Reduced serum albumin concentration in the elderly: a report from the Boston Collaborative Drug Surveillance Program, J. Am. Geriatr. Soc. **27**:20, 1979.

8. Hayes, M.J., Langman, M.J.S., and Short, A.H.: Changes in drug metabolism with increasing age. I. Warfarin binding and plasma protein, Br. J. Clin. Pharmacol. **2**:69, 1975.

9. Hooper, W.D., Bochner, F., Eadie, M.J., and Tyrer, J.H.: Plasma protein binding of diphenylhydantoin: effects of six hormones, renal and hepatic disease, Clin. Pharmacol. Ther. **15**:276, 1974.

10. O'Malley, K., Crooks, J., Duke, E., and Stevenson, I.H.: Effect of age and sex on human drug metabolism, Br. Med. J. **3**:607, 1971.

11. Richey, D.P., and Bender, D.A.: Pharmacokinetic consequences of aging, Annu. Rev. Pharmacol. Toxicol. **17**:49, 1977.

12. Vestal, R.E., Norris, A.H., Tobin, J.D., Cohen, B.H., Shock, N.W., and Andres, R.: Antipyrine metabolism in man: influence of age, alcohol, caffeine, and smoking, Clin. Pharmacol. Ther. **18**:425, 1975.

13. Vestal, R.E., Wood, A.J.J., Branch, R.A., Shand, D.G., and Wilkinson, G.R.: Effects of age and cigarette smoking on propranolol disposition, Clin. Pharmacol. Ther. **26**:8, 1979.

14. Wallace, S., Whiting, B., and Runcie, J.: Factors affecting drug binding in plasma of elderly patients, Br. J. Clin. Pharmacol. **3**:327, 1976.

Chapter 8

Effects of diet on drug disposition

Relationships between diet and drug response in human subjects were not even suspected, much less defined, until recent carefully designed and executed studies not only established a firm foothold on the subject, but also clearly pointed the way for future investigations.[5,7,8,13] At present a few examples exist that show how several dietary factors can alter rates of metabolism of test drugs such as antipyrine and theophylline.

EFFECTS OF
STARVATION
ON DRUG
DISPOSITION

Of all dietary manipulations, the extreme form—starvation—would be expected to produce the most marked pharmacokinetic alteration. When drugs were administered to fasting rodents, greatly reduced rates of hepatic metabolism of some drugs occurred,[4,9] but no major changes in rates of drug metabolism occurred in obese, otherwise healthy, human subjects after 7 to 10 consecutive days on a diet in which the total daily carbohydrate intake was less than 15 g.[15] This diet produced ketoacidosis as well as weight loss that ranged from 3.6 to 15 kg (8 to 33 pounds). When uncorrected for body weight, the apparent volume of distribution (aVd) of both antipyrine and tolbutamide was significantly lower after fasting than before, presumably because during fasting the early loss of body weight is mainly from body water rather than from fat stores or muscle mass. The extent of decrease in aVd was proportional in each subject to the loss of body weight. Therefore, when correction was made for body weight, fasting had no effect on aVd of either antipyrine or tolbutamide. Other hepatic microsomal oxidations were investigated, including those for sulfisoxazole, isoniazid, and procaine.[14] The results disclosed that when allowance was made for body weight, neither half-life nor clearance of these five drugs was changed in obese subjects on a diet containing a total caloric intake of less than 15 g/day of carbohydrates. Although fasting decreased sulfisoxazole excretion, this may be attributed to a decline in rate of urine flow and a fall in urinary pH, both favoring nonionic diffusion of the drug back into the circulation from the renal tubular lumen.

General conclusions regarding the failure of acute fasting to alter rates of hepatic metabolism were further extended by a study of seven female patients with confirmed, classical anorexia nervosa. In these patients prolonged refusal to eat had produced differing degrees of dehydration, hyponatremia, hypochloremia, hypokalemia, and anemia.[2] Compared with age- and sex-matched normal nurses who served as controls, the patients with anorexia nervosa had normal antipyrine pharmacokinetics when these values were corrected for body weight.

A study performed in India revealed that in 15 men suffering from nutritional edema—a severe manifestation of protein deficiency and resultant hypoalbuminemia—the mean plasma antipyrine half-life of 12.8 hours was not significantly different from that of age- and sex-matched nonsmoking controls (11.2 hours) but higher than that of age- and sex-matched smoking controls (8.9 hours).[10] This same study examined another group of 13 undernourished, hypoalbuminemic men without edema. Their short mean antipyrine half-life of 8.6 hours, similar to that of smoking controls (8.9 hours), could be due to the fact that some of them smoked cigarettes, some drank ethanol, and some were agricultural laborers exposed to pesticides known to induce hepatic drug-metabolizing enzymes. Thus in this study severe malnutrition did not by itself markedly alter antipyrine disposition.

A significant contribution to this topic from India measured phenylbutazone pharmacokinetics in four normal male controls (mean age 30) and five undernourished, hypoalbuminemic male subjects (mean age 36), none of whom smoked cigarettes or consumed ethanol chronically. Compared to controls, the malnourished group exhibited shorter mean plasma phenylbutazone half-lives but increased mean phenylbutazone apparent volume of distribution and metabolic clearance rate.[1] These changes in phenylbutazone disposition in undernutrition presumably arose from reduced binding of phenylbutazone to albumin, with a corresponding increase in availability of drug for metabolism and elimination. Because the conclusions could be important therapeutically, these results need to be confirmed in studies on larger groups of undernourished subjects. Nutritionally deprived hypoalbuminemic patients who receive drugs that are highly bound to albumin may require higher doses of these drugs because of their enhanced rates of elimination.

Renal elimination of certain drugs can be altered by fasting or starvation as mentioned for sulfisoxazole, whose renal excretion decreased during fasting. Also, since plasma free fatty acids (ffa) rise dramatically after 12 hours of fasting[18] and since these ffa bind albumin with an avidity capable of displacing many highly bound drugs, fasting for 24 to 72 hours would be expected to accelerate the rate of elimination of such highly bound drugs as bishydroxycoumarin, diazepam, phenylbutazone, phenytoin, and warfarin. Drug removal from the body would be hastened because displacement of drug from albumin by ffa makes the previously bound and hence sequestered drug immediately available for both metabolism and renal elimination, as in the case of undernutrition accompanied by hypoalbuminemia. This hypothesis remains to be established.

*MARKED
ALTERATIONS
IN DRUG
METABOLISM
CAUSED BY
DIETARY
MANIPULATION*
The most dramatic change in drug metabolism caused by dietary manipulation was described by Kappas and associates,[8] who showed that on an isocaloric diet the rate of antipyrine and theophylline metabolism was prolonged twofold as the percentage of total calories represented by carbohydrate doubled from 35% to 70% and the percentage of protein decreased from 44% to 10%. The percentage of total calories represented by fat remained constant in the two diets at approximately 20%. The pharmacokinetic values indicate that without alteration in total number of calories the switch from high to low protein with a reverse change in carbohydrate content affected only antipyrine and theophylline half-life and clearance, not their aVd (Fig. 8-1). This pattern suggests that this particular type of dietary manipulation affected antipyrine and theophylline metabolism rather than distribution.

FIG. 8-1   *Theophylline half-lives in six normal subjects maintained on their usual home diets and on two test-diet periods. Each bar represents mean ± SE for the six subjects. P, Protein; C, carbohydrate; F, fat. Values for diets 1, 3, and 4, are not significantly different from each other. Value for diet 2 is significantly different from that of diet 1 ($p = 0.05$) and diet 3 ($p = 0.01$).*

From Kappas, A., Anderson, K.E., Conney, A.H., and Alvares, A.P.: Clin. Pharmacol. Ther. 20:643, 1976.

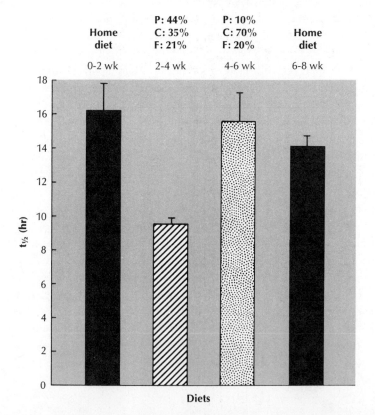

Many patients who receive drugs are debilitated and chronically ill; they may have inadequate nutrition and the proportion of their diet usually occupied by carbohydrate may be reversed because of intravenous therapy. For such patients the rate of drug elimination may be significantly changed. Furthermore, a certain percentage of the normal population is involved in various weight-reduction diets; these individuals could also be susceptible to the kinds of changes in drug-metabolizing capacity illustrated in Fig. 8-1. Drug dosage may also have to be changed according to new requirements in subjects who change their dietary patterns in ways similar to those shown in Fig. 8-1.

The question arises of why starvation produces negligible change in antipyrine metabolism, whereas with an isocaloric diet, simply switching the proportion of carbohydrate to protein exerts profound alterations on antipyrine metabolism. Possibly the body can detect the former dietary manipulation better than the latter type. Through detection of the gross dietary change of starvation, the body can compensate by providing from another source, at least for a limited time, the amino acids required for protein synthesis. By contrast, the body may not be able to detect and hence compensate for a much more subtle switch in the proportion of the total number of calories supplied in the diet as either carbohydrate or protein. If this change goes uncompensated, depletion of protein could reduce rates of synthesis of hepatic drug-metabolizing enzymes, which in turn could cause retention in the body of such drugs as antipyrine and theophylline.

EFFECTS OF CHARCOAL BROILING ON DRUG DISPOSITION

Food preparation can also affect drug concentrations and disposition. In rats charcoal-broiled beef (rather than beef cooked while covered with foil, which prevents formation of polycyclic hydrocarbons on the beef) increased by elevenfold intestinal metabolism of phenacetin in vitro.[11] Similarly designed studies were performed with eight healthy human volunteers in whom plasma antipyrine and theophylline half-lives were measured both before and after 7 days on a charcoal-broiled beef diet.[7] Later these drugs were also measured before and after another 7-day course on a diet containing the same amount of beef, but with the beef cooked while covered with foil. After eating charcoal-broiled beef, the subjects shortened their plasma antipyrine and theophylline half-lives by 22%. No change occurred in aVd of either drug, but clearance of both drugs increased. Charcoal broiling appeared to enhance hepatic oxidative metabolism of both drugs.[7]

STIMULATORY EFFECT OF BRUSSELS SPROUTS AND CABBAGE

In rats a diet containing certain cruciferous vegetables, such as brussels sprouts, cabbage, turnips, broccoli, cauliflower, or spinach, induced intestinal benzo[a]pyrene hydroxylase activity and the intestinal enzymes that metabolize 7-ethoxycoumarin, hexobarbital, and phenacetin.[12,17] It was demonstrated that certain indoles present in these cruciferous vegetables were potent inducers of the gut enzymes that metabolize these drugs. The stage was then set for a study in humans to determine whether a dietary regimen rich in these cruciferous vegetables could also exert an inductive effect on drug metabolism. The results obtained in a study on 10 healthy volunteers were positive and showed that on a 7-day diet rich in brussels sprouts and cabbage mean antipyrine half-lives were decreased by 13% and mean plasma phenacetin concentrations were decreased by 34% to 67%.[13]

Although statistically significant, very small changes in plasma antipyrine half-life (13%) and in antipyrine clearance (11%) after an intensive and unusual exposure for 1 week to cabbage and brussels sprouts raise the question of how clinically meaningful such dietary manipulations may be. Stated otherwise, could such dietary factors produce a toxic reaction in a patient by changing that patient's dosage requirement of commonly used drugs with low therapeutic indices? Probably they could. While the change in antipyrine clearance produced by a diet high in brussels sprouts and cabbage for 7 days was small, phenacetin plasma concentrations changed much more. For still other drugs, the change produced could be even larger.

| THEOBROMINE AS A METABOLIC INHIBITOR | Studies described previously established effects on drug disposition of chemically heterogeneous changes in diet. Work on the methylxanthine theobromine, a chemically homogeneous nutritional constituent of such dietary staples as chocolate and tea, revealed that because of daily dietary theobromine intake normal subjects are inhibited metabolically with respect to their capacity to eliminate theobromine.[5] |

After 2 weeks on a methylxanthine-free diet, each of six healthy male subjects increased his capacity to eliminate a test dose of theobromine (Fig. 8-2). Although theobromine is not used as a drug, closely related methylxanthines such as theophylline are.

In the same patient, during a single course of therapy, theophylline doses may need to be changed abruptly. We hypothesized, on the basis of our studies with theobromine previously described, that dietary theobromine intake might influence theophylline dosage requirements. The hypothesis was based on the assumption that theobromine intake in human subjects could inhibit theophylline metabolism. This assumption was recently supported by the demonstration that in human subjects theobromine inhibits rates of theophylline elimination.[3]

| COLA NUT INGESTION AND HEPATIC DRUG METABOLISM | A study performed on West African villagers identified, through multiple regression analysis, cola nut consumption to be the single best predictor of antipyrine clearance[6]; three other statistically significant predictive factors were sex, hemoglobin in women, and height in men. No attempt was made to determine effects on antipyrine clearance of cessation of cola nut chewing in chewers or of initiation of chewing in nonchewers. However, a carefully controlled study was performed to determine effects of cola nut chewing on antipyrine clearance in normal male volunteers living in a south central town in Pennsylvania.[16] In these subjects, no alteration in antipyrine clearance occurred after either 2 or 4 weeks of cola nut chewing. |

These results do not contradict the ones obtained in the study on West African villagers, because the genetic constitutions and environmental conditions of the subjects in each study was so different. Nevertheless, failure of chronic cola nut

Decay of a single oral dose of theobromine (6 mg/kg) before and after 2-week dietary   **FIG. 8-2**
abstention from methylxanthines.

From Drouillard, D.D., Vesell, E.S., and Dvorchik, B.H.: Clin. Pharmacol. Ther. 23:296, 1978.

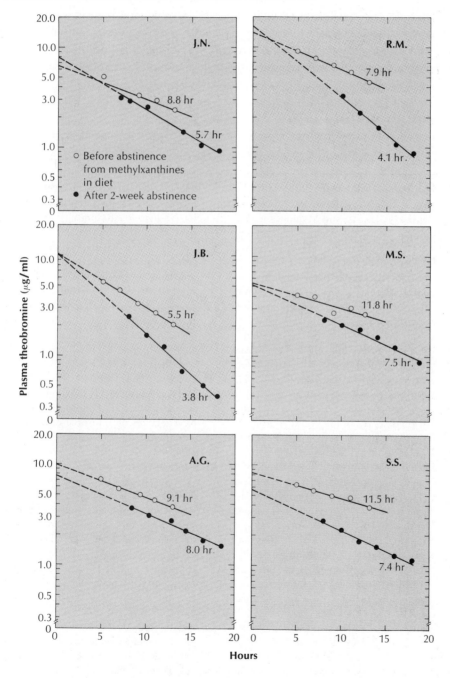

consumption to alter antipyrine clearance in normal volunteers in this country renders the West African investigation more difficult to interpret.

INTERACTIONS
BETWEEN DIET
AND OTHER
SIMULTANEOUSLY
OPERATING
CONDITIONS

Multiple, simultaneously acting factors can influence rates of drug elimination in either unselected normal volunteers or patients. Formidable difficulties interfere with accurate assessment of the relative contribution made by each of these simultaneously acting factors to large interindividual variations in rates of drug elimination.

REFERENCES

1. Adithan, C., Gandhi, I.S., and Chandrasekar, S.: Pharmacokinetics of phenylbutazone in undernutrition, Indian J. Pharmacol. **10**:301, 1978.
2. Bakke, O.M., Aanderud, S., Syversen, G., Bassoe, H.H., and Myking, O.: Antipyrine metabolism in anorexia nervosa, Br. J. Clin. Pharmacol. **5**:341, 1978.
3. Caldwell, J., Monks, T.J., Lawrie, S., and Smith, R.L.: Dietary methylxanthines (MXs) as determinants of theophylline (T) metabolism in man, Pharmacologist **21**:1973, 1979.
4. Dixon, R.L., Shultice, R.W., and Fouts, J.R.: Factors affecting drug metabolism by liver microsomes. IV. Starvation, Proc. Soc. Exp. Biol. Med. **103**:333, 1960.
5. Drouillard, D.D., Vesell, E.S., and Dvorchik, B.H.: Studies on theobromine disposition in normal subjects, Clin. Pharmacol. Ther. **23**:296, 1978.
6. Fraser, H.S., Bulpitt, C.J., Kahn, C., Mould, G., Mucklow, J.C., and Dollery, C.T.: Factors affecting antipyrine metabolism in West African villagers, Clin. Pharmacol. Ther. **20**:369, 1976.
7. Kappas, A., Alvares, A.P., Anderson, K.E., Pantuck, E.J., Pantuck, C.B., Chang, R., and Conney, A.H: Effect of charcoal-broiled beef on antipyrine and theophylline metabolism, Clin. Pharmacol. Ther. **23**:445, 1978.
8. Kappas, A., Anderson, K.E., Conney, A.H., and Alvares, A.P.: Influence of dietary protein and carbohydrate on antipyrine and theophylline metabolism in

man, Clin. Pharmacol. Ther. **20**:643, 1976.
9. Kato, R., and Gillette, J.R.: Sex differences in the effects of abnormal physiological states on the metabolism of drugs by rat liver microsomes, J. Pharmacol. Exp. Ther. **150**:285, 1965.
10. Krishnaswamy, K., and Naidu, A.N.: Microsomal enzymes in malnutrition as determined by plasma half-life of antipyrine, Br. Med. J. **1**:538, 1977.
11. Pantuck, E.J., Hsiao, K.C., Kuntzman, R., and Conney, A.H.: Intestinal metabolism of phenacetin in the rat: effect of charcoal-broiled beef and rat chow, Science **187**:744, 1975.
12. Pantuck, E.J., Hsiao, K.-C., Loub, W.D., Wattenberg, L.W., Kuntzman, R., and Conney, A.H.: Stimulatory effect of vegetables on intestinal drug metabolism in the rat, J. Pharmacol. Exp. Ther. **198**:278, 1976.
13. Pantuck, E.J., Pantuck, C.B., Garland, W.A., Min, B.H., Wattenberg, L.W., Anderson, K.E., Kappas, A., and Conney, A.H.: Stimulatory effect of brussels sprouts and cabbage on human drug metabolism, Clin. Pharmacol. Ther. **25**:88, 1979.
14. Reidenberg, M.M.: Obesity and fasting: effects on drug metabolism and drug action in man, Clin. Pharmacol. Ther. **22**:729, 1977.
15. Reidenberg, M.M., and Vesell, E.S.: Unaltered metabolism of antipyrine and tolbutamide in fasting man, Clin. Pharmacol. Ther. **17**:650, 1975.

16. Vesell, E.S., Shively, C.A., and Passananti, G.T.: Failure of cola-nut chewing to alter antipyrine disposition in normal male subjects from a small town in south central Pennsylvania, Clin. Pharmacol. Ther. 26:287, 1979.

17. Wattenberg, L.W.: Studies of polycyclic hydrocarbon hydroxylases of the intestine possibly related to cancer. Effect of diet on benzpyrene hydroxylase activity, Cancer 28:99, 1971.

18. Wood, F.C., Domenge, L., Bally, P.R., Renold, A.E., and Thorn, G.W.: Studies on the metabolic response to prolonged fasting, Med. Clin. North Am. 44:1371, 1960.

Chapter 9

Effects of occupation and disease on drug disposition

OCCUPATIONAL FACTORS THAT ALTER RESPONSE OF DRUG-METABOLIZING ENZYMES

In Chapter 6 it was shown that genetic factors contribute appreciably to large interindividual variations in rates of drug elimination among normal subjects under near basal conditions. However, in unselected subjects chronically exposed to numerous environmental compounds and conditions that can induce or inhibit the activity of hepatic mixed-function oxidases, rates of drug elimination are obviously not basal. In such subjects a dynamic interaction exists between the genes that control hepatic mixed-function oxidases and multiple environmental factors.

Although for convenience twin studies separate genetic from environmental contributions as though they were discrete unrelated entities, the transcriptional and translational mechanisms by which genetic information is expressed require environmental participation. Conversely, many environmental factors that alter rates of drug disposition in humans do so by affecting genetic mechanisms. Environmental chemicals, such as DDT, polychlorinated biphenyls, and polycyclic hydrocarbons, can alter, through induction, a subject's hepatic drug-metabolizing enzyme activity. As shown later in this chapter, disease states can also markedly change a subject's rate of drug elimination.

Physicians should recognize that chronic occupational exposure to the chemicals listed in Table 9-1 can alter a patient's basal rate of drug elimination, mainly by inducing or inhibiting the mixed-function oxidases responsible for hepatic drug metabolism.

OCCUPATIONAL CHEMICALS THAT ALTER DRUG-METABOLIZING CAPACITY

A partial list of chemicals encountered in a subject's occupation that are capable of accelerating or retarding rates of hepatic drug metabolism appears in Table 9-1. This list is suggestive rather than complete.

This aspect of occupational medicine (the influence of chemicals encountered at work on a subject's capacity to metabolize drugs) represents only a small portion of the entire subject. In recent years, the field of occupational medicine has expanded greatly because of recognition that various human diseases develop as a result of chronic exposure to certain chemicals during work. The association between certain

TABLE 9-1 Occupational chemicals that can alter rates of drug elimination, depending on intensity and duration of exposure

Number and sex of subjects*	Employed in	Chemical exposure	Test drug	Change in test drug produced by chemical	Reference
26 M	Insecticide plant	Lindane and DDT	Antipyrine	Shorter plasma $t_{1/2}$	Kolmodin, et al.†
15 M 18 F	Same insecticide plant as office workers	Unexposed (control)	—	—	—
18 M	DDT plant for more than 5 years	DDT and "DDT-related compounds"	Phenylbutazone and 6β-hydroxycortisol excretion in urine	Phenylbutazone $t_{1/2}$ ↓; urinary excretion of 6β-hydroxycortisol ↑	Poland et al.‡
18 M	Same DDT plant, same time	Unexposed (control)	—	—	—
14 M	Insecticide plant	Spray of solution containing 4% lindane, 0.1% pyrethrum, 2.5% malathion	Phenylbutazone	Phenylbutazone $t_{1/2}$ ↓	Kolmodin et al.†
9 M	Insecticide plant	Unexposed (control)	—	—	—
26 M	Tree nurseries	Spray of lindane 4%, 2.5% malathion	Antipyrine, phenylbutazone	Antipyrine $t_{1/2}$ ↓; Phenylbutazone $t_{1/2}$ ↓	Kolmodin-Hedman§
23 M	Tree nurseries	Spray of DDT	Oxazepam	Oxazepam $t_{1/2}$ unchanged	—
15 F 18 F	Office	Unexposed (control)	—	—	—
3 M 2 F	Capacitor manufacturing plant	Polychlorinated biphenyls	Antipyrine	Antipyrine $t_{1/2}$ ↓; clearance ↑; aVd unchanged	Alvares et al.∥
3 M 2 F	Same plant	Unexposed (control)	—	—	—
4 MC 4 FC	—	Chronic lead poisoning	Antipyrine, phenylbutazone	Antipyrine and phenylbutazone $t_{1/2}$ ↑; therapy for phenylbutazone poisoning decreased these values toward normal	Alvares et al.¶
2 ?C	—	Acute lead poisoning	—	—	—
1 MC 1 FC	—	Unexposed (control)	—	—	—

Continued.

*C, Children.
†Kolmodin, B., et al.: Clin. Pharmacol. Ther. 10:638, 1969.
‡Poland, A., et al.: Clin. Pharmacol. Ther. 11:724, 1970.
§Kolmodin-Hedman, B. In Morselli, P.L., et al., editors: Drug interactions. New York, 1974, Raven Press.
∥Alvares, A.P.: Clin. Pharmacokinet. 3:462, 1978.
¶Alvares, A.P.: Clin. Pharmacol. Ther. 19:183, 1976.
**Alvares, P.: Clin. Pharmacol. Ther. 22:140, 1977.
††Meredith, P.A., et al.: Br. J. Clin. Pharmacol. 3:960P, 1976.

TABLE 9-1 Occupational chemicals that can alter rates of drug elimination, depending on intensity and duration of exposure—cont'd

Number and sex of subjects	Employed in	Chemical exposure	Test drug	Change in test drug produced by chemical	Reference
8 M	Shipyard	Lead	Antipyrine	Antipyrine $t_{1/2}$ ↓	Alvares et al.[**]
10 M	Unspecified	Chronic lead poisoning	Antipyrine	Antipyrine $t_{1/2}$ ↓; clearance ↑; these reverted to normal with EDTA therapy	Meredith et al.[††]
23 ?	Anesthesia	OR gases; presumably volatile anesthetic agents (halothane, etc.)	Antipyrine	Antipyrine $t_{1/2}$ ↓ (measured once)	O'Malley et al.[27]
23 ?	Anesthesia	Unexposed (control)	—	—	—
7 M	Anesthesiology residency	Undefined volatile anesthetic agents	Warfarin	Warfarin $t_{1/2}$ ↑ measured before and after 4 months of exposure to OR	Ghoneim et al.[14]
5 M	Anesthesiology residency	Unexposed (control)	—	—	
26 M	Spray painting	Xylene, toluene, gasoline, benzene, butanol, butylacetate, methyl-isobutyl ketone, methyl-glycol acetate, isocyanates, epoxy resins, lead, zinc chromate, cadmium	Antipyrine	Antipyrine $t_{1/2}$ ↑	Døssing[12]
44 M	Herbicide plant	4-Chloro-2-methyl-phenoxyacetic acid, 4-chloro-2-methylphenoxy-propionic acid, 4,2-dichlorophenoxypropionic acid, 2,4,5-trichlorophenoxyacetic acid, 4,5-dichlorophenol, 2-methyl-4-chlorophenol, 2-methyl-4,6-dichlorophenol	Antipyrine	Antipyrine $t_{1/2}$ ↓	Døssing[12]
10 M	Greenhouse	Captan, diazinon, pirimicarb, methiocarb, permetrin, benomyl, dienichlor, parathion, aldicarb, lindane, xylene, trimethylbenzene, dimethylformamide	Antipyrine	Antipyrine $t_{1/2}$ ↓	

diseases and specific conditions at work was documented first in the eighteenth century by Percival Potts. He reported that English chimney sweeps were at high risk of developing cancer of the scrotum. In the twentieth century it was learned that exposure at work to asbestos, benzene, phenol, vinyl chloride, radium, and x rays also increased the risk of developing certain forms of cancer. Chronic intake of large doses of phenacetin by watchmakers in Switzerland to relieve the headaches produced by long hours of eyestrain greatly increased their risk of developing renal disease. Similarly, it was noted that coal miners had a much higher incidence of pulmonary disease than did age-matched controls who were not chronically exposed to the conditions of coal mines.

Although additional examples could be culled from the literature and fresh examples will undoubtedly be published soon, those enumerated in Table 9-1 illustrate clearly the general principle that many chemicals to which subjects are chronically exposed at work can change their basal rates of drug elimination.

Because this is a pill-oriented society, exposure to potent chemicals that can alter a subject's near basal rate of drug clearance is rarely limited to that subject's occupational exposure. Such chemicals are much more commonly ingested for medicinal, recreational, or nutritional purposes than ingested as a result of occupational exposure only.

A controlled experiment is necessary to assess the role of the chemicals listed in Table 9-1 with respect to their role in affecting a subject's capacity to metabolize drugs. In this experiment, only one factor is manipulated independently of the others. Subjects in a near basal state of drug clearance need to be selected for such a study. Then each subject's clearance of a test compound is determined several times before imposition of this factor and again several times after introduction of the factor. By constructing dose-response curves we can assess quantitatively the role exerted by each factor on drug clearance.

These essential points in experimental design are emphasized here because they may help explain the discrepant results in Table 9-1 for anesthetists. Table 9-1 shows that anesthetists in one study apparently had accelerated rates of antipyrine elimination,[27] whereas in another study their rates of warfarin elimination were prolonged.[14] In the former study, antipyrine was administered only once and the control group was not concurrent, whereas in the latter study anesthesiology residents served as their own controls with each subject's rate of warfarin elimination being measured on two separate occasions.

A single disease may exert different effects on the separate processes of drug absorption, distribution, metabolism, excretion, and receptor action. When each of these individual effects is measured and all effects summated, the net change in "drug response" may be negligible as a result of the balancing of one major effect by another acting in an opposite direction. Changes in the patient's condition or treatment may upset this balance and bring to light a major effect that the disease

EFFECTS OF DISEASE ON DRUG DISPOSITION

TABLE 9-2   A partial list of drugs whose half-lives have been reported to be altered by hepatic or renal dysfunction

Drug	Change in t½ — Hepatic dysfunction	Change in t½ — Renal dysfunction
Acetaminophen	↑	
Amiloride	↑	↑
Aminopyrine	↑	No change
Ampicillin		↑
Antipyrine	↑	No change
Carbenicillin	↑	↑
Cefazolin		↑
Cephacetrile		↑
Cephalexin		↑
Cephaloridine		↑
Cephalothin	↑	↑
Chloramphenicol		No change
Chlorpropamide	↑	↑
Clindamycin		↑
Cloxacillin	↑	↑
Colchicine	→	↑
Colistimethate	↑	↑
Diazepam		↓ or no change
Diazoxide		↑
Dicloxacillin		↑
Digitoxin	↑	↓ or no change
Digoxin		↑
Doxorubicin		
Erythromycin		↑
Ethambutol		↑
Flucytosine		↑
Furosemide		↑
Gentamicin		↑
Hydrocortisone	↑	
Indocyanine green	↑	
Isoniazid	↑	↑
Lidocaine	↑	
Meperidine	↑	No change
Methicillin		↑
Nafcillin	↑	↑
Niridazole	↑	↑
Oxacillin		↑
Oxazepam	No change	
Penicillin G		No change
Pentobarbital		
Phenacetin	No change	
Phenylbutazone	↑ or no change	
Phenytoin	↑ or no change	↑
Prednisone		
Procainamide		↑
Propranolol	↑	↓ or no change
Rifampicin	↑	↑
Streptomycin		↑
Sulfadimethoxine		↑
Sulfamethazine		↓ or no change
Sulfamethoxazole		↑
Sulfamethoxypyridazine		↑
Tetracycline		↑
Tobramycin		↑
Trimethoprim		↑
Vancomycin		↑
Warfarin	No change	No change

Data derived from reviews by Creasey,[9] Pagliaro and Benet,[28] Reidenberg,[36] and Vesell.[47]

exerts on a single pharmacokinetic or pharmacodynamic process by removing the offsetting effects of the disease on the other processes.

A critical point to remember is that a disease process may affect the disposition of different drugs in different ways. The reason is that each drug has a distinct pharmacological profile and the way a disease process alters the disposition of a particular drug depends on the specific pharmacological characteristics of the drug. For example, in hypoalbuminemia the disposition of drugs such as warfarin and phenylbutazone that are extensively bound to albumin will be changed, whereas the disposition of isoniazid and kanamycin that bind albumin negligibly will not be altered. As another example, hepatocellular disease changes the disposition of drugs biotransformed in the liver much more than it does the disposition of drugs such as barbital and the majority of antibiotics that are not.

Table 9-2 presents a partial list of drugs whose half-lives have been reported to be altered by diseases of the liver or kidney. Since changes in drug half-life can arise from alterations in rates of drug absorption, distribution, metabolism, or excretion, it is useful to consider effects of several prototypical disease states on each of these individual processes. One must also remember that changes in drug half-life do not necessarily indicate a change in rate of drug metabolism, since change in the volume of distribution of a drug can cause changes in drug half-life without a change in drug metabolism. Furthermore, large changes can occur in both the metabolism and volume of distribution of a drug without any change in drug half-life.

Many different disorders and pathological states can alter the normal rates and pathways for drug absorption, distribution, biotransformation, excretion, interaction with receptor sites, or various combinations of these. Since each drug has a distinct profile for these five processes, the extent to which a disease that affects these processes will alter the distribution of a drug depends on the particular drug. Therefore it is hazardous to extrapolate how pathological processes will affect other drugs on the basis of pathological effects that alter the distribution of one drug.

Clinical consequences of a change in drug distribution produced by disease will be determined also by the therapeutic index of the drug as well as by certain genetic and environmental characteristics of the patient. For example, a change of 200% in the plasma half-life of antipyrine, salicylates, or penicillin will probably have little or no clinical consequence, whereas a change of 20% in the plasma half-life of digoxin, procainamide, or lidocaine may prove critical. By the same token, a change of 1% in the albumin binding of warfarin, which normally is 99% bound, may have profound toxicological results; whereas a change of 1% in the albumin binding of probenecid, which normally is 75% bound, has negligible clinical consequences. Here the crucial factor is the percent change in the free, but not bound, portion of the drug.

Effects of disease states on the rate of absorption of a drug depend on many factors, including the site of drug administration. If the drug is administered orally, the influence of disease on rates of drug absorption will depend on the nature of the disease process, whether it affects the areas in the gut where the drug is normally

Drug absorption

absorbed, and how the disease alters the normal physiological volume, pH, temperature, viscosity, surface tension, and composition of the gastrointestinal secretions and contents.[22] Rates of drug absorption may also be influenced by whether food is present, the nature and quantity of bile salts and bacterial flora, the rate of splanchnic blood flow, prior diet, and food intake as well as gastrointestinal motility.[22] Until recently little was known about how disease states altered these factors in man; however, large interindividual differences in rates of absorption of many orally administered drugs occur in hospital patients[3,20,25] as well as in normal volunteers.[5,33,39] For example, a sevenfold range in the amount of tetracycline absorbed was reported in six fasting, healthy subjects.[32] Variations in gastric emptying may contribute significantly to large interindividual differences in drug absorption rate because numerous physiological conditions, such as posture and autonomic activity as well as the temperature, volume, viscosity, and tonicity of gastric contents, can change gastric emptying time. Grossly impaired absorption of paracetamol occurs in patients with delayed gastric emptying and pyloric stenosis.[15] In patients with slow gastric emptying, L-dopa may be ineffective.[7] Therapeutic failure of orally administered drugs usually accompanies gastric stasis.[15,26,30] In patients with achlorhydria, aspirin was absorbed significantly faster and plasma salicylate concentrations were higher than those in control subjects.[30] Acetaminophen plasma concentrations were significantly higher after oral administration of the drug to 12 convalescent hospital patients in bed than to 7 healthy ambulant volunteers matched for age and sex.[31]

Since rates of absorption of orally administered pills and capsules are dependent on rates of dissolution and dispersion, some of the factors enumerated above can alter such rates, thereby contributing to variations in drug absorption. It is interesting and somewhat surprising that the absorption of p-aminosalicylic acid and isoniazid was unchanged by gastrectomy performed for peptic ulcer, although complete failure to ethionamide absorption occurred in some patients.[24] Furthermore, gastrectomy failed to alter the absorption of sulfisoxazole, quinidine, or ethambutol unless vagotomy had been performed, thereby slowing gastric emptying.[45]

In jejunal disease folic acid absorption is diminished.[16] In ileal disease the transport of bile acids may be impaired, as well as the enterohepatic transport of many lipid-soluble drugs, since bile acids promote the gastrointestinal absorption of fat and certain fat-soluble compounds, including many drugs and vitamins A, D, K, and E. Ileal disease may be associated with impaired vitamin B_{12} absorption, since vitamin B_{12} is absorbed in the ileum after it forms a complex with intrinsic factor produced by the gastric parietal cell. Defective function of the ileum as a result of surgical removal or disease through interference with vitamin B_{12} absorption can lead to pernicious anemia. Vitamin B_{12} absorption can also be impaired in gastric diseases in which parietal cell function is abnormal, producing intrinsic factor deficiency and pernicious anemia. In some patients with pernicious anemia, precipitating or blocking antibodies to intrinsic factor have been identified.[13,38] In addition, regional enteritis as well as tropical sprue, celiac disease, and Whipple's disease, can produce vitamin B_{12} malabsorption. In steatorrhea, fat-soluble drugs and vitamins may be lost in the feces, producing deficiency of the fat-soluble vitamins, a deficiency of vitamin D being by far the most significant chronic problem in gastrointestinal disease.

Some active drugs are produced after metabolism of the inactive form by gut bacteria, the best example being cleavage of salicylazosulfapyridine, the drug of choice in the treatment of chronic ulcerative colitis. Diseases that change the nature of the gastrointestinal flora can affect the disposition of other drugs metabolized by gut bacteria. Possibly the effect of large doses of charcoal on gastrointestinal absorption of phenacetin is mediated by gut bacteria and induction of aryl hydrocarbon hydroxylase activity in these bacteria by charcoal.[29] Absorption of digoxin is reduced by neomycin administration.[23]

Drug distribution

Binding of many drugs to albumin is altered in several disease states, particularly in diseases of the liver and kidney associated with decreased concentrations of serum albumin. For example, phenytoin binding to albumin was decreased in plasma of 15 uremic patients.[34] The size of the unbound fraction correlated well with blood urea nitrogen, serum creatinine, and the clinical state of the patient. In addition to phenytoin, other organic acids including clofibrate, congo red, fluorescein, methyl red, phenytoin, sulfonamides, thyroxine, and tryptophan exhibited decreased protein binding in uremia. By contrast, most organic bases bind normally to plasma from uremic patients. A clinically significant neutral compound, digitoxin, exhibited decreased plasma binding in uremic patients.[40]

Disease states, including cirrhosis and nephritis, that are associated with hypoproteinemia and hypoalbuminemia exhibit elevations in the unbound fraction of most drugs compared with the unbound fraction present under conditions of normal protein and albumin concentrations. These situations illustrate the danger of selecting drug dose solely on the basis of total drug concentrations in plasma rather than on the free concentration, since only the free form is pharmacologically active. In cirrhosis, the plasma binding of the organic bases quinidine, diazepam, and triamterene, as well as of the organic acid fluorescein, are all decreased.

In addition to these disease-associated quantitative changes in drug binding to albumin, qualitative changes can occur in the nature of the binding. Such qualitative changes have been reported in uremia,[37] in which avidity of phenytoin binding to albumin is reduced.

Hepatic drug metabolism

An appropriate answer to the question of how liver disease affects the disposition of a drug normally eliminated primarily by hepatic metabolism requires consideration of several facts. Most drugs metabolized in the liver are converted by multiple reactions, including oxidations, reductions, and conjugations. It is not unusual for such drugs to have 10 to 20 distinctive metabolites, and for some as many as 30 or even 40 metabolites have been identified. Several enzymes responsible for these multiple reactions are cytoplasmic; others are associated with specific subcellular organelles. Under normal conditions the cytochrome P-450–dependent monooxygenases located in the smooth endoplasmic reticulum and responsible for many drug

FIG. 9-1 *Excretion of* $^{14}[CO_2]$ *in breath of patients with various forms of liver disease compared to control patients 2 hours after oral administration of a single tracer dose of* [^{14}C]*aminopyrine.*
From Hepner, G.W., and Vesell, E.S.: Ann. Intern. Med. **83**:632, 1975.

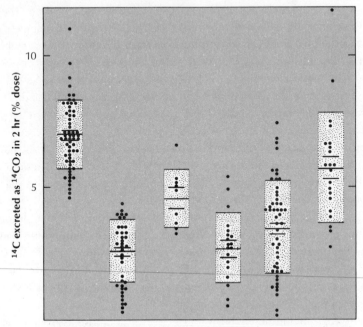

oxidations exist in at least three, and possibly six or more, molecular forms. Diseases of the liver can differentially affect these enzymes and isozymes.

Aside from these physiological considerations, pathophysiological changes in liver disease are relevant to the question at hand. The most common form of liver disease in this country, alcoholic cirrhosis, is a disease characterized by remissions and exacerbations, by a variable progression over time. During the early part of the disease, rates of metabolism of many drugs in alcoholic subjects may actually be faster than in normal subjects[47] because multiple doses of ethanol induce cytochrome P-450–dependent monooxygenases in hepatic smooth endoplasmic reticulum.[47] However, with time the disease process begins to convert functional hepatocytes into fibrous bands incapable of metabolizing drugs.

These facts are presented to show why it is difficult to predict precisely how a particular patient with alcoholic cirrhosis will be able to eliminate a drug whose disposition depends largely on hepatic metabolism. The best course for a physician to take is to give these patients slightly lower than normal doses of such drugs and to watch closely to make sure that the patient does not experience drug toxicity but derives the intended therapeutic benefit from the drugs administered. Such close initial observations after a drug is given may lead to subsequent modifications in the dose.

Fig. 9-1 shows how patients with different forms of liver disease metabolize a relatively safe test drug, aminopyrine, compared with patients with normal cardio-vascular, hepatic, and renal function. This test was developed to measure hepatic capacity to N-demethylate certain drugs.[17-19] In humans, aminopyrine is eliminated mainly by N-demethylation accomplished by cytochrome P-450–dependent mon-ooxygenases located in hepatic smooth endoplasmic reticulum. Subsequently, the methyl group removed by these enzymatic reactions is converted to CO_2, excreted in breath, and measurable as $^{14}CO_2$ if a single tracer dose of [dimethylamine-^{14}C]-aminopyrine (2 μCi) is initially administered. Fig. 9-1 shows that patients with certain forms of liver disease, such as fatty liver and cholestasis, do not exhibit marked reduction in their hepatic N-demethylating capacity. On the other hand, patients with hepatocellular diseases, such as cirrhosis, infectious hepatitis, and certain met-astatic cancers or hepatomas, do show reduced N-demethylating capacity.

These observations of reduced rates of aminopyrine elimination in almost all patients with parenchymal liver disease are in agreement with other observations that liver disease is also accompanied by reduced rates of hepatic antipyrine metab-olism.[1,2,8] These results can be harmonized with observations that warfarin disposition during acute viral hepatitis is unchanged[50] and that oxazepam disposition is normal during acute viral hepatitis and cirrhosis.[41] Between these extremes, a group of drugs of which clindamycin is an example apparently exhibit intermediate or moderate changes in disposition in liver disease.[4] A wide range, from no change what-ever in disposition to significant retardation, has been reported in liver disease, depending on the drug studied and its particular dispositional characteristics. For drugs with high hepatic extraction ratios (greater than 0.8), such as propranolol and lidocaine, alterations in blood flow accompanying liver disease can produce large changes in hepatic clearance of the compound. For drugs with very low hepatic extraction ratios (less than 0.2), such as antipyrine and aminopyrine, large variations in the extent to which hepatocellular disease alters their rates of metabolism cannot be caused by abnormal liver blood flow. These variations may be attributed in part to multiple molecular forms of hepatic cytochrome P-450 and to the differential effects that a particular hepatic disorder might exert on these forms.

In addition to the primary diseases of the liver shown in Fig. 9-1 that are associated with reduced aminopyrine N-demethylation, certain disorders of other organs may secondarily involve the liver. For example, in congestive heart failure, liver function may become impaired as a result of pooling of blood in the liver and reduced hepatic perfusion. Reduced blood flow to the liver would be expected to result in decreased hepatic uptake of drugs with a high hepatic extraction, whose clearance by the liver depends on liver blood flow. Therefore congestive heart failure was demonstrated to result in reduced rates of elimination of such drugs as lidocaine.[42,43] However, for drugs with low hepatic extraction, such as aminopyrine, whose clearance is not dependent on hepatic blood flow, it was not anticipated that reduced hepatic perfusion

resulting from congestive heart failure would exert any effect on their rates of elimination. Fig. 9-2 shows that patients admitted to the hospital because of acute congestive heart failure were unable to eliminate aminopyrine as rapidly as they could after
7 to 10 days of treatment for their heart failure. These results with aminopyrine
suggest that the hemodynamic changes associated with congestive heart failure impair
hepatic drug metabolism, thereby reducing the ability of the body to eliminate drugs
through this process.

FIG. 9-2   *Excretion of $^{14}[CO_2]$ 2 hours after an oral tracer dose of $[^{14}C]$aminopyrine in breath of 8
patients who received $[^{14}C]$aminopyrine before and 7 or 10 days after treatment of congestive heart failure. Note improvement in hepatic capacity to N-demethylate aminopyrine with
treatment of congestive heart failure as indicated by markedly increased $^{14}[CO_2]$ output in
breath after 7 or 10 days of treatment.*

From Hepner, G.W., Vesell, E.S., and Tatum, K.R.: Am. J. Med. 65:271, 1978.

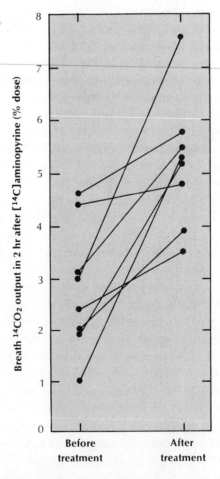

Only relatively few drugs are eliminated primarily by renal excretion. Obviously renal disease impairs the rate of removal of these drugs from the body. Therefore the dose of these drugs must be reduced, the extent of reduction in dose depending on the severity and duration of the renal disease. Drugs eliminated from the body primarily by renal excretion include colistin, penicillin, procainamide, digoxin, aminoglycoside antibiotics, barbital, cycloserine, ethambutol, methotrexate, and tetracycline.

Renal excretion of drugs

Since poor renal function is associated with decreased excretion of several drugs, it is important to modify normal drug dosage in uremic patients. Methods for this have been presented.[6,10,11,35] A linear relationship exists between the overall elimination rate constant (k_e) and the endogenous creatinine clearance (V'_{cr}):

$$k_e = k_{nr} + \delta \cdot V'_{cr}$$

In this equation, k_{nr} is the mean extrarenal elimination rate constant in anuric patients and δ is a constant relating V'_{cr} to the renal elimination rate constant (k_r) of the drug. This equation can be used for about 40 drugs; simple nomograms have been devised that allow estimation of rate of drug elimination in a patient with kidney disease from the value of V'_{cr}.[11,49] However, the apparent elimination rates of numerous drugs are unaltered by uremia, including antipyrine, histamine, phenacetin, phenytoin, phenobarbital, propranolol, quinidine, tolbutamide, and vitamin D.[34]

The information provided in Chapters 6 to 9 was selected to illustrate the extreme plasticity and sensitivity of human pharmacokinetic processes to perturbation by numerous factors. Five specific host factors were chosen because abundant evidence is available that clearly establishes the influence of each of these factors on rates of drug elimination in man: (1) genetic constitution, (2) age, (3) diet, (4) occupation, and (5) disease. The physician needs to be aware of certain details concerning each of these factors and to question the patient about them. In this way the physician will be more successful in selecting a dosage regimen that is therapeutic rather than toxic or ineffective. Furthermore, several steps are available to help the physician make the right choice: (1) close clinical observation of the patient for therapeutic, as well as toxic, signs of drug action; (2) quantitative endpoints for certain drugs (such as anticoagulants of antihypertensive agents) against which the dose can be titrated; and (3) measurement of drug concentrations in biological fluids of certain drugs whose therapeutic and toxic concentrations have been defined (Appendix A). Thus despite the fact that dynamic interactions occur among the many factors influencing rates of drug elimination in individual patients and render dosage selection difficult (Fig. 9-3), the physician can proceed in a rational, deliberate manner to make the correct choice of dose and to derive maximum therapeutic benefit from available drugs, while minimizing risks of toxicity.

PERSPECTIVE

FIG. 9-3   *Environmental factors affecting drug disposition in human subjects. Outer circle shows established or suspected environmental factors that can alter genetically controlled rates of drug elimination. A line joins environmental factors to suggest that several are associated and interdependent, rather than independent. Lines from each environmental factor to inner circle are wavy to suggest that modification of genetically controlled rates can occur at multiple levels. Such environmental effects need not occur directly at the genetic level.*

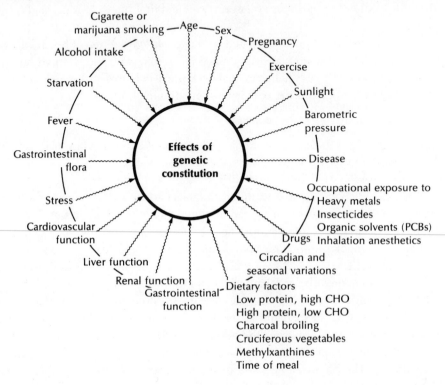

REFERENCES

1. Andreasen, P.B., Ranek, L., Statland, B.E., and Tygstrup, N.: Clearance of antipyrine-dependence of quantitative liver function, Eur. J. Clin. Invest. 4:129, 1974.
2. Andreasen, P.B., and Vesell, E.S.: Comparison of plasma levels of antipyrine, tolbutamide, and warfarin after oral and intravenous administration, Clin. Pharmacol. Ther. 16:1059, 1974.
3. Armstrong, B.K., Ukich, A.W., and Goatcher, P.M.: Plasma salicylate levels in rheumatoid arthritis produced by four different salicylate preparations, Med. J. Aust. 2:181, 1970.

4. Avant, G.R., Schenker, S., and Alford, R.H.: The effect of cirrhosis on the disposition and elimination of clindamycin, Am. J. Dig. Dis. 20:223, 1975.
5. Beermann, B., Hellstrom, K., and Rosen, A.: On the metabolism of propantheline in man, Clin. Pharmacol. Ther. 13:212, 1972.
6. Bennett, W.M., Singer, I., and Coggins, C.H.: Guide to drug usage in adult patients with impaired renal function, JAMA 223:991, 1973.
7. Bianchine, J.R., Calimlim, L.R., Morgan, J.P., Dujovne, C.A., and Lasagna, L.: Metabolism and absorption of L-3, 4-

dihydroxyphenylalanine in patients with Parkinson's disease, Ann. N.Y. Acad. Sci. **179:**126, 1971.

8. Branch, R.A., Herbert, C.M., and Read, A.E.: Determinants of serum antipyrine half-lives in patients with liver disease, Gut **14:**569, 1973.

9. Creasey, W.A.: Drug disposition in humans, New York, 1979, Oxford University Press.

10. Dettli, L.: Individualization of drug dosage in patients with renal disease, Med. Clin. North Am. **58:**977, 1974.

11. Dettli, L.: Translation of pharmacokinetics to clinical medicine. In Teorell, T., Dedrick, R., and Condliffe, P., editors: Pharmacology and pharmacokinetics, New York, 1974, Plenum Publishing Corp., pp. 69-86.

12. Døssing, M.: Changes in hepatic microsomal enzyme function in workers exposed to mixtures of chemicals, Clin. Pharmacol. Ther. **32:**340, 1982.

13. Fisher, J.M., Reese, C., and Taylor, K.B.: Intrinsic-factor antibodies in gastric juice of pernicious-anaemia patients, Lancet **2:**88, 1966.

14. Ghoneim, M.M., Delle, M., Wilson, W.R., and Ambre, J.J.: Alteration of warfarin kinetics in man associated with exposure to an operating-room environment, Anesthesiology **43:**333, 1975.

15. Hart, P., Farrell, G.C., Cooksley, W.G.E., and Powell, L.W.: Enhanced drug metabolism in cigarette smokers, Br. Med. J. **2:**147, 1976.

16. Hepner, G.W., Booth, C.C., Cowan, J., Hoffbrand, A.V., and Mollin, D.L.: Absorption of crystalline folic acid in man, Lancet **2:**302, 1968.

17. Hepner, G.W., and Vesell, E.S.: Assessment of aminopyrine metabolism in man by breath analysis after oral administration of ^{14}C-aminopyrine, N. Engl. J. Med. **291:**1384, 1974.

18. Hepner, G.W., and Vesell, E.S.: Quantitative assessment of hepatic function by breath analysis after oral administration of [^{14}C]-aminopyrine, Ann. Intern. Med. **83:**632, 1975.

19. Hepner, G.W., Vesell, E.S., Lipton, A., Harvey, H.A., Wilkinson, G.R., and Schenker, S.: Disposition of aminopyrine, antipyrine, diazepam, and indocyanine green in patients with liver disease or on anticonvulsant drug therapy: diazepam breath test and correlations in drug elimination, J. Lab. Clin. Med. **90:**440, 1977.

20. Koch-Weser, J.: Pharmacokinetics of procainamide in man, Ann. N.Y. Acad. Sci. **179:**370, 1971.

21. Kolmodin-Hedman, B.: Decreased plasma half-life of phenylbutazone in workers exposed to chlorinated pesticides, Eur. J. Clin . Pharmacol. **5:**195, 1973.

22. Levine, R.R.: Factors affecting gastrointestinal absorption of drugs, Am. J. Dig. Dis. **15:**171, 1970.

23. Lindenbaum, J., Maulitz, R.M., and Butter, V.P., Jr.: Inhibition of digoxin absorption by neomycin, Gastroenterology **71:**399, 1976.

24. Mattila, M.J., Friman, A., Larmi, T.K., and Koskinen, R.: Absorption of ethionamid, isoniazid and aminosalicylic acid from the postresection gastrointestinal tract, Ann. Med. Exp. Biol. Fenn. **47:**209, 1969.

25. Nelson, J.D., Shelton, S., Kusmiesz, H.T., and Haltalin, K.C.: Absorption of ampicillin and nalidixic acid by infants and children with acute shigellosis, Clin. Pharmacol. Ther. **13:**879, 1972.

26. Nimmo, J., Heading, R.C., Tothill, P., and Prescott, L.F.: Pharmacological modification of gastric emptying: effects of propantheline and metoclopramide on paracetamol absorption, Br. Med. J. **1:**587, 1973.

27. O'Malley, K., Stevenson, I.H., and Wood, M.: Drug metabolizing ability in operating theatre personnel, Br. J. of Anaesth. **45:**924, 1973.

28. Pagliaro, L.A., and Benet, L.Z.: Pharmacokinetic data. Critical compilation of terminal half-lives, percent excreted unchanged, and changes of half-life in renal and hepatic dysfunction for studies in humans with references, J. Pharmacokinet. Biopharm. **3:**333, 1975.

29. Pantuck, E.J., Hsiao, K.C., Kuntzman, R., and Conney, A.H.: Intestinal metabolism of phenacetin in the rat: effect of charcoal-broiled beef and rat chow, Science 187:744, 1975.

30. Prescott, L.F.: Gastrointestinal absorption of drugs, Med. Clin. North Am. 58:907, 1974.

31. Prescott, L.F.: Pathological and physiological factors affecting drug absorption, distribution, elimination and response in man. In Concepts in biochemical pharmacology. III. Berlin-Heidelberg-New York, 1975, Springer-Verlag, p. 241.

32. Prescott, L.F., and Nimmo, J.: Generic inequivalence—clinical observations, Acta Pharmacol. Toxicol. (Kbh) 29(suppl. 3):288, 1971.

33. Prescott, L.F., Steel, R.F., and Ferrier, W.R.: The effects of particle size on the absorption of phenacetin in man, a correlation between plasma concentration of phenacetin and effects on the central nervous system, Clin. Pharmacol. Ther. 11:496, 1970.

34. Reidenberg, M.M.: Kidney disease and drug metabolism, Med. Clin. North Am. 58:1059, 1974.

35. Reidenberg, M.M.: Renal function and drug action, Philadelphia, 1971, W.B. Saunders Co.

36. Reidenberg, M.M., and Drayer, D.E.: Effects of renal disease upon drug disposition, Drug Metab. Rev. 8:293, 1978.

37. Reidenberg, M.M., Odar-Cederlof, I., Von Bahr, C., Borga, O., and Sjoquist, F.: Protein binding of diphenylhydantoin and desmethylimipramine in plasma from patients with poor renal function, N. Engl. J. Med. 285:264, 1971.

38. Schade, S.G., Feick, P., Muckerheider, M., and Schilling, R.F.: Occurrence in gastric juice of antibody to a complex of intrinsic factor and vitamin B_{12}, N. Engl. J. Med. 275:528, 1966.

39. Schroder, H., and Campbell, D.E.S.: Absorption, metabolism, and excretion of salicylazosulfapyridine in man, Clin. Pharmacol. Ther. 13:539, 1972.

40. Shoeman, D.W., and Azarnoff, D.L.: The alteration of plasma proteins in uremia as reflected in their ability to bind digitoxin and diphenylhydantoin, Pharmacology 7:169, 1972.

41. Shull, H.J., Wilkinson, G.R., Johnson, R., and Schenker, S.: Normal disposition of oxazepam in acute viral hepatitis and cirrhosis, Ann. Intern. Med. 84:420, 1976.

42. Thompson, P.D., Melmon, K.L., and Richardson, J.A.: Lidocaine pharmacokinetics in advanced heart failure, Ann. Intern. Med. 78:449, 1973.

43. Thompson, P.D., Rowland, M., and Melmon, M.: The influence of heart failure, liver disease and renal failure on the disposition of lidocaine in man, Am. Heart J. 82:417, 1971.

44. Trenholme, G.M., Williams, R.L., Rieckmann, K.H., Frischer, H., and Carson, P.E.: Quinine disposition during malaria and during induced fever, Clin. Pharmacol. Ther. 19:459, 1976.

45. Venho, V.M.K., Jussila, J., and Aukee, S.: Drug absorption in man after gastric surgery, Fifth International Congress on Pharmacology, San Francisco, 1972, Abstract No. 1445, p. 241.

46. Vesell, E.S.: The antipyrine test in clinical pharmacology: conceptions and misconceptions, Clin. Pharmacol. Ther. 26:275, 1979.

47. Vesell, E.S., Page, J.G., and Passananti, G.T.: Genetic and environmental factors affecting ethanol metabolism in man, Clin. Pharmacol. Ther. 12:192, 1971.

48. Vesell, E.S.: Why individuals vary in their response to drugs, Trends in Pharmacological Sciences, pp. 349-351, Aug. 1980.

49. Wagner, J.G.: Biopharmaceutics and relevant pharmacokinetics, Hamilton, Ill., 1971, Drug Intelligence Publication.

50. Williams, R.L., Schary, W.L., Blaschke, T.F., Meffin, P.J., Melmon, K.L., and Rowland, M.: Influence of acute viral hepatitis on disposition and pharmacologic effect of warfarin, Clin. Pharmacol. Ther. 20:90, 1976.

section two

Drug effects on the nervous system and neuroeffectors

Chapter 10

General aspects of neuropharmacology

The more than 10 billion neurons that make up the human nervous system communicate with each other by means of chemical mediators. They exert their effects on peripheral structures by the release of these mediators and not by electrical impulses.

In the peripheral portions of the autonomic nervous system acetylcholine and norepinephrine play a predominant role. They act on postjunctional membranes, producing excitatory or inhibitory effects as a consequence of depolarization or hyperpolarization of these membranes.

Within the CNS the neurotransmitters and modulators are biogenic amines, certain amino acids, and numerous peptides. Among the biogenic amines, acetylcholine, norepinephrine, dopamine, serotonin, and probably histamine play a role. Amino acids, such as glutamic and aspartic acid, excite the postsynaptic membranes of many neurons. γ-Aminobutyric acid and glycine may be inhibitory transmitters. Among the peptides, about 20 are under consideration as transmitters of nerve signals. Substance P, the endorphins, and the enkephalins are some of the peptides of great current interest.

Numerous drugs mimic or influence the action of the chemical mediators and may be classified as neuropharmacological agents. Others act by unknown mechanisms but may be classified according to their clinical usage as hypnotics, analgesics, anticonvulsants, and general and local anesthetics.

The similarity between certain drug effects and those of nerve stimulation was noted before this century. Muscarine, from certain mushrooms, was known to slow the heart rate just like vagal stimulation. Adrenal extracts produced effects similar to those following stimulation of sympathetic nerves (Oliver and Shafer, 1895).

Definitive proof of chemical neurotransmission was provided in 1921 by the experiments of Loewi[18] and Cannon and Uridil.[6] In his classic experiment Otto Loewi

*THE CHEMICAL
NEUROTRANS-
MISSION
CONCEPT*

demonstrated that when the vagus nerve of a perfused frog heart is stimulated, a substance is released that is capable of slowing a second frog heart with no neural connections to the first. Cannon and Uridil[6] found that sympathetic nerve stimulation of the liver causes the release of a substance similar to epinephrine in many respects. This mediator, at first named "sympathin," is now believed to be norepinephrine. Identification of the neurotransmitter in adrenergic axons as norepinephrine was provided by von Euler.[29]

Acetylcholine was first studied systematically by Dale.[7] The "quantum hypothesis" of acetylcholine release and the role of synaptic vesicles in neuromuscular and synaptic transmission is a contribution of Katz and co-workers.[9,13] The discovery by Brodie and Shore[4] of monoamine release by reserpine led to a great expansion of knowledge regarding the metabolism and function of catecholamines in the nervous system. The uptake of catecholamines by sympathetic nerves is mainly a contribution of Axelrod.[1] The importance of these contributions is attested to by the Nobel prizes that have been awarded to most of the investigators just cited.

After these discoveries it became apparent that drugs need not necessarily act through nerves to influence an effector organ. In fact, it was then clearly seen that nerves could act by releasing chemical compounds, which in turn influenced the effector structures. Instead of classifying drugs as sympathomimetic and parasympathomimetic, it appeared more reasonable to classify nerves on the basis of the mediator released from them. This led to the concept of cholinergic and adrenergic nerve fibers.

SITES OF ACTION OF CHEMICAL MEDIATORS
The role of neurotransmitters at various anatomical sites is well established in some cases and is surmised in others. The generally accepted information on the site of action of these compounds may be summarized as follows:

1. Postganglionic parasympathetic nerve endings on smooth muscle, cardiac muscle, and exocrine glands: acetylcholine
2. Postganglionic sympathetic nerve endings on smooth muscle, cardiac muscle, and exocrine glands: norepinephrine (with the exception of nerve endings on sweat glands)
3. All autonomic ganglionic synapses: acetylcholine (although dopamine may modulate transmission)
4. Motor fiber terminals at skeletal neuromuscular junctions: acetylcholine
5. CNS synapses: acetylcholine, norepinephrine, dopamine, serotonin, histamine, glutamic and aspartic acid, γ-aminobutyric acid (GABA), glycine, and numerous peptides

The site of action of the various mediators in the autonomic nervous system is fairly well established. The situation is much more complex in the CNS where neurophysiological techniques are not sufficient for establishing the role of transmitter at a given site. Immunofluorescence and the biochemical identification of receptors in the brain for the selective localization of active agents are some of the newer approaches for establishing the transmitter role of various compounds.[24]

The neurotransmitters exert their effect on various membranes by interacting with specific receptors. The existence of these receptors may be deduced from structure-activity studies on congeneric series or from parallel shifts of dose-response curves in the presence of specific antagonists. The following receptors may be postulated for some of the neurotransmitters:

RECEPTOR CONCEPT IN NEUROPHARMA-COLOGY

1. Acetylcholine has muscarinic and nicotinic receptors. Muscarinic receptors are present in various smooth muscles, cardiac muscle, and exocrine glands. They are termed *muscarinic* because muscarine, a quaternary amine alkaloid, has actions similar to those of acetylcholine at the sites indicated. The muscarinic receptor is competitively blocked by atropine and related drugs.

The nicotinic receptors of acetylcholine are located in autonomic ganglia and at skeletal neuromuscular junctions. They are termed *nicotinic* because nicotine also acts on these receptors. The nicotinic receptors in the autonomic ganglia and in skeletal muscle are not identical. The effects of the acetylcholine in autonomic ganglia are blocked by hexamethonium, whereas the receptors at the skeletal neuromuscular junction are blocked by *d*-tubocurarine and related compounds.

There are muscarinic and nicotinic receptors in the CNS also.[3] Thus the synapse between the collaterals of motor axons and the Renshaw cell is nicotinic, whereas there is good evidence for the presence of muscarinic receptors also within the CNS.

2. Norepinephrine acts on adrenergic receptors that are classified as *alpha* (α) and *beta* (β). Drugs that block these receptors are known as α- and β-*adrenergic blocking agents*. In addition, α receptors are divided into α_1 and α_2 receptors, and β receptors are divided into β_1 and β_2 receptors (see pp. 156 to 157).

3. Dopamine acts on dopaminergic receptors in the CNS and probably in ganglia. The dopaminergic receptors are blocked specifically by antipsychotic drugs such as phenothiazines and butyrophenones. In addition to dopaminergic receptors, dopamine also acts on β_1 receptors in the heart and in higher doses on α receptors, where its action is blocked by phentolamine.

4. Serotonin acts on serotoninergic receptors in the CNS and in neuroeffector structures. Its actions are blocked by the antiserotonin compounds, such as methysergide.

5. Histamine acts on histaminergic receptors, which are classified as H_1 and H_2 receptors. The commonly used antihistamines are H_1-receptor antagonists, for example, pyrilamine. H_2-receptor antagonists have only been recently synthesized. A typical example is cimetidine.

Little is known about receptors for the hypothetical amino acid transmitters, but glycine appears to be antagonized by strychnine. Many other receptors are being investigated by radioligand binding techniques.[24]

Newer concepts on the cholinergic receptor

A partial isolation of the cholinergic receptor has been achieved as a result of studies on some snake venoms that combine irreversibly with such receptors. It was observed that the α toxin of *Bungarus multicinctus,* or bungarotoxin, exerts a post-synaptic blocking action similar to that of *d*-tubocurarine except that it is irreversible. The toxin can be labeled radioactively and serves admirably for the isolation and study of some cholinergic receptors. It has been estimated from such studies that in an end-plate of rat muscle there are about 3×10^7 receptor molecules.

> PROBLEM 10-1. *What accounts for the muscarinic or nicotinic nature of a cholinergic receptor? Crystallographic analysis of acetylcholine and related agonists provides a tentative answer to this question. Acetylcholine is a flexible molecule and rotation is possible at two different bonds. Muscarinic and nicotinic drugs differ from acetylcholine in the degree of rotation at the sites of torsion. Thus acetylcholine has both muscarinic and nicotinic effects, whereas the purely muscarinic or nicotinic congeners have constraints imposed on them by conformational factors.*

SYNAPSES AND NEUROMUSCULAR JUNCTIONS

The synapse is the site of transmission of the nerve impulse between two neurons. The axonal terminal is separated from the postsynaptic membrane by a synaptic cleft of about 200 Å in width. Electron micrographs show that the presynaptic element contains numerous vesicles, which are believed to store the transmitter. They also contain some mitochondria.

Transmission of the nerve impulse across the synapse is quite different from axonal conduction. First, transmission is unidirectional. Second, when the axon is stimulated electrically, there is a delay of about 0.2 second before the postsynaptic element is depolarized.

At somatic motor nerve endings the axon terminal lies within the synaptic gutters. Vesicles containing acetylcholine are present in the axon terminal. Nerve stimulation causes a release of acetylcholine that, diffusing across the gap, causes a change in permeability of the postjunctional membrane to Na^+ and K^+. The release process requires Ca^{++} and is inhibited by Mg^{++}. Botulinus toxin blocks acetylcholine release; hemicholinium, an experimental drug, blocks acetylcholine synthesis, presumably by interfering with the axonal uptake of choline (Fig. 10-1).

At the terminations of autonomic nerve fibers on smooth muscles, cardiac muscle, or exocrine glands, no specialized structures analogous to motor end-plates can be seen. The transmitters apparently are discharged at the terminal plexuses into the extracellular space and reach the receptors by diffusion.

EVIDENCE FOR CHOLINERGIC AND ADRENERGIC NEUROTRANS-MISSION

The role of a mediator in neurotransmission is suggested or established by some or all of the following:

1. The presence of the transmitter in the axon along with the enzyme responsible for its production and destruction
2. Similarity of the mediator's effect to that of nerve stimulation

Cholinergic nerve terminal depicting the synthesis, storage, and release of acetylcholine (ACh), its hydrolysis by cholinesterase, and its action on cholinergic receptors on the effector cell and presynaptic receptors.   *FIG. 10-1*

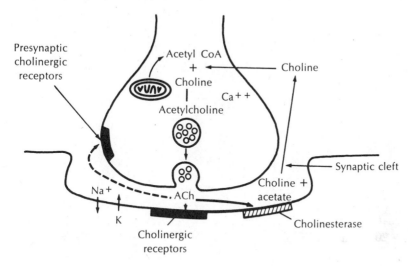

3. Release of the transmitter by nerve stimulation
4. Blockade of the effect of nerve stimulation by drugs that block the transmitter's action

Most of the criteria can be met in studies of neuromuscular transmission and ganglionic transmission. There are formidable difficulties in proving the transmitter role of a substance in the CNS by these same criteria.

Mediators to sweat glands and adrenal medulla

Two apparent exceptions exist to the statement that norepinephrine is the chemical mediator to sympathetically innervated structures. The sweat glands, while receiving sympathetic innervation, are known to be activated by cholinergic drugs and inhibited by anticholinergic drugs, atropine being the great inhibitor of sweating. This apparent anomaly has been explained in a satisfactory manner by demonstrating that the particular fibers innervating the sweat glands are cholinergic. In other words, on stimulation they release acetylcholine rather than norepinephrine.

The adrenal medulla is another apparent exception. This structure secretes epinephrine when cholinergic drugs are injected, but its response may be inhibited by ganglionic blocking agents. The explanation of this apparent anomaly is based on embryological considerations. The adrenal medulla is in reality a modified sympathetic ganglion, and it is therefore not surprising that it should respond to acetylcholine, which is the normal ganglionic mediator for both the sympathetic and parasympathetic nerves.

FIG. 10-2 *Autonomic innervation of various organs.*

Redrawn from a Sandoz Pharmaceuticals publication.

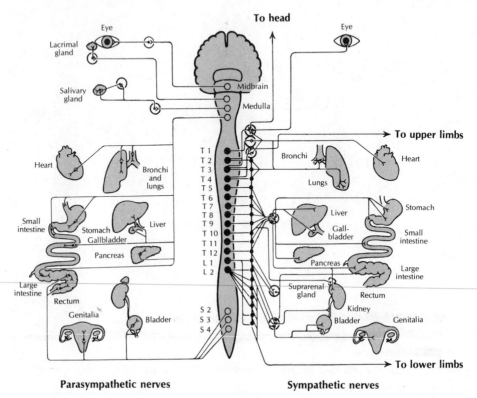

FIG. 10-3 *Schematic representation of autonomic innervation of neuroeffector cells.*

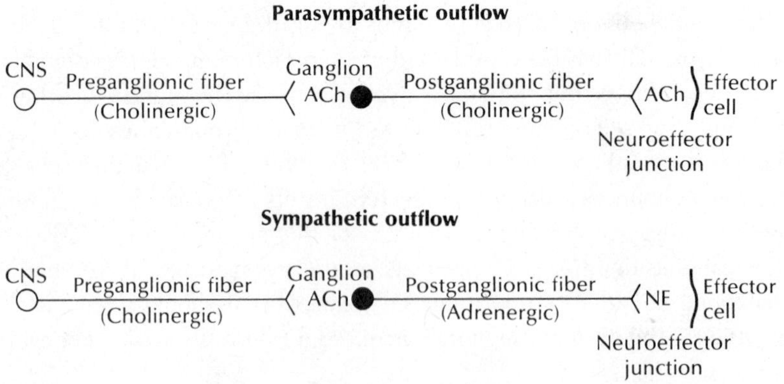

TABLE 10-1   Sites of drug action in relation to junctional transmission

Site of drug action	Mediator involved	
	Acetylcholine	Norepinephrine
Synthesis of mediator inhibited by	Hemicholinium*	Methyldopa† α-Methyltyrosine
Binding of mediator in granules inhibited by		Reserpine Guanethidine
Release of mediator enhanced by	Carbachol	Tyramine Amphetamine Reserpine Guanethidine
Release of mediator inhibited by	Botulinus toxin	Bretylium Monoamine oxidase (MAO) inhibitors (?)

Depolarization of postsynaptic membrane promoted by	A. Choline esters
	     Pilocarpine
	     Muscarine
	B. Nicotine
	     Dimethylphenylpiperazinium (DMPP)*
	C. Choline esters
	     Nicotine
	     Phenyltrimethylammonium (PTMA)*
		Catecholamine and related
		   amines

Depolarization of postsynaptic membrane inhibited by	A. Atropine and related drugs
	
	B. Hexamethonium nicotine
	
	C. *d*-Tubocurarine
	     Succinylcholine
		α-Receptor blocking agents:
		   phenoxybenzamine
		β-Receptor blocking agents:
		   propranolol

*Pharmacological tool only.
†Major clinical effect resulting from norepinephrine release rather than inhibition of synthesis.
A, Cholinergic neuroeffector site.
B, Ganglionic site.
C, Skeletal neuromuscular site.

The following steps may be distinguished in junctional transmission: (1) synthesis of the mediator, (2) binding of the mediator in a potentially active form, (3) release of the mediator substance, (4) depolarization of postsynaptic membrane, (5) elimination of the mediator, and (6) repolarization of the postsynaptic membrane. Theoretically, at least, drugs could influence junctional transmission by acting at any of the steps, and, indeed, we have examples of many such interactions, as shown in Table 10-1.

SEQUENCE OF CHEMICAL EVENTS IN JUNCTIONAL TRANSMISSION

Although in the foregoing discussion and in Table 10-1 the postjunctional site of action of drugs is emphasized, there is growing evidence of a presynaptic action of many drugs, particularly in relation to catecholamine release and also to neuromuscular transmission.[11]

Presynaptic actions of drugs

There is good evidence for the presence of α adrenoreceptors located prejunctionally on postganglionic adrenergic nerve endings, in addition to the α adrenoreceptors that are located postjunctionally. These prejunctional or α_2 receptors tend to reduce norepinephrine output when acted on by an adrenergic agonist.[2,15,16] Blockade of these receptors increases the release of norepinephrine. The α_1 and α_2 receptors are distinguished by their relative affinity for a series of agonists and antagonists. Thus clonidine is a more potent agonist for α_2 receptors than norepinephrine, methoxamine, or phenylephrine, whereas phentolamine and yohimbine are more potent α_2 antagonists than phenoxybenzamine or prazosin. Insulin release and intestinal hypersecretion are mediated by postsynaptic α_2 receptors.

FACTORS INFLUENCING RESPONSE OF EFFECTORS TO CHEMICAL MEDIATORS

The response of effector cells may be altered remarkably under certain circumstances. The two conditions that have received attention are sensitization following denervation and sensitization in the presence of other drugs.

Denervation supersensitivity

The supersensitivity of denervated structures is based on several mechanisms. Nonspecific supersensitivity may result from chronically reduced activity in a smooth muscle.[10] For example, chronic treatment of a guinea pig with a ganglionic blocking agent leads in a few days to an increased sensitivity of its isolated ileum to acetylcholine, histamine, potassium, and serotonin.[10] On the other hand, organs deprived of their adrenergic innervation become especially sensitive to catecholamines, probably because of absence of the uptake mechanism for the neurotransmitter (p. 108). Preganglionic denervation, also called *deafferentation*, is much less effective in increasing the susceptibility of various effectors to catecholamines. In this case the supersensitivity of smooth muscles may be nonspecific, resulting from chronically reduced activity.[10]

A very interesting mechanism appears to be operating in supersensitive skeletal muscle. A week or two following denervation the whole muscle fiber becomes responsive to externally applied acetylcholine, whereas only the end-plate region was sensitive before denervation. It appears as if new acetylcholine receptors had developed as a consequence of denervation.[22]

Sensitization by drugs

In contrast to the supersensitivity induced by denervation and prolonged inactivity, more rapid sensitization to mediators can be produced by certain drugs.

Enzyme inhibitors may be quite effective. The inhibitors of cholinesterase potentiate the actions of acetylcholine. Catechol and pyrogallol may increase the effectiveness of norepinephrine and epinephrine.

Drugs may also interfere with the buffer mechanisms and thereby may allow greater fluctuation in some physiological parameter such as blood pressure when a neuropharmacological agent is administered. It has been suggested that protovera-trine can have this action. The ganglionic blocking agents also increase the effectiveness of injected vasoactive drugs, probably by interfering with buffering responses.

The supersensitivity to catecholamines has been studied mostly on the nictitating membrane where two types of supersensitivity may exist.[27] A "presynaptic" supersensitivity develops after surgical denervation and is correlated with the degeneration of adrenergic nerve terminals. It is specific for catecholamines and related amines and develops within 48 hours after denervation. It is undoubtedly related to the absence of the catecholamine uptake mechanism. Another type of supersensitivity, which is nonspecific in that it applies not only to catecholamines but also to acetylcholine and other agonists, develops slowly after surgical denervation or decentralization. It appears to be postsynaptic and requires weeks for its development. This postsynaptic supersensitivity is a consequence of reduced levels of transmitter.

Cocaine,[19,27] antihistaminics, and tricyclic antidepressants cause presynaptic supersensitivity as a consequence of interference with catecholamine reuptake by the adrenergic terminals. On the other hand, chronic administration of reserpine leads to the postsynaptic type of supersensitivity by chronic depletion of the transmitters. Guanethidine interferes with catecholamine uptake and also produces a long-lasting supersensitivity. It probably exerts both presynaptic and postsynaptic effects.

In general, compounds that have a cocaine-like effect on the uptake of catecholamines sensitize effector cells to their pharmacological effects. The same compounds tend to block the actions of indirectly acting sympathomimetic drugs, such as those of tyramine.

In addition to the mechanisms of sensitization discussed, direct radioligand studies indicate that the *number* of receptors may change under various circumstances. An increase in receptor number is referred to as *up regulation* and a decrease in receptor number as *down regulation*.[17] Thus high concentrations of adrenergic agents lead to decreased numbers of receptors, whereas a reduction in the tissue or serum levels of catecholamines leads to the opposite effect.[17] These concepts may explain many observations on the changes in sensitivity to mediators in various disease states. They may also explain changes in sensitivity to various mediators induced by hormones and drugs. For example, it is tempting to attribute the propranolol withdrawal syndrome to an increase in receptor number and increased responsiveness to endogenous catecholamines.[17]

AMINE METABOLISM AND THE NERVOUS SYSTEM

The best known neurotransmitters are nitrogenous bases synthesized by the neuron from precursors and stored in vesicles ready to be released. The active amines do not cross the blood-brain barrier efficiently, whereas the precursor amino acids do. The importance of precursor availability and nutritional state in the control of brain neurotransmitter synthesis is receiving increasing attention.[32]

Acetylcholine   The important neurotransmitter acetylcholine is present in certain peripheral nerves and in nerve endings in brain (synaptosomes), where its vesicular localization has been demonstrated.

Acetylcholine is synthesized by the enzyme choline acetyltransferase, previously known as choline acetylase, according to the following schema:

Choline + Acetyl coenzyme A → Acetylcholine + Coenzyme A

Traditionally acetylcholine has been assayed by biological methods using a skeletal muscle such as the frog rectus abdominis or smooth muscle in the guinea pig ileum as test objects. There are now gas chromatographic techniques available for the same purpose.

During the nerve stimulation, *recently* synthesized acetylcholine may be preferentially released. The experimental compound *hemicholinium* blocks the synthesis of the mediator by interfering with the transport of choline across the neuronal membrane.

Acetylcholine released by a nerve impulse must be destroyed rapidly to allow the next impulse to act on a repolarized postsynaptic membrane within a few milliseconds. Hydrolysis of acetylcholine reduces the pharmacological activity of the compound a hundred-thousandfold.

Destruction of acetylcholine is accomplished by the *cholinesterases*, which are of two types. *Acetylcholinesterase*, or specific cholinesterase, hydrolyzes acetyl esters of choline more rapidly than butyryl esters. On the other hand, *pseudocholinesterase*, or nonspecific cholinesterase, is sometimes called butyrylcholinesterase because it hydrolyzes butyryl and other esters of choline more rapidly than the acetyl ester. Acetylcholinesterase is localized in neuronal membranes and surprisingly also in membranes of red cells and the placenta, where its function is unknown. Nonspecific cholinesterase is widely distributed in the body. Plasma cholinesterase is of the nonspecific type. Its presence in plasma is not related to neural activity, although its low titer after exposure to anticholinesterase pesticides is a useful method for diagnosing such poisonings. The titer of plasma cholinesterase is depressed also in advanced liver disease, since the enzyme is manufactured in the liver (p. 122).

Catecholamines   The collective term for norepinephrine, epinephrine, and dopamine is *catecholamine*, since these neurotransmitters are catechols (ortho-dihydroxybenzenes) and contain an amine group in their aliphatic side chain.

LOCALIZATION   The distribution of catecholamines in the body is well understood, thanks to the availability of suitable methods for their determination, such as the fluorometric assay. In addition, the histochemical fluorescence microscopy techniques developed by Swedish investigators allow an actual visualization of the catecholamine-containing structures (see Fig. 15-1), their precise localization, and their susceptibility to drug effects.

Norepinephrine is present in adrenergic fibers and in certain pathways within

TABLE 10-2   Distribution of norepinephrine and dopamine in the human brain (micrograms/gram)

	Norepinephrine	Dopamine
Frontal lobe	0.00-0.02	0.00
Caudate nucleus	0.04	3.12
Putamen	0.02	5.27
Hypothalamus (anterior part)	0.96	0.18
Substantia nigra	0.04	0.40
Pons	0.04	0.00
Medulla oblongata (dorsal part)	0.13	0.00
Cerebellar cortex	0.02	0.02

Based on data from Bertler, A.: Acta Physiol. Scand. **51**:97, 1961.

the CNS. *Epinephrine* constitutes most of the catecholamine present in the human adrenal medulla, although adrenal medullary tumors may contain largely norepinephrine. Small amounts of epinephrine may occur also in various organs and in the CNS, but its main function recognized so far has to do with the adrenal medulla. *Dopamine* is present in relatively high concentration in the brain and is particularly concentrated in the caudate nucleus and the putamen (Table 10-2).

The distribution of norepinephrine in various organs corresponds well with their adrenergic innervation. Although there is considerable species variation, the heart, arteries, and veins of most mammals contain norepinephrine of the order of 1 µg/g of tissue.[29] The liver, lungs, and skeletal muscle contain considerably less, whereas the vas deferens has about five to ten times as much.

BIOSYNTHESIS

The biosynthesis of catecholamines represents a small but very important portion of the metabolism of tyrosine. Other pathways lead to the formation of thyroxine, *p*-hydroxyphenylpyruvate, and melanin and to protein synthesis. Tyrosine itself may arise from hydroxylation of phenylalanine or may be taken up directly by the neurons for catecholamine synthesis.

The various steps in the biosynthesis of catecholamines are shown below (for structural formulas see Fig. 10-4):

$$\text{Tyrosine} \xrightarrow{\text{Tyrosine hydroxylase}} \text{Dopa} \xrightarrow[\text{acid decarboxylase}]{\text{L-Aromatic amino}} \text{Dopamine} \xrightarrow[\text{oxidase}]{\text{Dopamine-}\beta\text{-}}$$

$$\text{Norepinephrine} \xrightarrow[\text{N-methyltransferase}]{\text{Phenylethanolamine}} \text{Epinephrine}$$

Tyrosine hydroxylase,[28] a cytoplasmic enzyme, catalyzes the rate-limiting step in catecholamine biosynthesis. Thus inhibition of this enzyme by amino acid analogs such as α-methyltyrosine leads to a depletion of catecholamines in brain and various sympathetic nerves, with important functional consequences.

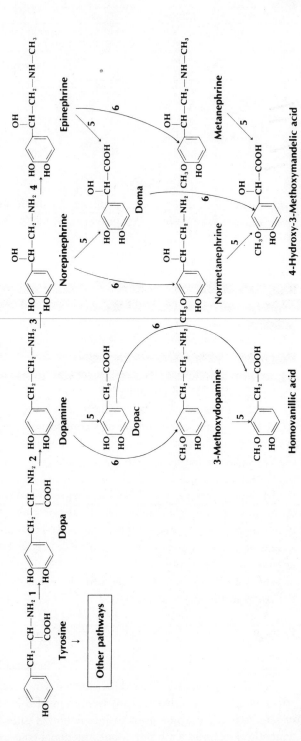

Pathways of synthesis and metabolism of catecholamines. Enzymes catalyzing various reactions are as follows: **FIG. 10-4**
1, tyrosine hydroxylase; 2, aromatic amino acid decarboxylase; 3, dopamine-β-hydroxylase; 4, phenylethanolamine-N-methyltransferase; 5, MAO plus aldehyde dehydrogenase; 6, catechol-O-methyltransferase. Dopa, 3,4-Dihydroxyphenylalanine; Dopac, 3,4-dihydroxyphenylacetic acid; Doma, 3,4-dihydroxymandelic acid.

From Crout, J.R.: Catecholamine metabolism. In Manger, C.W., editor: Hormones and hypertension, Springfield, Ill., 1966, Charles C Thomas, Publisher.

L-*Aromatic amino acid decarboxylase* is a cytoplasmic enzyme that decarboxylates a number of substrates in addition to dopa, for example, 5-hydroxytryptophan to serotonin.

Dopamine-β-oxidase, a copper-containing enzyme bound to the membranes of the exoplasmic granules, catalyzes the conversion of dopamine to norepinephrine. The enzyme is inhibited by copper reagents such as disulfiram and diethyldithiocarbamate. Because the enzyme is associated with the catecholamine vesicles, sympathetic stimulation leads to the appearance of dopamine-β-oxidase activity in the circulation.[30]

Phenylethanolamine-N-methyltransferase is a cytoplasmic enzyme present largely in the adrenal medulla where it catalyzes the transfer of a methyl group from S-adenosylmethionine to norepinephrine for the formation of epinephrine.

Negative feedback of catecholamine biosynthesis. Sympathetic nerve stimulation does not cause catecholamine depletion in the axon, suggesting that increased synthesis can keep up with loss. With the discovery of tyrosine hydroxylase as the rate-limiting enzyme in catecholamine biosynthesis, the relative constancy of catecholamine stores can be explained. Norepinephrine and dopamine inhibit tyrosine hydroxylase. It becomes understandable, then, that increased catecholamine release through sympathetic activity will lead to accelerated synthesis of catecholamines at nerve terminals. On the other hand, monoamine oxidase (MAO) inhibitors, which elevate catecholamine levels in adrenergic neurons, also lead to a slowdown in catecholamine biosynthesis.

The release and synthesis of catecholamines are influenced in an important way by a neuronal feedback, most clearly shown for dopamine in the brain.[5] It has been shown that dopamine receptor blockade by phenothiazines or haloperidol leads to a compensatory increase in the activity of dopaminergic cells by a neuronal feedback mechanism.

STORAGE AND RELEASE

Catecholamines are stored in vesicles in association with adenosine triphosphate and a soluble protein *chromogranin*. The vesicles are formed originally in the nerve cell body and are transported to the endings by axoplasmic flow. Constriction of an adrenergic nerve causes the accumulation of vesicles proximal to the ligature.

Release of catecholamines is believed to take place by a specialized form of exocytosis. During the release process adenosine triphosphate, chromogranin, and dopamine-β-oxidase appear in the perfusate of adrenal medullary tissue[8] in addition to catecholamines. Although these findings suggest that the vesicles empty their content, other evidence indicates that recently synthesized catecholamine is released preferentially.

In contrast with release by exocytosis, reserpine causes the release of the granular catecholamines into the axoplasm, where they are deaminated by the enzyme MAO present in the axonal mitochondria.

Catecholamine release requires calcium[8] and is in this respect similar to acetylcholine release from cholinergic nerves and to histamine release from mast cells.

DISPOSITION OF THE RELEASED CATECHOLAMINE

The relative constancy of catecholamine stores in adrenergic neurons is not only a consequence of feedback regulation of its biosynthesis. It is also an expression of a remarkable ability of these neurons to take up the amines after their release. More than half the released catecholamine may be conserved by this mechanism, which will be discussed in greater detail (p. 163).

The portion of the released catecholamine that escapes the amine pump reuptake is attacked by two enzymes: *catechol-O-methyltransferase* and *MAO*. The latter is widely distributed in the body, not only in adrenergic axonal mitochondria but also in nonneural structures. Catechol-*O*-methyltransferase is also widely distributed and is particularly concentrated in the liver and kidneys. Although the precise relationship of these enzymes to sympathetic function is not understood, it is clearly not as crucial as the acetylcholine-cholinesterase interdependence. For example, inhibition of catechol-*O*-methyltransferase by catechol or pyrogallol does not cause a significant increase in sympathetic activity or potentiation of the action of injected catecholamines. Similarly, drugs that inhibit MAO fail to potentiate the action of catecholamines and do not increase sympathetic functions in the periphery.

The detailed metabolic pathways of catecholamines are shown in Fig. 10-4. The role of many of these pathways may be appreciated from data on the urinary excretion of catecholamine metabolites in normal humans; the percentage of endogenous catecholamines and metabolites are as follows:

Norepinephrine + Epinephrine	1.1%
Normetanephrine + Metanephrine	7.6%
Vanillylmandelic acid (VMA)	91.0%

The 24-hour VMA excretion in normal individuals is 10 mg. Much larger amounts may be excreted by patients with adrenal medullary tumors (p. 166).

INTERACTION OF DRUGS WITH CATECHOLAMINE STORAGE AND RELEASE MECHANISMS

Numerous clinically useful drugs interact with the storage and release of catecholamines. They are listed in Table 10-3 and are discussed in some detail in the appropriate chapters.

Chemical sympathectomy: 6-hydroxydopamine

The administration of 6-hydroxydopamine, an interesting experimental tool, causes an extremely long-lasting depletion of catecholamines in organs innervated by the sympathetic division. Electron microscopic studies indicate that the drug causes a selective destruction of peripheral adrenergic nerve terminals. In newborn animals the whole neuron is destroyed irreversibly, whereas in adults only the terminals are affected so that the regeneration of the fibers is possible.[26] To destroy adrenergic terminals in the CNS, 6-hydroxydopamine must be injected into the ventricles because it does not cross the blood-brain barrier.

TABLE 10-3   Drugs interacting with catecholamine storage and release mechanisms

Drug	Clinical use	Site of action
Norepinephrine depletors Reserpine Guanethidine	Antihypertensive	Blockade of intraneuronal storage
False transmitters α-Methyldopa	Antihypertensive	Substitution of norepinephrine by false transmitter in storage granules
MAO inhibitors Pargyline	Antihypertensive	Inhibition of norepinephrine release by free norepinephrine or false transmitter
Neuron blockers Bretylium Debrisoquine	Antihypertensive	Prevention of norepinephrine release; also MAO inhibition
Amphetamine Ephedrine	Sympathomimetic	Norepinephrine release from granules
Tricyclic drugs Imipramine Amitriptyline	Antidepressant	Inhibition of adrenergic neuronal membrane amine carrier system

Modified from Shore, P.A. In Jones, R.J., editor: Proceedings of the Second International Symposium, New York, 1970, Springer-Verlag New York, Inc., p. 528.

Serotonin, or 5-hydroxytryptamine, is present in high concentrations in the en- *Serotonin* terochromaffin cells of the intestinal tract and in the pineal gland. It is also present in the brain, in platelets, and in mast cells of rats and mice. Serotonin occurs also in some fruits such as bananas.

The steps in the biosynthesis of serotonin are as follows:

$$\text{Tryptophan} \xrightarrow[\text{hydroxylase}]{\text{Tryptophan}} \text{5-Hydroxytryptophan} \xrightarrow[\text{decarboxylase}]{\text{L-Aromatic amino acid}} \text{5-Hydroxytryptamine}$$

Serotonin is degraded to 5-hydroxyindolacetic acid by the enzyme MAO. The daily excretion of 5-hydroxyindolacetic acid in humans is about 3 mg. It may increase greatly in patients with carcinoid tumor or after the administration of reserpine. The ingestion of bananas also results in elevated concentrations of 5-hydroxyindolacetic acid in the urine.

In the pineal gland there is not only a high concentration of serotonin but also a biosynthetic product of the amine, 5-methoxy-*N*-acetyltryptamine, also known as melatonin. This unique product lightens skin color by affecting melanocytes. It also exerts an effect on gonadal functions in female rats. Interestingly, melatonin synthesis is greatly influenced by light.

In addition to the previously discussed neurotransmitters, several endogenous compounds may play a role in neural function, although the available evidence is hardly sufficient for characterizing them as mediators of neurotransmission.

Histamine is present in the hypothalamus along with serotonin and catecholamines. Its presence in adrenergic nerves is interesting but may be related to the presence of mast cells close to these nerves. The brain can form histamine from histidine and is rich in the methylating enzyme that inactivates this biogenic amine. Unfortunately, no powerful inhibitors of the methylating enzyme are available.

Glutamic and *aspartic acids* are remarkably potent in causing depolarization of nerve cells when applied by iontophoresis. Furthermore, analogs of glutamic and aspartic acid, such as kainic acid, ibotenic acid, and *N*-methyl-*D*-aspartic acid, are also powerful agonists on central neurons.

Glycine is recognized increasingly as a probable inhibitory transmitter in the spinal cord. This simple amino acid is present in high concentration in the spinal cord and causes hyperpolarization of motoneurons.[31] Since strychnine is known to antagonize the effects of the naturally occurring inhibitory transmitter released from Renshaw cells to motoneurons, it was of great interest to examine the possible relationship between the alkaloid and glycine. Antagonism of the hyperpolarizing effect of glycine by strychnine applied by microelectrophoresis has been clearly demonstrated. Interestingly tetanus toxin in the same system does not antagonize the actions of glycine, implying a presynaptic site of action for the toxin.

γ-Aminobutyric acid (GABA) has also received some attention as a naturally occurring amine that may have a role in brain function. This compound is made by brain tissue through decarboxylation of glutamic acid.

$$\overset{\overset{\displaystyle NH_2}{\displaystyle |}}{HOOC-CH-CH_2-CH_2-COOH} \qquad H_2N-CH_2-CH_2-CH_2-COOH$$

Glutamic acid   **γ-Aminobutyric acid**

Brain tissue contains significant quantities of GABA. Its destruction is accomplished through transamination. The study of the effects of GABA on brain function has been greatly handicapped because it does not cross the blood-brain barrier effectively when injected.

Crustacean stretch receptors are inhibited by GABA, and studies of Purpura and co-workers[21] suggest that GABA and related omega amino acids may have inhibitory properties on central synaptic transmission when applied directly to the brain surface.

Peptides are suspected as important neurotransmitters in the CNS. Substance P, somatostatin, cholecystokinin, angiotensin II, and vasoactive intestinal peptide (VIP) are present in spinal-ganglion neurons, as shown by immunocytochemical studies. Substance P contains 11 amino acids and appears to be a sensory neurotransmitter that plays an important role in pain. Capsaicin, obtained from red pepper, causes a depletion of substance P from the spinal cord and elevates the threshold to painful stimuli.

The rational classification of neuropharmacological agents should be based on their site of action and mode of action, reflecting drug-receptor interactions. This can be done satisfactorily for drugs acting on autonomic end organs, autonomic nerve endings, autonomic ganglia, and skeletal neuromuscular junctions. At each site we have agonists and antagonists or drugs that promote or inhibit the release of neurotransmitters.

CLASSIFICATION OF NEUROPHARMACOLOGICAL AGENTS

AUTONOMIC AND RELATED DRUGS

Classification by *site of action* and *mode of action*

I. Drugs acting on autonomic receptors in end organs
  A. Agonists mimicking postganglionic transmitters
    1. Cholinergic drugs (parasympathomimetics)
      a. Direct action on effector cell (effective after denervation)—acetylcholine, pilocarpine
      b. Indirect action (potentiate endogenous ACh; ineffective after denervation)
        (1) Competitive cholinesterase inhibitors—physostigmine
        (2) Noncompetitive cholinesterase inhibitors—isoflurophate (DFP) (enzyme reactivated by pralidoxime)
    2. Adrenergic drugs (sympathomimetics)
      a. Direct action on effector cell (effective after denervation)—norepinephrine, epinephrine, isoproterenol
      b. Indirect action (release norepinephrine from adrenergic nerve endings; ineffective peripherally after denervation)—tyramine, amphetamine
      c. Mixed action (direct and indirect)—ephedrine, metaraminol
  B. Antagonists acting on end-organ receptors
    1. Cholinergic receptor antagonists (cholinergic blocking drugs)
      a. Competitive antagonists of "muscarinic" receptors—atropine
    2. Adrenergic receptor antagonists (adrenergic blocking drugs)
      a. Antagonize α-adrenergic receptors
        (1) Competitive—phentolamine
        (2) Noncompetitive—phenoxybenzamine
      b. Antagonize β-adrenergic receptors
        (1) Competitive—propranolol
II. Drugs acting on autonomic nerve endings
  A. Agonists that cause the release of transmitters
    1. Cholinergic neurons—none
    2. Adrenergic neurons—indirect and mixed acting sympathomimetics
  B. Drugs that inhibit the release of transmitters
    1. Cholinergic neurons—botulinum toxin
    2. Adrenergic neurons—bretylium, guanethidine
  C. Drugs that inhibit the synthesis of transmitters
    1. Cholinergic neurons (inhibits synthesis of ACh)—hemicholinium
    2. Adrenergic neurons (inhibits synthesis of norepinephrine)—α-methyl-*p*-tyrosine
  D. Drugs that inhibit the storage of transmitters in neurons
    1. Cholinergic neurons—none
    2. Adrenergic neurons (deplete norepinephrine)—reserpine, guanethidine
  E. Drugs that cause the formation of false transmitters in neurons
    1. Cholinergic neurons—none
    2. Adrenergic neurons—methyldopa, metaraminol, MAO inhibitors

F. Drugs that inhibit the uptake of transmitters into neurons
1. Cholinergic neurons—none
2. Adrenergic neurons—cocaine, desmethylimipramine and congeners
III. Drugs acting on autonomic ganglia
A. Agonists that stimulate postganglionic neurons ("nicotinic" stimulants)
1. Both cholinergic and adrenergic neurons—nicotine
B. Antagonists that inhibit "nicotinic" receptors or postganglionic neurons
1. Both cholinergic and adrenergic neurons (competitive antagonists)—hexamethonium, mecamylamine

NONAUTONOMIC DRUGS

I. Drugs acting on the skeletal muscle neuromuscular junction
A. Agonists mimicking the motor nerve transmitter, acetylcholine
1. Direct action on muscle cell—neostigmine
2. Indirect action (cholinesterase inhibitors)
a. Competitive—neostigmine, physostigmine
b. Noncompetitive—isoflurophate
B. Antagonists that block skeletal muscle receptors
1. Depolarizing—succinylcholine
2. Nondepolarizing (competitive)—*d*-tubocurarine
II. Drugs acting on sensory nerve endings
A. "Sensitize" stretch receptors monitoring blood pressure—Veratrum alkaloids
III. Drugs acting on all nerves to block conduction of action potentials
A. Local anesthetics
IV. Drugs acting on vascular smooth muscle
A. Vasoconstrictors—angiotensin, vasopressin
B. Vasodilators—nitrites, papaverine
C. Antihypertensive drugs—hydralazine, diazoxide
V. Other endogenous biologically active compounds
A. Serotonin, histamine, bradykinin, prostaglandins, etc.

For the sake of simplicity, autonomic drugs are classified in the succeeding chapters as cholinergic drugs, anticholinergic drugs (various types), adrenergic drugs, and adrenergic blocking drugs (alpha [α] and beta [β]).

REFERENCES

1. Axelrod, J.: The metabolism of catecholamines in vivo and in vitro, Pharmacol. Rev. **11**:402, 1959.
2. Berthelsen, S., and Pettinger, W.A.: A functional basis for classification of α-adrenergic receptors, Life Sci. **21**:595, 1977.
3. Brimblecombe, R.W.: Drug actions on cholinergic systems. In Bradley, P.B., editor: Pharmacology monographs, Baltimore, 1974, University Park Press.
4. Brodie, B.B., Spector, S., and Shore, P.A.: Interaction of drugs with norepinephrine in the brain, Pharmacol. Rev. **11**:548, 1959.

5. Bunney, B.J., Walters, J.R., Roth, R.H., and Aghajanian, G.K.: Dopaminergic neurons: effect of antipsychotic drugs and amphetamine on single cell activity, J. Pharmacol. Exp. Ther. **185**:560, 1973.
6. Cannon, W.B., and Uridil, J.E.: Studies on conditions of activity in endocrine glands: some effects on the denervated heart of stimulating nerves of the liver, Am. J. Physiol. **58**:353, 1921.
7. Dale, H.H.: The action of certain esters and ethers of choline and their relation to muscarine, J. Pharmacol. Exp. Ther. **6**:147, 1914.
8. Douglas, W.W.: Stimulus-secretion cou-

pling: the concept and clues from chromaffin and other cells, Br. J. Pharmacol. **34**:451, 1968.

9. Fatt, P., and Katz, B.: Spontaneous subthreshold activity at motor nerve endings, J. Physiol. **117**:109m 1952.

10. Fleming, W.W.: Nonspecific supersensitivity of the guinea-pig ileum produced by chronic ganglion blockade, J. Pharmacol. Exp. Ther. **162**:277, 1968.

11. Galindo, A.: The role of prejunctional effects in myoneural transmission, Anesthesiology **36**:598, 1972.

12. Hoffman, B.B., and Lefkowitz, R.J.: Radioligand binding studies of adrenergic receptors: new insights into molecular and physiological regulation, Annu. Rev. Pharmacol. Toxicol. **20**:581, 1980.

13. Katz, B., and Miledi, R.: Propagation of electric activity in motor nerve terminals, Proc. R. Soc. Biol. **161**:483, 1965.

14. Krieger, D.T., and Martin, J.B.: Brain peptides, N. Engl. J. Med. **304**:944, 1981.

15. Langer, S.Z.: Presynaptic regulation of catecholamine release, Biochem. Pharmacol. **23**:1793, 1974.

16. Langer, S.Z.: Presynaptic receptors and their role in the regulation of transmitter release, Br. J. Pharmacol. **60**:481, 1977.

17. Lefkowitz, R.J.: Direct binding studies of adrenergic receptors: biochemical, physiologic and clinical implications, Ann. Intern. Med. **91**:450, 1979.

18. Loewi, O.: Über humorale Übertragbarkeit der Herznervenwirkung, Arch. Ges. Physiol. **189**:239, 1921.

19. MacMillan, W.H.: A hypothesis concerning the effect of cocaine on the action of sympathomimetic amines, Br. J. Pharmacol. **14**:385, 1969.

20. Okamoto, M., Longenecker, H.E., and Riker, W.F.: Destruction of mammalian motor nerve terminals by black widow spider venom, Science **172**:733, 1971.

21. Purpura, D.P., Girado, M., Smith, T.G.,

Callan, D.A., and Grundfest, H.: Structure-activity determinants of pharmacological effects of amino acids and related compounds on central synapses, J. Neurochem. **3**:238, 1959.

22. Shore, P.A.: Release of serotonin and catecholamines by drugs, Pharmacol. Rev. **14**:531, 1962.

23. Shore, P.A.: Transport and storage of biogenic amines, Annu. Rev. Pharmacol. **12**:209, 1972.

24. Snyder, S.H., and Bennett, J.P., Jr.: Neurotransmitter receptors in the brain: biochemical identification, Annu. Rev. Physiol. **38**:153, 1976.

25. Snyder, S.H., Young, A.B., Bennett, J.P., and Mulder, A.H.: Synaptic biochemistry of amino acids, Fed. Proc. **32**:2039, 1973.

26. Thoenen, H., and Tranzer, J.P.: The pharmacology of 6-hydroxydopamine, Annu. Rev. Pharmacol. **13**:169, 1973.

27. Trendelenburg, U.: Mechanisms of supersensitivity and subsensitivity to sympathomimetic amines, Pharmacol. Rev. **18**:629, 1966.

28. Udenfriend, S.: Tyrosine hydroxylase, Pharmacol. Rev. **18**:629, 1966.

29. von Euler, U.S.: Noradrendine: chemistry, physiology, pharmacology and clinical aspects, Springfield, Ill., 1956, Charles C Thomas Publisher.

30. Weinshilboum, R.M., Thoa, N.B., Johnson, D.G., Kopin, I.J., and Axelrod, J.: Proportional release of norepinephrine and dopamine-β-hydroxylase from sympathetic nerves, Science **174**:1349, 1971.

31. Willis, W.D.: The case for the Renshaw Cell. In Riss, W., editor: Brain, behavior and evolution, vol. 5, Basel, 1971, S. Karger AG.

32. Wurtman, R.J., and Fernstrom, J.D.: Control of brain neurotransmitter synthesis by precursor availability and nutritional state, Biochem. Pharmacol. **25**:1691, 1976.

Chapter 11

Cholinergic (cholinomimetic) drugs

The various cholinergic drugs can be divided into two major groups: directly acting cholinergic drugs and cholinesterase inhibitors.

DIRECTLY ACTING
CHOLINERGIC
DRUGS
Choline esters

Although acetylcholine is an essential compound from the standpoint of its role in body physiology, two important considerations render it useless as a drug. First, even when it is injected intravenously, its actions are very brief because of its rapid destruction by the ubiquitous cholinesterases. Second, it has so many diverse effects that no selective therapeutic purpose can be achieved through its use. The various derivatives of acetylcholine, however, differ from the parent compound by being more resistant to the action of the cholinesterases and by having a certain amount of selectivity in their sites of action.

If we depict the acetylcholine-receptor combination in a manner similar to that postulated for acetylcholine-cholinesterase, as shown in Fig. 11-1, it can be seen that slight changes in the structure should alter the union of the drug with the receptor. Some of these changes can prevent an enzymatic attack on the molecule while still allowing an interaction of the drug with some of the receptors. Drugs in this group that have some importance are the following:

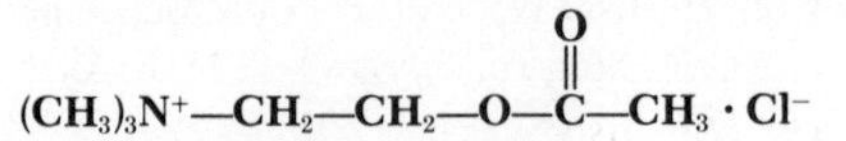

$$(CH_3)_3N^+ - CH_2 - CH_2 - O - \overset{\overset{\displaystyle O}{\|}}{C} - CH_3 \cdot Cl^-$$

Acetylcholine chloride

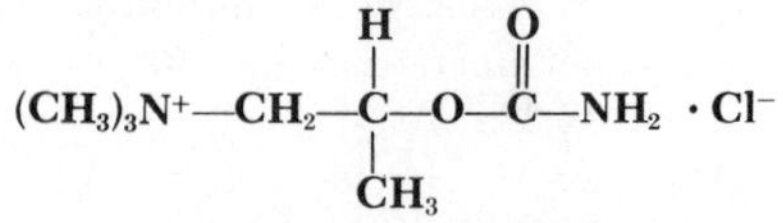

$$(CH_3)_3N^+ - CH_2 - \overset{\overset{\displaystyle H}{|}}{\underset{\underset{\displaystyle CH_3}{|}}{C}} - O - \overset{\overset{\displaystyle O}{\|}}{C} - NH_2 \cdot Cl^-$$

Bethanechol chloride

$$(CH_3)_3N^+ - CH_2 - \overset{\overset{\displaystyle H}{|}}{\underset{\underset{\displaystyle CH_3}{|}}{C}} - O - \overset{\overset{\displaystyle O}{\|}}{C} - CH_3 \cdot Cl^-$$

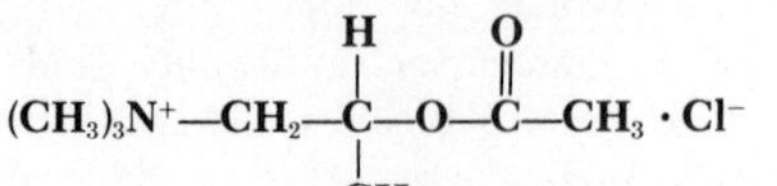

Methacholine chloride

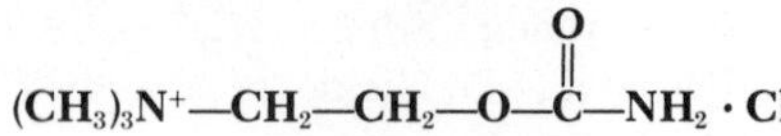

$$(CH_3)_3N^+ - CH_2 - CH_2 - O - \overset{\overset{\displaystyle O}{\|}}{C} - NH_2 \cdot Cl^-$$

Carbachol chloride

Interaction of acetylcholine and acetylcholinesterase.   *FIG. 11-1*

From Wilson, I.B.: Neurology 8(suppl. 1):41, 1958.

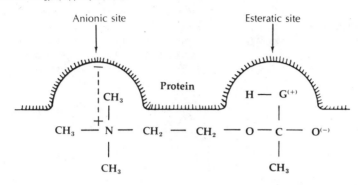

All drugs in this group are quaternary amines. Replacement of the acetyl group by carbamate protects the drug against cholinesterases and thus prolongs its half-life in the body. Substitution in the β carbon, as in acetyl-β-methylcholine, protects against the action of the nonspecific cholinesterase.

Bethanechol and methacholine have many of the actions of acetylcholine on smooth muscles and glands without significantly affecting ganglia and skeletal neuromuscular transmission.

Bethanechol (Urecholine) has selective effects on the gastrointestinal and urinary tracts and is the parasympathomimetic drug of choice for the treatment of postoperative abdominal distention and postoperative urinary retention. Bethanechol is not destroyed by cholinesterases and thus has prolonged effects. The usual cholinergic side effects are sweating, flushing, salivation, and aggravation of bronchial asthma. Hypotension may be caused by the drug but is not common. Contraindications to its use include bronchial asthma, severe cardiac disease, hyperthyroidism (atrial fibrillation may occur), and mechanical obstruction of the gastrointestinal and urinary tracts. Preparations include tablets of 5, 10, and 25 mg and solutions for subcutaneous injection, 5 mg/ml. The dosage for adults is 5 to 30 mg three or four times daily by mouth or 2.5 to 5 mg three or four times daily by subcutaneous injection.

Methacholine (Mecholyl) has few uses in medicine. It possesses mostly muscarinic activity, especially on the cardiovascular system. Because it is an acetyl ester, it is hydrolyzed by acetylcholinesterase, although more slowly than acetylcholine. Methacholine has been used in the treatment of paroxysmal atrial tachycardia because it abolishes the ectopic focus in the atrium, probably as a consequence of hyperpolarization. It is seldom used for this purpose because it can cause alarming syncopal attacks when injected by the subcutaneous route. Patients with adrenal medullary tumors respond to methacholine with a rise of blood pressure, since it stimulates the output of catecholamines from the tumor. The methacholine test for pheochromocytoma has had some popularity but is seldom used at present. Preparations include

FIG. 11-2   *Effect of acetylcholine on blood pressure before and after atropine. The following drugs were administered intravenously to a dog anesthetized with pentobarbital: A, acetylcholine, 10 µg/kg; between A and B, atropine, 1 mg/kg; B, acetylcholine, 10 µg/kg; C, acetylcholine, 100 µg/kg; between C and D, phentolamine, 5 mg/kg; D, acetylcholine, 100 µg/kg. Note that atropine prevented blood pressure lowering induced by small dose of acetylcholine. Large dose of acetylcholine actually caused elevation of blood pressure, the so-called nicotinic effect of acetylcholine. This response is blocked by phentolamine, an adrenergic blocking agent.*

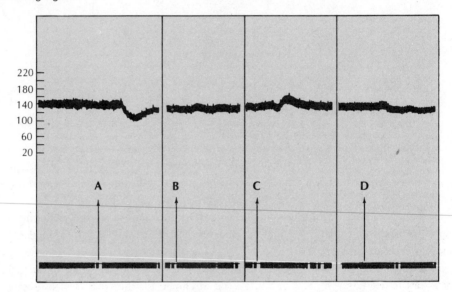

tablets containing 200 mg and powder for injectable solution, 25 mg. For adults the oral dosage is 50 to 600 mg three or four times daily; the subcutaneous dosage, 10 to 25 mg.

Carbachol is a very potent choline ester having both muscarinic and nicotinic effects. Its only use at present is in the treatment of glaucoma. Solutions of 0.5% to 1%, applied to the conjunctiva, cause miosis and reduction of intraocular pressure. The antidote to carbachol is atropine.

The muscarinic and nicotinic actions of the choline esters can be illustrated by a simple experiment. Fig. 11-2 shows the effect of injected choline esters on blood pressure responses of a dog before and after atropine administration.

In summary, the essential actions of the choline esters following subcutaneous injection are cutaneous vasodilatation with flushing, sweating, salivation, and increased tone of the smooth muscle of the gastrointestinal tract and urinary bladder. There are variable effects on heart rate and blood pressure. There is a precipitous fall in the blood pressure of some individuals, whereas in others the changes in blood pressure and heart rate are slight because compensatory reflexes remain active. It should always be kept in mind that asthmatic patients are particularly susceptible to the bronchoconstrictor action of these compounds. The antidote, atropine, should always be on hand before a choline ester is administered.

The two alkaloids pilocarpine and muscarine have the curious property of acting like acetylcholine on receptors of smooth muscles and glandular cells. Muscarine is present in the mushroom *Amanita muscaria*, along with toxic peptides,[23] whereas pilocarpine is found in the leaves of the plant *Pilocarpus jaborandi*.

Pilocarpine and muscarine

Muscarine

Pilocarpine

Both alkaloids show the so-called muscarin effects of acetylcholine without having significant nicotinic action. Atropine blocks these muscarinic effects. Muscarine, being a quaternary ammonium compound, shows some similarity to acetylcholine, but it is puzzling why pilocarpine, which is a tertiary amine, should also mimic the muscarinic effects of acetylcholine. It is well established, however, that this is not the result of cholinesterase inhibition.

Of these two drugs, muscarine has only academic interest. Pilocarpine, however, is employed in ophthalmology as a miotic and is occasionally used for stimulating the flow of saliva in patients who complain of dryness of the mouth during therapy with ganglionic blocking agents. For ophthalmological applications, pilocarpine is employed in a 1% solution. The usual dose for stimulating the secretion of saliva is 5 mg, given either orally or by subcutaneous injection. In addition to stimulating the flow of saliva, the drug greatly increases sweating. Its antidote is atropine.

PROBLEM 11-1. *The fixed dilated pupil may be an ominous sign caused by an involvement of the third nerve by an intracranial disease. How can this be distinguished from the accidental application to the eye of an anticholinergic (mydriatic) drug? In an interesting article,[21] topical application of pilocarpine is used to establish the diagnosis. The pupil responds well to pilocarpine in the case of nerve damage, whereas it is unresponsive if the dilated pupil is caused by the application of a mydriatic drug. Could an anticholinesterase such as physostigmine be substituted for pilocarpine in this diagnostic test?*

Some drugs inhibit the destruction of acetylcholine and thereby produce a higher concentration of the agent at those sites where it is released. They can also potentiate the action of some of the exogenous choline esters when these are administered.

ANTICHOLIN-ESTERASES

The cholinesterase inhibitors are of great interest in medicine. They have been found very useful in the treatment of myasthenia gravis and in the management of glaucoma. The group has also yielded some of our most potent insecticides, which are of great toxicological importance because of their widespread use. Cholinesterase inhibitors are valuable investigative tools. They are also potential chemical warfare agents. Physostigmine is also becoming useful in the treatment of atropine poisoning.

Physostigmine, *neostigmine, and* *related drugs*   Physostigmine and neostigmine are reversible anticholinesterases. Physostigmine is a tertiary amine used in the treatment of glaucoma and as an antidote in poisoning caused by atropine-like drugs. Neostigmine is a quaternary ammonium compound used in myasthenia gravis, in glaucoma, and as a gastrointestinal and urinary tract stimulant.

Physostigmine (eserine), an alkaloid obtained from the seeds of *Physostigma venenosum*, also known as calabar or ordeal bean, has been familiar to pharmacologists since the latter part of the nineteenth century. Synthesis of compounds related to physostigmine led to the development of neostigmine in 1931.[1]

Physostigmine   Neostigmine

Pharmacological investigations have shown that physostigmine is an antagonist of curare. In 1934 the British physician Mary Walker[22] tried physostigmine in the treatment of myasthenia gravis because of the clinical similarity of this disease to a curarized state. The results were impressive, and when neostigmine became available, it was tried also.

ACTION AND USES *OF PHYSOSTIGMINE*   The actions of physostigmine may be attributed entirely to cholinesterase inhibition on the basis of the following considerations. The drug inhibits cholinesterase in vitro. Its affinity for the enzyme may be 10,000 times greater than that of acetylcholine. After combination with the enzyme, it seems to be gradually dissociated and inactivated in the body. Consequently, the drug is a reversible inhibitor of the cholinesterases.

Physostigmine exerts no effect on the denervated pupil or on the denervated skeletal muscle, even when given by close intraarterial injection. It has potent effects on structures with normal innervation because of its ability to protect the endogenously released acetylcholine.

Physostigmine salicylate is the specific antidote for anticholinergic intoxication. Given intravenously or intramuscularly in doses of 1 mg, it counteracts the abnormal mental state caused by atropine or scopolamine. Physostigmine salicylate has also been used topically in the treatment of primary open-angle glaucoma, although pilocarpine is preferred. For open-angle glaucoma the drug is applied as a drop of 0.25% to 1% solution. Effects of physostigmine on long-term memory processes are interesting but still investigational.[5]

Some of the actions of neostigmine are caused by cholinesterase inhibition, where-as others are the result of a combination of enzyme inhibition plus a direct acetyl-choline-like effect. On the denervated eye, for example, neostigmine acts like phy-sostigmine, producing no pupillary constriction. On the other hand, intraarterially injected neostigmine will elicit an effect at the neuromuscular junction even when the nerves are degenerated and all cholinesterase has been previously destroyed by diisopropyl fluorophosphate. This evidence suggests that the muscarinic actions of neostigmine are produced by cholinesterase inhibition, whereas the nicotinic actions, at least at the neuromuscular site, are in part a result of a direct effect.

The intramuscular injection of 0.5 to 1 mg of neostigmine methylsulfate (Pro-stigmin methylsulfate) into a normal human being will produce the usual cholinergic effects: elevation of skin temperature, sweating, salivation, intestinal contractions with a desire to defecate, contraction of smooth muscles of the urinary tract with an urgency to micturate, some slowing of the heart rate with possible hypotension, and muscle fasciculations. Atropine will antagonize the muscarinic effects but not the neuromuscular nicotinic actions of neostigmine. This antidote should be available whenever neostigmine is employed.

In addition to the injectable methylsulfate, neostigmine can be given by mouth as the bromide salt. Much larger doses are given orally, 15 to 30 mg, because much of the drug is inactivated in the gastrointestinal tract. Absorption may be variable, and untoward reactions may occur if too much of the drug is suddenly absorbed.

Drugs related to neostigmine. **Edrophonium** (Tensilon) has a structure that is similar to that of neostigmine. This drug has been introduced as an anticurare agent. It also has diagnostic and investigative uses in myasthenia.

$$\text{OH} \quad \underset{\diagdown \text{CH}_3}{\overset{\diagup \text{CH}_3}{\text{N}^+\!\!-\!\text{C}_2\text{H}_5}} \cdot \text{Cl}^-$$

Edrophonium chloride

The essential feature of edrophonium is its short duration of action. From a practical standpoint it may be considered an extremely short-acting neostigmine. In the myasthenic patient the intravenous injection of 2 to 5 mg of edrophonium will cause rapid and transient improvement of muscular strength. This may be used for diagnostic purposes and also for "titrating" the degree of effectiveness of other treat-ment. The physician may be in doubt as to whether to increase or decrease the dosage of neostigmine for a myasthenic patient. If intravenous edrophonium causes further improvement in the patient, it is likely that previous therapy has been inadequate. On the other hand, if the reaction to this edrophonium test is unfavor-able, indicating overtreatment, increasing the neostigmine dosage would be unde-sirable. The action of edrophonium in this test lasts only a few minutes.

The drug is a potent antidote to curare. It acts more rapidly than neostigmine, and its action is more transient. Although the drug has some cholinesterase inhibitory properties, its neuromuscular effect is probably a direct one.

Neostigmine substitutes. **Pyridostigmine** (Mestinon) is used in the treatment of myasthenia gravis, in single doses of 60 mg orally. Its duration of action is 4 hours.

Ambenonium (Mytelase) is also used in the treatment of myasthenia gravis in single doses of 10 mg orally. Its duration of action is 8 hours.

Organophosphorus anticholinesterases

Diisopropyl fluorophosphate (DFP; isoflurophate) and a variety of other alkyl phosphates are highly toxic compounds that produce irreversible inactivation of the cholinesterases. They were developed as potential chemical warfare agents and have had some therapeutic applications, but their principal interest is toxicological because of their widespread use as insecticides.

The structural formulas of some of the organophosphorus compounds are:

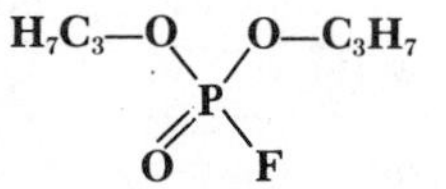

Diisopropyl fluorophosphate

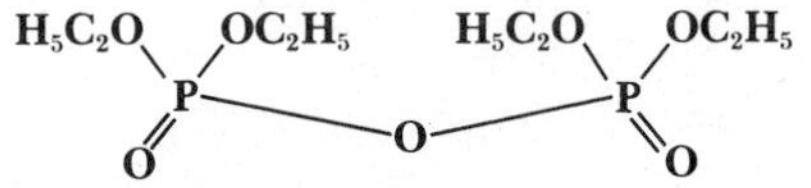

Tetraethyl pyrophosphate

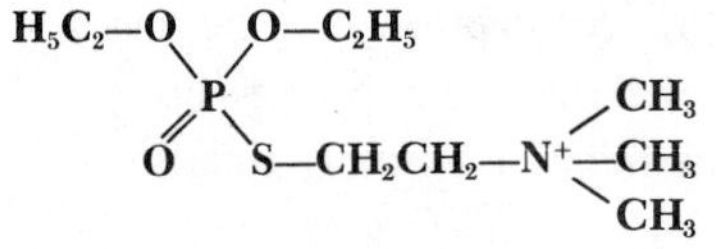

Echothiophate

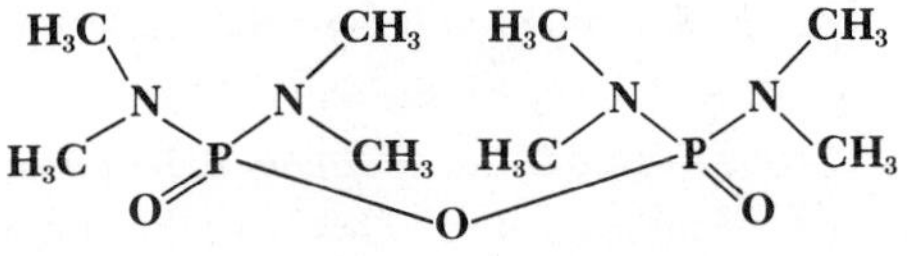

Octamethyl pyrophosphoramide

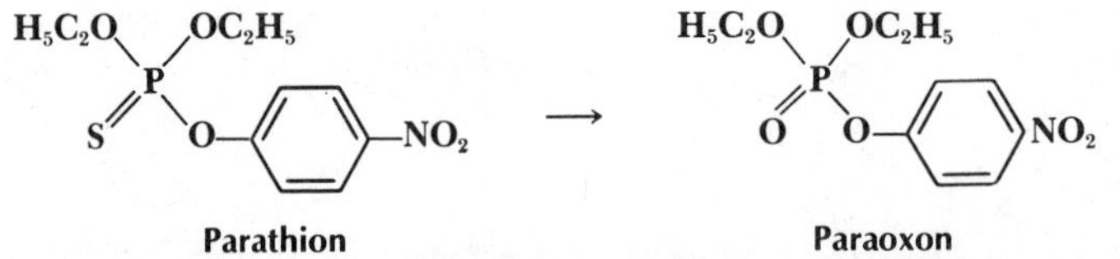

Parathion

Paraoxon

Whereas the reversible anticholinesterases depress enzymatic activity for a few hours following a single administration, the organophosphorus compounds produce an effect that may persist for weeks or months. The difference may be attributed to the fact that the organophosphorus compounds combine with the cholinesterases, which then become phosphorylated. The phosphorylated enzyme is stable, does not hydrolyze, and is inactive against acetylcholine. As a consequence, enzymatic activity will remain reduced until new enzyme material is synthesized, unless some reactivator of cholinesterase is employed as an antidote.

The nonspecific cholinesterase of plasma is affected preferentially and primarily by the alkyl phosphates. With sufficient doses, however, there is increasing destruction of acetylcholinesterase in red cells and in neural tissue. Nonspecific cholinesterase of plasma is regenerated by the liver in about 2 weeks. It may take 3 months to regenerate acetylcholinesterase activity at synapses and neuromuscular junctions.

TABLE 11-1   Signs and symptoms of organophosphate poisoning

Muscarinic manifestations	Nicotinic manifestations	CNS manifestations
Bronchoconstriction	Muscular fasciculation	Restlessness
Increased bronchial secretions	Tachycardia	Insomnia
Sweating	Hypertension	Tremors
Salivation		Confusion
Lacrimation		Ataxia
Bradycardia		Convulsions
Hypotension		Respiratory depression
Miosis		Circulatory collapse
Blurring of vision		
Urinary incontinence		

Modified from Namba, T., Nolte, C.T., Jackrel, J., and Grob, D.: Am. J. Med. **50**:475, 1971.

PHARMACOLOGICAL EFFECTS

When DFP or other alkyl phosphate anticholinesterases are injected or inhaled, the clinical picture that develops is a combination of peripheral cholinergic effects and involvement of the CNS (Table 11-1). Muscle fasciculations, constricted pupils, salivation, sweating, abdominal cramps, and respiratory distress are consequences of cholinesterase inactivation in the periphery. Anxiety, restlessness, electroencephalographic changes, and perhaps even terminal convulsions may be related to the actions of the inhibitor on the CNS. Atropine protects against the peripheral muscarinic effects and the involvement of the CNS. It exerts no protective effect against muscle fasciculations and skeletal muscle weakness.[11] The cause of death in organophosphate poisoning is respiratory paralysis.

ANTIDOTAL ACTION OF PRALIDOXIME

Pralidoxime (pyridine-2-aldoxime-methiodide; PAM) is a tailor-made molecule developed on the basis of a mechanism postulated by Wilson[24] to explain the action of the alkyl phosphate anticholinesterases. Experimental studies have shown that hydroxylamine and oximes are capable of regenerating the enzyme when it is presumably phosphorylated by the alkyl phosphates. With this knowledge, a molecule was designed in which the distance between the quaternary nitrogen and the oxime is the same as that postulated for acetylcholine. It was predicted that such a compound would fit into the cholinesterase enzyme and would act as a more efficient regenerator than would an ordinary oxime. This work led to the synthesis of pralidoxime.

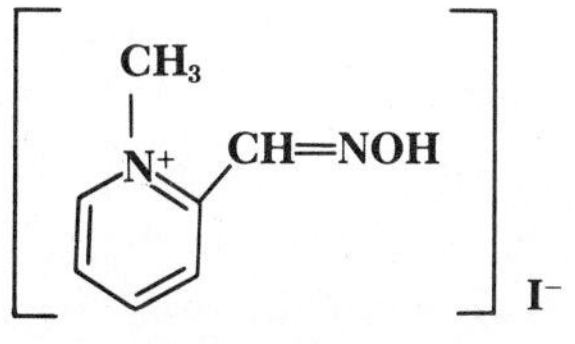

Pralidoxime iodide

The interactions of organophosphates, cholinesterases, and reactivators such as pralidoxime may be visualized in the following manner:

$$\underset{\text{Organophosphate}}{R_2\underset{\text{Acyl}}{\overset{\displaystyle R_1\quad O}{\diagdown P \diagup}}} + \underset{\text{Cholinesterase}}{H \cdot \text{Esterase}} \longrightarrow \underset{\substack{\text{Phosphorylated} \\ \text{esterase}}}{R_2\underset{\text{Esterase}}{\overset{\displaystyle R_1\quad O}{\diagdown P \diagup}}} \xrightarrow{\text{Pralidoxime}} \underset{\substack{\text{Reactivated} \\ \text{esterase}}}{H \cdot \text{Esterase}}$$

Pralidoxime must be administered parenterally. It is usually given by intravenous infusion, 50 mg/kg of body weight dissolved in 1000 ml of saline solution. The drug has some depolarizing effect of its own in addition to reactivation of the phosphorylated cholinesterases.

Other reactivator oximes such as diacetylmonoxime (DAM) and bisquaternary oximes have been studied.

MEDICAL USES
OF ORGANO-
PHOSPHATES

Although the organophosphates are used most widely as insecticides (Malathion, Diazinon) and are potential chemical warfare agents, some have medical uses.

Isoflurophate, echothiophate, and demecarium are used in the treatment of glaucoma. When applied locally, the action of the drugs remains localized. They may produce a prolonged decrease of intraocular pressure over a period of weeks. The effect of the organophosphorus compounds may be partially blocked in glaucoma by the prior application of physostigmine or neostigmine.

A very high percentage of presently available insecticides contain organophosphorus anticholinesterases. Acute and chronic poisoning resulting from these pesticides is not uncommon.

The *treatment of organophosphorus poisoning* is as follows. Atropine sulfate, 1 to 2 mg, should be administered as symptoms appear. This antidote may be given every hour up to 25 to 50 mg in a day. The skin, stomach, and eyes should be decontaminated. Pralidoxime is administered by slow intravenous infusion in a dose of 1 g for adult if the patient fails to respond to atropine. Certain drugs are contraindicated in organophosphorus poisoning. These include morphine, theophylline, or aminophylline. If the patient is cyanotic, artificial respiration should be administered even before atropine.

General features of
cholinesterase
inhibition

Much has been learned about the importance of the cholinesterases from studies on the action of anticholinesterases. It appears from these studies that serum cholinesterase is probably of no great physiological importance but may have a significant effect when exogenous labile choline esters are administered. Serum cholinesterase can be reduced to very low levels with DFP treatment without important consequences. Measurements of serum cholinesterase activity may be altered by disease of the liver or by the previous administration of anticholinesterases. Such measurements are of importance in industrial medicine to evaluate the extent of exposure to anticholinesterases, thus preventing inadvertent poisoning.

The specific acetylcholinesterase appears to exist in excess at the various junctions at which acetylcholine functions as a mediator of neural transmission. Moderate decreases of acetylcholinesterase have little physiological consequence. On the other hand, a severe reduction of brain cholinesterase, down to 10% of normal, has been observed in animals when death occurs from the administration of an anticholinesterase.

The presence of acetylcholinesterase in the red cell is puzzling, since no obvious physiological reason for it seems to exist. It has been suggested that the acetylcholine-cholinesterase system has a much broader significance than that expected from its neuroeffector function.

Cholinesterase activity of the red cell mass can reflect hematopoietic activity. The regeneration of acetylcholinesterase activity of red blood cells following the administration of irreversible anticholinesterases is directly proportional to the production of new cells.

Myasthenia gravis is a neuromuscular disease characterized by muscle fatigability. The density of the acetylcholine receptor at the neuromuscular junction is reduced by humoral and possibly cell-mediated immune factors, resulting in impairment of neuromuscular transmission.[7]

PHARMACO-LOGICAL ASPECTS OF MYASTHENIA GRAVIS

Repetitive stimulation of a motor nerve in a myasthenic patient rapidly leads to fatigue of the muscles innervated by that particular nerve. Intraarterial injection of acetylcholine, neostigmine, or edrophonium increases the strength of the fatigued muscles. In normal persons the intraarterial injection of these drugs produces fasciculation and weakness, probably as a result of persistent depolarization of the neuromuscular end-plates. Also, myasthenic patients are susceptible to doses of *d*-tubocurarine or quinine that scarcely affect normal persons.

Various anticholinesterases are useful for the diagnosis and management of myasthenia. For diagnostic purposes, neostigmine in a dose of 1 to 2 mg may be injected by the intramuscular route with atropine, 0.6 mg. Smaller doses (0.5 mg) of neostigmine may be used by the intravenous route. Endrophonium may be given for diagnosis in a dose of 2 to 8 mg intravenously.

For the management of weakness, neostigmine and related drugs are most useful. Neostigmine bromide is administered orally in doses of 15 to 30 mg, sometimes as often as every 3 hours (Table 11-2). Much smaller doses of neostigmine as the methylsulfate suffice when given by the intramuscular route.

Neostigmine bromide   **Pyridostigmine bromide**   **Ambenonium chloride**

TABLE 11-2	Anticholinesterase preparations	
Drug	Preparations	Usual route of administration
Physostigmine (eserine)	0.1% to 1% solution	Topical (eye)
Neostigmine bromide (Prostigmin bromide)	Tablets, 15 mg	Oral
Neostigmine methylsulfate (Prostigmin methylsulfate)	Injectable solutions, 0.25, 0.5, and 1 mg/ml	Subcutaneous or intramuscular
Pyridostigmine (Mestinon)	Tablets, 60 mg	Oral
Ambenonium (Mytelase)	Tablets, 10 and 25 mg	Oral
Demecarium (Humorsol)	0.25% solution	Topical (eye)
Edrophonium (Tensilon)	Injectable solution, 10 mg/ml	Intravenous
Echothiophate (Phospholine)	0.25% solution	Topical (eye)

Cholinergic crisis   Excessive doses of anticholinesterases produce what is often called a cholinergic crisis. Its muscarinic signs are miosis, sweating, salivation, lacrimation, and a hyperactive bowel. Its nicotinic signs are revealed by muscle fasciculations and paralysis. The diagnosis of anticholinesterase poisoning can be made on the basis of these symptoms and signs, since there are essentially no other diagnostic possibilities.[9]

An intravenous injection of 2 mg of edrophonium may be useful in distinguishing between cholinergic crisis and myasthenic crisis. If the injection is followed by increased strength, it is an indication of undertreatment rather than overtreatment.[19]

Drug interactions   The following drugs require caution in myasthenic patients, since they may aggravate the symptoms of the disease:

1. Antibiotics, such as streptomycin, kanamycin, tobramycin, gentamicin, polymyxin, and tetracycline
2. Antiarrhythmics, such as quinidine, quinine, and procainamide
3. Local anesthetics, such as procaine and lidocaine
4. General anesthetics, particularly ether
5. Muscle relaxants, such as curare and succinylcholine
6. Analgesics, including morphine and meperidine

1. Aeschlimann, J.A., and Reinert, M.: Pharmacological action of some analogues of physostigmine, J. Pharmacol. Exp. Ther. **43**:413, 1931.

2. Becker, B., and Ballin, N.: Glaucoma, Annu. Rev. Med. **17**:235, 1966.

3. Brimblecombe, R.W.: Drug actions on cholinergic systems. In Bradley, P.B., editor: Pharmacology monographs, Baltimore, 174, University Park Press.

4. Cohen, J.B., and Changeux, J.P.: The cholinergic receptor protein in its membrane environment, Annu. Rev. Pharmacol. **15**:83, 1974.

5. Davis, K.L., Mohs, R.C., Tinklenberg, J.R., Pfefferbaum, A., Hollister, L.E., and Kopell, B.S.: Physostigmine: improvement of long-term memory processes in normal humans, Science **201**: 272, 1978.

6. Duvoison, R.C., and Katz, R.: Reversal of central anticholinergic syndrome in man by physostigmine, JAMA **206**: 1963, 1968.

7. Elias, S.B., and Appel, S.H.: Recent advances in myasthenia gravis, Life Sci. **18**:1031, 1976.

8. Fambrough, D.M., Drachman, D.B., and Satyamurti, S.: Neuromuscular junction in myasthenia gravis: decreased acetylcholine receptors, Sciece **182**:293, 1973.

9. Hallett, M., and Cullen, R.F.: Intoxication with echothiophate iodide, JAMA **222**:1414, 1972.

10. Hofmann, W.W.: The treatment of myasthenia gravis, Ration. Drug Ther. **13**: No. 2, Feb. 1979.

11. Kanagaratnam, K., Boon, W.H., and Hoh, T.K.: Parathion poisoning from contaminated barley, Lancet **1**:538, 1960.

12. Koelle, G.B.: Acetylcholine—current status in physiology, pharmacology and medicine, N. Engl. J. Med. **286**:1086, 1972.

13. Leopold, I.H., and Keates, E.: Drugs used in the treatment of glaucoma. I. Clin. Pharmacol. Ther. **6**:130, 1965.

14. Leopold, I.H., and Keates, E.: Drugs used in the treatment of glaucoma. II. Clin. Pharmacol. Ther. **6**:262, 1965.

15. Lindstrom, J., and Dau, P.: Biology of myasthenia gravis, Annu. Rev. Pharmacol. Toxicol. **20**:337, 1980.

16. Lisak, R.P.: Myasthenia gravis: mechanisms and management, Hosp. Pract. March 1983, p. 101.

17. Moore, H.: Advantages of pyridostigmine bromide (Mestinon) and edrophonium chloride (Tensilon) in the treatment of transitory myasthenia gravis in the neonatal period, N. Engl. J. Med. **253**:1075, 1955.

18. Namba, T., Nolte, C.T., Jackrel, J., and Grob, D.: Poisoning due to organophosphate insecticides, Am. J. Med. **50**:475, 1971.

19. Osserman, K.E., and Kaplan, L.I.: Studies in myasthenia gravis: use of edrophonium chloride (Tensilon) in differentiating myasthenic from cholinergic weakness, Arch. Neurol. Psychiatr. **70**:385, 1953.

20. Quinby, G.E., Loomis, T.A., and Brown, H.W.: Oral occupational parathion poisoning treated with 2-PAM iodide, N. Engl. J. Med. **268**:639, 1963.

21. Thompson, H.S., Newsome, D.A., and Loewenkfeld, I.E.: The fixed dilated pupil, Arch. Ophthalmol. **86**:21, 1971.

22. Walker, M.B.: Case showing effect of prostigmine on myasthenia gravis, Proc. R. Soc. Med. **28**:759, 1935.

23. Wieland, T.: Poisonous principles of mushrooms of the genus Amanita, Science **159**:946, 1968.

24. Wilson, I.B.: A specific antidote for nerve gas and insecticide (alkylphosphate) intoxication, Neurology **8**(suppl. 1):41, 1958.

REFERENCES

Chapter 12

Atropine group of cholinergic blocking drugs

GENERAL CONCEPT   Atropine and related drugs are important therapeutic agents and have widespread uses as pharmacological tools. They are competitive antagonists of acetylcholine on organs innervated by postganglionic nerves. Atropine, scopolamine, and related drugs find important applications in ophthalmology, anesthesia, and cardiac and gastrointestinal diseases. In addition to their peripheral anticholinergic effects, most of these drugs act on the CNS and are used in the treatment of Parkinson's disease and vestibular disorders, as proprietary hypnotics, and as antidotes for the anticholinesterases. In this last instance both peripheral and central actions of the drugs are of great benefit. The receptors blocked by atropine are muscarinic.

ATROPINE AND SCOPOLAMINE   Atropine and scopolamine are among the oldest drugs in medicine. Many solanaceous plants have been used for centuries because of their active principles of *l*-hyoscyamine and *l*-hyoscine. The name *hyoscyamine* is derived from *Hyoscyamus niger* (henbane). It is of some toxicological interest to know that the common jimsonweed, *Datura stramonium*, also contains these alkaloids. These drugs also are often called the belladonna alkaloids because they are found in the deadly nightshade, *Atropa belladonna*.

Chemistry   The alkaloids as they occur in the plants are *l*-hyoscyamine and *l*-hyoscine (scopolamine). Atropine is *dl*-hyoscyamine, with racemization occurring during the extraction process. Just as acetylcholine is an ester of an amino alcohol, the blocking drugs of the belladonna group are esters of complex organic bases with tropic acid. Atropine and scopolamine differ only slightly in the structure of the organic base part of the molecule, as is evident from comparison of their structural formulas.

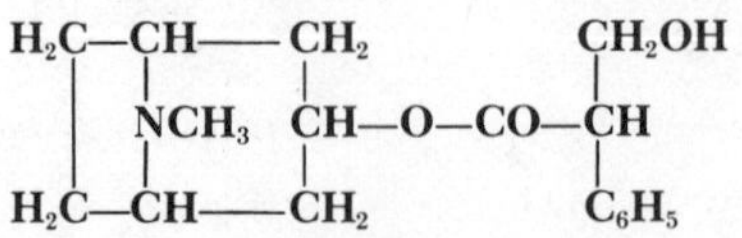

$$H_2C-CH——CH_2 \qquad CH_2OH$$
$$| \qquad NCH_3 \quad CH-O-CO-CH$$
$$H_2C-CH——CH_2 \qquad C_6H_5$$

Atropine

$$HC-CH——CH_2 \qquad CH_2OH$$
$$O\triangleleft \quad NCH_3 \quad CH-O-CO-CH$$
$$HC-CH——CH_2 \qquad C_6H_5$$

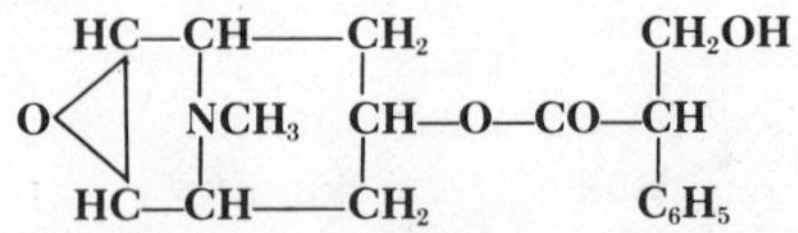

Scopolamine

Atropine and scopolamine are competitive antagonists of acetylcholine at receptor sites in smooth muscles, cardiac muscle, and various glandular cells (see Fig. 2-2, p. 12). The effectiveness of this competition is greatest against the muscarinic effects of injected cholinergic drugs and against the tonic effect of the vagus nerve on the heart. These drugs are less effective in blocking the actions of parasympathetic nerves on the gastrointestinal tract and urinary bladder.

Mode of action

The actions of atropine and scopolamine on the cardiovascular system and on the eye are very similar. The two drugs differ mainly in their CNS effects. In therapeutic doses, given parenterally, scopolamine tends to produce considerable sleepiness, whereas atropine is not likely to produce this evidence of CNS depression. While it is generally believed that scopolamine is a CNS depressant and atropine is a stimulant, in reality the effect depends on the dose. In low doses both drugs tend to cause sedation. In larger doses both cause stimulation, which may progress to delirium. Finally, after very high doses of either drug, coma may supervene.

There is definite gradation in the sensitivity of various functions mediated by acetylcholine to inhibition by atropine and scopolamine. Therapeutic doses of 0.6 mg of atropine or 0.3 mg of scopolamine may cause dryness of the mouth and inhibit sweating. Blockade of the cardiac vagus requires somewhat larger doses. Gastrointestinal and urinary tract smooth muscle is even more resistant to the action of atropine and scopolamine. Finally, the inhibition of gastric secretion requires such large doses in humans that side effects on the more susceptible sites would make that therapeutic objective completely impractical.

Cardiovascular system effects. The effects of atropine and scopolamine on blood pressure are not impressive. Most vascular areas in the body do not receive parasympathetic innervation. It is common experience in the laboratory to inject atropine intravenously into a dog, 1 mg/kg of body weight, without observing a significant change in the mean pressure.

Pharmacological effects

The effect of atropine on the heart rate in humans is complex. With large enough doses, tachycardia develops, as expected, from blockade of vagal influences on the heart. With smaller doses, paradoxical as it may seem, the heart rate may be slowed. Ablation experiments have shown that atropine stimulates vagal nuclei in the medulla, an action that results in bradycardia unless large enough doses are used to prevent such an action at the muscarinic receptors. In one study the final effect of scopolamine on heart rate was found to be the result of two separate actions, one tending to produce tachycardia, the other bradycardia.[10]

A distinctly anomalous vascular effect of atropine is its production of cutaneous dilatation. In warm environments, atropine may promote cutaneous vasodilatation because it tends to block sweating, thus causing body temperature to rise. However, atropine has an additional cutaneous vasodilator action that cannot be explained on this basis. Flushing of the skin may be very noticeable following moderately large doses of atropine.

FIG. 12-1 *Autonomic innervation of iris.*

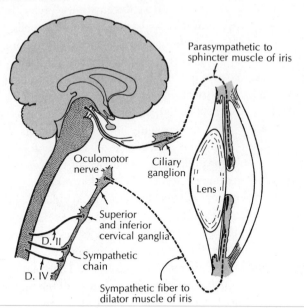

Gastrointestinal effects. In large enough doses the belladonna alkaloids will reduce motility and tone of the gastrointestinal tract and may even reduce the volume of its various secretions. Motility is more easily reduced by therapeutic doses than is gastric secretion, particularly if a peptic ulcer is present.

Effect on urinary tract. Atropine has little effect on the ureters. It relaxes the fundus of the bladder but promotes contraction of the sphincter, thus favoring urinary retention.

Effect on eye. The actions of atropine on the eye are straightforward. When it is applied directly to the conjunctiva (0.5% to 1% solutions), the drug will produce mydriasis and paralysis of accommodation (cycloplegia). In addition, in patients subject to glaucoma it may precipitate an acute attack with catastrophic increases in intraocular pressure.

The circular muscle of the iris receives cholinergic innervation through fibers traveling in the third nerve (Fig. 12-1). Atropine blocks the actions of acetylcholine on this sphincter muscle, and the resulting predominance of the radial fibers produces mydriasis. The atropinized pupil does not react to light. Cycloplegia is caused by paralysis of the ciliary muscles, which are normally innervated by cholinergic fibers. Increased intraocular pressure is generally attributed to impeded drainage of aqueous humor through the canals of Schlemm.

It should be recalled that the adrenergic drugs also can produce mydriasis. They act, however, by contracting the radial muscle of the iris. Accommodation is not paralyzed by the adrenergic drugs, in contrast to the atropine-like compounds.

CNS effects. In atropine poisoning the CNS effects are very striking; patients become excited and maniacal. Large therapeutic doses stimulate respiration and may prevent death from respiratory depression in poisoning caused by the alkyl phosphate cholinesterase inhibitors.

There are additional reasons for believing that the belladonna alkaloids affect the CNS. Scopolamine in particular is valuable in the management of Parkinson's disease and in the prevention of motion sickness.[2] When it is given by injection, the drug promotes a state of sedation and twilight sleep and may cause amnesia.[9]

Atropine and scopolamine are well absorbed from the gastrointestinal tract and following subcutaneous injection. They may even be absorbed following topical application. Accidents may occur in ophthalmological use, particularly in children, if the drug is allowed to reach the nasal mucosa through the nasolacrimal duct after its application to the conjunctival sac.

Atropine is rapidly excreted from the body and about 50% of an injected dose appears in the urine within 4 hours. The remainder is excreted within 24 hours in the form of metabolites and the unchanged drug.[12] The duration of the pharmacological effects reflects the rapidity of excretion except for the dilatation of the pupils and paralysis of accommodation, which may persist for a long time, particularly when atropine is applied topically to the conjunctiva.

Absorption, excretion, and metabolism

The belladonna alkaloids are used either in galenic preparations* or in a pure form. Belladonna tincture is given orally in a dose of 0.6 ml, which is equivalent to 0.2 mg of atropine. Atropine sulfate tablets are available in several different sizes. The usual dose is 0.6 mg. Scopolamine hydrobromide tablets are available in sizes of 0.3 to 0.6 mg. The usual dose is 0.6 mg. Solutions of atropine sulfate are available for instillation into the conjunctival sac. The usual strength of these solutions is 0.5% to 1%.

Preparations and clinical uses

Ophthalmological use. The anticholinergic drugs are applied topically for producing mydriasis and cycloplegia. Atropine itself has such a long duration of action that its use in ophthalmology is impractical. Homatropine and cyclopentolate are much more commonly employed and have a much shorter duration of action.

Preoperative uses. It is customary to administer atropine or scopolamine before operative procedures and general anesthesia. The drug protects the patient from excessive salivation and bradycardia. Scopolamine is often used in obstetrics because it produces sedation and amnesia. The anticholinergics were particularly important when ether was widely employed. With the newer anesthetics, excessive tracheobronchial secretions are not produced and the need for routine preanesthetic anticholinergics is questioned by some.[12]

---

*Galenic preparations contain one or several organic ingredients as contrasted with pure chemical substances.

Cardiac uses. Atropine is being used increasingly after myocardial infarction for reversing bradycardia caused by excessive vagal activity. The drug is also useful in digitalis-induced heart block. Although many physicians will use atropine after myocardial infarction if the heart rate falls below 60,[12] there is no certainty about the need or safety of this procedure unless hypotension or arrhythmias justify it. Large intravenous doses of atropine may cause dangerous tachycardia and ventricular arrhythmias in cardiac patients.

Uses in gastrointestinal disease. Anticholinergic drugs are used widely in the treatment of peptic ulcer. The drugs may diminish vagally mediated secretion, relieve spasm, and prolong the time during which antacids remain in the stomach by slowing down gastric emptying. To be effective, the anticholinergics must often be administered in large enough doses to cause discomfort, such as difficulty of vision and urination. Although there is no evidence for a favorable effect of anticholinergics on the long-term progress of ulcer disease, these drugs are unquestionably of considerable symptomatic benefit. The quaternary anticholinergics are preferred by many gastroenterologists. In large doses they may cause postural hypotension in addition to other predictable atropine-like effects. In addition to the usual contraindications, atropine should not be used in the presence of obstructive lesions, since it promotes retention.

Antiparkinsonian drugs. These drugs are discussed on p. 134. *Atropine-like drugs for vestibular disorders* are discussed along with the antihistaminic drugs on p. 221. The use of scopolamine as a hypnotic in combination with antihistaminics is unimportant except from a commercial standpoint. The presence of scopolamine in such over-the-counter preparations should be kept in mind in relation to possible drug interactions and in cases in which atropine-like drugs are contraindicated.

Toxicity and antidotes

The belladonna alkaloids and atropine-like drugs are generally safe medications. Large doses in a normal individual may cause unpleasant effects but are not life-threatening. Blurred vision, tachycardia, dry mouth, constipation, and urinary retention are among these unpleasant effects. Patients with glaucoma and prostatic hypertrophy may have disastrous reactions even to therapeutic doses of these drugs. Normal individuals have survived doses as high as 1 g taken by mouth.

Full-blown atropine poisoning is characterized by excitement and maniacal tendencies, hot and dry skin, dilated pupils, and tachycardia. The subcutaneous injection of 25 mg of methacholine will not elicit cholinergic effects in such patients.

Patients with atropine poisoning should be managed with supportive care. Sedatives such as chlordiazepoxide or diazepam may be helpful in controlling violent excitement.

Physostigmine has been found remarkably effective as an antidote in atropine poisoning. The drug may be injected subcutaneously in doses of 1 to 4 mg.[13] The injection may be repeated in 1 hour if necessary. Although the effectiveness of physostigmine in atropine poisoning has been known for years on the basis of animal experiments, its clinical usefulness became obvious more recently as a consequence of clinical observations made on patients with Parkinson's disease who received excessive amounts of atropine-like drugs.[13]

PROBLEM 12-1. Why is physostigmine preferable to neostigmine in reversing the CNS effects of atropine? The answer undoubtedly has some connection with the relative rates of penetration of the two drugs across the blood-brain barrier. Physostigmine is not a quaternary compound, but neostigmine is.

Numerous drugs, such as antihistamines and tricyclic antidepressants, have atropine-like effects and may contribute to atropine poisoning. Atropine-like drugs counteract the extrapyramidal side effects of the phenothiazines.

The atropine substitutes will be classified on the basis of their primary usefulness, which to a certain extent reflects their selectivity. On this basis they fall into three groups: the atropine-like mydriatics, the antispasmodics, and the antiparkinsonian drugs.

ATROPINE SUBSTITUTES

Atropine itself is a powerful mydriatic and cycloplegic, but its long duration of action is generally a disadvantage except in the treatment of iritis. For examination of the fundus and measurement of refractive errors, a number of shorter-acting agents are preferred. Some of these are homatropine, eucatropine, cyclopentolate, and tropicamide. In addition, adrenergic drugs such as phenylephrine (Neo-Synephrine) produce mydriasis without cycloplegia when applied topically to the eye.

Atropine-like mydriatics

Homatropine is the oldest of the atropine-like mydriatic drugs. It differs from atropine only in the fact that it is an ester of mandelic rather than of tropic acid. Homatropine is applied to the eye in 2% solutions. It produces mydriasis fairly rapidly, but its action lasts only 1 or 2 days. It is a less potent cyclopegic than atropine and is commonly used in ophthalmology.

$$H_2C-CH-\!\!-\!\!-CH_2 \quad\quad OH$$
$$\quad\quad | \quad\quad\quad | \quad\quad\quad\quad |$$
$$\quad\quad NCH_3 \quad CH-O-CO-CH$$
$$\quad\quad | \quad\quad\quad |$$
$$H_2C-CH-\!\!-\!\!-CH_2 \quad\quad C_6H_5$$

Homatropine

Eucatropine (Euphthalmine) is a weaker drug than homatropine. It produces mydriasis in 30 minutes, which lasts only about 12 hours. The drug has little cycloplegic action. It is used in 2% to 5% solutions.

Cyclopentolate hydrochloride (Cyclogyl) produces mydriasis in 30 to 60 minutes, with return of normal vision in less than 24 hours. It is used in 0.5% and 1% solutions, although for deeply pigmented eyes a 2% solution may be necessary.

FIG. 12-2 *Effect of atropine sulfate and atropine methylbromide on maternal and fetal heart rates. The lesser effect of the quaternary anticholinergic drug on fetal heart rate illustrates a basic difference between the two types of drugs as regards their passage across biological membranes.*

From dePadua, C.B., and Gravenstein, J.S.: JAMA 208:1022, 1969.

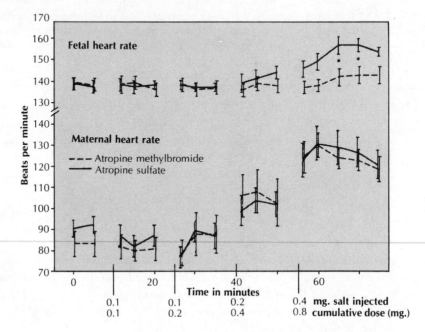

Tropicamide (Mydriacyl) is a very rapidly acting mydriatic and cycloplegic. It produces mydriasis in less than 30 minutes, and its action lasts only 15 to 20 minutes. It is used in 0.5% and 1% solutions.

Anticholinergic smooth muscle relaxants

A large group of atropine substitutes has been synthesized for the purpose of obtaining some selective action on the gastrointestinal tract. The great incentives for this search are the prevalence of peptic ulcer and the belief that desirable objectives in its management are relief of smooth muscle spasm and hypersecretion.

Conversion of the usual tertiary atropine-like drugs to quaternary amines introduces a number of important changes into their pharmacology. (1) Quaternary amines are less lipid soluble and do not penetrate the CNS. (2) The quaternary atropine-like drugs exert some ganglionic blocking effect that may reinforce their actions on the gastrointestinal tract. Thus the quaternary atropine methylbromide would not be expected to penetrate into the CNS as efficiently as atropine sulfate. The difference between the two in regard to penetration across biological membranes is shown in Fig. 12-2.

QUATERNARY ANTICHOLINERGIC DRUGS

Quaternary anticholinergic drugs used in 2 to 15 mg doses include methscopolamine (Pamine), homatropine methylbromide (Novatran), propantheline (Pro-Banthine), oxyphenonium (Antrenyl), penthienate (Monodral), valethamate (Murel), pipenzolate (Piptal), and poldine (Nacton). Quaternary anticholinergics used in doses of 50 to 100 mg or more include methantheline (Banthine), tridihexethyl (Pathilon), mepiperphenidol (Darstine), tricyclamol (Elorine), diphemanil (Prantal), amolanone (Amethone), and hexocyclium (Tral).

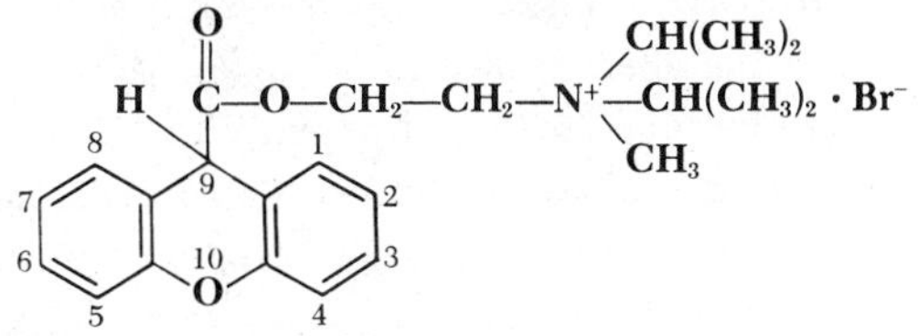

Propantheline bromide

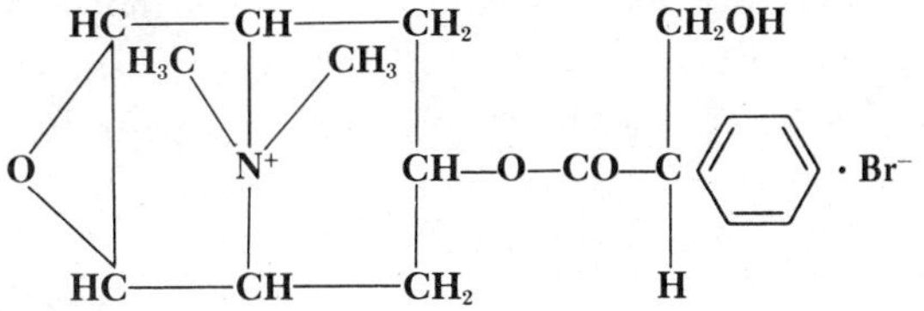

Methscopolamine bromide

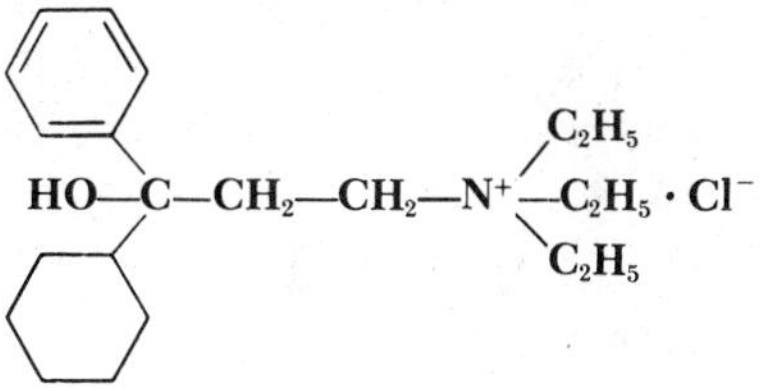

Tridihexethyl chloride

TERTIARY ANTICHOLINERGIC DRUGS

Among these synthetic atropine substitutes the most potent, used in doses of 10 mg, are dicyclomine (Bentyl) and oxyphencyclimine (Daricon). Drugs of this group used in doses of 50 mg or more are piperidolate (Dactil), aminocarbofluorene (Pavatrine), and amprotropine (Syntropan). Adiphenine (Trasentine), largely obsolete, also belongs to this group.

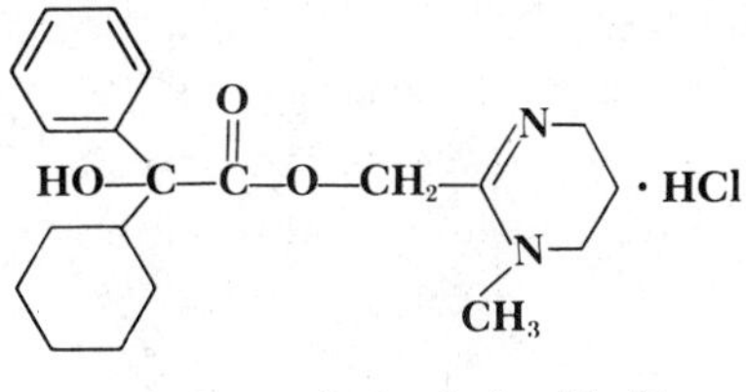

Oxyphencyclimine hydrochloride

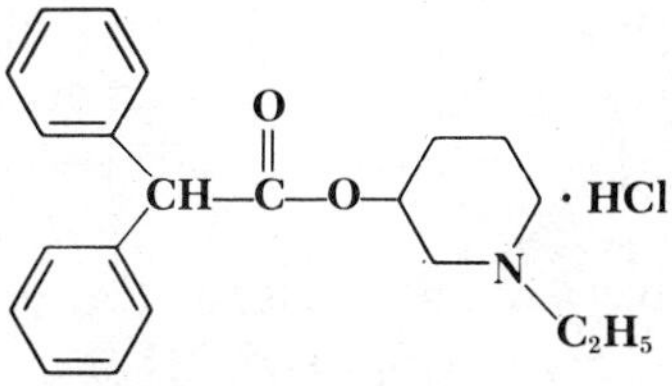

Piperidolate hydrochloride

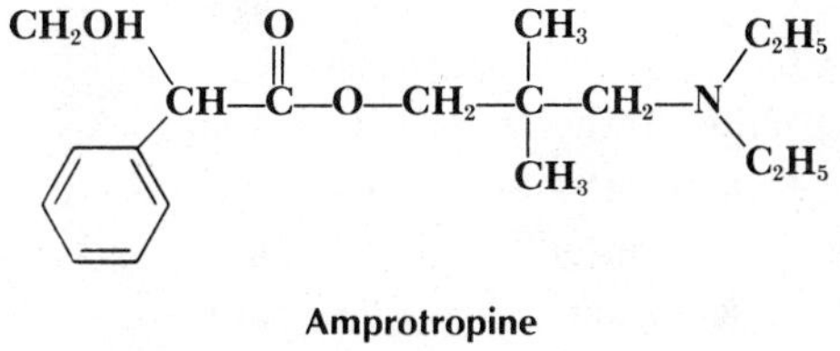

Amprotropine

DUAL
ANTISPASMODIC
ACTION

Some anticholinergics, such as dicyclomine hydrochloride (Bentyl), are not only parasympatholytic but possess a direct depressant action on the intestinal smooth muscle. The evidence for this statement is based on the ability of dicyclomine to counteract not only the effects of acetylcholine but also those of bradykinin on the intestinal smooth muscle. The clinical significance of this *musculotropic* antispasmodic action is difficult to evaluate.

*Antiparkinsonian
drugs*

The pharmacology of parkinsonism has been revolutionized during the last few years by the discovery of the effectiveness of L-dopa in its treatment and the role of dopamine in extrapyramidal function. Until recently the treatment of this common and disabling condition was based on the empiric use of (1) belladonna alkaloids and their synthetic congeners, (2) antihistamines, (3) drugs with both anticholinergic and antihistaminic properties (benztropine), and (4) dextroamphetamine for some manifestations of postencephalitic parkinsonism, such as oculogyric crisis and rigidity.

Parkinsonism, characterized by tremor, rigidity, and akinesia, includes idiopathic paralysis agitans, postencephalitic parkinsonism, and other disturbances of the extrapyramidal system. It may also be caused by drugs. It was suggested more than 100 years ago that the belladonna alkaloids might be useful in the management of the syndrome, and drug studies have contributed greatly to current concepts of its pathophysiology (Table 12-1).

CHOLINERGIC AND
DOPAMINERGIC
MECHANISMS IN
PARKINSONISM

The effectiveness of belladonna alkaloids in the treatment of parkinsonism called attention to the possible role of cholinergic mechanisms in its causation. It seemed reasonable to theorize that some brain centers must have become supersensitive to acetylcholine in the parkinsonian patient, perhaps as a form of denervation supersensitivity or as a consequence of removal of an inhibitory influence.

The role of cholinergic mechanisms in parkinsonism was supported by experiments that showed that *tremorine*, a cholinomimetic drug, produces a syndrome in animals resembling parkinsonism.[14] The injection of acetylcholine into the globus pallidus of patients undergoing stereotaxic surgery resulted in increased tremor contralaterally. Furthermore, the anticholinesterase physostigmine was found to exacerbate the symptoms of parkinsonian patients.[8] In this last study the suggestion was made that the role of the cholinergic system may be a result of the involvement of a dopaminergic mechanism.[8]

Histochemical fluorescence techniques have shown[1] that the characteristic green fluorescence of catecholamines is present in the nerve cell bodies of the *substantia nigra* and in the nerve terminals of the *striatum*, both areas being rich in dopamine. Furthermore, lesions placed in the substantia nigra of rats resulted in a decrease in dopamine in the ipsilateral striatum.[1]

The nigrostriatal dopaminergic system probably plays an important pathogenetic role in parkinsonism. In idiopathic parkinsonism the most conspicuous lesions are found in the substantia nigra, and the level of dopamine is found to be decreased in the striatum where the axonal terminations of the striatal neurons are located. The

---

TABLE 12-1 Drug effects in parkinsonism

Drugs that aggravate or cause parkinsonism	Drugs that relieve parkinsonism
Reserpine	Belladonna alkaloids
Chlorpromazine (phenothiazines)	Synthetic anticholinergic drugs
Haloperidol	Antihistamines
α-Methyldopa	Drugs having both anticholinergic and antihistaminic properties
	Levodopa
	Amantadine
	Dextroamphetamine
	Apomorphine

---

effectiveness of L-dopa in the treatment of parkinsonism suggests also that this precursor of dopamine, when administered in large doses, may overcome the deficiency of dopamine that is known to exist in the nigrostriatal dopaminergic pathway.

Drugs that aggravate parkinsonism. Both reserpine and chlorpromazine aggravate the symptoms of parkinsonism. Reserpine causes a depletion of dopamine in the striatum and thus, according to the theory, would remove an inhibitory influence on a cholinergic system. L-Dopa reverses the effect of reserpine, since it is converted to dopamine.

Drugs that relieve parkinsonism. The anticholinergic drugs would be expected to be effective if the cholinergic system is hyperactive as a consequence of removal of dopaminergic inhibitory influences. Most of the antihistaminics also have anticholinergic actions, which may account for their effectiveness.

Dextroamphetamine may be useful in the treatment of certain manifestations of postencephalitic parkinsonism, such as rigidity and oculogyric crisis. Dextroamphetamine promotes presynaptic dopamine release and blocks its reuptake.

Amantadine, an antiviral drug, has been reported to be beneficial in parkinsonism. Although the mode of action of this drug is uncertain, dopamine release from neuronal storage sites following its injection has been claimed on the basis of animal experiments.[11]

Apomorphine, a dopaminergic amine, and related aporphines appear promising in the treatment of parkinsonism.[6]

MAJOR ANTIPARKINSONIAN AGENTS

The available antiparkinsonian drugs fall into the following groups on the basis of their pharmacological properties:
1. Belladonna alkaloids, including atropine and scopolamine
2. Synthetic anticholinergics, such as trihexyphenidyl hydrochloride (Artane), biperiden hydrochloride (Akineton), cycrimine hydrochloride (Pagitane), and procyclidine hydrochloride (Kemadrin)

3. Antihistamines such as diphenhydramine hydrochloride (Benadryl) and orphenadrine citrate (Norflex) or orphenadrine hydrochloride (Disipal)
4. Drugs with both anticholinergic and antihistaminic properties, such as benztropine mesylate (Cogentin mesylate)
5. Phenothiazines with anticholinergic and antihistaminic actions, such as ethopropazine (Parsidol)
6. Levodopa (L-dopa), acting on dopaminergic mechanisms
7. Miscellaneous drugs probably acting on dopaminergic mechanisms, such as amantadine and dextroamphetamine

Trihexyphenidyl hydrochloride

Diphenhydramine hydrochloride

Benztropine mesylate

Orphenadrine hydrochloride

Belladonna alkaloids and synthetic anticholinergics. The naturally occurring belladonna alkaloids atropine and scopolamine have been used for years in treatment of parkinsonism. They have been replaced by the newer synthetics because the latter do not produce as powerful peripheral anticholinergic symptoms for a given amount of relief of parkinsonian disability.

The action and uses of the synthetic anticholinergics are similar. All are chemically related to trihexyphenidyl, and all produce atropine-like untoward effects such as dryness of the mouth, blurred vision, dizziness, and dysuria.

Trihexyphenidyl hydrochloride (Artane) is available in tablets of 2 and 5 mg, timed-release capsules of 5 mg, and elixir, 2 mg/5 ml. Dosage ranges from 1 mg initially to a maximum of 20 mg daily.

Biperiden hydrochloride (Akineton hydrochloride) is available in 2 mg tablets for oral administration; **biperiden lactate** (Akineton lactate) is available as a solution, 5 mg/ml, for injection.

Cycrimine hydrochloride (Pagitane hydrochloride) is available in tablets of 1.25 and 2.5 mg.

Procylidine hydrochloride (Kemadrin) is available in tablets of 2 and 5 mg.

Antihistamines. Diphenhydramine and the closely related orphenadrine have some usefulness in the treatment of parkinsonism including that induced by drugs such as the phenothiazines. They are not as effective as the anticholinergics but produce fewer atropine-like untoward effects. On the other hand, they produce considerable drowsiness.

Diphenhydramine hydrochloride (Benadryl) is available in 25 and 50 mg capsules, elixirs of 12.5 mg/5 ml, and solutions for intravenous and intramuscular injections containing 10 or 50 mg/ml.

Orphenadrine citrate (Norflex) is available in tablets, 100 mg, and solutions for injection, 30 mg/ml.

Orphenadrine hydrochloride (Disipal) is available in tablets, 50 mg.

Drugs with both anticholinergic and antihistaminic properties. The major representative of this class is benztropine mesylate. An examination of its chemical structure reveals similarities to atropine and a typical antihistaminic. Its pharmacological properties resemble those of atropine not only with regard to untoward effects but also from the standpoint of duration of action, which is long.

Benztropine mesylate (Cogentin mesylate) is available in tablets of 0.5, 1, and 2 mg and in solution for intramuscular or intravenous injection, 1 mg/ml.

Ethopropazine hydrochloride (Parsidol), a phenothiazine with both anticholinergic and antihistaminic actions, may be useful as an adjunct to the anticholinergic drugs. It causes considerable drowsiness, muscle cramps, and paresthesia and may cause agranulocytosis and hypotension. Its preparations include tablets of 10, 50, and 100 mg.

Levodopa. Levodopa is considered the most effective medication for parkinsonism. When administered orally in increasing doses, it is likely to benefit at least 50% of the patients, although it may take several weeks for the improvement to become manifest. Fortunately, it is not necessary to discontinue the usual anticholinergic medications while the dosage is being built up. The initial daily dose is 300 mg to 1 g. Dosage is built up gradually until marked improvement occurs or adverse reactions make further increases impractical.

MAO inhibitors, when used concomitantly with levodopa, may cause hypertensive crises. Pyridoxine in large doses (more than 5 mg) reverses the effects of levodopa by promoting its peripheral decarboxylation. Sympathomimetic amines may have exaggerated effects in patients treated with levodopa. Anticholinergics should be used cautiously and in reduced dosages. Antihypertensive drugs should also be used with caution because postural hypotension may occur as a reaction to levodopa. Phenothiazines may cause parkinsonian-like symptoms that are usually resistant to levodopa. Many antihistamines have anticholinergic effects and should be used with caution in association with levodopa.

Levodopa (Dopar, Larodopa) is available in capsules containing 100, 250, and 500 mg.

Levodopa has been combined with an inhibitor of aromatic amino acid decarboxylase, carbidopa, and introduced under the trade name of **Sinemet.** Carbidopa is the hydrazino derivative of methyldopa. Carbidopa inhibits the decarboxylation of peripheral levodopa, but it does not enter the CNS. As a consequence more levodopa is available for transport to the brain and the amount of levodopa required is reduced by about 75%. Sinemet is available in tablets of two strengths: Sinemet 10/100 contains 10 mg of carbidopa and 100 mg of levodopa; Sinemet 25/250 contains 25 mg of carbidopa and 250 mg of levodopa.

Patients receiving levodopa must discontinue their medication at least 8 hours before taking the levodopa-carbidopa combination. Common serious adverse effects of the combination are choreiform and other involuntary movements, mental changes, nausea, arrhythmias, postural hypotension, and many others. Dosage must be determined by careful titration for each patient.

Amantadine. This antiviral agent produces clinical improvement in some patients having parkinsonian symptoms and does so more rapidly than levodopa. The mode of action of amantadine is not understood, although there is a highly suggestive experimental finding of an amantadine-dopamine interaction.[11]

Adverse effects of amantadine include hyperexcitability, slurred speech, ataxia, insomnia, and gastrointestinal disturbances. Convulsions have occurred after the administration of excessive doses.

Amantadine hydrochloride (Symmetrel) is available in capsules of 100 mg and as a syrup containing 50 mg/ml. Initial dose for adults is 100 mg once daily for 5 to 7 days.

REFERENCES

1. Anden, N.E., Carlsson, A., Dahlstrom, A., Fuxe, K., Hillarp, N.A., and Larsson, K.: Demonstration and mapping out of nigro-neostriatal dopamine neurons, Life Sci. 3:523, 1964.
2. Brand, J.J., and Perry, W.L.M.: Drugs used in motion sickness. A critical review of methods available for the study of drugs of potential value in its treatment and of the information which has been derived by these methods, Pharmacol. Rev. 18:895, 1966.
3. Calne, D.B., Laurence, D.R., and Stern, G.M.: L-Dopa in postencephalitic parkinsonism, Lancet 1:744, 1969.
4. Cotzias, G.C., and Papavasiliou, P.S.: Blocking the negative effects of pyridoxine on patients receiving levodopa, JAMA 215:1504, 1971.
5. Cotzias, G.C., Papavasiliou, P.S., and Gellene, R.: Modification of parkinsonism—chronic treatment with L-dopa, N. Engl. J. Med. 280:337, 1969.
6. Cotzias, G.C., Papavasiliou, P.S., Tolosa, E.S., Mendez, J.S., and Bell-Midura, M.: Treatment of Parkinson's disease with aporphines, N. Engl. J. Med. 294:567, 1976.
7. DePadua, C.B., and Gravenstein, J.S.: Atropine sulfate vs atropine methyl bromide: effect on maternal and fetal heart rate, JAMA 208:1022, 1969.
8. Duvoisin, R.C.: Cholinergic-anticholinergic antagonism in parkinsonism, Arch. Neurol. 17:124, 1967.
9. Frumin, M.J., et al.: Amnesic actions of diazepam and scopolamine in man, Anesthesiology 45:406, 1976.
10. Gravenstein, J.S., and Thornby, J.I.: Scopolamine in heart rates in man, Clin. Pharmacol. Ther. 10:395, 1969.
11. Grelak, R.P., Clark, R., Stump, J.M., and Vernier, V.G.: Amantadine-dopamine interaction: possible mode of action in parkinsonism, Science 169:203, 1970.

12. Greenblatt, D.J., and Shader, R.I.: Anticholinergics, N. Engl. J. Med. **288:** 1215, 1973.

13. Heiser, J.F., and Gillin, J.C.: The reversal of anticholinergic drug-induced delirium and coma with physostigmine, Am. J. Psychiatry **127**;1050, 1971.

14. Ingelfinger, F.J.: Anticholinergic therapy of gastrointestinal disorders, N. Engl. J. Med. **268:**1454, 1963.

15. Lieberman, A., Estey, E., Kupersmith, M., Gopinathan, G., and Goldstein, M.:

Treatment of Parkinson's disease with lergotrile mesylate, JAMA **238:**2380, 1977.

16. Schwab, R.S., England, A.C., Jr., Poskanzer, D.C., and Young, R.R.: Amantadine in the treatment of Parkinson's disease, JAMA **208:**1168, 1969.

17. Schwartz, B.: The glaucomas, N. Engl. J. Med. **299:**182, 1978.

18. Yahr, M.D., and Duvoisin, R.C.: Drug therapy of parkinsonism, N. Engl. J. Med. **287:**20, 1972.

Chapter 13

Ganglionic blocking agents

**GENERAL
CONCEPT**

Neurotransmission within autonomic ganglia can be blocked either by compounds that prevent the depolarizing actions of acetylcholine or by drugs that produce persistent depolarization. In concentrations that have little effect at other sites, ganglionic blocking agents depress the actions of acetylcholine on ganglionic neurons.

Nicotinic receptors for acetylcholine are mainly responsible for transmission through intact, functional ganglia. Under certain experimental circumstances, muscarinic and catecholamine receptors can also be demonstrated (Fig. 13-1). Although pharmacological blockade of muscarinic and catecholamine receptors alters ganglion potentials, fast excitation of autonomic neuroeffectors is unimpeded.

Sympathetic ganglia have been remarkably productive tissues for research on how neurons respond to transmitters and drugs. Neuron interactions there provide evidence of facilitation (addition of excitations), occlusion (signal block by simultaneous competition), and recruitment (one pathway directing many neurons). These neuronal properties suggest that electrical information entering ganglia is "interpreted" within the ganglionic neuropil before it is conducted to neuroeffectors.[7]

**GANGLIONIC
STIMULANTS**

Certain ganglionic stimulants such as tetramethylammonium, small doses of nicotine, and the experimental drug dimethylphenylpiperazinium (DMPP)[8] will cause vasoconstriction and blood pressure elevations as a consequence of their stimulant action on ganglia. This type of drug effect has not yet found therapeutic applications. It should be remembered, however, that some of the drugs used in the diagnosis of pheochromocytoma (for example, methacholine) cause catecholamine release. This is analogous to ganglionic or adrenomedullary stimulation.

**GANGLIONIC
BLOCKING
AGENTS**

140   *Development*

The curious ability of nicotine to block ganglionic transmission following initial stimulation has been known for many years. During the latter part of the nineteenth century, Langley charted the distribution of fibers emanating from sympathetic ganglia by selectively blocking the ganglia with local applications of nicotine.

Impulse transmission in sympathetic autonomic ganglia. ACh interacts with a nicotinic **FIG. 13-1**
receptor on the ganglionic neuron to cause a rapid depolarization, resulting in a fast
excitatory postsynaptic potential (EPSP). ACh also binds to muscarinic receptors on prin-
cipal cells to cause a late EPSP and on interneurons that release dopamine. Dopamine
interactions with catecholamine receptors initiate an inhibitory postsynaptic potential
(IPSP). Sites of action for receptor antagonist drugs are shown.

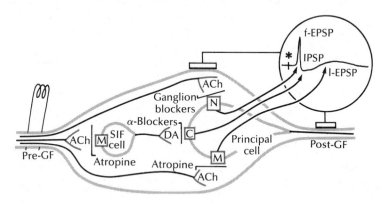

The ability of tetraethylammonium to block the effect of ganglionic stimulants was also known for many years. Such blocking agents received little attention, however, until 1946, when the mode of action of tetraethylammonium on the mammalian circulation was thoroughly investigated.[1] These studies suggested the possibility of blocking ganglionic transmission in a fairly selective manner.

A variety of ganglionic blocking agents was developed for practical use, particularly in treating hypertension and in producing controlled hypotension. Some of the more widely used compounds were hexamethonium chloride, pentolinium tartrate, chlorisondamine chloride, and trimethaphan camphosulfonate. More recently, mecamylamine hydrochloride and pempidine tartrate were tried clinically.[5]

The chemical formulas of some of the ganglionic blocking agents are as follows: *Chemistry*

$(C_2H_5)_3N^+{-}CH_2{-}CH_3 \cdot Cl^-$ $(CH_3)_3\,N^+{-}CH_2{-}(CH_2)_4{-}CH_2{-}N^+(CH_3)_3 \cdot 2Cl^-$

Tetraethylammonium chloride   **Hexamethonium chloride**

$N^+{-}CH_2{-}CH_2{-}CH_2{-}CH_2{-}CH_2{-}N^+ \cdot 2C_4H_5O_6$

$\overset{|}{C}H_3$ $\overset{|}{C}H_3$

Pentolinium tartrate

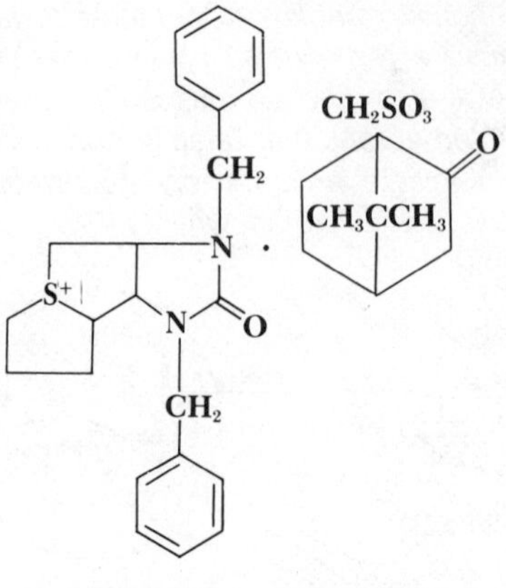

Trimethaphan camphorsulfonate

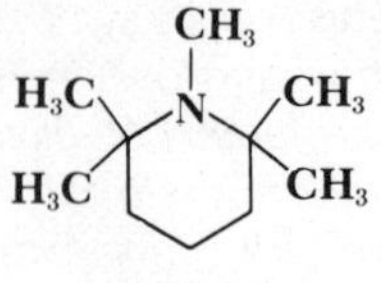

Pempidine

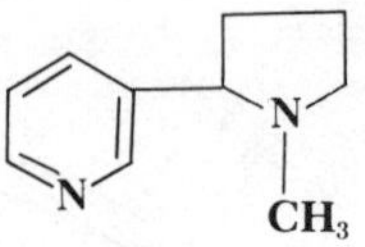

Nicotine

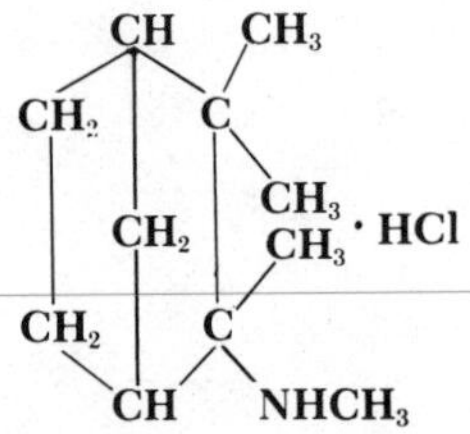

Mecamylamine hydrochloride

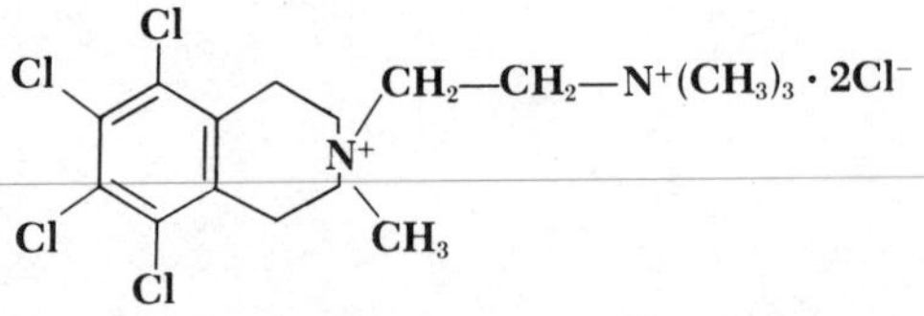

Chlorisondamine chloride

Most ganglionic blocking drugs are quaternary ammonium compounds, just as acetylcholine has a quaternary nitrogen. Mecamylamine and pempidine, however, are not quaternary amines.

Clinical pharmacology

The pharmacological effects of ganglionic blocking agents depend on the autonomic tone prevailing in an organ at the time of administration, since the drugs block both sympathetic and parasympathetic ganglia.

The ganglionic blocking agents are used principally for decreasing the influence of the sympathetic division of the autonomic nervous system on the circulation. Ganglionic blockers were "first-line" drugs for the management of hypertension before more "specific" compounds became available. Ganglionic blockers are "nonspecific" by comparison because they diminish body activities controlled by both branches of the autonomic nervous system.

A very picturesque description of a person without a functioning autonomic nervous system was given by Paton in his account of the "hexamethonium man."

He is a pink complexioned person, except when he has stood in a queue for a long time, when he may get pale and faint. His handshake is warm and dry. He is a placid and relaxed companion; for instance he may laugh, but he can't cry because the tears cannot come. Your rudest story will not make him blush, and the most unpleasant circumstances will fail to make him turn pale. His collars and socks stay very clean and sweet. He wears corsets and may, if you meet him out, be rather fidgety (corsets tend to compress his splanchnic vascular pool, fidgety to keep the venous return going from his legs). He dislikes speaking much unless helped with something to moisten his dry mouth and throat. He is long-sighted and easily blinded by bright light. The redness of his eyeballs may suggest irregular habits and in fact his head is rather weak. But he always behaves like a gentleman and never belches nor hiccups. He tends to get cold and keeps well wrapped up. But his health is good; he does not have chilblains and those diseases of modern civilization, hypertension and peptic ulcer, pass him by. He is thin because his appetite is modest; he never feels hunger pains and his stomach never rumbles. He gets rather constipated so that his intake of liquid paraffin is high. As old age comes on, he will suffer from retention of urine and impotence, but frequency, precipitancy, and strangury will not worry him. One is uncertain how he will end, but perhaps if he is not careful, by eating less and less and getting colder and colder, he will sink into a symptomless, hypoglycemic coma and die, as was proposed for the universe, a sort of entropy death.*

Circulatory effects. The ganglionic blocking drugs tend to lower blood pressure by decreasing sympathetic tone to various vascular areas. The intensity of this hypotensive action depends on a number of factors. The position of the patient has a great influence. There may be only slight lowering of the pressure while the patient is in the recumbent position. When the patient stands, however, the mean pressure may fall precipitously to the point of faintness. This is known as postural hypotension and undoubtedly results from pooling of blood in the extremities in the absence of compensatory vasoconstriction there.

Side effects and complications. In addition to the unavoidable postural hypotension, smooth muscle tone of the gastrointestinal and urinary tracts may be relaxed by ganglionic blocking agents, resulting in constipation or difficulty in voiding. As one might expect, the pupils may dilate and there can be interference with accommodation for near vision. Salivary secretion may be inhibited, and the resulting dry mouth may be sufficiently uncomfortable to require administration of pilocarpine. Sweating is also reduced, not by an atropine-like effect, but because of decreased sympathetic activity as a consequence of the ganglionic block.

The quaternary ammonium ganglionic blocking agents are poorly absorbed from the gastrointestinal tract. Drugs such as tetraethylammonium or trimethaphan camphorsulfonate cannot be used by mouth because of poor absorption. Although chlorisondamine and pentolinium are given by oral administration, their absorption is far from complete. The oral-intravenous LD_{50} ratio of these drugs in mice is about 20:1. On the other hand, the secondary amine, mecamylamine, is much better absorbed, giving an oral/intravenous LD_{50} ratio of about 4:1.[6]

The ganglionic blocking agents of the quaternary ammonium group are eliminated through renal excretion. Their distribution in the body is largely extracellular.

Metabolism

---

*From Paton, W.D.M.: The principles of ganglionic block. In Scientific basis of medicine, vol. 2, London, 1954, Athlone Press.

Differences among various ganglionic blocking agents

The various ganglionic blocking drugs differ with respect to potency, oral absorption, and duration of action.

Mecamylamine hydrochloride (Inversine) is a potent drug that is well absorbed from the gastrointestinal tract and has a duration of action of 4 to 12 hours. The initial oral dose is 2.5 mg twice daily. This dose is gradually increased until a satisfactory effect is obtained, usually at a dose level of 30 mg/day.

The drug may cause CNS stimulation and neuromuscular blockade in large doses.

Pempidine (Perolysen) is similar in action to mecamylamine. It is well absorbed from the gastrointestinal tract and is used in doses of 2.5 mg twice daily by mouth. In large doses it may cause CNS stimulation and neuromuscular blockade.

Hexamethonium (Methium), at the other end of the spectrum, is poorly and irregularly absorbed and is now obsolete.

Pentolinium (Ansolysen) is about five times as potent as hexamethonium in lowering blood pressure. The subcutaneous injection of 3 mg of pentolinium has about the same effect as 15 mg of hexamethonium by the same route.

Chlorisondamine (Ecolid) appears to be a potent ganglionic blocking agent that has a long duration of action. The recommended daily dose is about 100 to 200 mg, usually given in two doses (only by intravenous infusion).

Trimethaphan camphorsulfonate (Arfonad) is a very short-acting ganglionic blocking agent. It is chiefly used for producing controlled hypotension during special surgical operations. Although it is a potent histamine-releasing agent in dogs, no adverse effects that could be attributed to histamine release have occurred in human beings. Intravenous infusion of a solution containing 1 mg/ml will significantly lower blood pressure. When the infusion is stopped, blood pressure returns to its normal levels in about 5 minutes. Trimethaphan camsylate (Arfonad) is available as a 50 mg/ml solution that is diluted to 1 mg/ml for intravenous infusion.

REFERENCES

1. Acheson, G.H., and Moe, G.K.: The action of tetraethylammonium ion on the mammalian circulation, J. Pharmacol. Exp. Ther. **87**:220, 1946.
2. Aviado, D.M.: Hemodynamic effects of ganglion blocking drugs, Circ. Res. **8**:304, 1960.
3. Eränkö, O.: Small intensely fluorescent (SIF) cells and nervous transmission in sympathetic ganglia, Annu. Rev. Pharmacol. Toxicol. **18**:417, 1978.
4. Paton, W.D.M.: The principles of ganglionic block. In Scientific basis of medicine, vol. 2, London, 1954, Athlone Press.
5. Salem, M.R.: Therapeutic uses of ganglionic blocking drugs, Int. Anesthesiol. Clin. **16**:171, 1978.
6. Stone, C.A., Torchiana, M.L., Navarro, A., and Beyer, K.H.: Ganglionic blocking properties of 3-methylaminoisocamphane hydrochloride (mecamylamine): a secondary amine, J. Pharmacol. Exp. Ther. **117**:169, 1956.
7. Volle, R.L.: Modification by drugs of synaptic mechanisms in autonomic ganglia, Pharmacol. Rev. **18**:839, 1966.
8. Winbury, M.M.: Comparison of the vascular actions of 1-1-dimethyl-4-piperazinium (DMPP), a potent ganglionic stimulant, J. Physiol. **147**:1, 1959.

Chapter 14

Neuromuscular blocking agents and muscle relaxants

The clinically useful neuromuscular blocking drugs act postsynaptically by one of two major mechanisms: (1) competition with acetylcholine for the end-plate receptor (nondepolarizing blocking agents) and (2) initial depolarization followed by desensitization to the transmitter despite repolarization. An example of a nondepolarizing blocking agent is *d*-tubocurarine; succinylcholine acts by the second mechanism. Neuromuscular blocking drugs act on nicotinic receptors.

Skeletal muscle relaxation may be achieved by other mechanisms also. The centrally acting agents, such as mephenesin, meprobamate, and other antianxiety agents including diazepam, produce muscle relaxation by a primary action on the CNS. Finally, drugs such as dantrolene act on the skeletal muscle itself to cause relaxation.

In addition to the therapeutically useful muscle relaxants, many drugs cause disorders of neuromuscular transmission as an unwanted side effect. For example, antibiotics such as the aminoglycosides and polymyxins, local anesthetics, and others may cause postoperative respiratory depression or may aggravate myasthenia gravis.

GENERAL CONCEPT

Experimentation with the South American arrow poison, *curare*, was one of the earliest examples of scientific work in pharmacology. In the nineteenth century Magendie and his pupil Claude Bernard studied the effects of curare on nerve-muscle preparations. Claude Bernard was able to show that the drug prevented the response of the muscle to nerve stimulation. Surprisingly, it did not prevent the muscle from responding to direct stimulation, and it failed to block conduction in the nerve. It therefore seemed to exert its effect at the junction of nerve and muscle.

The active principle of *Chondodendron tomentosum* roots is *d*-tubocurarine, which has been isolated and its structure established. It is a fairly large molecule in which two quaternary ammonium structures appear to be separated by an estimated distance of 14 Å, compared with the critical distance of 7 Å in acetylcholine.

The neuromuscular blocking agents are of two types: *nondepolarizing* and *depolarizing*. The nondepolarizing agents are *d*-tubocurarine, gallamine, benzoquinonium, and pancuronium. Depolarizing drugs are succinylcholine and decamethon-

NEUROMUSCULAR BLOCKING AGENTS Development

145

ium. This second category of drugs produces initial depolarization followed by desensitization of the receptors to acetylcholine.

Clinical pharmacology	The intravenous injection of 5 to 10 mg of *d*-tubocurarine produces flaccid paralysis of the extremities. Doubling these doses may produce apnea. The effects last for 10 minutes, with muscle strength returning in 40 minutes. There is a characteristic progression of effects, with the extrinsic muscles of the eye being affected first and then those of the face, the extremities, and finally the diaphragm.

The usual therapeutic doses of *d*-tubocurarine are unlikely to produce significant CNS action, since the blood-brain barrier represents a considerable defense against quaternary ammonium compounds. The beneficial effect on pain in certain clinical conditions is ascribed to the relaxation of contracted muscles and not to primary analgesic or hypnotic effect.

Drug interactions with nondepolarizing muscle relaxants such as *d*-tubocurarine are of great importance. General anesthetics such as ether, halothane, cyclopropane, and methoxyflurane intensify the action of nondepolarizing agents, making a reduction of their dosage necessary. Antibiotics such as neomycin, streptomycin, polymyxin B, colistin, kanamycin, and viomycin potentiate neuromuscular blockade. Quinine and quinidine also potentiate the action of neuromuscular blocking drugs. Anticholinesterase insecticides such as parathion, malathion, and tetraethyl pyrophosphate have some properties similar to those of the depolarizing blocking agents, and prolonged apnea may result when the patient exposed to such insecticides is treated with neuromuscular blocking drugs. Finally, patients with myasthenia gravis, acidosis, or severe renal disease react excessively to the usual doses of *d*-tubocurarine.

Adverse reactions to the nondepolarizing neuromuscular blocking drugs include prolonged apnea, bronchospasm, and hypotension, the last two being partly a consequence of histamine release.[11] Ganglionic blockade may contribute to the hypotension. Neostigmine and edrophonium (Tensilon) are antagonists of the early nondepolarizing actions of *d*-tubocurarine. Nevertheless, the most important antidotal measure is artificial respiration.

Mode of action	It is generally believed that acetylcholine is released from synaptic vesicles with passage of the nerve impulse.[5] The mediator produces a small electrical charge known as the *end-plate potential*. Under normal circumstances this produces in turn the propagated *action potential*. In a partially curarized preparation the small end-plate potential is clearly visible, since it is not followed by the larger action potential. The effect of curare on the end-plate potential and the anticurare action of physostigmine are shown in Fig. 14-1.

The administration of the depolarizing agents results in muscle fasciculations as the initial response, whereas the competitive blocking agents do not have this effect.

Effect of curarine on the end-plate potential of the frog sartorius and the antagonistic action **FIG. 14-1**
of physostigmine. 1, After 6 μM of curarine; 2, after 9 μM of curarine; 3, after 9 μM of
cuplus physostigmine 10^{-5}.

From Eccles, J.C., et al.: J. Neurophysiol. 5:211, 1942.

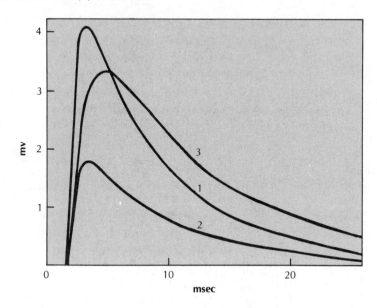

Mixed block. Initial depolarization followed by block is referred to as mixed block.

When a depolarizing drug is applied to a muscle, the depolarization is not sustained but tends to fade. It appears as if the acetylcholine receptors become inactive. The term *receptor inactivation* has been introduced to describe this phenomenon, which is probably of great importance in the second phase of the action of succinylcholine.

The various neuromuscular blocking agents differ with respect to potency, mode of action, and the nature of their side effects.

d-**Tubocurarine** is injected intravenously in the form of solutions containing 3 or 15 mg/ml. *d*-Tubocurarine chloride (Tubarine) is available for injection in a solution, 3 mg/ml. Its action is transient. About one third of the amount administered is excreted unchanged in the urine, whereas the rest is metabolically altered. It is probably still the most important competitive neuromuscular blocking agent, although the newer **dimethyltubocurarine chloride** (Mecostrin) has a potency about three times as great. A solution of dimethyltubocurarine iodide (Metubine iodide), 2 mg/ml, is available for injection.

Differences among more common neuromuscular blocking agents

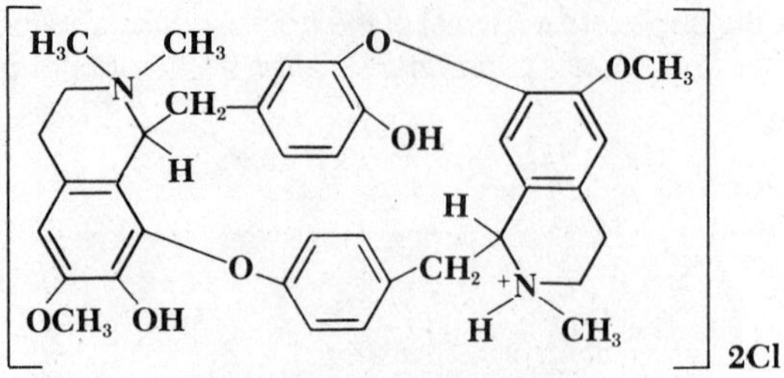

d-Tubocurarine chloride

Pancuronium dimethobromide is a recently introduced nondepolarizing neuro-muscular blocking agent that differs from *d*-tubocurarine in its greater potency and lack of histamine-releasing or ganglionic blocking actions. As indicated in its structural formula, the drug has a steroid nucleus with two quaternary amines attached. Its potency is such that, administered intravenously, 2 mg of pancuronium dimetho-bromide produces about the same effect as 10 to 15 mg of *d*-tubocurarine.[10]

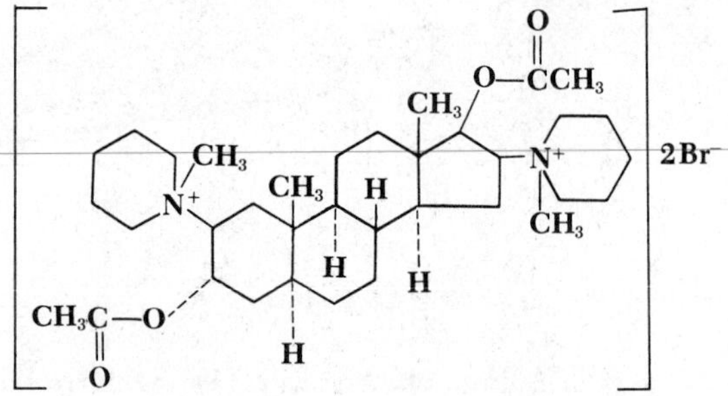

Pancuronium dimethobromide

Gallamine triethiodide (Flaxedil triethiodide) and **benzoquinonium** (Mytolon) are also neuromuscular blocking drugs of the competitve type. They have certain side effects that are not observed following the use of *d*-tubocurarine. Gallamine has an atropine-like effect on the cardiac branch of the vagus nerve and can produce considerable tachycardia. Gallamine triethiodide is available in solutions for injec-tion of 20 and 100 mg/ml. The actions of gallamine triethiodide are very similar to those of tubocurarine. It may have a slightly shorter duration of action, and it does not cause histamine release. This may be an advantage in asthmatic persons. On the other hand, its tendency to cause tachycardia by its vagolytic and perhaps cate-cholamine-releasing action may be a disadvantage in patients in whom tachycardia may represent a hazard.

Decamethonium bromide (Syncurine; C-10), one of the methonium compounds, is a depolarizing blocking agent that has been largely replaced by succinylcholine. Decamethonium bromide solution, 1 mg/ml is available for injection.

$$Br^- \cdot N(CH_3)_3 \!-\! (CH_2)_{10} \!-\! N^+(CH_3)_3 \cdot Br^-$$

Decamethonium bromide

It is interesting to note that the difference between this drug and hexamethonium consists of four additional methylene groups in decamethonium. This change in the distance between the two quaternary ammonium groups is sufficient to change the drug from a primary ganglionic blocking agent to one that is principally active on the neuromuscular junction.

Succinylcholine (Anectine) has the following structural formula:

$$Cl^- \cdot \underset{H_3C}{\overset{H_3C}{\underset{\diagup}{\overset{\diagdown}{N^+}}}}\!\!-\!\!CH_2CH_2O\overset{O}{\overset{\|}{C}}CH_2CH_2\overset{O}{\overset{\|}{C}}OCH_2CH_2\overset{CH_3}{\underset{CH_3}{\overset{\diagup}{\underset{\diagdown}{N^+}}}}\!\!-\!\!CH_3 \cdot Cl^-$$

Succinylcholine chloride

When succinylcholine chloride, 0.5 to 1 mg/kg of body weight, is injected intravenously, there may be considerable muscular contraction for several seconds before paralysis develops. The muscles remain paralyzed for about 5 minutes and resume their function in another 5 minutes.

The drug has a selective action on the neuromuscular receptor sites, although in large doses it may cause some effects similar to those of acetylcholine on the heart and circulation.

The actions of succinylcholine are prevented by *d*-tubocurarine, whereas neostigmine is definitely not an antidote and may even aggravate the muscle paralysis caused by succinylcholine.

The short duration of action of succinylcholine may be attributed to its rapid metabolic degradation. The compound is hydrolyzed by plasma cholinesterase to succinylmonocholine and choline. In a second step, succinylmonocholine is hydrolyzed to succinic acid and choline by the cholinesterases.

In some patients, succinylcholine has produced prolonged apnea caused by quantitative or qualitative differences in cholinesterase, a genetic abnormality (p. 57).

Succinylcholine is a valuable agent for producing short periods of muscular relaxation. It may be given in single intravenous doses or by intravenous infusion. Preparations of succinylcholine chloride (Anectine chloride) for injection include powder, 500 mg and 1 g, and solutions of 20, 50, and 100 mg/ml. Facilities for artificial respiration are essential, since this appears to be the only effective antidotal measure to apnea.

Usefulness

The greatest usefulness of the neuromuscular blocking agents is in anesthesia, in which they contribute to muscular relaxation. They also are employed for facilitating endotracheal intubation.

Succinylcholine is employed for protecting patients against severe convulsions in electroconvulsive therapy. Curare-like drugs have also been used in the treatment of tetanus, but they are not the drugs of choice for this condition.

SKELETAL MUSCLE DEPRESSANTS THAT ACT ON THE SPINAL CORD
Centrally acting skeletal muscle relaxants

In addition to those acting at the neuromuscular junction, other drugs can cause muscle relaxation by acting on internuncial spinal neurons to depress polysynaptic pathways (Fig. 14-2). These centrally acting muscle relaxants also act on higher centers and are commonly used as antianxiety agents. Although experimentally these drugs can depress the spinal cord at dose levels that do not cause sleep or anesthesia, in clinical practice it is difficult to say how much of their muscle-relaxing power is simply a consequence of the antianxiety effects. Although some drugs in this series are promoted as centrally acting muscle relaxants, others almost identical in structure are widely used for their antianxiety properties.

Indications for these drugs include the treatment of muscle spasm resulting from sprains, arthritis, myositis, and fibrositis. Drugs in this group can cause adverse effects such as drowsiness, lethargy and ataxia, allergic manifestations, and psychic dependence, particularly to the meprobamate and chlordiazepoxide group of compounds.

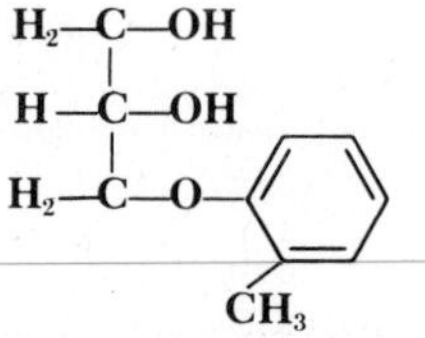

Mephenesin 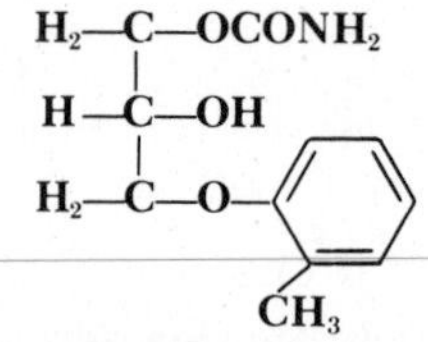   Mephenesin carbamate 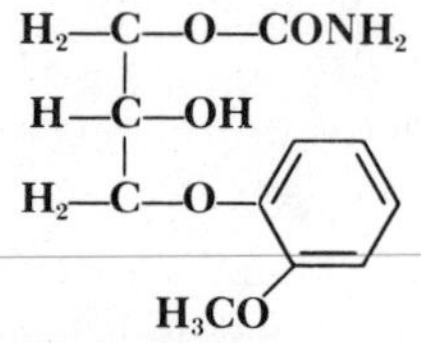   Methocarbamol

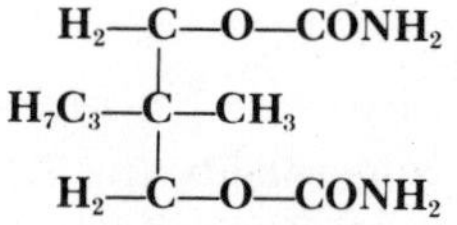

Meprobamate 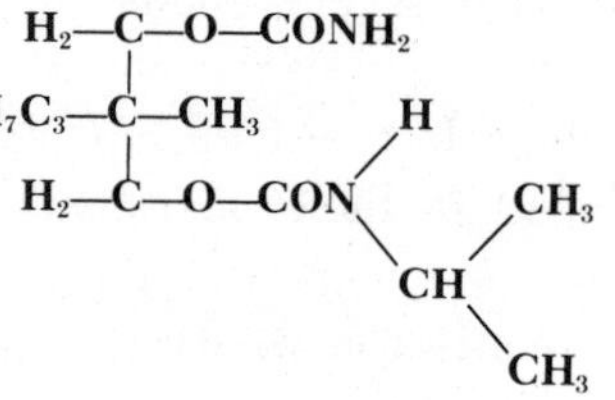   Carisoprodol 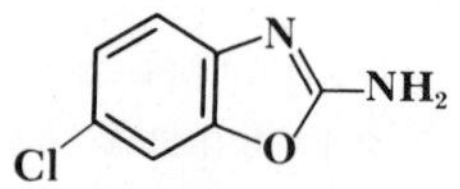   Zoxazolamine

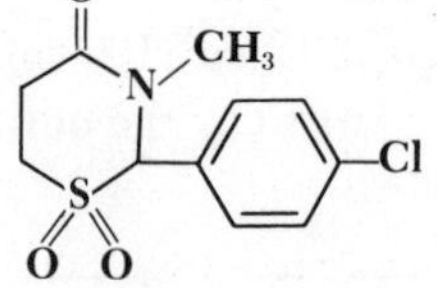

Chlormezanone 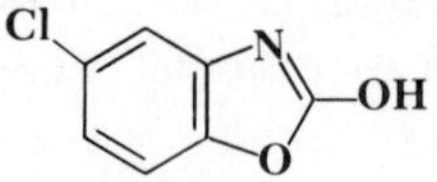   Chlorzoxazone

Mephenesin and mephenesin carbamate. These propanediol derivatives were the first drugs introduced as centrally acting muscle relaxants. Their selective action on spinal neurons was shown by abolition of strychnine convulsions in animals at dose levels that, in contrast to general anesthetics, did not cause sleep. These drugs are rather weak and must be given in large doses to obtain an effect. Preparations for mephenesin (Tolserol) include tablets, 500 mg, and elixir, 500 mg/5 ml. Mephenesin carbamate (Tolseram) is available in tablets, 500 mg, and elixir, 1 g/5 ml.

Innervation of skeletal muscle. FIG. 14-2

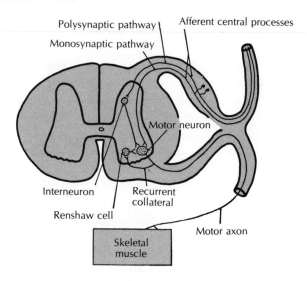

Polysynaptic pathway
Monosynaptic pathway
Afferent central processes
Motor neuron
Interneuron
Recurrent collateral
Renshaw cell
Motor axon
Skeletal muscle

Methocarbamol. Closely related to mephenesin carbamate, the drug has the same indication, uses, and limitations. Methocarbamol (Robaxin) is available in tablets, 500 and 750 mg, and, for injection, in solution of 100 mg/ml in 50% polyethylene glycol.

Chlorphenesin carbamate. This drug is closely related to mephenesin and has the same moderate effectiveness as a centrally acting muscle relaxant. Chlorphenesin carbamate (Maolate) is available in tablets, 400 mg.

Meprobamate. Another drug closely related to mephenesin, this propanediol has become extremely popular as a so-called minor tranquilizer. Its use and abuse are discussed on p. 266. Preparations of meprobamate (Miltown, Equanil) include capsules and tablets containing 200 and 400 mg.

Carisoprodol. Closely related to meprobamate, this drug has some limited usefulness in the treatment of muscle spasms. Preparations of carisoprodol (Soma) include tablets, 350 mg, and capsules, 250 mg.

Benzoxazole derivatives. The centrally acting muscle relaxants zoxazolamine (Flexin) and chlorzoxazone (Paraflex) were developed on the basis of the observation that benzimidazole had depressant effects on polysynaptic pathways of the spinal cord. Zoxazolamine turned out to be hepatotoxic and was removed from the market. The closely related chlorzoxazone has some usefulness in muscle spasms caused by neurological diseases. It also may cause jaundice in an occasional patient. It is available in tablets, 500 mg.

Chlormezanone. Chlormezanone (Trancopal) is used more as an antianxiety agent and has no specific effects on muscle rigidity. It is available in tablets, 100 and 200 mg.

Metaxalone. Chemically unrelated to the propanediols, this drug is 5-[3,5,(-di-methylphenoxyl)methyl]-2-oxazolidinone. Its usefulness in spastic conditions is probably related to its sedative effect. Metaxalone (Skelaxin) is available in tablets, 400 mg.

The diazepoxides. Chlordiazepoxide (Librium) and diazepam (Valium) are generally viewed as antianxiety agents and are discussed in Chapter 24. These drugs may be useful for reducing spasm in musculoskeletal disorders and may be considered as centrally acting skeletal muscle relaxants. They are available in tablet form and also as injectable solutions.

Baclofen. Baclofen (Lioresal) is a new skeletal muscle relaxant related to GABA (γ-aminobutyric acid). It appears to be useful in muscle spasm associated with multiple sclerosis and may be of value in conditions related to spinal cord injuries. Baclofen is 4-amino-3 (*p*-chlorophenyl) butyric acid. It is supplied in tablets, 10 mg.

Cyclobenzaprine. Cyclobenzaprine hydrochloride (Flexeril) is chemically and pharmacologically related to the tricyclic antidepressants. It is indicated for the short-term treatment of acute, painful musculoskeletal conditions. The drug has numerous side effects just as the tricyclic antidepressants. It should not be used in patients receiving MAO inhibitors. Cyclobenzaprine hydrochloride is available in tablets, 10 mg.

Dantrolene: a new approach to spasticity. Dantrolene sodium (Dantrium) is a new hydantoin derivative that acts on the skeletal muscle beyond the neuromuscular junction. The drug may act by interfering with the release of calcium. Although quite new, dantrolene has produced some improvement in patients with strokes, multiple sclerosis,[8] and postencephalitic athetosis and dystonia.

The drug is useful in the treatment of anesthetic-induced malignant hyperthermia probably because it uncouples excitation and contraction in skeletal muscle by interfering with calcium release from the sarcoplasmic reticulum.

Dantrolene may cause numerous serious reactions and side effects. When used chronically, hepatic damage, seizures, pleural effusion with pericarditis, and skin reactions suggesting hypersensitivity have been noted. Gastrointestinal, neurological, psychiatric, and cardiovascular adverse effects have also been reported.

The starting dose in adults is 25 mg twice a day orally. This dosage may have to be increased gradually to a maximum of 400 mg daily. Beneficial effects may require treatment for a week. Dantrolene sodium (Dantrium Intravenous) is available in vials containing 20 mg of the drug. It is indicated, along with other supportive measures, for the management of malignant hyperthermia crisis.

REFERENCES

1. Argov, Z., and Mastaglia, F.L.: Disorders of neuromuscular transmission caused by drugs, N. Engl. J. Med. **301**:409, 1979.

2. Baclofen (Lioresal): new muscle relaxant for multiple sclerosis, Med. Lett. **20**:43, 1978.

3. Bridenbaugh, P.O., and Churchill-Davidson, H.C.: Response to tubocurarine chloride and its reversal by neostigmine methylsulfate in man, JAMA **203**:541, 1968.

4. Comroe, J.H., Jr., and Dripps, R.D.: The histamine-like action of curare and tubocurarine injected intracutaneously and intraarterially in man, Anesthesiology **7**:260, 1946.

5. Eccles, J.C.: The physiology of nerve cells, Baltimore, 1957, The Johns Hopkins University Press.

6. Ellis, K.O., and Bryant, S.H.: Excitation-contraction uncoupling in skeletal muscle by dantrolene sodium, Naunym-Schmiedebergs Arch. Pharmacol. **274**:107, 1972.

7. Ellis, K.O., and Carpenter, J.F.: Studies on the mechanism of action of dantrolene sodium, a skeletal muscle relaxant, Naunyn-Schmiedebergs Arch. Pharmacol. **275**;83, 1972.

8. Gelenberg, A.J., and Poskanzer, D.C.: The effect of dantrolene sodium on spasticity in multiple sclerosis, Neurology **23**:1313, 1973.

9. Henneman, E., Kaplan, A., and Unna, K.: A neuropharmacological study on the effect of myanesin (Tolserol) on motor systems, J. Pharmacol. Exp. Ther. **97**:331, 1949.

10. Kariss, J.H., and Gissen, A.J.: Evaluation of new neuromuscular blocking agents, Anesthesiology **35**:149, 1971.

11. Mongar, J.L., and Whelan, R.F.: Histamine release by adrenaline and *d*-tubocurarine in the human subject, J. Physiol. **120**:146, 1953.

12. Van Winkle, W.B.: Calcium release from skeletal muscle sarcoplasmic reticulum: site of action of dantrolene sodium? Science **193**:1130, 1976.

13. Young, R.R., and Delwaide, P.J.: Spasticity, N. Engl. J. Med. **304**:96, 1981.

Chapter 15

Adrenergic (sympathomimetic) drugs

The adrenergic or sympathomimetic drugs comprise a large group of compounds that act *directly* on adrenergic receptors or that release catecholamines from nerve endings and thus act *indirectly*. Some of these drugs have a *mixed effect*, acting directly on receptors and also releasing the catecholamines.

The adrenergic group includes the endogenous biogenic amines norepinephrine, epinephrine, dopamine, and the related synthetic catecholamines, such as isoproterenol. It also includes ephedrine and miscellaneous adrenergic vasoconstrictors, bronchodilators, CNS stimulants, and anorexians.

The effect of these drugs can be predicted from a knowledge of (1) the type of adrenergic receptor with which they interact, (2) the direct, indirect, or mixed nature of their action, and (3) their penetration or lack of penetration into the CNS.

CATECHOLAMINES
Norepinephrine, epinephrine, and dopamine are the endogenous catecholamines, whereas isoproterenol is a synthetic, chemically related analog. These substances are termed *catecholamines* because their structure consists of catechol (*o*-dihydroxybenzene) and an amino group on the side chain.

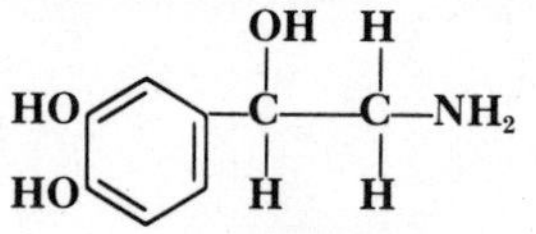

Norepinephrine

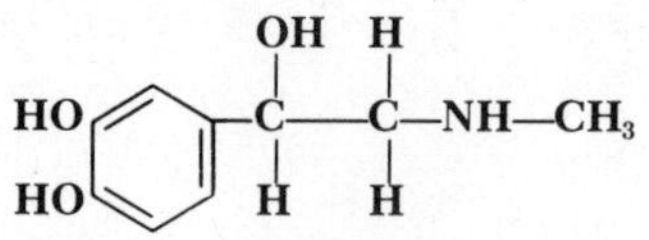

Epinephrine

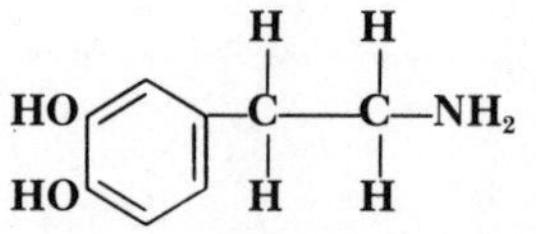

Dopamine

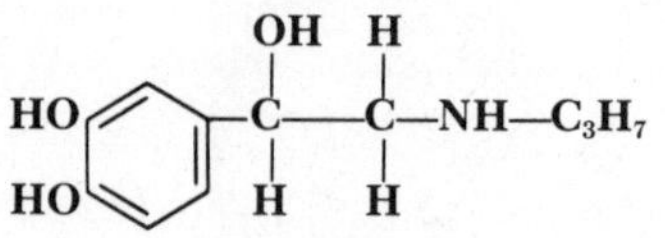

Isoproterenol

As shown in their structural formulas, epinephrine differs from norepinephrine in having a methyl group on the nitrogen, isoproterenol has an isopropyl group on

Fluorescent adrenergic terminals around small arteries and a vein in the rat mesentery.   *FIG. 15-1*

From Falck, B.: Acta Physiol. Scand. 56(suppl. 197):19, 1962.

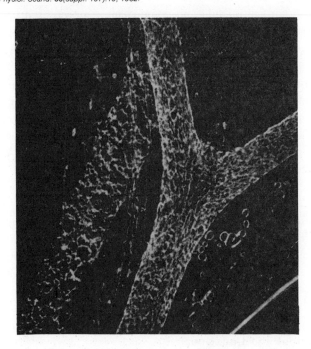

the nitrogen, and dopamine lacks the β-hydroxyl on the side chain. The prefix *nor-* in norepinephrine is derived from German chemical terminology. It is the abbreviation of *Nitrogen ohne Radikal*, which means nitrogen without radical.

Occurrence and physiological functions

The presence of norepinephrine in adrenergic nerve fibers was demonstrated by von Euler in 1946. It had been suspected that the "sympathin" released following adrenergic nerve stimulation was norepinephrine.

The relationship between adrenergic nerves and blood vessels and the presence of catecholamines in the nerves is strikingly demonstrated by the fluorescence technique of the Swedish investigators Falck, Hillarp, and Carlsson, as shown in Fig. 15-1.

Epinephrine is highly concentrated in the granules of the adrenal medulla. It is also present in many other organs, probably in chromaffin cells. Sympathetic denervation affects the norepinephrine content of an organ without a significant decrease in epinephrine concentration. From this observation it is suspected that epinephrine is present in chromaffin cells, which have nothing to do with adrenergic innervation.

The adrenal medullary granules and probably the adrenergic axonal vesicles contain catecholamines along with adenosine triphosphate in the proportion of 4:1.

They also contain a special soluble protein, *chromogranin*, and the enzyme dopamine-β-oxidase.

In the human adrenal medulla, norepinephrine may represent as much as 20% of the total catecholamine content. It may constitute a much higher percentage in the adrenal medulla of the newborn infant and in tumors of the adrenal medulla.

The main functions of norepinephrine appear to be the maintenance of normal sympathetic tone and adjustment of circulatory dynamics. Epinephrine appears to be the great emergency hormone that stimulates metabolism and promotes blood flow to skeletal muscles, preparing the individual for "fight or flight."

Dopamine is localized in certain areas of the CNS where it serves as an important transmitter. Dopamine is also the precursor of norepinephrine and epinephrine at other sites. The role of dopamine in Parkinson's disease and in the actions of psychoactive drugs is discussed on pp. 134 and 247.

Adrenergic and dopaminergic receptors

The classification of adrenergic receptors as *alpha* (α) and *beta* (β), originally proposed by Ahlquist[1] in 1948, is now generally accepted. The concept was based on the order of activity of a series of sympathomimetic drugs at various effector sites and was greatly strengthened when specific blocking agents were developed for each receptor. As shown in Table 15-1, the functions associated with α receptors are vasoconstriction, mydriasis, and intestinal relaxation. β Receptors mediate adrenergic influences for vasodilatation, cardioacceleration, bronchial relaxation, positive inotropic effect, and intestinal relaxation.

Norepinephrine acts on both α and β receptors. Epinephrine also acts on both receptors, but its β effects predominate. Isoproterenol is a pure β agonist and its actions are blocked by propranolol, a β-adrenergic blocking agent. Other drugs such as methoxamine and phenylephrine act on α receptors, and their effects are blocked by phenoxybenzamine or by phentolamine, both α-adrenergic blocking agents. Thus we have a graduation from pure α agonists to pure β agonists.

SUBCLASSES OF α AND β RECEPTORS

Although α receptors mediate mostly vasoconstriction and are postsynaptic, there are also presynaptic α receptors that mediate inhibition of norepinephrine release. This finding, based on relative affinity for a series of agonists, led to the subclassification of α receptors into α_1 and α_2 receptors. The α_2 receptor is most susceptible to the agonists clonidine, epinephrine, norepinephrine, methoxamine, and phenylephrine. The order of potency of antagonists on the α_2 receptor is phentolamine, yohimbine, phenoxybenzamine, and prazosin. This is in marked contrast with the α_1 receptor, where norepinephrine is a potent agonist and phenoxybenzamine is a potent antagonist. These facts may seem academic but acquire practical importance in antihypertensive therapy and may explain why phentolamine causes postural hypotension, whereas prazosin does not.

In addition to the presynaptic action of the α_2 receptor, inhibiting norepinephrine release, it also mediates other effects, such as insulin release by glucose and intestinal hypersecretion.

TABLE 15-1   Receptors mediating various adrenergic drug effects

Effector organ	Receptor	Response
Heart		
Sinoatrial node	β	Tachycardia
Atrioventricular node	β	Increase in conduction rate and shortening of functional refractory period
Atria and ventricles	β	Increased contractility
Blood vessels		
To skeletal muscle	α and β	Contraction or relaxation
To skin	α	Contraction
Bronchial muscle	β	Relaxation
Gastrointestinal smooth muscle		
To stomach	β	Decreased motility
To intestine	α and β	Decreased motility
Gastrointestinal sphincters		
To stomach	α	Contraction
To intestine	α	Contraction
Urinary bladder		
Detrusor	β	Relaxation
Trigone and sphincter	α	Contraction
Eye		
Radial muscle, iris	α	Contraction (mydriasis)
Ciliary muscle	β	Relaxation

Based on data from Epstein, S.E., and Braunwald, E.: N. Engl. J. Med. 275:1106, 1966.

β receptors are also of two types, β_1 and β_2. The β_1 receptors mediate the cardiac effects of catecholamines and also lipolysis. The β_2 receptors mediate bronchodilatation and adrenergic vasodilatation. The β_2 agonists are especially useful in the treatment of asthma (see p. 168) and in the prevention of premature labor. Antagonists may be nonselective for β_1 and β_2 receptors such as propranolol or they may have a greater effect on β_1 receptors in the heart, like metoprolol.

Dopamine acts on dopaminergic receptors in the mesenteric and renal blood vessels, where it causes selective vasodilatation and is antagonized by haloperidol and the phenothiazines. In addition, it acts on β_1 receptors in the heart, where its action is blocked by propranolol. In larger doses it also acts on peripheral blood vessels, where it produces vasoconstriction and its action is antagonized by phentolamine.

From a biochemical standpoint, the α_2 and β receptors mediate actions on adenylate cyclase, the α_2 receptor causing inhibition and the β receptor causing stimulation.

The various aspects of the pharmacology of norepinephrine (levarterenol; Levophed) and epinephrine (adrenaline) will be discussed first, followed by those of dopamine, ephedrine, and other adrenergic, sympathomimetic drugs.

The differences between the pharmacological effects of norepinephrine and epi-

Norepinephrine and epinephrine

TABLE 15-2   Cardiovascular effects of small dose of norepinephrine in humans

Systolic pressure	Increased
Diastolic pressure	Increased
Mean pressure	Increased
Heart rate	Slightly decreased
Cardiac output	Slightly decreased
Peripheral resistance	Increased

TABLE 15-3   Cardiovascular effects of small dose of epinephrine in humans

Systolic pressure	Increased
Diastolic pressure	Decreased (increased by large dose)
Heart rate	Increased
Mean pressure	Unchanged
Cardiac output	Increased
Peripheral resistance	Decreased

nephrine are a consequence of the generally greater influence of norepinephrine on α receptors, whereas epinephrine has a stronger action on β receptors. Nevertheless, both drugs have effects on both receptors.

CARDIOVASCULAR
EFFECTS

The actions of norepinephrine and epinephrine on the cardiovascular system may be quite different when both drugs are administered in small doses. They are not very different if large unphysiological doses are used.

Net effects of small doses in humans. When norepinephrine is infused intravenously into a normal person, it is generally given in a solution containing 4 mg of the drug in 1 L of isotonic fluid. If this solution containing 4 μg/ml is infused at such a rate that the patient receives about 10 μg/min, the hemodynamic changes listed in Table 15-2 will be observed. If a similar infusion of epinephrine were to be given to an individual, the changes listed in Table 15-3 would generally be observed. The differences in heart rate elicited by the two drugs are illustrated in Fig. 15-2.

The difference between the circulatory effects of epinephrine and norepinephrine reflects their different potency at various sites within the cardiovascular system. Norepinephrine has widespread vasoconstrictor properties, whereas epinephrine constricts some vascular areas and dilates others. The blood pressure elevation pro-

Effect of norepinephrine and epinephrine infusion on blood pressure and heart rate in   *FIG. 15-2*
humans. Note increased mean pressure and decreased heart rate following infusion of
norepinephrine and also essentially unchanged mean pressure, increase in pulse pressure,
and elevated heart rate following infusion of epinephrine.

From Barcroft, H., and Konzett, H.: Lancet 1:147, 1949.

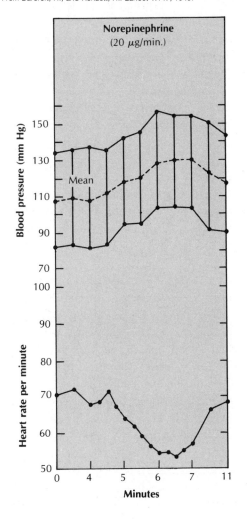
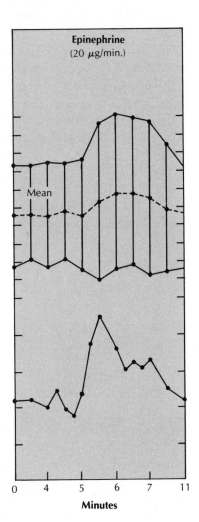

duced by norepinephrine brings into play reflexes that will cause bradycardia, which can be eliminated by the administration of atropine.

Epinephrine, on the other hand, stimulates the heart, and since there is no elevation of mean pressure, no reflex mechanisms come into play to slow the heart. The differences observed in humans following the infusion of dilute solutions of the two drugs may be attributed to their different peripheral actions, which affect the heart through reflex mechanisms.

Response of heart and various vascular areas. The actions of epinephrine on the heart consist of increased rate,* increased force of contraction, increased irritability, and increased coronary blood flow.

Norepinephrine has cardiac accelerator action also, but this inherent chronotropic effect is opposed by reflex slowing secondary to vasoconstriction and elevated blood pressure.

The increased coronary blood flow following the injection of epinephrine is largely a result of the increased cardiac work and metabolism. It has no usefulness in relieving precordial pain and may even precipitate anginal attacks in patients with coronary atherosclerosis.

The differences between epinephrine and norepinephrine tend to disappear when they are injected in large doses. Under these circumstances both will elevate diastolic pressure, increase peripheral resistance, and reduce blood flow through skeletal muscles.

The effects of epinephrine on renal hemodynamics have received considerable attention. It is generally accepted that the drug decreases renal plasma flow but does not influence glomerular filtration, the net effect being an increased filtration fraction. Large doses of epinephrine, however, may decrease the filtration fraction by stopping blood flow through some nephrons.

Cerebral blood flow is affected in a complex manner by norepinephrine and epinephrine. Through their direct action these drugs cause constriction of the cerebral vessels. The elevation of systemic pressure however, can oppose this direct action to such an extent that no significant change in cerebral blood flow may occur.

| BRONCHODILATOR EFFECT | Epinephrine is a dilator of the bronchial smooth muscle; norepinephrine is a much weaker dilator on this particular effector, whereas isoproterenol is a more active bronchodilator than epinephrine. The bronchodilator effect is not important when these drugs are administered to a normal individual. It becomes prominent when the bronchi are constricted by some pharmacological agent such as histamine or methacholine or in disease states such as bronchial asthma. Epinephrine is a time-honored remedy in the latter condition. |

| OTHER SMOOTH MUSCLE EFFECTS | Under special circumstances epinephrine causes mydriasis by contracting the radial muscle of the iris. This effect does not usually occur with direct application of the drug, but cocaine sensitizes the radial muscle to topically applied epinephrine. Norepinephrine has less effect on the eye. |

The capsule of the spleen is contracted by epinephrine in some animals such as the dog. It is questionable that this effect occurs in humans.

The catecholamines have some slight inhibitory actions on the gastrointestinal smooth muscle. This action has little physiological and no therapeutic importance.

---

*Heart rate may be decreased by epinephrine as a consequence of reflex vagal activity, which can be blocked by atropine.

The same may be said for the complex and variable effects of epinephrine on the uterus.

It is believed at present that injected catecholamines do not cross the blood-brain barrier efficiently. Alterations in norepinephrine content in the CNS may be associated with altered brain function and behavior, but injected catecholamines do not exert prominent effects. Nevertheless, the injection of epinephrine into normal humans produces anxiety and weakness.

Certain adrenergic drugs such as amphetamines have a marked stimulant action on the CNS.

Oxygen consumption may be increased by 25% following the injection of a therapeutic dose of epinephrine. Norepinephrine has considerably weaker effects on both oxygen consumption and lactic acid production in man.

Epinephrine and isoproterenol, and to a lesser degree norepinephrine, exert complex effects on carbohydrate metabolism. They elevate blood sugar by glycogenolysis and also inhibit glucose utilization. By stimulating glycogenolysis, glucose is released from the liver and lactic acid from muscle. The influence on phosphorylase has been studied extensively by Sutherland and Rall.[11-13] It appears that epinephrine in many tissues promotes the formation of a cyclic adenylic acid, adenosine-3',5'-monophosphate.

Adenosine-3',5'-monophosphate
(cyclic adenylic acid)

The formation of cyclic adenylate and some of its functions are shown in Fig. 15-3.

Catecholamines promote the release of fatty acids from adipose tissue and elevate the level of unesterified fatty acids in the blood. Thus the sympathetic nervous system, through catecholamine release, provides not only glucose but also free fatty acids as energy sources. The important effect on fatty acid release can be blocked by adrenergic blocking agents.

Marked elevations of plasma potassium may occur following the injection of epinephrine. It is believed that the source of this potassium is the liver.

FIG. 15-3 Cyclic AMP and phosphorylase activation. Site of action of epinephrine, glucagon, and methylxanthines.

From Butcher, R.W.: N. Engl. J. Med. **279**:1378, 1968.

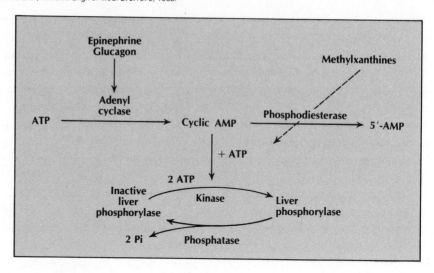

FIG. 15-4 Norepinephrine metabolism in the postganglionic sympathetic neuron.

From Abrams, W.B.: Dis. Chest **55**:148, 1969.

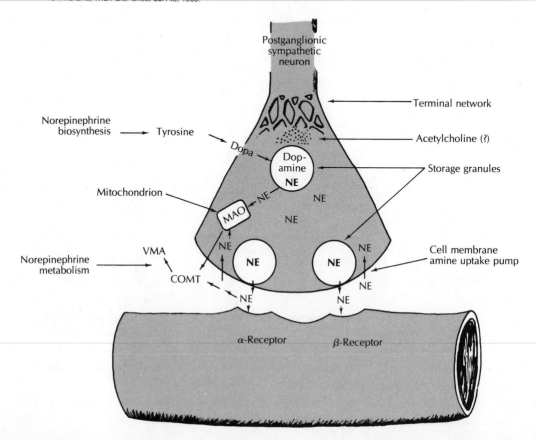

Catecholamines are made in the body from tyrosine through a series of steps involving dopa (3,4-dihydroxyphenylalanine), dopamine, norepinephrine, and finally epinephrine (p. 105). It is believed that these catecholamines are synthesized at the sites at which they are stored before their release. BIOSYNTHESIS

The steps in the synthesis of norepinephrine by sympathetic nerves are shown in Fig. 15-4. Norepinephrine synthesis varies directly in relation to nerve stimulation. Catecholamine synthesis is regulated by *tyrosine hydroxylase*, the rate-limiting enzyme. An inhibitor of tyrosine hydroxylase, α-methyltyrosine, blocks the increased catecholamine synthesis that results from nerve stimulation.

There is much evidence to indicate that norepinephrine inhibits tyrosine hydroxylase. Thus the regulation of norepinephrine synthesis in adrenergic nerves is achieved by end-product inhibition.

The termination of action of norepinephrine and epinephrine is largely a consequence of reuptake by adrenergic nerves. This reuptake is achieved by an amine pump in the nerve membrane that requires sodium and is inhibited by cocaine, the tricyclic antidepressants (such as desipramine), and also ouabain. That portion of norepinephrine and epinephrine that escapes the reuptake is attacked by the enzymes catechol-*O*-methyltransferase (COMT) and MAO (Fig. 15-5). TERMINATION OF ACTION

The normal urinary excretion of catecholamines and metabolites in man is as follows:

Norepinephrine + Epinephrine	1.1%
Normetanephrine + Metanephrine	7.6%
4-Hydroxy-3-methoxymandelic acid (VMA)	91%

The 24-hour VMA excretion in normal individuals is 10 mg. Much larger amounts may be excreted by patients with adrenal medullary tumors (p. 166).

A number of experimental facts suggest that uptake of catecholamines by nerves is the most important mechanism for the termination of the action of catecholamines. First, the injection of small physiological doses of tritiated norepinephrine results in its rapid clearance from the blood by the heart and other organs innervated by adrenergic fibers. That this uptake is in adrenergic fibers has been demonstrated by histochemical techniques in vitro. Furthermore, sympathetic nerve stimulation or reserpine treatment causes release of tritiated catecholamine.

Denervated structures take up only very small quantities of tritiated norepinephrine. Such structures, of course, are supersensitive to the action of catecholamines. Cocaine, imipramine, and certain antihistaminics block the uptake of norepinephrine and potentiate the action of catecholamines. These relationships may become clear by an examination of Fig. 15-6 (see also p. 108).

The neuronal uptake of norepinephrine is often referred to as *uptake*$_1$.[4] In addition, there is a second uptake system in various smooth muscles and glandular tissues, called *uptake*$_2$. The significance of uptake$_2$ is not at all clear. It is not blocked by cocaine or desipramine.

FIG. 15-5   *Major pathways of norepinephrine metabolism. MAO actually changes norepinephrine and normetanephrine to the corresponding mandelic aldehydes. These products are then transformed to mandelic acids by aldehyde dehydrogenase. (For other details see text.)*

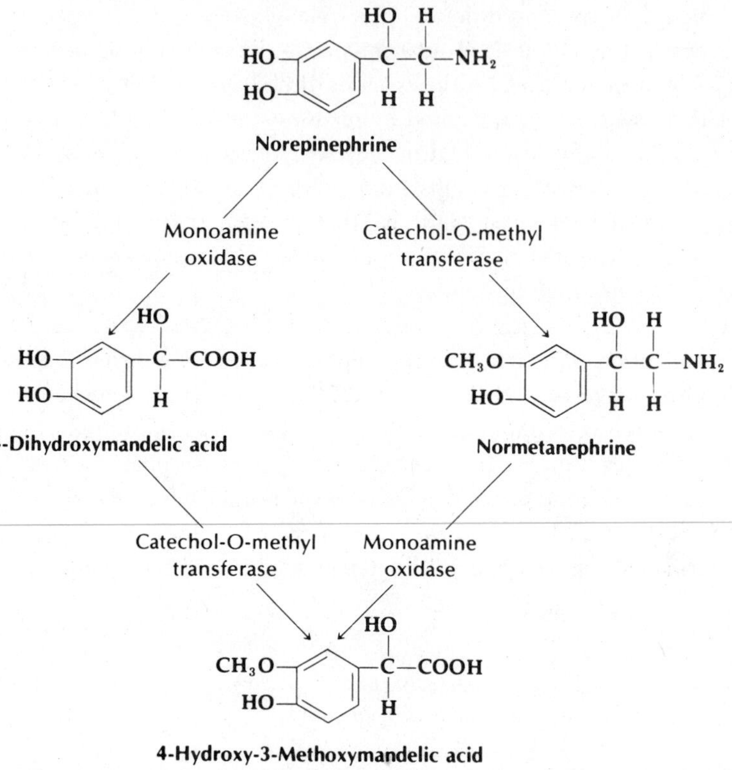

Norepinephrine

Monoamine oxidase

Catechol-O-methyl transferase

3,4-Dihydroxymandelic acid

Normetanephrine

Catechol-O-methyl transferase

Monoamine oxidase

4-Hydroxy-3-Methoxymandelic acid

FIG. 15-6   *Fate of norepinephrine released from adrenergic nerve. 1, Release and interaction with receptor on effector cell; 2, reuptake into the nerve of a portion of released norepinephrine; 3, metabolism by COMT and to a lesser extent by MAO; 4, metabolic degradation within the nerve by MAO of norepinephrine released within the axoplasm (such as following ingestion of reserpine).*

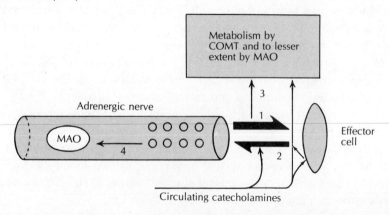

The relatively nonspecific amine pump of the adrenergic neuron transports not only catecholamines but also tyramine, metaraminol, α-methylnorepinephrine, and even serotonin. Some of these, such as metaraminol, may be held by the axon terminal and released on nerve stimulation, thereby acting as *false transmitters*. The antihypertensive drug α-methyldopa is taken up by the neuron and transformed to α-methylnorepinephrine, which also acts as a false transmitter when released.

Despite the low specificity of the amine pump, the adrenergic neuron is protected against the accumulation of all sorts of amines by the much greater specificity of the granular storage mechanism. Thus when tyramine is taken up, it is not only deaminated by MAO but the amine is also rejected by the granules, since only β-hydroxylated amines are held there. After the use of MAO inhibitors, however, tyramine, which is protected against deamination, is transformed by the fairly nonspecific dopamine-β-oxidase into the β-hydroxy derivative *octopamine*, which can be stored in the granules and acts as a false transmitter.

Adrenergic nerve terminals can take up compounds that may be injurious to them. The experimental drug *6-hydroxydopamine* causes degenerative changes in adrenergic nerve terminals, leading to *chemical sympathectomy*. Desipramine, a known blocker of the amine pump, prevents these effects.

THE AMINE PUMP AND FALSE TRANSMITTERS

The therapeutic uses of epinephrine and norepinephrine are based on the vasoconstrictor, cardiac stimulant and bronchodilator properties of these compounds.

THERAPEUTIC APPLICATIONS

Vasoconstrictor uses. Epinephrine is commonly added to local anesthetic solutions because its vasoconstrictor action delays the absorption of the local anesthetic and thereby restricts its effect to a given area. Because of its vasoconstrictor ability, epinephrine is widely used in the treatment of urticaria and angioneurotic edema.

Norepinephrine (Levophed) infusions have been widely used in the management of hypotension and shock. The initial enthusiasm decreased considerably once it was realized that in shock there is already a greatly increased sympathetic activity and that correction of underlying abnormalities such as decreased blood volume or fluid balance disturbances is more important.

Cardiac uses. Either epinephrine or the newer drug isoproterenol is indicated in the management of heart block or Adams-Stokes syndrome. These drugs act partly to improve atrioventricular conduction but mostly by stimulating ventricular automaticity, thus producing an increased ventricular rate. Caution should be exercised in the so-called states of prefibrillation, since the drug may precipitate ventricular arrhythmias. It is permissible to inject epinephrine directly into the heart in asystole in an attempt to achieve resuscitation. Cardiac massage is gaining much favor over the simple epinephrine resuscitation.

Bronchodilator action. Epinephrine is a time-honored remedy in the treatment of bronchial asthma. For this purpose it may be given subcutaneously in the amount of 0.2 to 0.5 ml of a 1:1000 solution. It may also be given by inhalation. For this purpose a stronger solution (up to 1:100) is employed in a nebulizer. Isoproterenol has been replacing epinephrine in this type of treatment.

Overdoses of norepinephrine or epinephrine may cause severe hypertension, pulmonary edema, and arrhythmias (particularly following the use of certain general anesthetics). In addition, extravasation ischemia may result at the site of intravenous infusions of levarterenol. This can be treated by the local infiltration of phentolamine (Regitine), an α-adrenergic blocking agent.

Patients receiving tricyclic antidepressants or guanethidine, which block the amine uptake mechanism in adrenergic nerves, may show exaggerated responses to norepinephrine and epinephrine.

CATECHOLAMINES AND DISEASE STATES

Hypertension. Hypertension is clearly not caused solely by an increase in sympathetic activity. No significant increase in catecholamine excretion has been found in persons with essential hypertension. On the other hand, plasma catecholamines may be elevated in this condition.

Pheochromocytoma. A rare form of hypertension is caused by tumors of adrenomedullary tissue that secrete norepinephrine with variable amounts of epinephrine. Although pheochromocytoma is a rare tumor, its diagnosis is most important because it represents one of the few forms of completely curable hypertension.

Several tumors have been examined by chemical methods. It appears that most of them contain very high concentrations of norepinephrine and smaller amounts of epinephrine. There may be as much as 10 to 15 mg/g of tissue, and the total catecholamine content of a large tumor may be more than 1 g.

Several methods have been introduced during the last few years for the diagnosis of pheochromocytoma. Some of these are based on neuropharmacological principles and others on the determination of catecholamines in the urine. Although pharmacological tests are inaccurate and hazardous as compared with chemical tests, they illustrate interesting principles.

Pharmacological tests. Drug tests for pheochromocytoma are of two types: those that can promote the secretion of catecholamines from the tumor and cause blood pressure elevation, and those that inhibit the actions of norepinephrine and thereby cause lowering of the elevated blood pressure.

Among those drugs that elevate blood pressure in patients with pheochromocytoma are histamine, methacholine, and tetraethylammonium. Drugs that lower blood pressure in patients with pheochromocytoma are phenoxybenzamine and phentolamine.

The most widely used drug in diagnosis of pheochromocytoma is phentolamine (Regitine). A dose of 5 mg is injected intravenously or intramuscularly. If systolic blood pressure falls more than 35 mm Hg and diastolic pressure more than 25 mm Hg, the test is considered positive.

Chemical tests. The diagnosis of pheochromocytoma may be established by the determination of normetanephrine plus epinephrine or norepinephrine plus epinephrine or VMA in a 24-hour urine specimen. There is a rapid screening procedure for VMA in many laboratories, but its diagnostic accuracy is not as great as that of other procedures. Methyldopa, tetracycline, and quinidine may falsely increase nor-epinephrine plus epinephrine values. MAO inhibitors will increase normetanephrine plus metanephrine. Anxiety and excitement do not elevate the excretion of cate-cholamines sufficiently to cause diagnostic errors. On the other hand, acute myo-cardial infarction, surgical trauma, and shock may cause abnormally high urinary output of the catecholamines and their metabolites.

Levarterenol bitartrate (Levophed bitartrate) is available for injection in a 0.2% solution equivalent to 1 mg of base per milliliter in 2 and 4 ml ampules. For intra-venous infusion in adults 4 to 8 ml of the 0.2% solution is added to 500 ml of 5% dextrose injection. The injection rate is regulated to keep the systolic blood pressure somewhat below normal. *PREPARATIONS*

Epinephrine hydrochloride (Adrenalin chloride) is a solution containing for in-jection, 1 mg/ml, and for inhalation, 10 mg/ml.

Epinephrine bitartrate is available in special devices (Medihaler-epi) for inha-lation, deliver 0.3 mg per dose.

Epinephrine suspension, aqueous or in oil, for injection contains 2.5 or 2 mg/ml.

Epinephrine bitartrate and epinephrine hydrochloride are also available for ophthalmic uses in 1% and 2% solutions.

This catecholamine has important functions as a chemical mediator in some parts of the CNS. In addition it has been introduced as a therapeutic agent under the trade name Intropin. *Dopamine*

Dopamine acts on β receptors in the heart, causing increased contractility and heart rate. In large enough doses it acts on α receptors in blood vessels, causing vasoconstriction. Dopamine exerts some unusual vasodilator effects on the renal, mesenteric, coronary, and intracerebral vessels, which suggest the existence of spe-cific dopaminergic receptors. These are not blocked by propranolol but are inhibited by haloperidol and the phenothiazines.[3] These dopamine vascular receptors may be similar to the dopaminergic receptors in the basal ganglia (p. 134).

The hemodynamic effects of dopamine depend on the dose with some individual variations. Intravenous infusion of 1 to 10 μg/kg/min leads to increased cardiac contractility, cardiac output, and renal blood flow. Heart rate and mean blood pres-sure do not change significantly. With higher infusion rates arterial pressure rises and heart rate decreases.

Dopamine infusions are used in some cases of shock and in chronic refractory congestive failure. In shock, dopamine should not be administered until blood volume becomes adequate as reflected by a central venous pressure of 10 to 15 cm H_2O.

Ventricular arrhythmia is the most serious adverse effect. Nausea, vomiting, and hypotension may also occur. If the blood pressure becomes elevated, it is comforting to know that the action of the drug is dissipated in a few minutes.

The cardiac actions of dopamine are antagonized by propranolol, its hypertensive effects are inhibited by phentolamine, and dopaminergic vasodilation is blocked by haloperidol or the phenothiazines. Furthermore, MAO inhibitors cause exaggerated responses to dopamine.

Dopamine hydrochloride (Intropin) is available in 5 ml ampules that contain 200 mg of dopamine. The drug should be diluted in a 250 or 500 ml sterile intravenous solution. Infusion rates should be adjusted so that 2 to 5 μg/kg/min of the drug are given.

Dobutamine is related to dopamine but it has a selectivity for β_1 receptors in the heart. It is used in acute myocardial infarction and in coronary bypass operations. Since the half-life of the drug is very short, it is given by intravenous infusion, in doses of 2.5 to 15 μg/kg/min. Dobutamine (Dobutrex) is available in 20 ml vials, containing 250 mg.

MISCELLANEOUS ADRENERGIC DRUGS

The various sympathomimetic drugs may act *directly* on α and β receptors, or they may act *indirectly* by releasing endogenous catecholamines. Some also have a *mixed* action, both direct and indirect. Some important examples are as follows.

	α AGONISTS	β AGONISTS
Direct acting drugs	Methoxamine	Isoproterenol
Mixed acting drugs	Metaraminol	Ephedrine (indirect on α receptors)
Indirect acting drugs	Tyramine	
	Amphetamine	

The evidence for this classification is based on various considerations. It has been demonstrated that tyramine, ephedrine, amphetamine, and phenylethylamine, now considered to be indirectly acting agents, had less effect in animals in whose tissue the norepinephrine content had been depleted by reserpine (Fig. 15-7).

The infusion of norepinephrine restored the capacity of the animals to react to these drugs. In a reserpinized animal the *responses* to some adrenergic drugs are normal or augmented. Other adrenergic drugs are suppressed, and still others are partly antagonized by reserpine. Drugs of the first type include norepinephrine, epinephrine, and phenylephrine. They are direct acting. Among those suppressed by norepinephrine depletion are tyramine, amphetamine, phenylethylamine, and hydroxyamphetamine. Partially suppressed and having presumably a mixed effect are ephedrine and phenylpropanolamine.

Another line of evidence that suggests norepinephrine release as the mode of action of many sympathomimetic drugs is the observation that indirectly acting amines are ineffective on chronically denervated structures.

Classification based on clinical usage

A discussion of the sympathomimetic amines may be simplified by placing them into categories based on their clinical usage. There are three such categories: the vasoconstrictors, the bronchodilators, and the CNS stimulants. Despite some overlap in these activities, it is possible to select sympathomimetics for therapeutic purposes on the basis of predominant action. Ephedrine, a prototype of the sympathomimetic

Blood pressure response to tyramine. A, Reserpinized cat. B, Control cat. Dose of reser-   **FIG. 15-7**
pine: 7 mg/kg subcutaneously. Dose of tyramine: 0.5 mg/kg intravenously. Arrows indicate
times of injection.

From Carlsson, A., Rosengren, E., Bertler, Å., and Nilsson, J.: Psychotropic drugs, Amsterdam, 1957, Elsevier Publishing Co.

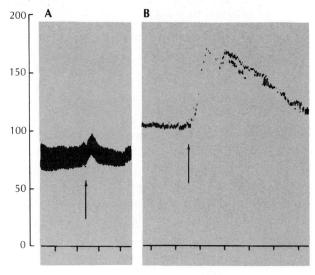

Tyramine (0.5 mg/kg)

amines, belongs to a special category. It is used for its cardiovascular, bronchodilator, and stimulant properties.

Adrenergic vasoconstrictors are phenylephrine, methoxamine, mephentermine, metaraminol, and the nasal vasoconstrictors phenylephrine hydrochloride, hydroxy-amphetamine, phenylpropranolamine, propylhexedrine, cyclopentamine, tuamino-heptane, methylhexaneamine, naphazoline, and tetrahydrozoline. Dopamine is also being advocated in the treatment of hypotension.

Adrenergic bronchodilators are isoproterenol, protokylol, isoetharin, and me-thoxyphenamine. Related vasodilators are nylidrin and isoxsuprine. The newer β_2 bronchodilators such as terbutaline and metaproterenol will be discussed in Chapter 40.

Adrenergic vasodilators include nylidrin, isoxsuprine, and isoproterenol.

Adrenergic CNS stimulants and anorexiants are amphetamine sulfate, dextroam-phetamine, methamphetamine, and the related appetite suppressants phenmetrazine and diethylpropion.

Used in China for centuries and introduced into the United States in 1923, *Ephedrine* ephedrine is a naturally occurring sympathomimetic drug. Its action is similar to that of epinephrine and norepinephrine except for a much longer duration of action, effectiveness after oral administration, CNS stimulation, and occurrence of tachyphylaxis on frequent administration. On a weight basis it is about 100 times weaker; thus it is administered in doses of about 25 mg. Its action lasts for hours, and it is well absorbed from the gastrointestinal tract. From the standpoint of intestinal absorption of sympathomimetic drugs, the generalization may be made that the *phenyl* amines are much better absorbed than are the catechol derivatives.

Ephedrine

Ephedrine is an indirectly acting phenylisopropylamine. Its peripheral actions are reduced by intensive pretreatment with reserpine or by sympathetic denervation.

In addition to its vasopressor effects, ephedrine acts on the heart, with the heart rate usually increasing. Ephedrine dilates the bronchi and is useful in the treatment of asthma. It causes mydriasis when applied to the eye, produces CNS stimulation with anxiety and wakefulness, and has some slight anticurare action on the skeletal muscles. It is occasionally useful in myasthenia gravis.

Ephedrine sulfate USP is available for oral administration in the form of capsules containing 25 and 50 mg and also as an elixir containing 5 and 10 mg/5 ml. For injection, solutions containing 20, 25, or 50 mg/ml are available.

Adrenergic vasoconstrictors related to epinephrine or ephedrine

Phenylephrine (Neo-Synephrine) is a direct-acting α-receptor agonist. Subcutaneous injection of 5 mg has been used for the prevention of hypotension during spinal anesthesia and for the treatment of orthostatic hypotension. It is also a nasal decongestant.

Methoxamine (Vasoxyl) is a direct-acting α-receptor agonist lacking cardiac stimulant properties. It is available for injection as a solution containing 10 and 20 mg/ml.

Mephentermine (Wyamine) is both a direct and indirect vasoactive drug acting on both α and β receptors. The duration of its vasoconstrictor and myocardial stimulant action is 60 minutes following subcutaneous injection of 10 to 30 mg.

Metaraminol (Aramine) resembles phenylephrine in its properties, but it acts both directly and indirectly. It is taken up by sympathetic fibers and released as a false transmitter. The drug is administered subcutaneously or intramuscularly in doses of 2 to 10 mg. It is available as metaraminol bitartrate in injectable solutions containing 10 mg/ml.

Hydroxyamphetamine (Paredrine) resembles ephedrine in its action except for having little CNS effect. The drug is available in tablet form, 20 mg, for oral administration and as an ophthalmic preparation in a 1% solution.

Phenylpropanolamine is used almost entirely as an oronasal decongestant.

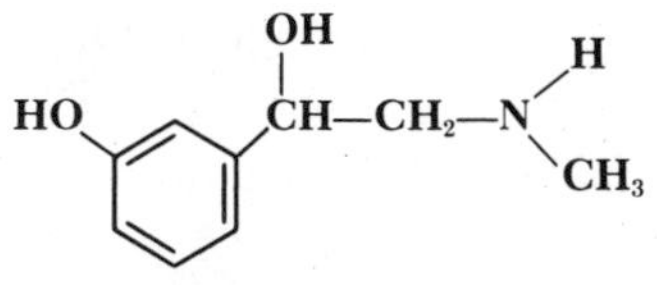

Phenylephrine

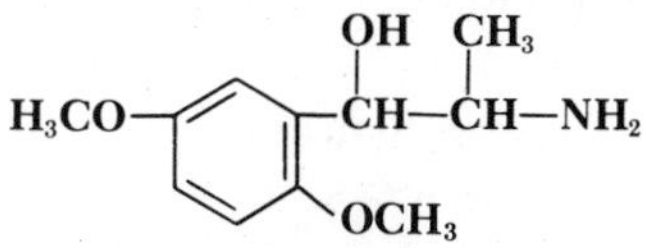

Methoxamine

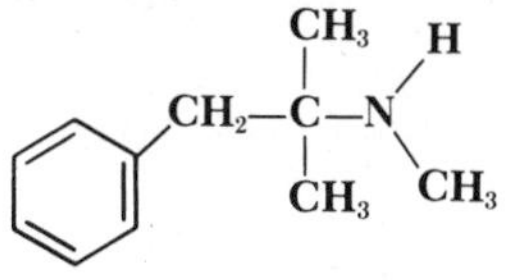

Mephentermine

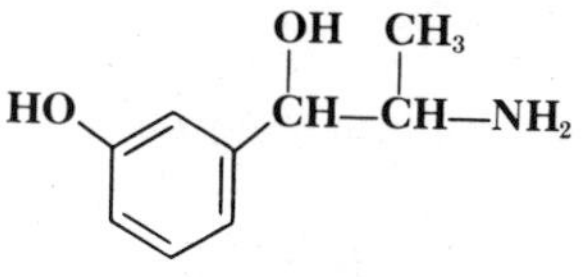

Metaraminol

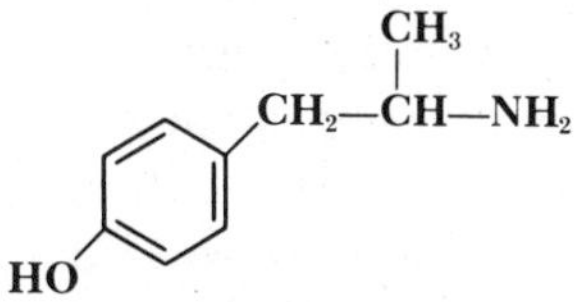

Hydroxyamphetamine

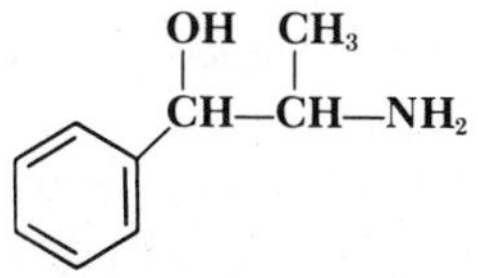

Phenylpropanolamine

Some of the commonly used nasal decongestants are the following.

Phenylephrine hydrochloride (Neo-Synephrine hydrochloride) is available in solutions of 0.125% for topical application; it may cause rebound swelling of the nasal mucosa. Oral administration of the drug in capsules of 10 and 25 mg is somewhat unpredictable in its effect.

Phenylpropanolamine hydrochloride (Propadrine hydrochloride) is available in capsules of 25 mg; it has also been used as an anorexiant but is ineffective.

Propylhexedrine (Benzedrex) is commonly administered by inhalation. It has many of the properties of amphetamine but with lesser pressor effect and much less CNS stimulation.

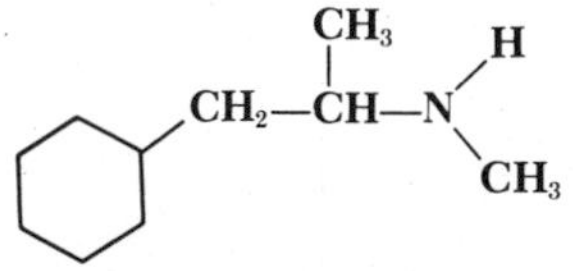

NASAL VASOCON-STRICTORS

Propylhexedrine

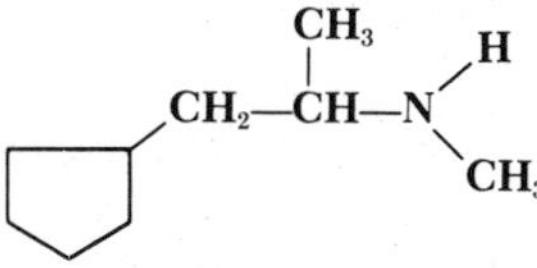

Cyclopentamine

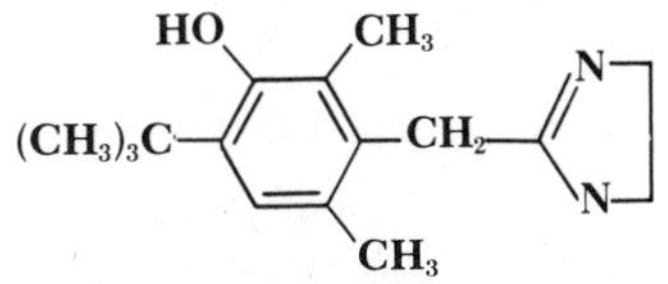

Oxymetazoline

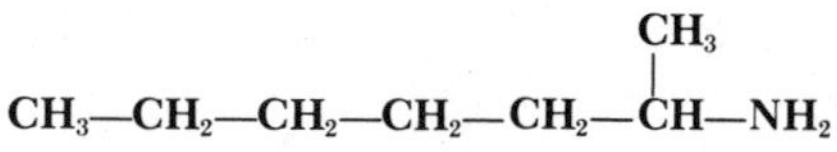

Tuaminoheptane

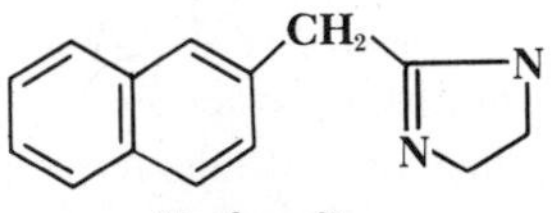

Naphazoline

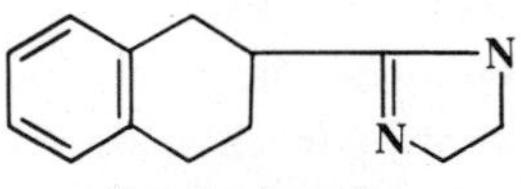

Tetrahydrozoline

Cyclopentamine hydrochloride (Clopane hydrochloride) is applied topically as a 0.5% solution.

Oxymetazoline hydrochloride (Afrin) is available in 0.05% solution as nose drops and spray.

Tuaminoheptane (Tuamine) is available as a 1% solution and also as an inhalant.

Naphazoline hydrochloride (Privine hydrochloride), an imidazoline derivative, is available in 0.05% solutions as nose drops and a spray. It may cause profound drowsiness and coma in children and also rebound swelling of the mucosa and cardiac irregularities when used excessively.

Tetrahydrozoline hydrochloride (Tyzine) is similar to naphazoline chemically and in its adverse effects.

Currently, nasal vasoconstrictors or decongestants are considered to be symptomatic medications that have some usefulness but are not harmless. Continued use of these medications may actually induce chronic congestion of the nasal mucosa, probably because ischemia leads to rebound swelling. In excessive doses the nasal decongestants produce the usual adrenergic effects such as increased blood pressure, dizziness, palpitation, and in some cases CNS stimulation. In addition, the imidazoline derivatives naphazoline and tetrahydrozoline have produced drowsiness and coma in children.

The nasal decongestants are frequently combined with antihistamines. Thus preparations containing phenylephrine and an antihistamine have become very popular as nasal decongestants that are taken orally.

Adrenergic bronchodilators
ISOPROTERENOL

Isoproterenol (isopropylnorepinephrine) is a potent activator of β receptors. It dilates the bronchial smooth muscle and has powerful effects on the heart. It also dilates blood vessels, particularly in skeletal muscle. When used in the treatment of bronchial asthma, it may cause tachycardia, arrhythmias, and hypotension. Some instances of sudden death in asthmatic persons have been attributed to excessive use of isoproterenol.[10]

Isoproterenol

Isoproterenol is used primarily in the treatment of bronchial asthma, atrioventricular block, and cardiac arrest.

Palpitations, arrhythmias, anginal pain, and headache may occur following the use of isoproterenol. The drug may intensify arrhythmias caused by digitalis. Cyclopropane, halogenated anesthetics, and propellants may sensitize the myocardium to isoproterenol. The effects of the drug are blocked by propranolol.

Isoproterenol hydrochloride (Isuprel hydrochloride) is available in solutions of 1:100 (10 mg:ml), 1:200 (5 mg/ml), and 1:400 (2.5 mg/ml) for oral inhalation; solutions containing 0.2 mg/ml for injection; and sublingual tablets of 10 and 15 mg. The effects of the tablets are somewhat unpredictable because of erratic absorption.

In addition to isoproterenol, several adrenergic drugs and theophylline derivatives are used as bronchodilators. Epinephrine and ephedrine are widely used and have already been discussed (pp. 157 and 160). Protokylol, isoetharine, and methoxyphenamine are additional adrenergic bronchodilators. Among the theophylline derivatives, aminophylline (theophylline ethylenediamine), oxtriphylline, theophylline in 20% alcohol, and theophylline sodium glycinate are commonly used in asthmatic individuals. The corticosteroids, although not primarily bronchodilators, are also of great importance in the treatment of severe asthma. *OTHER BRONCHODILATORS*

In addition to these bronchodilators, certain β-receptor agonists, such as metaproterenol sulfate (Alupent), terbutaline (Brethine), and salbutamol, are being employed in the treatment of asthma because they have fewer cardiac side effects.

The bronchodilators are discussed in Chapter 40 in connection with drug effects on the respiratory tract.

Isoproterenol is a β-adrenergic stimulant that dilates blood vessels while it stimulates the heart. Certain vasodilators have been developed that probably act through a similar mechanism. These are **nylidrin** (Arlidin) and **isoxsuprine** (Vasodilan). Although these drugs can dilate peripheral blood vessels experimentally, their effectiveness in the management of peripheral vascular disease is not universally accepted among clinical investigators. Nylidrin is used orally in doses of 6 mg and isoxsuprine is also used orally in doses of 10 to 20 mg. Although the action of these drugs resembles that of isoproterenol, they probably act indirectly by releasing catecholamines. *Adrenergic vasodilators*

Nylidrin

Isoxsuprine

The amphetamines are powerful stimulants of the CNS. *Dextro*amphetamine has relatively greater central, and less cardiovascular, effects than the *levo* isomer. The drug is used and also abused mainly in relation to its anorexiant effect, and even this use is questioned by many authorities. In addition to being an anorexiant, dextroam- *Adrenergic CNS stimulants and anorexiants* *AMPHETAMINES* phetamine finds some application as an analeptic in the treatment of narcolepsy, as an antidepressant, in the management of hyperkinetic children, and in postencephalitic reactions.

Numerous anorexiants have been developed and are used by the medical profession, often without the realization that these drugs are essentially relatives of dextroamphetamine without significant advantages over the anorexiant prototype. Some of the drugs are methamphetamine (Desoxyn), phenmetrazine (Preludin), diethylpropion (Tenuate; Tepanil), phenylpropanolamine (Propadrine), phentermine (Ionamin; Wilpo), chlorphentermine (Pre-Sate), benzphetamine (Didrex), and phendimetrazine (Plegine). In addition, numerous mixtures of adrenergic stimulants with barbiturates and other depressants have been prepared and are used widely. Despite their popularity, such mixtures are generally not recommended.

The disadvantages in the use of anorexiants are related to the development of psychic dependence and to untoward effects resulting from adrenergic actions. Toxic psychosis may result from large doses of many of these drugs.

$$CH_2-CH-NH_2$$
$$| $$
$$CH_3$$

Amphetamine

The vascular effects of the amphetamines may be attributed to endogenous catecholamine release, since they do not elevate blood pressure in a reserpinized animal.

The central stimulant effects of amphetamine are not inhibited by catecholamine depletion by reserpine, but blockade of catecholamine synthesis quickly inhibits the behavioral actions of amphetamine. These findings suggest that although the drug's cardiovascular effects stem from the release of preformed peripheral norepinephrine, the drug's behavioral actions are mediated through a newly synthesized fraction of brain catecholamines.

Certain central stimulants, such as methylphenidate, while mimicking amphetamine's central effects, clearly act by a different mechanism, since the effects of such drugs are blocked by reserpine but not by catecholamine synthesis blockade, unless synthesis inhibition is prolonged until catecholamine depletion occurs.

Habituation and tolerance develop to the central effects of amphetamine. Large and repeated doses may produce a psychosis that has many of the characteristics of paranoid schizophrenia.

Amphetamine is well absorbed from the gastrointestinal tract. The main metabolite of amphetamine is phenylacetone, a product of microsomal deamination. A minor metabolite, *p*-hydroxyamphetamine, is taken up by adrenergic nerves and transformed to *p*-hydroxynorephedrine, which is stored in vesicles, thus forming a false transmitter.

Amphetamine (Benzedrine) is available in tablets, 5, 10, and 15 mg; sustained action capsules; and injectable solutions containing 20 mg/ml.

Dextroamphetamine (Dexedrine) is available in tablets 5, 10, and 15 mg; sustained action capsules; elixir, 5 mg/5 ml; and injectable solutions containing 20 mg/ml.

Methylphenidate (Ritalin) is available in tablets, 5, 10, and 20 mg, and in injectable solutions containing 10 mg/ml.

Methamphetamine (*d*-deoxyephedrine) is closely related from a structural standpoint to both ephedrine and amphetamine. It is a potent CNS stimulant and has a considerable pressor effect on blood vessels. It is used for the same purposes as amphetamine in approximately the same dosage.

Phenmetrazine (Preludin) is used as an appetite suppressant, a questionable approach to the treatment of obesity. It has considerable CNS effects.

Diethylpropion (Tenuate; Tepanil) is employed as an anorexigenic agent. It is basically an amphetamine-like drug, although it is claimed that it causes less jitteriness and insomnia and also fewer cardiovascular effects than does amphetamine. The drug is considerably weaker than dextroamphetamine and is used in doses of 25 mg orally.

Phenmetrazine   Diethylpropion

MISCELLANEOUS ANOREXIANTS

Clortermine hydrochloride (Voranil), **fenfluramine hydrochloride** (Pondimin), and **mazindol** (Sanorex) are additional anorexiants that have been recently evaluated.[2] They are comparable to other anorexiants in suppressing appetite. They may be used as short-term adjuncts to other measures that include caloric restriction, exercise, and psychotherapy. Of these drugs, mazindol (Sanorex) is not a phenethylamine and is claimed to have a different mode of action from the others. Fenfluramine (Pondimin) is unusual in causing CNS depression along with appetite suppression.

Clortermine and fenfluramine are said to affect the appetite control centers in the hypothalamus. This is also true for all phenethylamines. Mazindol reportedly facilitates the electric activity in the septal region of the brain.

DRUG INTERACTIONS

All the CNS stimulants and anorexiants may cause hypertensive crises in patients taking MAO inhibitors. All, except fenfluramine, antagonize the antihypertensive action of guanethidine (Ismelin). Fenfluramine may potentiate the antihypertensive action of guanethidine and methyldopa (Aldomet). Fenfluramine, being a sedative, may increase the effects of alcohol and other CNS depressants. Mazindol potentiates the vasopressor effect of levarterenol in dogs and probably should not be combined with vasopressor medications.

Structure-activity relationships in adrenergic series

A great deal is known about the relationships between structure and activity in adrenergic drugs. Such knowledge in general is important to the pharmaceutical chemist as a guide in synthetic work on new drugs. Structure-activity relationships are also of fundamental importance in that they should reflect basic characteristics of receptor mechanisms. In the case of adrenergic drugs the problem is complicated by the fact that many sympathomimetic drugs act indirectly through the release of endogenous catecholamines. The differences in action of these drugs may be related to the predominant site of catecholamine release.

A few generalities may serve to illustrate the concept of structure-activity relationships.

The basic adrenergic structure is phenylethylamine.

$$CH_2-CH_2-NH_2$$

Phenylethylamine

Hydroxyl groups on the benzene ring or on the side chain influence the metabolic rate and absorption of the drugs as well as their actions on receptors. Sympathomimetics that are not catechols are generally absorbed better and are, of course, not attacked by O-methylation.

Substitutions on the nitrogen have a great influence on the type of receptor with which the drug will interact. Thus norepinephrine, lacking substitutions, acts on α receptors, epinephrine with one methyl group acts on both receptors, and isoproterenol acts almost entirely on β receptors.

Substitutions on the α carbon tend to prolong the action of the drug, probably because of protection against enzymatic destruction. The OH group on the β carbon is necessary for granular storage in adrenergic neurons.

REFERENCES

1. Ahlquist, R.P.: A study of the adrenotropic receptors, Am. J. Physiol. **153**:586, 1948.
2. Dykes, M.H.: Evaluation of three anorexiants, JAMA **230**:270, 1974.
3. Goldberg, L.I.: Dopamine—clinical uses of an endogeneous catecholamine, N. Engl. J. Med. **21**:707, 1974.
4. Iversen, L.L.: Uptake mechanisms for neurotransmitter amines, Biochem. Pharmacol. **23**:1927, 1974.
5. Langer, S.Z.: Presynaptic regulation of catecholamine release, Biochem. Pharmacol. **23**:1793, 1974.
6. Lefkowitz, R.J.: β-Adrenergic receptors: recognition and regulation, N. Engl. J. Med. **295**:323, 1976.
7. Lefkowitz, R.J.: Direct binding studies of adrenergic receptors: biochemical, physiologic, and clinical implications, Ann. Intern. Med. **91**:450, 1979.
8. Shore, P.A.: Transport and storage of biogenic amines, Annu. Rev. Pharmacol. **12**:209, 1972.
9. Steer, M.L., Atlas, D., and Levitzki, A.: Interrelations between β-adrenergic receptors, adenylate cyclase and calcium, N. Engl. J. Med. **292**:409, 1975.

10. Stolley, P.D.: Asthma mortality, Am. Rev. Respir. Dis. **105**:883, 1972.

11. Sutherland, E.W.: The effect of the hyperglycemic factor and epinephrine on enzyme systems of liver and muscle, Ann. N.Y. Acad. Sci. **54**:693, 1951.

12. Sutherland, E.W., and Rall, T.W.: The relationship of adenosine-3′,5′-phosphate to the action of catecholamines. In Adrenergic mechanisms, Ciba Foundation and Committee for Symposium on Drug Action, Boston, 1960, Little, Brown & Co.

13. Sutherland, E.W., and Rall, T.W.: The relation of adenosine-3′,5′-phosphate and phosphorylase to the actions of catecholamines and other hormones, Pharmacol. Rev. **12**:265, 1960.

14. Weil, M.H., Shubin, H., and Carlson, R.: Treatment of circulatory shock, JAMA **231**:1280, 1975.

Chapter 16

Adrenergic blocking agents

**GENERAL
CONCEPT**
 Adrenergic blocking agents are drugs that competitively inhibit the actions of catecholamines and other adrenergic agonists on their specific receptors. They are effective against catecholamines released from sympathetic nerve endings.

Adrenergic blocking drugs are classified as *alpha* (α) and *beta* (β) adrenergic blocking agents, reflecting the existence of two types of receptors. In tissues that possess both types of receptors, such as most blood vessels, α stimulation causes contraction and β stimulation causes relaxation. The α-adrenergic blocking drugs in such a tissue cause vasodilation. In organs whose receptors are almost entirely β such as the heart, the β blockers oppose the excitatory effects of norepinephrine released from sympathetic nerve endings.

Drugs that deplete catecholamines or prevent their release in adrenergic nerves should be called *catecholamine depleters* and *adrenergic neuronal blocking drugs*, respectively, and should not be confused with the *adrenergic blocking agents* that act on α and β receptors. Certain imprecise older terms such as *adrenolytic*, *sympatholytic*, and *sympathoplegic* should be abandoned.

**α-ADRENERGIC
BLOCKING
AGENTS**
General features
 The α-adrenergic blocking drugs inhibit the effect of various agonists on the α receptor. They reverse the actions of epinephrine on the blood pressure, oppose the actions of norepinephrine, but do not prevent β receptor–mediated effects of adrenergic drugs such as cardiac effects and vasodilatation.

The single most characteristic feature of the α-adrenergic blocking agents is their ability to convert the pressor effect of epinephrine into a depressor response. This epinephrine reversal by phentolamine is shown in Fig. 16-1. Vascular smooth muscle has both α and β receptors. Since epinephrine acts on both receptors, it causes vasodilatation if the α receptors are blocked. On the other hand, norepinephrine has no effect on β receptors in vascular smooth muscle; thus its pressor effects are decreased by the α blockers but are not converted to a depressor response.

FIG. 16-1

Epinephrine reversal by phentolamine. Effect of epinephrine on blood pressure before and after injection of phentolamine. Dog was anesthetized with pentobarbital sodium. At A, epinephrine was injected intravenously, 1 µg/kg. At B, phentolamine was injected, 5 mg/ kg. At C, epinephrine injection was repeated. Time is given in seconds. Note lowering of mean pressure by epinephrine following adrenergic blocking agent. Increased pulse pressure under these circumstances is an indication that adrenergic blocking agent does not prevent the cardiac stimulant effect of epinephrine.

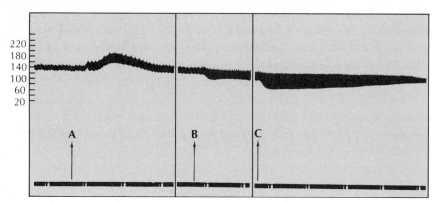

The various drugs in this group differ from each other in potency and duration of action. They may also possess pharmacological properties entirely unrelated to adrenergic blockade.

Differences among various α-adrenergic blocking agents

Phenoxybenzamine hydrochloride

Phenoxybenzamine (Dibenzyline), when administered in doses of 20 to 100 mg, produces lowering of blood pressure and orthostatic hypotension. The effects of the drug last more than 24 hours. It is available in capsules of 10 mg.

PHENOXY-BENZAMINE

The long duration of action of phenoxybenzamine is probably a consequence of a stable combination between the drug and the α receptor. In this case, although competition exists between the drug and catecholamines for the receptor during the early stages of blockade, such competition becomes ineffective as the blockade develops fully. The term *nonequilibrium blockade* has been applied to such an interaction between agonist and antagonist.

Occasional indications for the use of phenoxybenzamine include peripheral vascular diseases in which vasospasm is an important feature (such as Raynaud's disease) and the management of pheochromocytoma both before and during the operation.

Among the many adverse effects that may be caused by phenoxybenzamine, orthostatic hypotension, tachycardia, nasal congestion, and miosis are common and predictable.

TOLAZOLINE HYDROCHLORIDE

Tolazoline hydrochloride (Priscoline), a weak α blocker, causes peripheral vaso-dilatation largely by a direct relaxant effect on vascular smooth muscle. In addition, the drug is a direct cardiac stimulant and its use is often accompanied by tachycardia.

Tolazoline is used in the treatment of peripheral vascular diseases for the relief of vasospasm. It is available in tablets of 25 mg, timed-release tablets of 80 mg, and solution for injection, 25 mg/ml.

Adverse effects of the drug include pilomotor stimulation (gooseflesh), tachycardia, and increased gastrointestinal motility and hydrochloric acid secretion. Tolazoline is related structurally to histamine.

Tolazoline hydrochloride   Phentolamine hydrochloride

PHENTOLAMINE

Phentolamine is an α blocker used almost exclusively for the diagnosis of pheo-chromocytoma and for the prevention of hypertension during operative removal of the tumor. Preparations include phentolamine hydrochloride (Regitine hydrochloride) in tablets, 50 mg, and phentolamine mesylate (Regitine mesylate) in powder for injection, 5 mg. In addition to its blocking action on receptors, the drug has other pharmacological actions similar to those of tolazoline, to which it is chemically related.

Adverse effects include orthostatic hypotension, tachycardia, nasal stuffiness, and gastrointestinal disturbances such as nausea, vomiting, and diarrhea.

In patients having an adrenal medullary tumor, the intravenous injection of 5 mg of phentolamine generally causes a rapid fall of blood pressure, 25 mm Hg diastolic and 33 mm Hg systolic. False positive and false negative reactions may occur, how-ever, and the pharmacological tests for pheochromocytoma are being replaced by the more reliable chemical tests (p. 166).

AZAPETINE PHOSPHATE

Azapetine phosphate (Ilidar), an α-adrenergic blocking drug with additional smooth muscle–relaxing actions on the peripheral vasculature, is used in vasospastic diseases. It is available in tablets, 25 mg.

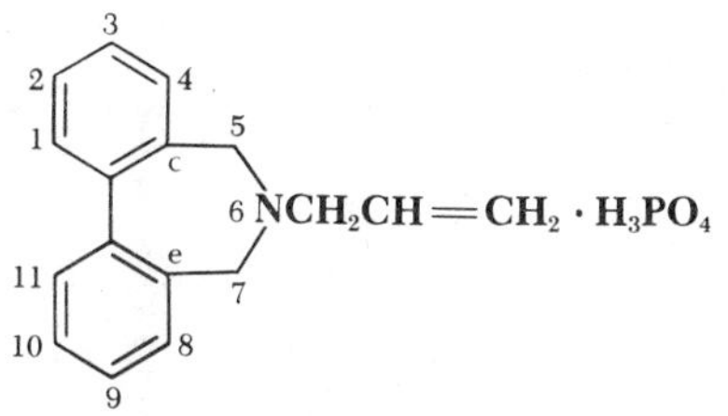

Azapetine phosphate

Prazosin is a recently introduced antihypertensive drug, which initially was thought to act by a direct relaxant effect on vascular smooth muscle. It was later found, however, that prazosin is a powerful but unusual α-blocking agent.[9] It is a useful antihypertensive, which has fewer side effects than the other available α blockers, probably because of its selective action on postsynaptic α receptors. The drug does not cause the marked tachycardia as seen, for example, with phenoxybenzamine. The reason for the difference may lie in the action of phenoxybenzamine in blocking both presynaptic and postsynaptic α receptors. Blockade of the presynaptic receptor prevents released norepinephrine from acting on this receptor to inhibit further transmitter release. Consequently, enhanced norepinephrine release occurs with phenoxybenzamine and can then stimulate unprotected cardiac β receptors. The weak action of prazosin on presynaptic receptors would result in less cardiac stimulation.

PRAZOSIN

Prazosin hydrochloride (Minipress) is available in 1, 2, and 5 mg capsules. Adverse effects include a marked postural hypotension following the first dose. Fortunately, this effect does not generally persist with continued drug use.

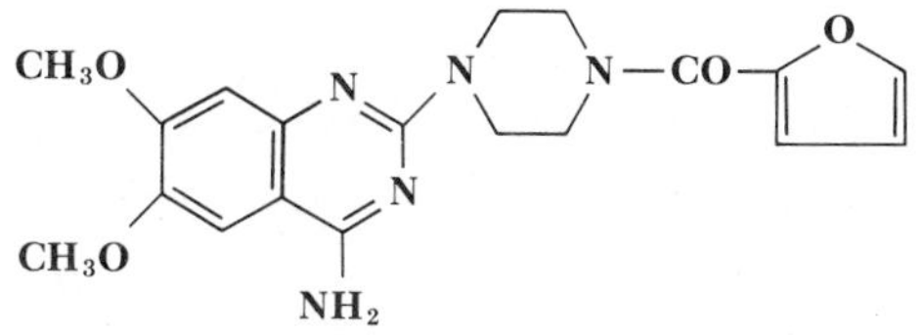

Prazosin

Certain alkaloids of ergot, such as ergotamine, have some α-adrenergic blocking action. They are not used as adrenergic blocking agents. Their pharmacology is discussed in Chapter 21.

ERGOT ALKALOIDS

β-Adrenergic blockers are competitive inhibitors of catecholamines at the β adrenoreceptor. Some of these drugs have relatively greater effect on the β_1 receptor in the heart and differ from each other in their duration of action (Table 16-1). The currently approved β blockers in this country are atenolol (Tenormin), metoprolol (Lopressor), nadolol (Corgard), pindolol (Visken), propranolol (Inderal), and timolol (Timolide). A summary of their properties is shown in Table 16-2.

β-ADRENERGIC BLOCKING AGENTS

TABLE 16-1   Effects of β-adrenergic receptor blockade

Heart rate	Decreased
Myocardial contractility	Decreased
Cardiac output	Decreased
Arterial blood pressure	Unaffected or decreased
Effect of exercise on heart rate and cardiac output	Decreased
Effects of isoproterenol	Blocked
β-Adrenergic drug effects (myocardial, arterial, bronchial, metabolic)	Blocked

TABLE 16-2   Pharmacological properties of some β blockers

Drug	Relative cardioselectivity (β_1)	Sympathomimetic activity	Membrane stabilizing effect
Propranolol	0	0	+ +
Metoprolol	+	0	0
Nadolol	0	0	0
Atenolol	+	0	0
Timolol	0	0	0
Pindolol	0	+	+

Although β blockers were originally developed for the treatment of angina pectoris, they have numerous other clinical indications. These include hypertension, arrhythmia, thyrotoxicosis, hypertrophic cardiomyopathy, migraine, and glaucoma.

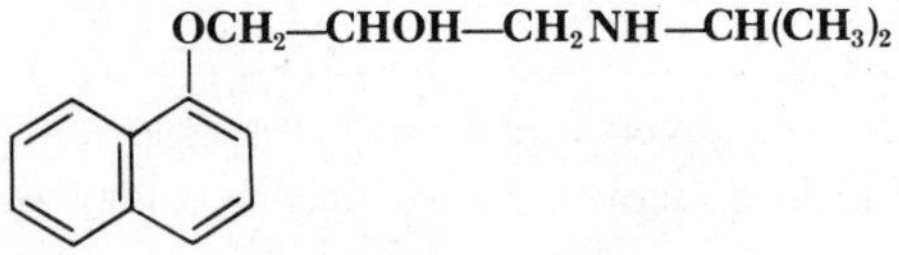

$$OCH_2\!-\!CHOH\!-\!CH_2NH\!-\!CH(CH_3)_2$$

Propranolol

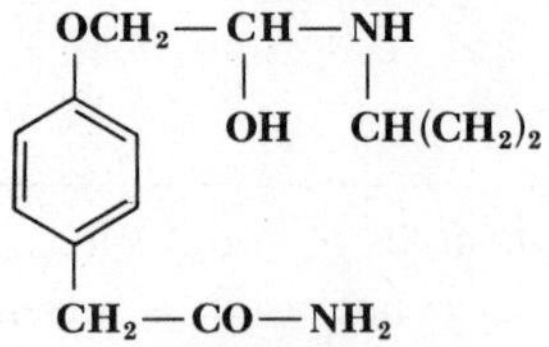

$$OCH_2\!-\!CH\!-\!NH$$
$$OH \quad CH(CH_2)_2$$
$$CH_2\!-\!CO\!-\!NH_2$$

Atenolol

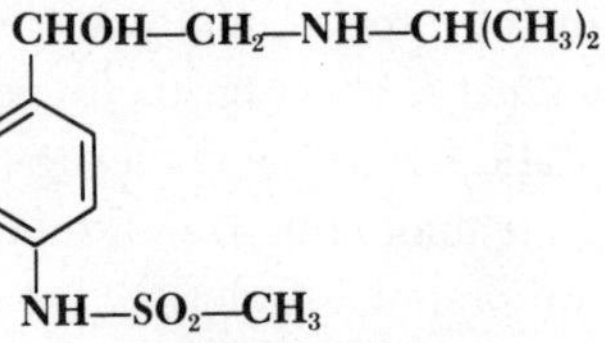

$$CHOH\!-\!CH_2\!-\!NH\!-\!CH(CH_3)_2$$
$$NH\!-\!SO_2\!-\!CH_3$$

Sotalol

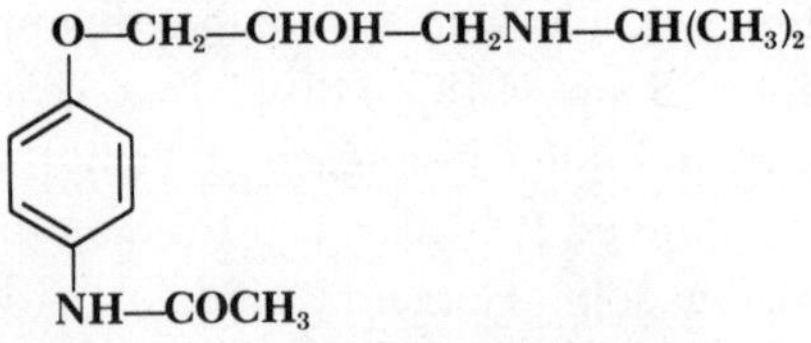

$$O\!-\!CH_2\!-\!CHOH\!-\!CH_2NH\!-\!CH(CH_3)_2$$
$$NH\!-\!COCH_3$$

Practolol

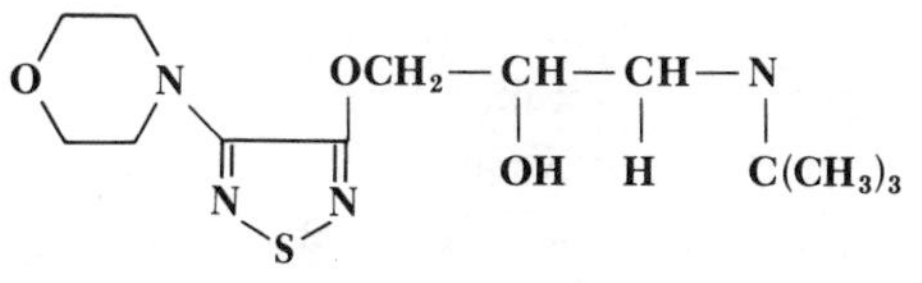

Timolol

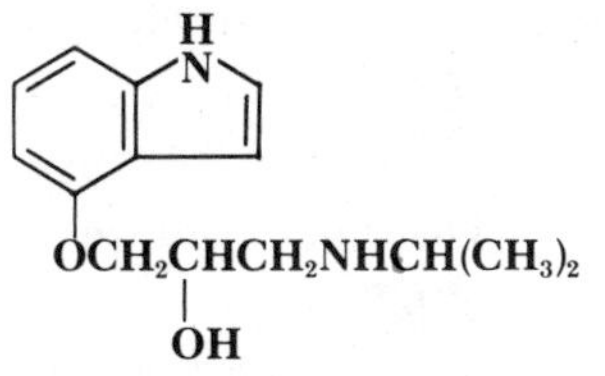

Pindolol

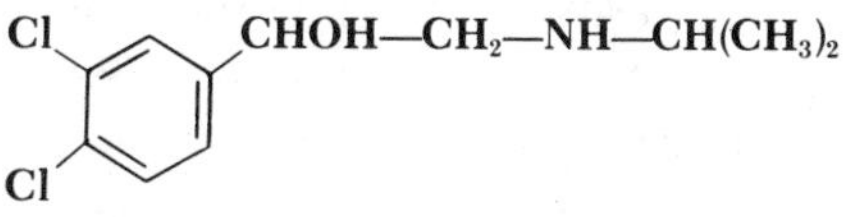

Dichloroisoproterenol

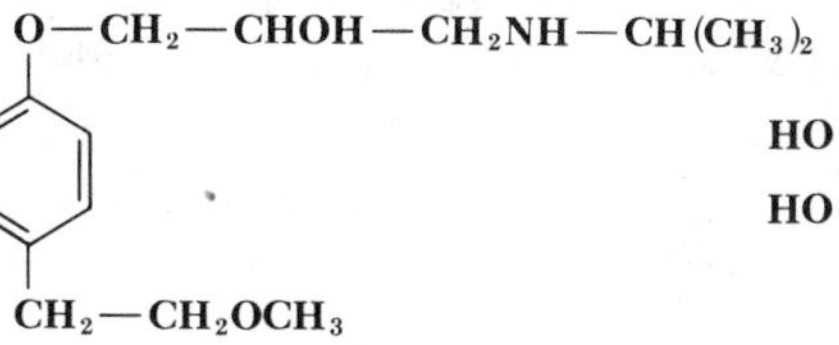

Metoprolol

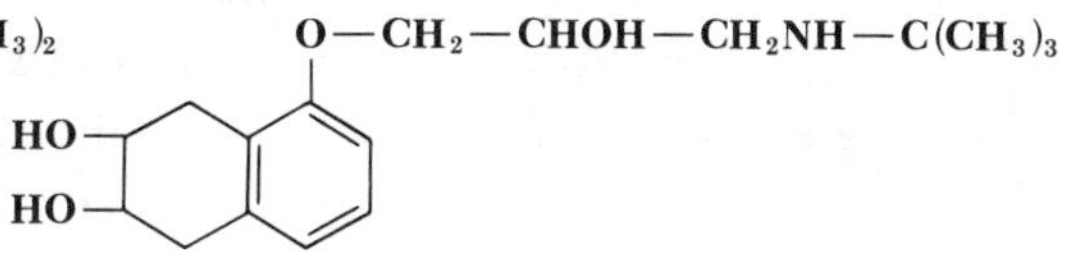

Nadolol

Pharmacological effects. Propranolol antagonizes competitively the effects of catecholamines released from adrenergic nerves or from the adrenal medulla on all β receptors. As a consequence the drug exerts negative chronotropic and inotropic effects on the heart, slows atrioventricular conduction, promotes bronchoconstriction, lowers plasma renin activity, and may cause hypoglycemia. It also exerts some quinidine-like actions on the heart.

Propranolol

The effects of propranolol may be overcome by sufficiently large doses of isoproterenol, which is a β agonist, or by glucagon, which acts on a different receptor but also activates adenyl cyclase.

Pharmacokinetics. Propranolol is absorbed completely from the gastrointestinal tract. About 50% is extracted by the liver as the drug is being absorbed, the so-called first-pass effect. Plasma concentrations are low and variable. The half-life of the drug is 3 hours. The major metabolite, 4-hydroxypropranolol, is active as a β blocker but has a short half-life.[1,3]

Despite its short half-life, propranolol may be administered at 6- to 8-hour intervals to achieve therapeutic effects. Altered renal function has little effect on the dosage regimens. On the other hand, phenobarbital decreases the half-life of the drug.

Clinical uses. Action tremors and *migraine* also respond to propranolol. Glaucoma is especially responsive to the action of timolol.

The *antiarrhythmic effect* of propranolol results largely from β blockade. Its quinidine-like effect may contribute to its effectiveness in digitalis-induced arrhythmias. Propranolol is a racemic mixture. The *levo* form is the β blocker, but the *dextro* form has a greater membrane effect. Propranolol is used in supraventricular tachyarrhythmias such as in thyrotoxicosis. Ventricular tachycardias caused by catecholamines or digitalis are also important indications, but in other types of ventricular tachycardias propranolol is not the first choice.

Angina pectoris is benefited by propranolol in selected patients who do not respond to conventional measures such as sublingual nitroglycerin. The drug should not be used in patients in whom angina is precipitated only by great effort because of the adverse effects of the drug on some properties of the myocardium.

The *antihypertensive effect* of propranolol has not been explained in a completely satisfactory manner.[3] Reduction of cardiac output, inhibition of renin release, and some CNS effects have all been suggested as possible mechanisms of the antihypertensive action of propranolol, but there are arguments against each one of these suggestions.[3] When propranolol is used in combination with a peripheral vasodilator such as hydralazine, its beneficial effect is more easily understandable. Peripheral vasodilation leads to reflex cardiac stimulation, which is blocked by propranolol.

Hypertrophic subaortic stenosis is accompanied by symptoms such as angina, which are made worse by increased cardiac contractility. The usefulness of propranolol then becomes obvious.

Hyperkinetic cardiocirculatory states are benefited by propranolol as a consequence of the ability of the drug to depress cardiac function.

Propranolol is used both before and during surgical intervention for *pheochromocytoma*. By itself, propranolol may cause a rise in arterial pressure in these patients. Thus α-receptor blocking agents must be used simultaneously.

Myocardial infarction. A Norwegian multicenter study showed that timolol reduced mortality in acute myocardial infarction and the rate of reinfarction. Similar results have been reported by other investigators for propranolol and metoprolol. This effect seems to be a general property of the β blockers.

Adverse effects and drug interactions. The major adverse effects of propranolol result from depression of cardiac contractility, heart block, and bronchial constriction.

Propranolol may cause hypoglycemia and interfere with the recovery from hypoglycemia following insulin administration. Propranolol may increase the hypotensive actions of the phenothiazines, and it inhibits the β-adrenergic effects of dopamine administered or formed from levodopa. Propranolol may aggravate the negative inotropic effects of quinidine. The β blocker is used in the treatment of digitalis-induced arrhythmias but may exaggerate bradycardia caused by digitalis. Bradycardia induced by propranolol responds to atropine.

Propranolol withdrawal. Abrupt withdrawal of propranolol and other β blockers leads to increased cardiac excitability and exacerbation of angina or even myocardial infarction. These changes begin in 2 days, and the patient's condition returns to normal in 10 to 14 days. This is generally attributed to up regulation of the β receptors as a consequence of prolonged suppression by the drugs. It is important to withdraw the β blockers very gradually.

Preparations. Propranolol (Inderal) is available in tablets, 10 and 40 mg, and injectable solutions containing 1 mg/ml in 1 ml containers.

Metoprolol (Lopressor) differs from propranolol in its relative cardioselectivity and lack of membrane-stabilizing effect. It has an elimination half-life of 3 to 4 hours.

Nadolol (Corgard) is not cardioselective, but it has an elimination half-life of 14 to 24 hours.

Atenolol (Tenormin) is cardioselective and has a half-life of 6 to 9 hours.

Timolol (Timoptic, Timolide) is not cardioselective, has a favorable effect on glaucoma, and has an elimination half-life of 3 to 4 hours.

Pindolol (Visken) is not cardioselective and has some intrinsic sympathomimetic and membrane-stabilizing effects. Its elimination half-life is 3 to 4 hours.

Newer β-blocking drugs

REFERENCES

1. Evans, G.H., and Shand, D.G.: Disposition of propranolol. V. Drug accumulation and steady-state concentrations during chronic oral administration in man, Clin. Pharmacol. Ther. **14**:487, 1973.
2. Frishman, W.H.: β-adrenoceptor antagonists: new drugs and new indications, N. Engl. J. Med. **305**:500, 1981.
3. Holland, O.B., and Kaplan, N.M.: Propranolol in the treatment of hypertension, N. Engl. J. Med. **294**:930, 1976.
4. Kosinski, E.J., and Malindzak, G.S.: Glucagon and isoproterenol in reversing propranolol toxicity, Arch. Intern. Med. **132**:840, 1973.
5. Prichard, B.N.C.: β-Adrenergic receptor blockade in hypertension, past, present, and future, Br. J. Clin. Pharmacol. **5**:379, 1978.
6. Rangno, R.E.: Stopping beta blockers in patients with angina, Ration. Drug. Ther. **15**:1, 1981.
7. Schelling, J.L., Scazziga, B., Dufour, R.J., Milinkovic, N., and Weber, A.A.: Effect of pindolol, a beta receptor antagonist, in hyperthyroidism, Clin. Pharmacol. Ther. **14**:158, 1973.
8. Stallworth, J.M., and Jeffords, J.V.: Clinical effects of azapetine (Ilidar) on peripheral vascular disease, JAMA **161**:840, 1956.
9. Stokes, G.S., and Oates, H.F.: Prazosin—new alpha adrenergic blocking agent in treatment of hypertension, Cardiovasc. Med. **3**:41, 1978.
10. Winkler, G.F., and Young, R.R.: Efficacy of chronic propranolol therapy in action tremors of the familial, senile or essential varieties, N. Engl. J. Med. **290**:984, 1974.

Chapter 17

Drugs acting on the adrenergic neuron

<table>
<tr><td>

**GENERAL
CONCEPT**

</td><td>

Drugs can influence sympathetic functions by affecting the storage and release of catecholamines, thus providing tools for an entirely new pharmacological approach to the nervous system. Such drugs have found wide application as *antihypertensive agents* and in the field of *psychopharmacology*.

</td></tr>
</table>

This field was opened up by the discovery that reserpine, a *Rauwolfia* alkaloid, caused a release of serotonin (5-hydroxytryptamine) from its binding sites in various tissues. Subsequently, it was shown that reserpine also releases norepinephrine and dopamine. Decreased sympathetic functions induced by reserpine, such as hypotension and bradycardia, are now generally attributed to the catecholamine depletion at the adrenergic nerve endings.

Other drugs can influence catecholamine stores also. Guanethidine causes depletion of peripheral amine stores. On the other hand, bretylium blocks adrenergic fibers without depleting their catecholamine content.

The monoamine oxidase (MAO) inhibitors raise the catecholamine content of neural tissues in several species. This finding suggests that the enzyme may have a regulatory function on the concentration of bound catecholamines. Hypotension that follows the use of MAO inhibitors may be related to the accumulation of norepinephrine or some other amine in ganglia and adrenergic fibers.

**MECHANISMS OF
CATECHOLAMINE
RELEASE**

Drugs may release catecholamines by one of two mechanisms, and these mechanisms may be further influenced by at least four additional pharmacological actions.

The *two basic* mechanisms of release and the drugs that illustrate them are as follows:

    Interference with granular storage mechanism
        Reserpine
        Guanethidine

Schematic representation of nerve ending and effector cell. (For details see text.)   *FIG. 17-1*

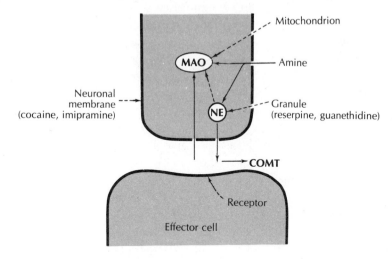

Displacement of catecholamines
   Tyramine
   Amphetamine
   Metaraminol
   Methyldopa (through its metabolite α-methylnorepinephrine)

1. *Interference with granular storage mechanism*. As shown in Fig. 17-1, when catecholamines are released physiologically, a small granule is extruded and its amine acts on the receptor. On the other hand, when the amine is released by drugs such as reserpine or guanethidine, it is freed from the granule within the axoplasm, making it subject to attack by MAO. Instead of the active amine, mostly its inactivated products appear outside the nerve. This is probably the reason why the injection of reserpine, although causing massive depletion of catecholamines, does not result in an elevation of blood pressure.

2. *Displacement of catecholamines*. The indirectly acting sympathomimetic drugs such as tyramine and amphetamine can cause a release of catecholamines. Other amines not only displace catecholamines but also are incorporated into the granule. These include metaraminol and α-methylnorepinephrine. The latter is a metabolite of methyldopa, which undoubtedly causes amine depletion by this indirect mechanism.

The basic mechanisms of catecholamine release can be modified by at least four pharmacological influences.

The *MAO inhibitors* protect the intraneuronally released catecholamines from inactivation.

Certain drugs, the *adrenergic neuronal blocking agents*, prevent catecholamine release induced by nerve stimulation or by the indirectly acting amines such as tyramine. The best known example of such drugs is bretylium. Conceptually, these drugs behave as if they anesthetized the adrenergic fibers. Indeed, they have local anesthetic properties and concentrate in adrenergic fibers.

Drugs that act at the neuronal membrane (Fig. 17-1) such as cocaine and imipramine have several important actions on catecholamine release. They block the action of tyramine and other indirectly acting amines. They do not block the action of reserpine, a point in favor of a difference in the site of action of tyramine and reserpine. Cocaine and other drugs that inhibit the membrane pump for amines cause an apparent "sensitization" of the receptor by allowing the local accumulation of catecholamine.

Drugs may act on presynaptic α or β receptors that modulate catecholamine release.[5]

Basic differences between the actions of reserpine and guanethidine	Although both reserpine and guanethidine deplete nerves of their catecholamine by acting on the granular storage mechanism, guanethidine has additional effects. Its intravenous injection regularly leads to a transient elevation of blood pressure, caused by a *tyramine-like* effect that can be blocked by cocaine. To make matters more complex, guanethidine has an early *bretylium-like* effect that somehow interferes with norepinephrine release after nerve stimulation.

An additional difference between reserpine and guanethidine is of great importance. Reserpine depletes catecholamines and serotonin from many sites, including the brain. Guanethidine apparently fails to cross the blood-brain barrier and thus has no effect on brain amines. |
| *Mechanism of decreased sympathetic activity induced by catecholamine depletion* | When the catecholamine content of a nerve is decreased to below 50%, stimulation of the nerve results in a lessened response. The rate of depletion varies in different organs. Cardiac catecholamine declines rapidly, and adrenal stores are more resistant. The rate of depletion is a function not only of the dose of reserpine but also of the rate of turnover of the amine at the various sites. It has been estimated that the half-time of catecholamines in the heart is 4 to 8 hours, in contrast with their half-time of 7 days in the adrenal medulla. Depletion must be rapid in arterioles and venules. This is why reserpine is useful as an antihypertensive drug. |
| *RESERPINE* | Alkaloids of *Rauwolfia serpentina* have antihypertensive and tranquilizing properties. Reserpine and some other *Rauwolfia* alkaloids produce depletion of norepinephrine, dopamine, and also serotonin from various binding sites in the brain and peripheral nerves. The drug not only causes a release of amines but also blocks their granular uptake. It does not, however, block the action of catecholamines. It may have some blocking effect on norepinephrine synthesis by preventing the uptake of dopamine into storage granules that contain dopamine-β-oxidase. |

The antihypertensive drug guanethidine (Ismelin) causes decreased sympathetic activity by a dual mechanism, depleting norepinephrine at peripheral nerve endings in the manner of reserpine and also causing early sympathetic neuronal blockade at a time when catecholamines are not yet depleted in the nerve. It is not a ganglionic blocking agent and does not prevent the action of catecholamines (p. 201). *GUANETHIDINE*

Debrisoquine (Declinax) is structurally related to guanethidine, but it produces adrenergic neuronal blockade by the same mechanisms as bretylium. It is a potent antihypertensive agent when used in the same dosage as guanethidine.[7] *DEBRISOQUINE*

The studies showing that debrisoquine as well as bretylium inhibits MAO and is apparently concentrated in the adrenergic neurons throw new light on the mode of action of these drugs.

Bretylium (Darenthin) produces a selective block on the peripheral sympathetic nervous system without opposing the action of injected or released catecholamines. *BRETYLIUM*

Bretylium tosylate

Bretylium blocks the adrenergic fiber without depleting its catecholamine content and may act as a local anesthetic that concentrates in adrenergic fibers.

Bretylium blocks the enzyme MAO; perhaps this action in the adrenergic nerves explains its action.

Although bretylium is basically a very interesting drug, its clinical use has been attended by so many toxic effects, including muscular weakness and mental confusion, that it is no longer available. There is some interest in its experimental use as an antiarrhythmic drug.

Methyldopa (Aldomet), an analog of dihydroxyphenylalanine, competes with this precursor of norepinephrine for the enzyme that decarboxylates aromatic L-amino acids. Although it inhibits the synthesis of both norepinephrine and serotonin, norepinephrine levels in the brain remain low for a much longer time than serotonin levels. This and other evidence suggests that much of the catecholamine depletion induced by methyldopa is caused by the drug's being metabolized to form α-methylnorepinephrine that replaces norepinephrine and acts as a "false transmitter." The various consequences of the presence of false transmitters are summarized in Fig. 17-2. *METHYLDOPA*

MAO inhibitors were introduced as antidepressants. One of their surprising side effects was orthostatic hypotension, which suggested interference with sympathetic functions. *MAO INHIBITORS*

FIG. 17-2 *Catecholamine metabolism in the adrenergic neuron, indicating the possible role of false transmitters.*

From Kopin, I.J.: In Adrenergic neurotransmission, Ciba Foundation Study Group No. 33, Boston, 1968, Little, Brown & Co.

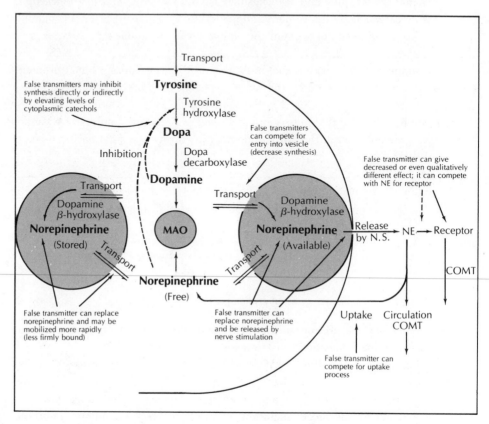

Experimentally, the MAO inhibitors elevate the levels of norepinephrine and serotonin in the brain, ganglia, and other peripheral tissues. In addition, they prevent many of the actions of reserpine, including its ability to lower amine levels.

One of the serious disadvantages of the MAO inhibitors is the increased likelihood of adverse reactions to ingested foods and to drugs that may release monoamines in the body. The ingestion of aged cheese, beer, or certain wines has caused hypertensive emergencies in patients who were being treated with MAO inhibitors. These serious reactions have been traced to the presence of tyramine in these foods and beverages. Tyramine would normally be deaminated by MAO. When its deamination is inhibited by drugs, it releases catecholamines in the body. Adverse reactions to indirectly acting sympathomimetic drugs have also occurred under similar circumstances.

Although most MAO inhibitors are used as antidepressants, one of these, pargyline (Eutonyl), was introduced as an antihypertensive agent.[3]

REFERENCES

1. Anderson, J.L., Popat, K.D., and Pitt, B.: Paradoxical ventricular tachycardia and fibrillation after intravenous bretylium therapy, Arch. Intern. Med. **141**:301, 1981.

2. Brodie, B.B., Olin, J.S., Kuntzman, R.G., and Shore, P.A.: Possible interrelationships between release of brain norepinephrine and serotonin by reserpine, Science **125**:1293, 1957.

3. Bryant, J.M., Torosdag, S., Schvartz, N., Fletcher, L., Fertig, H., Schwartz, S., and Quan, R.B.F.: Antihypertensive properties of pargyline hydrochloride, JAMA **178**:406, 1961.

4. Heisenbluttel, R.H., and Bigger, J.T.: Bretylium tosylate: a newly available antiarrhythmic drug for ventricular arrhythmias, Ann. Intern. Med. **91**:229, 1979.

5. Langer, S.Z.: Presynaptic regulation of catecholamine release, Biochem. Pharmacol. **23**:1793, 1974.

6. Maxwell, R.A., and Wastila, W.B.: Adrenergic neuron blocking drugs, Handbook Exp. Pharmacol. **39**:161, 1977.

7. Moe, R.A., et al.: Cardiovascular effects of 3,4,-dihydro-2(1H) isoquinoline carboxamidine (Declinax), Curr. Ther. Res. **6**:299, 1964.

8. Shore, P.A.: Release of serotonin and catecholamines by drugs, Pharmacol. Rev. **14**:531, 1962.

9. Shore, P.A.: Transport and storage of biogenic amines, Annu. Rev. Pharmacol. **12**:209, 1972.

10. Starke, K., and Montel, H.: Alpha-receptor mediated modulation of transmitter release from central noradrenergic neurones, NaunynSchniedebergs Arch. Pharmacol. **279**:53, 1973.

Chapter 18

Antihypertensive drugs

GENERAL
CONCEPT

Effective treatment of hypertension is one of the major developments in medicine. Beginning in 1949 when ganglionic blocking agents were introduced, a series of important discoveries occurred, which led to the present availability of numerous antihypertensive drugs that are capable of exerting a favorable effect on life expectancy and the complications of hypertension.[9,17,18]

Some of the most significant developments that led to the present state of antihypertensive treatment were the introduction of hydralazine in 1952, reserpine in 1953, the thiazide diuretics in 1959, guanethidine in 1960, methyldopa and clonidine in 1967, β-adrenergic blocking drugs in 1968, and recently, prazosin, an α-adrenergic blocking drug. It appears at present that the introductions of the thiazide diuretics and the β-adrenergic blocking drugs have had the greatest impact on the management of hypertension.

The antihypertensive drugs act by many different mechanisms, as summarized in Table 18-1. An understanding of these mechanisms is essential for tailoring antihypertensive therapy to the individual patient's requirement. A diagrammatic representation of blood pressure–regulating mechanisms is shown in Fig. 18-1.

RELATION OF
ANGIOTENSIN AND
ALDOSTERONE TO
HYPERTENSION

The demonstration that renal ischemia leads to hypertension resulted in the discovery of a kidney enzyme, renin, which is in the granules of the juxtaglomerular apparatus. When this enzyme is released by ischemia or perhaps by a decreased caliber of the afferent arteriole, it acts on a substrate in blood and eventually yields angiotensin, a potent vasopressor polypeptide. This sequence of events is shown in Table 18-2.

The amino acid composition of angiotensin I is as follows:

Asp-Arg-Val-Tyr-Ileu-His-Pro-Phe-His-Leu

The converting enzyme removes the terminal histidyl-leucine to form angiotensin II. Angiotensin I has little or no biological activity, although it may have some effect

TABLE 18-1   Site of action of antihypertensive drugs

Site of action	Mode of action	Drug	Trade name
Arteriolar smooth muscle	Direct vasodilatation	Hydralazine Diazoxide Minoxidil Nitroprusside	Apresoline Hyperstat Loniten Nipride
α-Adrenergic receptors	Receptor blockade	Phentolamine Phenoxybenzamine Prazosin	Regitine Dibenzyline Minipress
β-Adrenergic receptors	CNS effect Myocardial depression Renin release inhibition	Propranolol Metoprolol	Inderal Lopressor
Sympathetic fibers	Blockade of norepinephrine release (also depletion) Inhibition of MAO	Guanethidine Pargyline	Ismelin Eutonyl
Paravertebral ganglia	Ganglionic blockade	Chlorisondamine Hexamethonium Mecamylamine Pentolinium Trimethaphan	Ecolid Inversine Ansolysen Arfonad
CNS	Depression of cardiovascular control center False neurotransmitter Norepinephrine depletion	Clonidine Methyldopa Reserpine	Catapres Aldomet Many
Carotid sinus	Reflex sympathetic depression	Veratrum Electric stimulation	
Kidney	Sodium excretion Volume depletion	Many diuretics	

TABLE 18-2   Metabolism of angiotensin

Sequence	Inhibitors
Renin in kidney ↓	β Blockers
Renin released + Angiotensinogen ↓	
Angiotensin I (decapeptide) +	
Converting enzyme ↓	Inhibitors (captopril)
Angiotensin II (octapeptide) +	Antagonists (saralasin)
Angiotensinases A, B, C ↓ ↘	
Angiotensin III Split product (heptapeptide)	

FIG. 18-1   *Diagrammatic representation of blood pressure–regulating mechanisms.*
From Abrams, W.B.: Dis. Chest **55**:148, 1969.

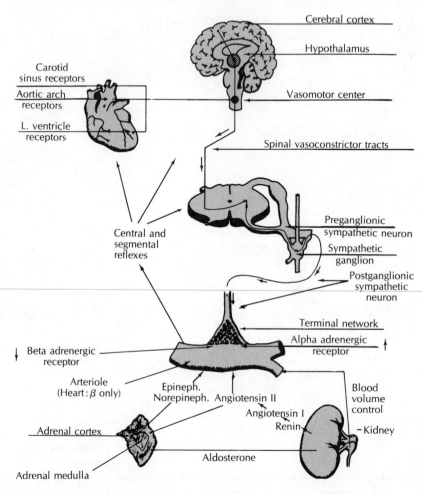

on aldosterone release, as does angiotensin III. Oral contraceptives increase the renin substrate concentrations and promote angiotensin formation.

Saralasin (1-sarcosyl-8-alanyl-angiotensin II) is a specific angiotensin antagonist with essentially no other pharmacological action. Given intravenously it serves as an investigational tool for determining the contribution of angiotensin to the blood pressure elevation.

Renin release   The release of renin from the juxtaglomerular apparatus of the kidney is under intensive investigation. Lowering of blood pressure and renal perfusion pressure promotes the release of the enzyme. Some of the effect of lowered blood pressure on renin release may be mediated through sympathetic fibers. In fact, catecholamines can cause renin release. They do this apparently by acting on β receptors, since propranolol blocks catecholamine-induced renin release.

The pharmacological effects of angiotensin II (hereafter referred to as angiotensin) are as follows: (1) elevation of blood pressure, (2) contraction of isolated smooth muscle preparations, (3) release of aldosterone, and (4) release of catecholamines from adrenal medulla and adrenergic nerves. Not only does angiotensin release catecholamines but it also prevents their reuptake by adrenergic nerves. *Pharmacological effects*

The vasopressor effects of angiotensin are exerted primarily on peripheral resistance vessels in the skin, splanchnic area, and kidney. It has little cardiac stimulant action. The capacitance vessels are not greatly affected by it, differing in this respect from the response to catecholamines.

Several features of the action of angiotensin are of great interest in research on hypertension. This polypeptide has an effect on the vasomotor centers, resulting in increased sympathetic activity. It also potentiates the actions of catecholamines. It causes sodium retention by promoting the release of aldosterone from the adrenal cortex. Angiotensin is a potent central dipsogenic agent in animals and can alter vasopressin secretion.

The renin-angiotensin system along with the sympathetic nervous system plays a role in many hypertensive states. Since both plasma renin activity and catecholamine concentrations can be measured, the selection of antihypertensive medications is increasingly influenced by these measurements.

The various antihypertensive drugs may be classified according to their mode of action as shown in Table 18-1. They will be discussed under the headings of direct vasodilators, α-adrenergic blocking drugs, β-adrenergic blocking drugs, MAO inhibitors, ganglionic blocking agents, central depressants of sympathetic functions, reflex inhibitors of central sympathetic function, and antihypertensive drugs that promote salt excretion. *CLASSIFICATION OF ANTIHYPERTENSIVE DRUGS*

Direct vasodilators act on the vascular smooth muscle. They include hydralazine (Apresoline) and minoxidil (Loniten) for chronic use. Diazoxide (Hyperstat) and sodium nitroprusside (Nipride) are reserved for active hypertensive emergencies. *DIRECT VASODILATORS*

Hydralazine hydrochloride (1-hydrazinophthalazine hydrochloride) (Apresoline) is a direct relaxant of the vascular smooth muscle that is used commonly in chronic hypertension. Although the drug relaxes the vascular smooth muscle, it often produces considerable cardiac stimulation through reflex mechanisms. The cardiac effects may be prevented by β-adrenergic blocking agents. *Hydralazine*

Headache, palpitations, and gastrointestinal disturbances are not uncommon after taking the drug. A unique and more serious adverse effect is seen frequently when doses larger than 200 mg daily are administered. Many such patients develop a *ADVERSE EFFECTS* syndrome resembling systemic lupus erythematosus. This syndrome is reversible in most cases.

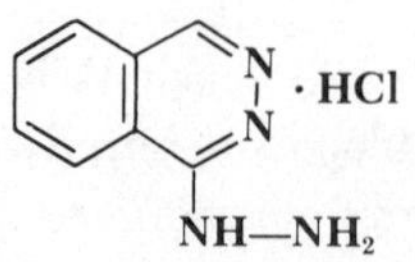

Hydralazine hydrochloride

The combined use of hydralazine and β blockers is becoming widely accepted in the management of hypertension. With the addition of a diuretic, the combination is quite effective.

PREPARATIONS   Hydralazine hydrochloride (Apresoline) is obtainable in tablets of 10, 25, 50, and 100 mg and in a solution for injection, 20 mg/ml.

Minoxidil   Minoxidil (Loniten) is a recently introduced powerful vasodilator, which is administered orally. It is indicated only for patients with severe hypertension who do not respond to other drugs. Minoxidil causes considerable sodium retention and edema, tachycardia, and hirsutism. The sodium retention may be controlled by the use of potent diuretics, and the tachycardia responds to β blockers. Minoxidil has produced hemorrhagic right atrial lesions in dogs, an effect that apparently does not occur in humans.[13]

Minoxidil (Loniten) is available in tablet form. The initial dose should be 5 mg, and the dosage is increased gradually to 40 mg a day in single or divided doses. The antihypertensive effect of the drug lasts at least 12 hours.

Diazoxide   Diazoxide (Hyperstat) is a nondiuretic congener of the thiazide drugs. Administered intravenously, it can be used for the rapid lowering of blood pressure in hypertensive emergencies. The effect lasts about 12 hours. Injection of diazoxide causes hyperglycemia as a consequence of inhibition of insulin release.

PREPARATION AND DOSAGE   Diazoxide (Hyperstat) is supplied in a 20 ml ampule containing 300 mg of the drug. The preparation is injected intravenously and rapidly. Blood pressure decreases within 2 minutes to its lowest level. Then it increases fairly rapidly for 30 minutes and more slowly for the next 2 to 12 hours.

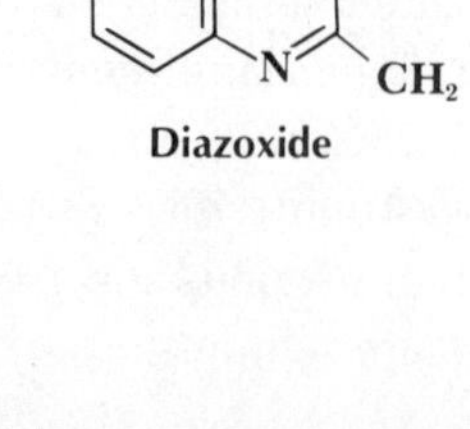

Diazoxide

Sodium nitroprusside (Nipride) is a direct vasodilator that has been approved for use in hypertensive crises. A dose of 1 μg/kg/min administered by intravenous infusion produces a rapid lowering of the blood pressure. The infusion rate must be adjusted by monitoring the blood pressure. The drug is very sensitive to light, and the infusion system should be protected against light.

Sodium nitroprusside

Adverse effects of nitroprusside include nausea, disorientation, and muscle spasms. The metabolic product of nitroprusside, thiocyanate, is excreted by the kidney. Toxic effects may develop in patients who have renal impairment. Also, patients with hepatic impairment will detoxify the drug more slowly. When infused for prolonged periods to create a bloodless field in surgical procedures, thiocyanate and cyanide concentrations in the blood may become elevated, and delayed metabolic acidosis may supervene. The dosage of sodium nitroprusside should probably not exceed 500 μg/kg to avoid these toxic effects.

Sodium nitroprusside (Nipride) is available in 5 ml amber-colored vials containing the equivalent of 50 mg sodium nitroprusside dihydrate for reconstitution with dextrose in water for intravenous infusion.

The α-adrenergic blocking drugs, such as phenoxybenzamine and phentolamine (Chapter 16), have not been useful in the management of hypertension because of their tendency to produce postural hypotension and marked reflex tachycardia. A relatively new α-adrenergic blocking drug, prazosin (Minipress), does not cause as much tachycardia as the other drugs of the same class or as hydralazine.

α-ADRENERGIC BLOCKING DRUGS

Prazosin hydrochloride (Minipress) exerts its antihypertensive action by blocking postsynaptic α_1-adrenergic receptors in blood vessels. Its superiority over other α-blocking drugs is attributed to its greater affinity for postsynaptic receptors than for presynaptic α_2-adrenergic receptors. Blockade of presynaptic receptors by phenoxybenzamine or phentolamine results in increased release of norepinephrine. Prazosin has little effect on presynaptic receptors.[6]

Prazosin

Prazosin

Following oral administration, plasma concentrations of prazosin peak between 1 and 3 hours, the drug having a half-life of about 4 hours. Prazosin is excreted mainly through biliary excretion in the form of inactive metabolites.

Prazosin is an effective antihypertensive drug, particularly when combined with a diuretic. It may be especially useful in patients who do not respond well to a β blocker–diuretic combination. Prazosin dilates both the systemic arterial and venous beds and has been found useful in the treatment of heart failure, since it reduces preload and afterload without causing cardiac acceleration.

UNTOWARD EFFECTS A commonly encountered effect of prazosin is often called the *first-dose phe-nomenon*,[6] characterized by weakness often progressing to syncope, which occurs within 1 hour after the first dose is taken. It is probably caused by postural hypotension and is aggravated by exercise and sodium depletion. The drug may aggravate angina. Prazosin hydrochloride (Minipress) is available in 1 and 5 mg tablets. The initial dose should be 1 mg two or three times a day.

> PROBLEM 18-1. *Why is it necessary to use an α blocker during the operation for pheochromo-cytoma when a β blocker is being administered? Manipulation of the tumor results in the release of norepinephrine and epinephrine from the tumor. These catecholamines would produce excessive hypertension in the presence of a β blocker. Thus an α blocker must be added.*

β-ADRENERGIC BLOCKING DRUGS The β-adrenergic blocking drugs are widely used in the treatment of hypertension. In combination with a diuretic they are quite effective and produce fewer adverse effects than most antihypertensive drugs. For several years propranolol (Inderal) was the only β blocker available in this country. The antihypertensive effect of this drug was quite unexpected and was discovered accidentally when patients with hypertension and angina were treated with β blockers in England. With the recognition of the existence of β_1, or cardiac, receptors efforts were made to develop specific blocking drugs for these receptors that would not effect the β_2 receptors mediating catecholamine effects on the bronchial tree and vasodilator influences. Such a cardioselective β_1-receptor blocker is now available in the form of metoprolol (Lopressor). Nadolol (Corgard) is a longer acting nonselective β blocker. Atenolol (Tenormin) and pindolol (Visken) are other drugs in this class.

Mechanism of action Despite extensive investigations, the mechanism of the antihypertensive action of the β-blocking drugs is not known.[7] A single statement explaining the mechanism of action of *all* β blockers in *all* hypertensive patients cannot be made. Main theories for this drug class center on (1) *CNS effects*, (2) *decreased renin release*, and (3) *reduced cardiac output*. One or more of these actions is probably relevant in individual patients.

The following issues illustrate the difficulty that exists when trying to make one of these theories encompass all patients. (1) *CNS effects:* Some β blockers are thought not to penetrate the CNS but are fully effective. On the other hand, whether CNS penetration occurs with chronic use or small amounts of drug reach a localized site in the CNS are unresolved possibilities. Animal studies with CNS administration of β blockers have shown interaction with cardiovascular integrating sites. (2) *Decreased renin release:* Reductions in blood pressure can occur when plasma renin activity is unaffected by β blockers; thus, this action alone cannot be an *absolute* necessity for hypotension. Reports exist that document no change in blood pressure control in patients switched from one β blocker to another having some intrinsic activity. Plasma renin activity rose after the drug switch, but blood pressure control was unaffected. On the other hand, there are patients who respond to β-blocking drugs with a clear fall in plasma renin activity and decreased daily aldosterone output. (3) *Reduced cardiac output:* β Blockers reduce cardiac output in *essentially all subjects,* but only a portion will respond with a chronic hypotensive effect. Why? One possibility is that the baroreceptors do not neutralize the fall in cardiac output in some patients who thus "respond" with a fall in blood pressure. "Nonresponders" may be those whose baroreceptor function effectively neutralizes the fall in cardiac output.

Propranolol

Propranolol (Inderal) is the most widely used β blocker in hypertension. Its mechanism of action is still poorly understood. Although the drug blocks renin release and reduces cardiac output,[8] these effects cannot explain the usefulness of the drug as an antihypertensive agent.

PHARMACOKINETICS

Propranolol is well absorbed from the intestine, but 50% to 70% of an oral dose is extracted and metabolized by the liver during the first pass. The major metabolite, 4-hydroxypropranolol, is active but has a shorter half-life. Propranolol as a half-life of 4 to 6 hours. Despite its short half-life, twice-daily dosage may be sufficient in most patients.

EFFECTIVENESS

It has been shown in a cooperative study[18] that blood pressure was well controlled in only 52% of patients when propranolol was taken alone. In combination with a diuretic this percentage increased to 81%, and the addition of hydralazine to the propranolol-diuretic combination produced good results in 92% of the patients. Propranolol then has a major role in combination therapy, particularly because it can counteract some of the adverse hemodynamic effects of other antihypertensive agents. Propranolol is very useful in patients who have anginal pain.

ADVERSE EFFECTS

Propranolol does not cause orthostatic hypotension. It may produce congestive failure and asthmatic attacks in susceptible individuals. Bradycardia is common but is not a contraindication to continued therapy. Gastrointestinal side effects, Raynaud's phenomenon, and worsening of claudication are rare. The drug has a disadvantage in insulin-dependent diabetic patients, since it may mask the symptoms of hypoglycemia. The majority of patients taking propranolol show no adverse effects of any kind.

DOSAGE AND ADMINISTRATION

Propranolol (Inderal) is available in 10, 20, 40, 60, and 80 mg tablets. Dosage for the treatment of hypertension must be individualized. Initial dosage is 80 mg daily in divided doses. The usual effective dose range is 160 to 480 mg daily.

Metoprolol

Metoprolol (Lopressor) is a cardioselective agent, since it blocks β receptors in the heart preferentially.[10] The drug can be used in patients with asthma and in those having intermittent claudication. The plasma half-life of metoprolol is 3 to 6 hours, but the antihypertensive effect is longer, and the drug may be given twice daily in a total daily dose of 50 to 200 mg. The drug is available in 50 and 100 mg tablets.

Nadolol

Nadolol (Corgard) is a β blocker characterized by slow elimination, having a plasma half-life of 12 hours. Thus it may be used once a day in the chronic management of hypertension. The drug is excreted unchanged in the urine and stool.

Atenolol

Atenolol (Tenormin) is a relatively cardioselective β blocker, which has a half-life of 6 to 9 hours.

Pindolol

Pindolol (Visken) is not cardioselective but has some intrinsic sympathomimetic activity. Its half-life is 3 to 4 hours.

• • •

Generally the antihypertensive action of the β blockers is very similar. Their great popularity is due to the fact that they produce relatively few undesirable side effects. Side effects of β-blocker therapy include bronchospasm, congestive heart failure, bradyarrhythmia, sedation, abnormal response to hypoglycemia, hyperglycemia, acute withdrawal syndrome, blood lipid changes, and gastrointestinal symptoms.

ADRENERGIC NEURONAL BLOCKING DRUGS

A number of drugs, such as guanethidine, other guanidine compounds, and bretylium, can block the release of catecholamines from adrenergic nerve fibers.

Guanethidine

Guanethidine sulfate (Ismelin) is an adrenergic neuronal blocking agent, which is a highly effective antihypertensive drug. In addition to blocking adrenergic neurons, guanethidine causes catecholamine release and depletion. In this respect it resembles reserpine with the important difference that it does not cross the blood-brain barrier.

MODE OF ACTION

Guanethidine blocks adrenergic neurons selectively because it is concentrated within the neurons by the same membrane transport system that pumps norepinephrine into the nerves following its release. The tricyclic antidepressants oppose the antihypertensive actions of guanethidine because they block its uptake into the adrenergic neurons.

In addition to its adrenergic neuronal blocking actions, guanethidine causes some catecholamine depletion, which may be termed a *reserpine-like effect*. Other less important actions consist of a tyramine-like effect, meaning that the drug can cause release of catecholamines, and a *cocaine-like effect*, which refers to blockade of the membrane amine pump. The adrenergic neuronal blocking action is sometimes referred to as a *bretylium-like effect*.

CLINICAL PHARMACOLOGY

The onset of action of guanethidine is slow. Maximum effects may not develop for 2 or 3 days after initiation of treatment. For this reason patients are started on small doses such as 10 mg once daily, which are maintained for 5 to 7 days before the amount of drug administered is increased. Guanethidine is a drug with long duration of action. Its effect may persist for 7 days after its administration has been discontinued.

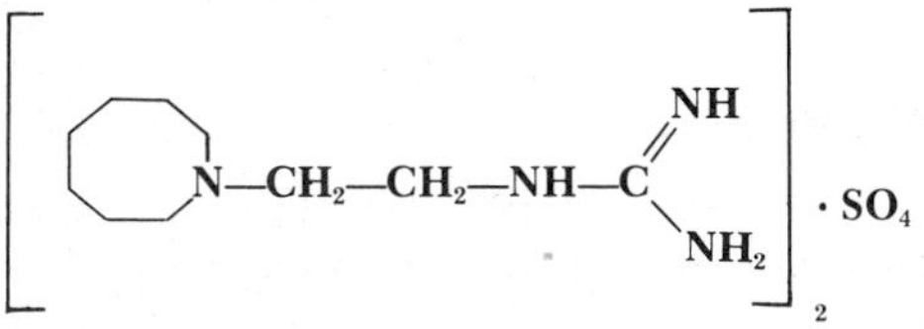

Guanethidine sulfate

The absorption of guanethidine is only about 50% of the orally administered dose. The drug is largely excreted by the kidney.

Guanethidine has a great advantage over reserpine in that it does not cross the blood-brain barrier and thus does not cause sedation and depression. It has replaced the ganglionic blocking agents because it does not inhibit parasympathetic ganglia. It has a strange effect on male sexual function, preventing ejaculation without affecting erection.

PREPARATIONS

Guanethidine sulfate (Ismelin) is available in tablets containing 10 and 25 mg. No parenteral forms are available because the drug is not useful for the treatment of hypertensive emergencies. In fact, it could aggravate them.

MAO INHIBITORS

One of the common side effects of MAO inhibitors is postural hypotension (p. 270). Although the mechanism of this is not well understood, at least one member of the series has been introduced as an antihypertensive agent.

Pargyline (Eutonyl) is administered orally in doses of 25 to 50 mg once daily. Side effects consist of orthostatic hypotension, gastrointestinal disturbances, insomnia, and headaches.

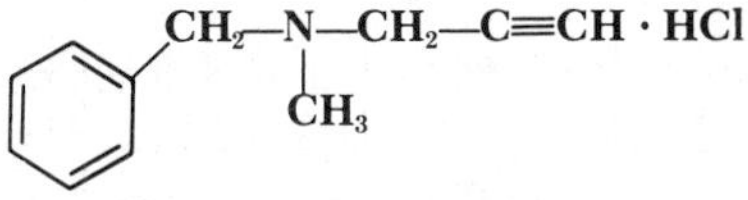

Pargyline hydrochloride

Probably the greatest disadvantage of the MAO inhibitors is their incompatibility with a large variety of drugs. Thus in patients receiving pargyline the indirect sympathomimetics would be contraindicated, as shown by the violent reaction to foods containing tyramine in such patients. Also, combinations of antidepressants are strictly contraindicated (p. 271). It is difficult to see why the drug should be used in the face of so many dangers.

Pargyline (Eutonyl) comes in tablets containing 10, 25, and 50 mg of the drug.

GANGLIONIC BLOCKING AGENTS

The ganglionic blocking agents (Chapter 13) such as hexamethonium, pentolinium, and mecamylamine have received extensive trial in hypertensive diseases. Reductions of blood pressure, particularly in the standing position, can be achieved, but again the inevitable side effects of orthostatic hypotension and parasympathetic ganglionic blockade complicate this approach to the management of hypertension.

CENTRAL DEPRESSANTS OF SYMPATHETIC FUNCTIONS
Clonidine

Clonidine hydrochloride (Catapres) acts by α_2-receptor stimulation in the CNS to lower blood pressure. In combination with a diuretic, clonidine is suitable for long-term therapy. A rebound increase in blood pressure has been reported following rapid withdrawal of clonidine.[11,12]

Clonidine

MODE OF ACTION

The intravenous administration of clonidine is followed by a transient pressor response and a more sustained depressor effect accompanied by bradycardia. It is believed that the initial pressor response is exerted on peripheral α receptors. The antihypertensive action is probably the result of an action of the drug on α receptors within the CNS and on cardiovascular centers in the medulla.

It is believed that there is a noradrenergic component in the central baroreceptor reflex pathway.[11] Norepinephrine lowers the blood pressure when injected into the cisterna magna. Clonidine may act on the same receptors as norepinephrine, thus mimicking the actions of baroreceptor stimulation. Clonidine is a potent α_2 agonist.

ADVERSE REACTIONS AND DRUG INTERACTIONS

Drowsiness and dryness of the mouth are common adverse effects. Constipation occurs in some patients. Postural hypotension is rare. Withdrawal symptoms on discontinuation of clonidine therapy include restlessness, tachycardia, and a rebound increase in blood pressure. Desipramine and other tricyclic antidepressants may interfere with the antihypertensive effects of clonidine.

METABOLISM

Clonidine is absorbed well after oral administration. Plasma levels reach their peak within 3 to 5 hours and the half-life is 12 to 16 hours. Following oral administration, 60% of the drug is excreted by the kidney, mostly in the form of metabolites.

Clonidine hydrochloride (Catapres) is available in the form of tablets, 0.1 and 0.2 mg. The initial dose for adults is 0.1 mg two or three times daily. The usual maintenance dose is 0.2 to 0.8 mg daily. Dosage must be adjusted to the patient's requirement. The drug is more effective if it is given in association with a diuretic. It is also more potent for reducing the blood pressure in the upright position. Withdrawal symptoms are more likely to occur if larger doses (more than 1.2 mg daily) are employed.

PREPARATIONS AND DOSAGES

Methyldopa (Aldomet) was introduced as an antihypertensive drug on the theory that, being an inhibitor of aromatic amino acid decarboxylase, it would lower catecholamine concentrations in the body by that mechanism. It was found, however, that the drug is taken up and metabolized to α-methylnorepinephrine.

Methyldopa

The mode of antihypertensive action of methyldopa is not completely understood. It appears to act on central adrenergic mechanisms through its metabolite α-methylnorepinephrine.

$$HO-\!\!\!\!\!\!\bigcirc\!\!\!\!-CH_2-\underset{\underset{CH_3}{|}}{\overset{\overset{NH_2}{|}}{C}}-COOH$$

Methyldopa

Methyldopa is recommended for the treatment of most types of hypertension. It is preferred by some for patients with chronic renal disease and in hypertensive emergencies. For the latter, the drug may be injected intravenously—in contrast with guanethidine, which is only used orally. Methyldopa causes much less orthostatic hypotension than guanethidine, ganglionic blocking drugs, or MAO inhibitors.

Adverse reactions to methyldopa include marked drowsiness in many patients, depression, and nightmares. In some individuals the administration of methyldopa is followed in about a week by an influenza-like reaction that may be caused by sensitization to the drug. In some of these individuals, subsequent administration of small doses of methyldopa will elicit the same reaction. This syndrome is accompanied rarely by alterations in serum glutamic oxaloacetic transaminase levels and mild hepatitis.

ADVERSE REACTIONS

Methyldopa is absorbed well from the gastrointestinal tract. Its elimination is largely renal, with a half-life of 2 hours. Some of the drug is eliminated much more slowly, however, and cumulation may occur when renal function is inadequate. The drug and its metabolites may give false positive tests in the diagnosis of pheochromocytoma.

PHARMACOKINETICS

PREPARATIONS	Methyldopa (Aldomet) is available in 250 and 500 mg tablets. Methyldopa hydrochloride (Aldomet ester hydrochloride) is available as a solution for intravenous injection, 250 mg/5 ml.

Reserpine

Reserpine is the prototype of several alkaloids present in *Rauwolfia serpentina*, or Indian snakeroot. Used in India for centuries, it was introduced into Western medicine in the 1950s. At first reserpine seemed as important for its tranquilizing properties as for its usefulness in the treatment of hypertension. It was gradually replaced as an antipsychotic drug by the phenothiazines. It is still important as an antihypertensive drug and as a fascinating pharmacological tool.

BASIC ACTION AND EFFECTS

Reserpine has one basic action responsible for most, if not all, of its pharmacological effects. The drug causes a depletion of catecholamines and serotonin in the central and peripheral nervous system and some other sites. Depletion is a consequence of amine release. Not only are the amines released from their binding sites, but their reaccumulation is also prevented. Some interference by reserpine with catecholamine synthesis has been reported.

Parasympathetic effects of reserpine are in part a result of decreased sympathetic activity. Bradycardia, aggravation of peptic ulcer, increased gastrointestinal motility, and miosis may all be explained as results of parasympathetic predominance.

The *CNS effects* of the drug are among its greatest disadvantages in the treatment of hypertension. An unpleasant type of drowsiness and lethargy is particularly disliked by individuals who must be intellectually alert and creative. Depression and suicides have occurred during chronic reserpine administration. Reserpine increases the CNS depressant actions of other drugs such as barbiturates and alcohol. It predisposes patients to severe hypotension during surgery and anesthesia.

Various derivatives of reserpine are very similar in action to the parent compound. Syrosingopine produces fewer central effects in relation to its antihypertensive action. This selectivity has been attributed to the fact that its norepinephrine-depleting action is largely limited to the peripheral nervous system. It is also much less potent.

Reserpine

The dried root of *Rauwolfia serpentina* Benth (Raudixin) is available in tablets containing 50 and 100 mg. Preparations of *reserpine* include tablets of 0.1, 0.25, and 1 mg; an elixir containing 0.25 mg/4 ml; and solution for injection, 2.5 mg/ml.

Syrosingopine (Singoserp) is available in tablets of 1 mg.

PREPARATIONS

The veratrum alkaloids, protoveratrines A and B, act through the remarkable mechanism of promoting the activity of afferent nerves from the carotid sinus and aortic arch and thereby causing a reflex inhibition of central sympathetic activity with subsequent parasympathetic predominance. Unfortunately, the protoveratrines cause considerable nausea in many patients, and their dosage must be carefully adjusted to obtain a good hypotensive effect. These disadvantages have limited the usefulness of these compounds, but their pharmacology illustrates some unique mechanisms of drug action.

A number of alkaloids occur in plants of the species *Veratrum viride* and *Veratrum album*. They are classified as (1) tertiary amine esters and (2) secondary amines and their glycosides. The various alkaloids are polycyclic ring structures showing some resemblance to the cardiac glycosides.

REFLEX INHIBITORS OF CENTRAL SYMPATHETIC FUNCTION

If a small dose (less than 2 mg) of a mixture of protoveratrines A and B (Veralba) is injected intravenously into a human being, the characteristic effect consists of bradycardia and drop in blood pressure. When proportionately larger doses are given to animals, temporary apnea is produced in addition to the circulatory effects.

It has been suggested that these veratrum alkaloids may sensitize the afferent endings in the baroreceptors of the carotid sinus and other areas so that they have greater response to the normally effective stretch stimulus.

Effects of protoveratrines A and B

Drugs that promote salt secretion, such as the thiazides, are important in the treatment of hypertension because sodium is involved in some way in the pathogenesis of the disease.

Rats on a high salt intake develop hypertension. Also, the hypertensive effect of deoxycorticosterone and aldosterone is probably attributable to salt retention. Conversely, the antihypertensive action of a low salt diet is generally accepted at present. The mechanism whereby an excess of salt in the body contributes to hypertension is not definitely known. Expansion of extracellular fluid volume and alterations in the salt concentration in arteriolar walls have been suggested as important factors.

ANTIHYPERTEN-SIVE DRUGS THAT PROMOTE SALT EXCRETION

Most investigators believe that thiazide diuretics exert their antihypertensive action through salt depletion. Isolated observations suggest that these drugs may also have extrarenal effects. In any case, they have been a welcome addition to antihypertensive therapy because it is much easier to accomplish salt depletion through this means than by strict limitation of salt intake.

The most useful oral diuretics, discussed in greater detail in Chapter 38, are the thiazides and the related drugs chlorthalidone (Hygroton) and quinethazone (Hy-

Chlorothiazide and related drugs

dromox). They are widely used in the treatment of hypertension because of their safety and effectiveness and their ability to increase the antihypertensive action of other unrelated drugs.

Another potent diuretic, metolazone (Zaroxolyn), has also been introduced recently as an antihypertensive agent administered once daily.

The aldosterone antagonist spironolactone is sometimes combined with the thiazide diuretics, mainly to reduce potassium loss. The same is true for triamterene (Dyrenium).

The adverse effects of the thiazide diuretics, such as hypokalemia, hyperuricemia, and aggravation of diabetes, are discussed in Chapter 38. On the whole, these drugs are very useful in the treatment of hypertension.

Captopril

Captopril (Capoten) is an inhibitor of the converting enzyme, which changes angiotensin I to angiotensin II. It is used in patients who have not responded to other antihypertensive drugs, such as combinations of β blockers and vasodilators. The drug has many adverse effects. It can cause proteinuria, neutropenia, excessive hypotension, and a false positive test for acetone in the urine. Captopril is started with doses of 25 mg three times a day. The dose may be increased every 1 to 2 weeks. The drug has a greater antihypertensive effect if one of the thiazides is added to the treatment. Captopril (Capoten) is supplied in tablets, 25, 50, and 100 mg.

REFERENCES

1. Blythe, W.B.: Captopril and renal autoregulation, N. Engl. J. Med. **308**:390, 1983.
2. Curtis, J.J., Luke, R.G., Whelchel, J.D., Diethelm, A.G., Jones, P., and Dustan, H.P.: Inhibition of angiotensin-converting enzyme in renal transplant recipients with hypertension, N. Engl. J. Med. **308**:377, 1983.
3. DeCharme, D.W., Freyburger, W.A., Graham, B.E., and Carlson, R.G.: Pharmacologic properties of minoxidil: a new hypotensive agent, J. Pharmacol. Exp. Ther. **184**:662, 1973.
4. Erdös, E.G.: Angiotensin I converting enzyme, Circ. Res. **36**:247, 1975.
5. Freis, E.D.: Salt in hypertension and the effects of diuretics, Annu. Rev. Pharmacol. Toxicol. **18**:13, 1979.
6. Graham, R.M., and Pettinger, W.A.: Prazosin, N. Engl. J. Med. **300**:232, 1979.
7. Hammond, J.J., and Kirkendall, W.M.: Beta blocking drugs and the treatment of hypertension, Tex. Med. **74**:43, 1978.
8. Holland, O.B., and Kaplan, N.M.: Propranolol in the treatment of hypertension, N. Engl. J. Med. **294**:930, 1976.
9. Hypertension Detection and Follow-up Program Cooperative Group: Five-year findings of the hypertension detection and follow-up program. I. Reduction in mortality of persons with high blood pressure, including mild hypertension, JAMA **242**:2562, 1979.
10. Koch-Weser, J.: Metoprolol, N. Engl. J. Med. **301**:698, 1979.
11. Kosman, M.E.: Evaluation of clonidine hydrochloride (Catapres), JAMA **233**:174, 1975.
12. Pettinger, W.A.: Recent advances in the treatment of hypertension, Arch. Intern. Med. **137**:679, 1977.
13. Pettinger, W.A., and Mitchell, H.C.: Minoxidil—an alternative to nephrectomy for refractory hypertension, N. Engl. J. Med. **289**:167, 1973.
14. Pettinger, W.A., and Mitchell, H.C.: Renin release, saralasin and vasodilator-

beta-blocker drug interaction in man, N. Engl. J. Med. **292**:1214, 1975.

15. Schirger, A., and Sheps, S.G.: Prazosin—new antihypertensive agent, JAMA **237**:989, 1977.

16. Scriabine, A.: β-Adrenoceptor blocking drugs in hypertenson, Annu. Rev. Pharmacol. Toxicol. **19**:269, 1979.

17. Veterans Administration Cooperative Study Group on Antihypertensive Agents: Effects of treatment on morbidity in hypertension. II. Results in patients with diastolic blood pressure averaging 90 through 114 mm. Hg, JAMA **213**:1143, 1970.

18. Veterans Administration Cooperative Study Group on Antihypertensive Agents: Propranolol in the treatment of essential hypertension, JAMA **237**:2303, 1977.

19. Yeh, B.K., Nantel, A., and Goldberg, L.I.: Antihypertensive effect of clonidine, Arch. Intern. Med. **127**:233, 1971.

20. Zacest, R., Gilmore, E., and Koch-Weser, J.: Treatment of essential hypertension with combined vasodilation and beta-adrenergic blockade, N. Engl. J. Med. **286**:617, 1972.

Chapter 19

Histamine

Histamine is of interest in pharmacology and medicine because of its potent pharmacological activity and its wide distibution in tissues. When released from its binding sites, histamine can elicit reactions that range in intensity from mild itching to shock and death.

It would seem that such a potent and easily released endogenous compound would have important functions in the body. There is indeed evidence for a local role of histamine in inflammation. It is also quite certain that the amine plays a role in anaphylaxis, allergies, and drug reactions.

The role of histamine in normal physiology is not clearly established. It is probably one of the neurotransmitters, and it undoubtedly functions in the process of gastric secretion. Many other "local hormonal functions" have been attributed to it.

HISTAMINE RECEPTORS

Histamine acts on two separate and distinct receptors, termed H_1 and H_2 receptors (Table 19-1). Contraction of the smooth muscle of the bronchi and intestine is mediated by H_1 receptors and is antagonized by a typical antihistamine. On the other hand, H_2 receptors mediate the actions of histamine on gastric secretion, cardiac acceleration, and inhibition of the contractions of the rat uterus. These actions are antagonized by a new type of antihistamine exemplified by burimamide[2] and the related drugs metiamide, cimetidine, and ranitidine.

Both H_1 and H_2 receptors mediate the vasodilator effects of histamine.[14] The H_1 receptors are generally more important, except for certain areas. For example, vasodilatation along the distribution of the temporal artery in humans is more strongly influenced by H_2 receptors.

DEVELOPMENT OF CONCEPTS

Histamine was first synthesized in 1906 by Windaus. It was also found to occur naturally in ergot as the product of bacterial contamination. The pharmacological properties of histamine were extensively studied by Sir Henry Dale, who was impressed with the similarities in the actions of histamine and the manifestations of anaphylaxis in several species such as the guinea pig, rabbit, and dog. Once histamine

TABLE 19-1	Distribution of histamine receptors in the body	
Histamine receptor	Tissue	Antagonist
H_1	Smooth muscle of intestine, bronchi, blood vessels	Classical antihistamines (diphenhydramine)
H_2	Gastric parietal cell	Cimetidine
	Smooth muscle of some blood vessels	Ranitidine
	Guinea pig atria	Metiamide
	Rat uterus	Burimamide

was found widely distributed in mammalian tissues, numerous roles were assigned to it, often uncritically. Studies by Thomas Lewis on the release of "H substance" from the skin in response to injury had a great influence.

When the antihistaminic drugs were developed in the 1940s, many of the histaminic theories of various physiological functions and pathological processes were abandoned because of the inability of these drugs to modify them.

The demonstration in the 1950s of a close association between mast cells and histamine created much interest, and research concerning histamine focused on mechanisms of its release from mast cells. It was soon realized, however, that there is also an important non–mast cell pool of histamine, the function of which is still being investigated.

Histamine is widely distributed in the body. Its concentration varies in different species; in humans the highest concentrations are found in the lungs, skin, and stomach. Details of its distribution are given in Table 19-2.

TISSUE DISTRIBUTION AND FORMATION

It is generally believed that most of the histamine present in tissues arises locally as a consequence of decarboxylation of histidine. Various foods may contain histamine and intestinal bacteria may form large amounts, but whatever histamine is absorbed is rapidly altered and does not contribute to the body's stores of this amine.

With the availability of experimental drugs that destroy mast cells, such as compound 48/80, it has become possible to identify two pools of histamine in the body. The mast cell pool is widely distributed in the connective tissue and is depleted experimentally by the mast cell–destroying agents.

The circulating basophils behave like the mast cells and contain very high concentrations of histamine. The non–mast cell pool includes the gastric mucosa and the small amounts present in the brain, heart, and other organs. It is not known with certainty what the cellular localization of non–mast cell histamine is, but it is suspected that with the exception of the gastric mucosa, it is present in neural elements.[12] It differs from mast cell histamine in its more rapid turnover rate and its resistance to the usual histamine releasers such as compound 48/80.

TABLE 19-2   Histamine content of human tissues

Tissue	Histamine content
Lung	33 ± 10 μg/g*
Mucous membrane (nasal)	15.6 μg/g
Stomach	14 ± 4.0 μg/g*
Duodenum	14 ± 0.9 μg/g*
Skin	6.6 μg/g (abdomen)
	30.4 μg/g (face)
Spleen	3.4 ± 0.97 μg/g*
Kidney	2.5 ± 1.2 μg/g*
Liver	2.2 ± 0.76 μg/g*
Heart	1.6 ± 0.07 μg/g*
Thyroid	1.0 ± 0.13 μg/g*
Skeletal muscle	0.97 ± 0.13 μg/g*
Central nervous tissue	0-0.2 μg/g
Plasma	2.6 μg/L
Basophils	1,080 μg/10^9 cells
Eosinophils	160 μg/10^9 cells
Neutrophils	3.0 μg/10^9 cells
Lymphocytes	0.6 μg/10^9 cells
Platelets	0.009 μg/10^9 platelets
Whole blood	16-89 μg/L

Based on data from Van Arsdel, P.P., Jr., and Beall, G.N.: Arch. Intern. Med. **106**:192, 1960.
*Mean ± Standard error.

HISTIDINE DECARBOXYLASES

Chemically, histamine is 2(4-imidazolyl) ethylamine. Its structure is as follows:

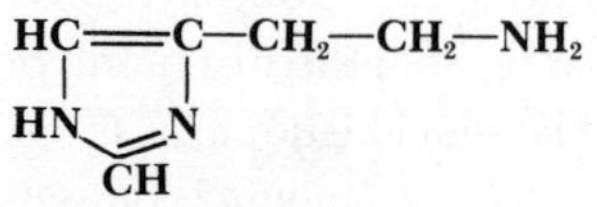

$$HC = C - CH_2 - CH_2 - NH_2$$
$$HN \quad N$$
$$CH$$

Histamine

Mammalian tissues contain two different histidine decarboxylases. The one known as specific histidine decarboxylase, present in mast cells, is inhibited by methylhistidine and the hydrazine analog of histidine, but not by methyldopa. The other enzyme, also known as aromatic L-amino acid decarboxylase, decarboxylates several aromatic L-amino acids (dopa, for example). It is inhibited by methyldopa. There is every reason to believe that specific histidine decarboxylase is more important physiologically.

DEGRADATION OF HISTAMINE IN THE BODY

The degradation of histamine in the body takes place through two main pathways, with considerable species variation in their relative importance. In humans, histamine is primarily methylated to 1-methylhistamine. This product is converted to 1-methyl-

Known pathways of histamine metabolism. Relative importance of the different pathways **FIG. 19-1**
in human males is indicated by figures at bottom, which are expressed as percent of the
total ^{14}C excreted in the urine during 12 hours after intradermal injection of ^{14}C histamine.
Of the injected ^{14}C, 74% to 93% was excreted in 12 hours.

From Nilsson, K., Lindell, S.-E., Schayer, R.W., and Westling, H.: Clin. Sci. *13:*313, 1959.

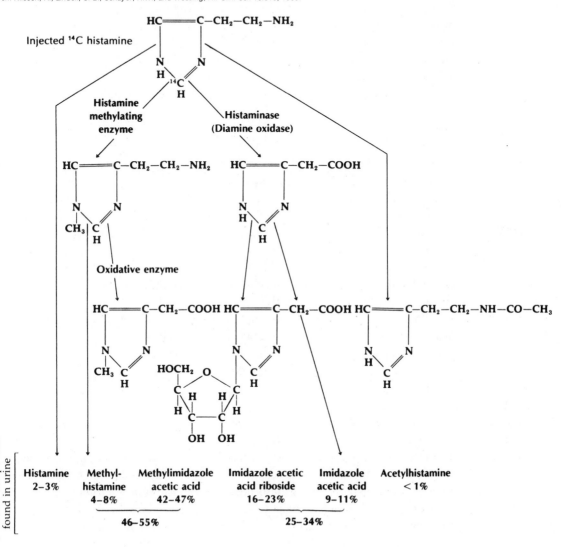

imidazole-4-acetic acid by the enzyme MAO. In the other pathway, which also occurs in humans, histamine is oxidized by diamine oxidase to imidazole-4-acetic acid, much of which is conjugated with ribose and is excreted as the riboside. The known pathways are shown in Fig. 19-1.

In addition to these compounds, some *N*-acetylhistamine also appears in the urine. The acetyl compound appears to reflect orally ingested histamine and amine formed by intestinal bacteria. The exact site of acetylation is still in doubt. There are suggestions that intestinal bacteria can acetylate histamine, and some investigators believe that no acetylation occurs outside the gastrointestinal tract.

It has been estimated that about 1% of histamine slowly injected intravenously appears in the urine in the free form, whereas most orally ingested histamine is found in the conjugated form in the urine. It has been estimated that in a normal person 2 to 3 mg of histamine may be released daily from the tissues. Urticaria in humans or the injection of histamine-releasing agents into animals causes an increase in the urinary excretion of histamine.

BINDING AND RELEASE OF MAST CELL HISTAMINE

Histamine is highly concentrated in the granules of the mast cell. These granules also contain large amounts of heparin, proteolytic enzymes, and, in some species (rats and mice), serotonin. Histamine release is visualized as a two-step process. In the first step the granules are suddenly extruded; in the second, as the granules are exposed to the cations in the extracellular environment, histamine is released by ion exchange. The amine is held within the granule by electrostatic forces.

Although granule release generally accompanies histamine release, it is possible that release of the amine could occur within the cell also. The appearance of granules within the mast cell is shown in Fig. 19-2.

Histamine is released from mast cells by physical and chemical agents, antigen-antibody reactions, and a variety of drugs.

Release by chemicals and drugs

Many early isolated observations suggested that simple chemicals can cause release of histamine in the body. Intracutaneous morphine injections in humans produces the "triple response of Lewis," consisting of localized redness, localized edema, and a diffuse redness. This was suspected of being an example of a chemical causing release of H substance. It has also been shown that curare alkaloids can liberate histamine, and this was thought to explain the episodes of bronchial constriction accompanying intravenous curare injections. With the discovery of adverse reactions to certain diamidines and polypeptide antibiotics (licheniformin, polymyxin), interest in this problem increased greatly.

The chemical histamine-releasing agents may be divided into two classes: small-molecule amines and certain large-molecule compounds such as dextran, polyvinyl-pyrrolidone, and ovomucoid, which are active only in some species.

A variety of organic bases can cause release of histamine from mast cells. The most active compound known is compound 48/80, a condensation product of *p*-methoxyphenylethylmethylamine with formaldehyde (Fig. 19-2).

Mast cells of rat mesentery 3 hours after intraperitoneal injection of compound 48/80.   *FIG. 19-2*

From Riley, J.F., and West, A.B.: J. Pathol. Bacteriol. **69**:269, 1955.

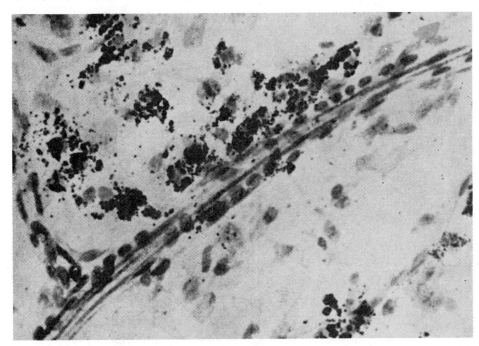

Compound 48/80

It has been suggested that histamine release can be caused not only by the curare alkaloids but also by such commonly used drugs as morphine, codeine, papaverine, meperidine, atropine, hydralazine, and even sympathomimetic amines. Histamine release by these drugs may not be significant unless they are administered intravenously in fairly large doses.

A characteristic feature of histamine release by chemical compounds is the development of tachyphylaxis to subsequent injections. When one obtains a marked fall in blood pressure following intravenous injection of 100 to 200 µg/kg of compound 48/80 in a dog, a second injection of the drug may have no effect whatever for several hours.

Histamine release plays an important role in the symptomatology of experimental anaphylactic shock in several species. In 1910 Dale and Laidlaw[4] observed that the symptoms elicited by histamine in guinea pigs, dogs, and rabbits were very similar to the manifestations of anaphylactic shock in these species. In guinea pigs the dominant symptom is bronchial constriction and asphyxial death from intravenous doses as small as 0.4 mg/kg. In dogs profound hypotension and acute enlargement of the liver are caused by both histamine and anaphylaxis. In the rabbit the pulmonary arterioles are constricted and acute dilatation of the right side of the heart ensues when either histamine is injected or antigen is administered to the previously sensitized animal.

In addition, in the dog the blood may become incoagulable in anaphylaxis but not after histamine injection. Much was made of this difference until it was demonstrated that anaphylaxis in the dog also releases heparin, presumably from the mast cells, which are abundant in the dog's liver.

The release of histamine by injecting antigens into the sensitized animal has been demonstrated also by perfusion experiments of the skin and on addition of the antigen in vitro to sensitized minced tissues.

In acute anaphylactic reactions in humans, histamine probably plays an important role. In anaphylaxis the human being reacts like the dog and the guinea pig, exhibiting profound hypotension, bronchial constriction, or laryngeal edema.

Important new observations have been made on histamine release from human leukocytes by specific antigens such as ragweed extract.[13] These studies suggest that the cyclic AMP and drugs that activate adenyl cyclase have an inhibitory action on histamine release. There is a possibility that drugs widely used in allergic diseases, such as the catecholamines and theophylline, may exert an inhibitory effect on histamine release in addition to their well-known antagonism to many of its pharmacological actions. Anaphylactically induced histamine release is inhibited by the drug disodium cromoglycate (Intal) in vitro (p. 714).[11] It is enhanced by phosphatidylserine in rat mast cells.

Histamine taken by mouth has essentially no effect because it is altered by the intestinal bacteria, the gastrointestinal wall, and also the liver.

If injected intravenously, however, as little as 0.1 mg of histamine phosphate causes a sharp decline in the blood pressure, acceleration of the heart rate, elevation of the cerebrospinal fluid pressure, flushing of the face, and headache. There is also stimulation of gastric hydrochloric acid secretion. All these effects last only a few minutes. If a similar injection is given to an asthmatic individual, even while he or she is free of demonstrable breathing difficulty, there will be a marked decrease in vital capacity, and a severe attack of asthma may be precipitated.

When larger doses of histamine are administered intravenously, which can be done only in animals, the blood pressure remains low for a considerable length of time, and there is marked elevation of the hematocrit reading. Histamine shock may ensue, with possibly fatal termination. The lethal dose in species such as the dog, in which the circulatory action of histamine predominates, may be as high as several milligrams per kilogram of body weight.

The two factors involved in the circulatory actions of histamine are arteriolar dilatation and increased capillary permeability. These cause loss of plasma from the circulation.

Circulatory effects

A striking demonstration of the histamine effect on capillaries is seen when very low concentrations are injected intracutaneously in humans. The injection of as little as 10 μg of the drug produces the "triple response of Lewis." The sequence of events consists of localized redness, localized edema or wheal, and diffused redness or flare.

The localized redness and wheal are the consequences of vasodilatation and increased capillary permeability. The diffuse flare involves neural mechanisms, perhaps axon reflexes, since it can be abolished by previous sectioning of sensory nerves.

The triple response is interesting because human skin seems to respond to a variety of injuries in the same manner as it does to histamine injections. This similarity led Sir Thomas Lewis to suggest that perhaps various injuries may cause release of a histamine-like substance, or H substance, from the skin; this substance then mediates the manifestations of evanescent skin inflammations.

Histamine increases the rate and force of contraction of the heart in several species.[15] Both H_1 and H_2 receptors are present in the heart, and species variations in their distribution are great. Histamine stimulates adenylate cyclase in the human heart. This is not blocked by propranolol. The significance of cardiac histamine receptors is not entirely clear. Large doses of histamine cause norepinephrine release from the heart.

Human beings and guinea pigs are very susceptible to the bronchoconstrictor action of histamine. Persons with a previous history of asthma are particularly vulnerable and may respond with an acute asthmatic attack to a dose of histamine that would only cause minor decreases in vital capacity in a normal person. This is generally interpreted as increased susceptibility to histamine of the bronchial smooth muscle in asthmatic persons. Asthmatic individuals are highly susceptible not only to histamine but also to methacholine.

Other smooth muscle effects

In view of the ineffectiveness of the antihistaminic drugs in asthmatic patients, other mediators have been looked for. Slow reacting substance of anaphylaxis (SRS-A) was found to be a potent stimulant of the bronchial smooth muscle. It is released from IgE-sensitized fragments of human lung. It is an acidic lipid formed from arachidonic acid by the enzyme lipoxygenase. It is a leukotriene and a member of the eicosanoid family. It has powerful effects on the human bronchial smooth muscle.

Histamine is a potent stimulant of gastric hydrochloric acid secretion. As little as 0.025 mg of the drug injected subcutaneously in humans will cause marked increase in hydrochloric acid secretion but few other effects in the body. This response to

Effect on secretions

histamine is used in tests for complete achlorhydria. Histamine-resistant achlorhydria has diagnostic importance in conditions such as addisonian pernicious anemia.

The polypeptide gastrin is an extremely potent stimulant of gastric acid secretion, being 500 times as potent as histamine. Its actions are also antagonized by the H_2 antihistamines, which raises interesting speculations on the relationship between gastrin and histamine.

Histamine stimulates to a slight extent the secretory activities of many other glandular cells. Effects on salivary and bronchial secretions can be demonstrated, but these actions are not important in a normal person. Its effect on catecholamine secretion has been mentioned before.

ROLE IN HEALTH AND DISEASE

Very little is known about the possible physiological roles of histamine. The presence of this potent capillary and arteriolar dilator in mast cells, which are in intimate contact with blood vessels, suggests some role more significant than causation of hives. Just what this role may be cannot be stated at present.

In one interesting experiment,[5] normal rats exposed to ultraviolet light, after having been injected previously with hematoporphyrin, reacted in about a day with edema of the skin. When these rats were pretreated for a week with the histamine-releasing agent compound 48/80 to deplete the histamine content of their skin, they did not react to the ultraviolet light.

Histamine undoubtedly plays a role in gastric secretion. It acts on H_2 receptors and may have a "permissive" enhancing effect on the actions of gastrin and acetylcholine. This will be discussed further in relation to cimetidine (p. 224).

Histamine probably plays an important role in neural function. The brain has receptors for this amine, and the enzymes for its synthesis and inactivation by methylation are also present. A ganglionic stimulant effect of histamine has been demonstrated. Histamine releases catecholamines in pheochromocytoma and in animal experiments. Drugs used in parkinsonism and the tricyclic antidepressants have potent antihistaminic effects.

It has also been suggested that certain types of vascular headaches may be caused by histamine. The evidence for the histaminic cause in this instance is largely indirect. It is based on the facts that injected histamine can reproduce the symptoms and that repeated administration produces "desensitization" and symptomatic improvement.

MEDICAL USES

Histamine is useful as a diagnostic adjunct for differentiating pernicious anemia from other diseases of the stomach on the basis of achlorhydria. It is also used occasionally in the diagnosis of pheochromocytoma, since it stimulates the output of catecholamines from the adrenal medullary tumor. Intracutaneous injections of histamine may be used for revealing the integrity of blood supply and innervation to an area. Other medical uses based on its vasodilator action are obsolete.

$$CH_2-CH_2-NH_2 \cdot 2HCl$$

Histamine dihydrochloride

$$CH_2-CH_2-NH_2 \cdot HCl$$

Betazole hydrochloride

Betazole is an isomer of histamine that stimulates gastric secretion but has only $\frac{1}{50}$ the potency of histamine. Furthermore, it has relatively less effect than histamine on the cardiovascular system and may be safer for determination of gastric acidity. However, the drug may be dangerous in asthmatic persons.

Histamine preparations include histamine phosphate solutions for injection, containing 0.275, 0.55, and 2.75 mg/ml. Betazole hydrochloride (Histalog) is available as a solution for injection, 50 mg/ml.

REFERENCES

1. Beaven, M.A.: Histamine, N. Engl. J. Med. **294**:30, 1976.

2. Black, J.W., Duncan, W.A.M., Durant, C.J., Ganellin, C.R., and Parsons, E.M.: Definition and antagonism of histamine H_2-receptors, Nature **236**:385, 1972.

3. Copenhaver, J.H., Jr., Nagler, M.E., and Goth, A.: The intracellular distribution of histamine, J. Pharmacol. Exp. Ther. **109**:401, 1953.

4. Dale, H.H., and Laidlaw, P.P.: The physiological action of β-iminozolethylamine, J. Physiol. **41**:318, 1910.

5. Feldberg, W., and Talesnik, J.: Reduction of tissue histamine by compound 48/80, J. Physiol. **120**:550, 1953.

6. Ginsburg, R., Bristow, M.R., Stinson, E.B., and Harrison, D.C.: Histamine receptors in the human heart, Life Sci. **26**:2245, 1980.

7. Goth, A.: Histamine release by drugs and chemicals. In Schachter, M., editor: International encyclopedia of pharmacology and therapy: histamine and antihistamines, vol. 1, New York, 1973, Pergamon Press Inc.

8. Goth, A.: On the general problem of the release of histamine. In Rocha e Silva, M., editor: Handbook of experimental pharmacology, 18/2:57, Berlin, 1978, Springer-Verlag.

9. Goth, A.: Adams, H.R., and Knoohuizen, M.: Phosphatidylserine: selective enhancer of histamine release, Science **173**:1034, 1971.

10. Goth, A., and Johnson, A.R.: Current concepts on the secretory function of mast cells, Life Sci. **16**:1201, 1975.

11. Kusner, E.J., Dunnick, B., and Herzog, D.J.: The inhibition by disodium cromoglycate in vitro of anaphylactically induced histamine release from rat peritoneal mast cells, J. Pharmacol. Exp. Ther. **184**:41, 1973.

12. Levine, R.J., Sato, T.L., and Sjoerdsma, A.: Inhibition of histamine synthesis in the rat by hydrazino analog of histidine and 4-bromo-3-hydroxy benzyloxyamine, Biochem. Pharmacol. **14**:139, 1965.

13. Lichtenstein, L.M., and Margolis, S.: Histamine release in vitro: inhibition by catecholamines and methylxanthines, Science **161**:902, 1968.

14. Powell, J.R., and Brody, M.J.: Participation of H_1 and H_2 histamine receptors in physiological vasodilator responses, Am. J. Physiol. **231**:1002, 1976.

15. Verma, S.C., and McNeill, J.H.: Cardiac histamine receptors and cyclic AMP, Life Sci. **19**:1797, 1976.

16. Weissman, G.: The eicosanoids of asthma, N. Engl. J. Med. **308**:454, 1983.

Chapter 20

Antihistaminic drugs

Drugs that block the effects of histamine competitively at various receptor sites are referred to as antihistaminic drugs. The actions of histamine on bronchial and intestinal smooth muscles can be blocked by the conventional antihistamines, as exemplified by mepyramine. On the other hand, the effects of histamine on gastric secretion are not blocked by the usual antihistamines but are prevented by the newer type of competitor, as exemplified by cimetidine.

The antihistaminics are classified as H_1- and H_2-receptor antagonists. Diphenhydramine and tripelennamine were the first H_1 antihistaminics introduced in this country many years ago. Cimetidine and ranitidine, congeners of burimamide and metiamide,[1] were introduced fairly recently and are H_2-receptor antagonists.

The H_1 antihistaminic drugs are useful not only in allergic diseases but also for the prevention of motion sickness and in the treatment of parkinsonism. Also, their sedative effect may be of some benefit. The H_2 antihistamines, such as cimetidine and ranitidine, are useful in the treatment of peptic ulcer disease.[2]

ANTIHISTAMINES: H_1-RECEPTOR ANTAGONISTS

Development

The field of antihistaminics was opened up by the discovery that certain phenolic ethers could protect guinea pigs against anaphylactic shock and histamine. The response of the guinea pig to the inhalation of histamine aerosol has been used widely in subsequent development of new antihistaminics.

Chemistry

The basic structure of the antihistaminics may be represented as a substituted ethylamine:

$$X\text{—}CH_2CH_2N{<}^{R_1}_{R_2}$$

If it is recalled that histamine is 2-(4-imidazolyl)ethylamine, it is apparent that some relationship may exist between the ethylamine portion of the histamine molecule and the fact that the antihistamines are substituted ethylamines. Perhaps this portion of the histamine molecule is essential for its attachment to some of the receptor structures.

The R groups in the ethylamine structure are in most cases CH_3. If the X in the basic structure is nitrogen, the compound may be looked on as a substituted ethylenediamine. Examples of this type of antihistaminic drugs are tripelennamine (Pyribenzamine; PBZ), methapyriline (Thenylene; Histadyl), thonzylamine (Neohetramine), pyrilamine (Neo-Antergan), and many others. The structural formulas of tripelennamine and methapyrilene are shown below.

If a recommended dose of one of the antihistaminics is taken orally by a normal person, the only noticeable effects will be on the CNS. Drowsiness is quite common, and barbiturates taken simultaneously appear to be synergistic in causing sleepiness. There is no relationship between the antihistaminic potency of these drugs and their central depressant action. Chlorpheniramine produces less sedation for an equivalent antihistaminic action than diphenhydramine. An unusual antihistaminic, phenindamine (Thephorin), may even have CNS stimulant properties.

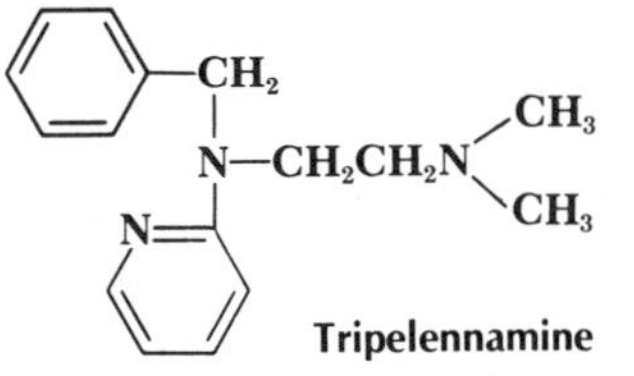

Clinical pharmacology

Tripelennamine

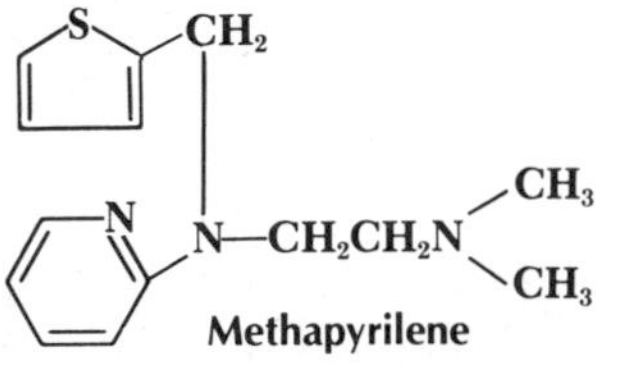

Methapyrilene

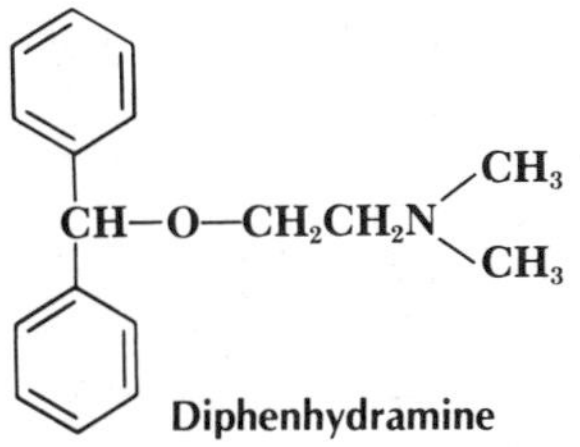

Diphenhydramine

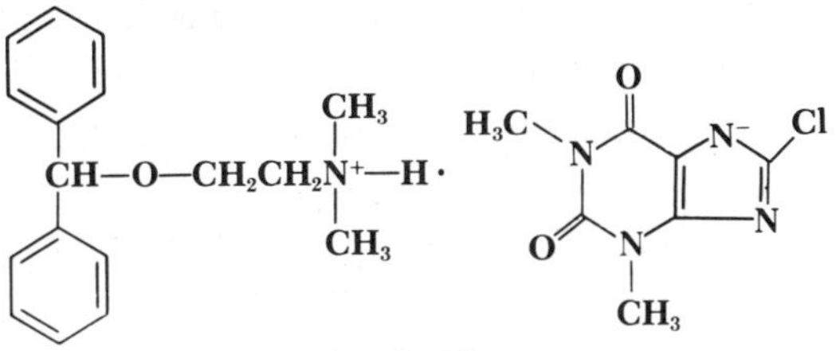

Dimenhydrinate

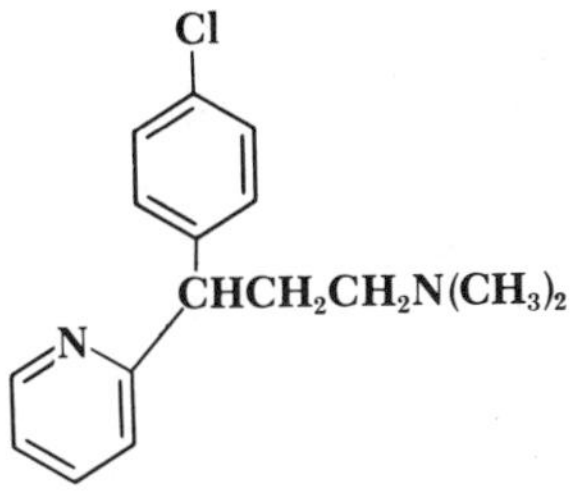

Chlorpheniramine

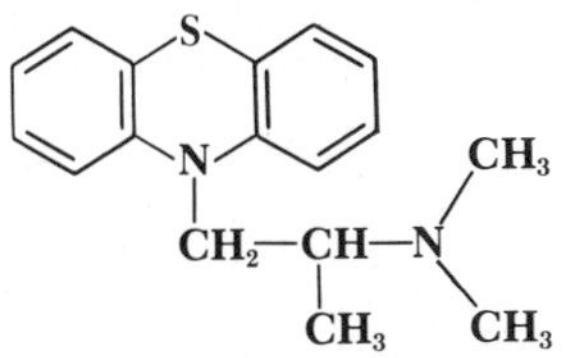

Promethazine

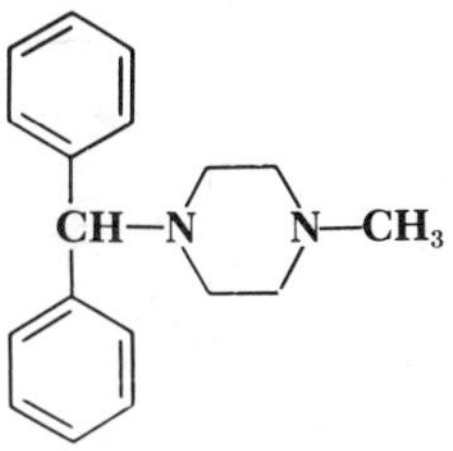

Cyclizine

FIG. 20-1   Effect of histamine on blood pressure and its antagonism by an antihistaminic drug. A, Histamine, 1 μg/kg IV. B, Histamine, 5 μg/kg IV. C, Diphenhydramine, 5 mg/kg IV. D, Histamine, 1 μg/kg IV. E, Histamine, 5 μg/kg IV. Blood pressure recording of dog anesthetized with pentobarbital sodium. Time in 15 seconds. Note that the antihistaminic drug, although exerting considerable protection against vasodepressor action of histamine, failed to eliminate it completely.

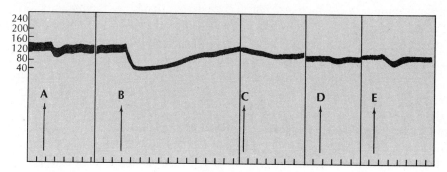

If the patient suffers from urticaria or hay fever, the various antihistaminics will produce considerable relief with variable sedation. Surprisingly, these drugs have very little benefit in the treatment of asthma, and this ineffectiveness has led to some doubt concerning the role of histamine in asthma.

With the recognition of two separate receptors for histamine and the discovery of H_2-receptor antagonists, many puzzling aspects of the pharmacology of antihistamines can be clarified. Gastric secretion is mediated by H_2 receptors and is not blocked by the commonly available antihistamines, which are H_1-receptor antagonists.[1] It appears also that vasodilatation and increased capillary permeability are mediated by both types of receptors and that such actions of histamine can be blocked completely only by a combination of H_1- and H_2- receptor antagonists[1] (Fig. 20-1).

Antihistaminics are often applied topically to obtain symptomatic improvement in itching skin conditions, but in several cases contact dermatitis developed as a consequence of sensitization of the patient to the topically applied antihistaminics.

Miscellaneous actions

Besides being competitive antagonists of histamine, the antihistaminics have a number of additional actions. These are (1) CNS effect, (2) anticholinergic effect, (3) local anesthetic properties, and (4) antiserotonin action.

Antihistaminics produce a *sedative CNS effect* different from the actions of barbiturates and other sedative-hypnotics. The sedative effect of the antihistaminics is not pleasant. Furthermore, if the dose of the antihistamine is increased, sedation is replaced by marked irritability, leading to convulsions, hyperpyrexia, and even death. Toxic doses are likely to produce excitation in children. Additional CNS effects are probably related to anticholinergic properties.

The *anticholinergic effect* manifests itself as a drying of salivary and bronchial secretions, similar to the effect of atropine. For the same reason these drugs may have adverse effects in the treatment of bronchial asthma by increasing the viscosity of secretions in the respiratory tract.

The anticholinergic effect of the antihistaminics may be related to their usefulness in the prevention of motion sickness. Dimenhydrinate is widely used for this. There is good indication from clinical studies that the drug owes its antimotion sickness properties to diphenhydramine, one of its components. Certain antihistaminics such as cyclizine and meclizine are especially recommended for the prevention of motion sickness. The effectiveness of diphenhydramine in Parkinson's disease may also result from its anticholinergic properties.

The *local anesthetic properties* of antihistaminics make them suitable as antipruritic agents in topical applications. Unfortunately, they may cause sensitization, and their use as topical agents is best avoided.

Antiserotonin properties are quite common in antihistaminic drugs. At least one, cyproheptadine (Periactin), is generally viewed as a combined antihistamine-antiserotonin. There is no reason to believe, however, that antagonism to serotonin confers any special advantages in an antihistaminic.

Therapeutic uses

There are many conditions in which antihistaminics are helpful. There are others in which they are used but perhaps should not be.

Conditions in which the antihistaminics are helpful include allergic rhinitis, urticaria, some types of asthma, and motion sickness. Conditions in which antihistaminics are not the drugs of choice include acute anaphylactic emergencies (epinephrine is much more useful), most cases of asthma, diseases of the skin, eyes, and nose, and the common cold.

In the selection of antihistaminics, their sedative action is a major consideration. Potency is not so important, since it only influences the size of the tablets used. The duration of action of most antihistamines when given in a therapeutic dose is about 4 hours and is greatly influenced by the dose. The usual adult doses and sedative potencies of a number of antihistamines are shown in Table 20-1.

Absorption and metabolism

The H_1 antagonists are absorbed rapidly and completely from the gastrointestinal tract. They cause systemic effects in less than 30 minutes, and absorption is complete in 4 hours. In the case of diphenhydramine, peak blood levels occur in 1 hour, declining to essentially zero in 6 hours. The H_1 antagonists are metabolized in the liver by hydroxylation, and these drugs may stimulate the hepatic microsomal enzymes.

Toxicity

On the whole the antihistaminics are remarkably nontoxic compounds when used in the recommended doses. It is possible that the widespread use of these drugs may contribute to automobile accidents because of their sedative properties. It is also likely that the simultaneous use of antihistaminics and other depressant drugs

TABLE 20-1	Doses and sedative properties of various antihistamines		
Generic name	Trade name	Usual adult dose (mg)	Degree of sedation
Carbinoxamine	Clistin	4	+
Chlorothen	Tagathen	25	+
Phenindamine	Thephorin	25	+ *
Chlorpheniramine	Chlor-Trimeton	4	+ +
Brompheniramine	Dimetane	4	+ +
Triprolidine	Actidil	2.5	+ +
Doxylamine	Decapryn	12.5	+ +
Chlorcyclizine	Di-Paralene	50	+ +
Methapyrilene	Histadyl	25	+ +
Dimethindine	Forhistal	1	+ +
Pyrilamine	Neo-Antergan	25	+ +
Cyproheptadine	Periactin	4	+ +
Tripelennamine	Pyribenzamine	50	+ +
Diphenhydramine	Benadryl	50	+ + +
Promethazine	Phenergan	12.5	+ + +

Based on data from Feinberg, S.M.: Pharmacol. Phys. 1(12):1, 1976.
*Stimulation possible.

such as barbiturates or alcohol may exert synergistic depressant actions. A few cases of skin sensitization have been reported following topical use of antihistaminics.

Acute poisoning has occurred following ingestion of very large doses of the antihistaminics, particularly in children. Surprisingly, the symptoms consisted of CNS excitation and convulsive phenomena. The management of acute poisoning is purely symptomatic. The anticonvulsant barbiturates must be tried very cautiously because there is experimental evidence that their toxicity may be additive to that of the antihistaminics.

Some of the antihistaminics commonly used for the prevention of motion sickness have been found to be teratogenic in rats. As a consequence, meclizine, cyclizine, and chlorcyclizine should not be used in pregnant women, and preparations offered for self-medication must bear a warning to that effect. The teratogenic effect is not related to an antihistaminic effect but seems related to a structural feature, all of these drugs being piperazines.

Antihistaminics with antiserotonin action

Among the antihistaminic drugs, promethazine has considerable antiserotonin action on smooth muscles, approaching LSD in this activity. Chlorpromazine, a tranquilizer, is about half as active. A relatively new antihistaminic, cyproheptadine hydrochloride, is a potent antiserotonin drug as well.

Cyproheptadine hydrochloride

Administered in doses of 4 to 20 mg daily, cyproheptadine hydrochloride (Periactin) is available for the same indications as other antihistaminics. In addition, there are claims for its effectiveness in the postgastrectomy dumping syndrome and other conditions, but further experience is needed for evaluating these claims.

The H_1-receptor antagonists or classical antihistamines do not block the gastric secretory effect of histamine. To explain this anomaly it was proposed in 1966 that there were two histamine receptors. In 1972 Black and co-workers described the first antagonist, burimamide, which competitively antagonized the effects of histamine on gastric parietal cells, guinea pig atria, and rat uterus. These histamine receptors were called H_2-receptor antagonists. Further studies led to the synthesis of metiamide, which had effects similar to those of burimamide, but which was better absorbed from the gastrointestinal tract. Following extensive clinical use, several patients developed agranulocytosis while on metiamide. Because of this a newer H_2 antagonist, cimetidine, was introduced,[4] which so far has not caused serious hematological toxicity. In cimetidine, the thiourea in the side chain is changed to cyanoguanidine. Ranitidine was introduced more recently.

H_2-RECEPTOR ANTAGONISTS

These two groups of drugs differ in their chemistry, pharmacokinetics, and clinical uses, in addition to acting on different receptors.

In the H_1 antihistamines the imidazole ring structure is extensively modified or replaced by other substituents. In the H_2 antagonists the side chain is extensively modified. More than 700 compounds had to be synthesized before burimamide was obtained.

In contrast with the H_1 antagonists, the H_2 antihistamines are generally less lipid-soluble compounds, do not cross the blood-brain barrier, and do not cause sedation.

Differences between H_1 and H_2 antihistamines

Cimetidine (Tagamet) causes a significant reduction in diurnal gastric acid secretion.[2] After 6 weeks of treatment most ulcer patients were cured, as compared with members of the placebo group. When the drug was administered in doses of 200 mg three times a day, even stimulated gastric secretion was inhibited.

Cimetidine

MECHANISM OF INHIBITION OF GASTRIC SECRETION	The H_2-receptor antagonists, such as cimetidine, inhibit gastric secretion caused by histamine, gastrin, acetylcholine, and food.[10] There are several possible explanations for this apparent lack of specificity of the inhibitory action. Histamine could be the final common pathway for the various stimuli. Or there could be separate receptors on the parietal cell for histamine, gastrin, and acetylcholine, but occupation of the histamine receptor interferes in some way with the others. Finally, histamine could have a "permissive" effect on the actions of the other stimuli.

CLINICAL PHARMACOLOGY, INDICATIONS, AND TOXICITY	A 300 mg dose of cimetidine at bedtime causes a significant reduction of gastric acidity for at least 8 hours. The drug is well absorbed when given orally, has a plasma half-life of 2 hours, and is excreted in the urine, 70% unchanged.

Approved indications for cimetidine are active duodenal ulcer disease and hypersecretory states in Zollinger-Ellison syndrome and mastocytosis. Investigational uses include reflux esophagitis, pancreatic insufficiency, stress ulcers, and upper gastrointestinal hemorrhage.

Adverse effects of cimetidine are rare. The drug is not very lipophilic and does not cause drowsiness because of poor penetration into the CNS. In very large doses, the drug has caused renal and hepatic damage in dogs, but the doses required were of the order of 500 mg/kg.

ADVERSE EFFECTS AND DRUG INTERACTIONS	Considering the large number of patients taking cimetidine, adverse reactions have been few. Mental confusion is seen occasionally in elderly patients, perhaps because the drug may have crossed the blood-brain barrier. Meningitis and encephalitis are considered contraindications to the use of cimetidine. In large doses the drug may cause some antiandrogenic effects, and reversible gynecomastia has been reported. Minor changes in serum creatinine concentrations and transaminases may occur, and hepatic drug metabolism may slow down.

Warfarin and phenindione are potentiated by cimetidine because their hepatic metabolism is slowed. Cimetidine may also slow the metabolism of chlordiazepoxide and diazepam. Phenytoin clearance is reduced because of the inhibitory effect of cimetidine on hepatic microsomal oxidation. The dosage of β blockers should be reduced when cimetidine is added to the treatment, since the H_2 blocker may reduce the hepatic first-pass effect on propranolol and probably other β blockers.

Histamine

Burimamide

Ranitidine

Cimetidine

The newer histamine H_2 receptor antagonist is very similar in its actions and indications to cimetidine. It differs from cimetidine in a greater potency and a longer duration of action so that twice daily dosage is sufficient. Early experience indicates that the drug does not inhibit the hepatic drug metabolizing microsomal enzymes. As a consequence, the action of warfarin and other drugs is not prolonged. It probably does not inhibit the androgen receptor at the usual doses.

Ranitidine

Ranitidine hydrochloride (Zantac) is available in 150 mg tablets.

REFERENCES

1. Black, J.W., Duncan, W.A.M., Durant, C.J., Ganellin, C.R., and Parsons, E.M.: Definition and antagonism of histamine receptors, Nature **236**:385, 1972.
2. Bodemar, G., and Walan, A.: Cimetidine in treatment of active duodenal and pre-pyloric ulcers, Lancet **2**:161, 1976.
3. Brand, J.J., and Perry, W.L.M.: Drugs used in motion sickness, Pharmacol. Rev. **18**:895, 1966.
4. Brimblecombe, R.W., Duncan, W.A.M., Durant, G.J., et al.: Cimetidine: a non–thiourea H_2-receptor antagonist, J. Int. Med. Res. **3**:86, 1975.
5. Danilevicius, Z.: A new star: how brightly will it shine? JAMA **237**:2224, 1977.
6. Finkelstein, W., and Isselbacher, K.J.: Cimetidine, N. Engl. J. Med. **299**:992, 1978.
7. Goth, A.: Antihistamines. In Middleton, E., Jr., Reed, C.E., and Ellis, E.F.: Allergy: principles and practice, St. Louis, 1978, The C.V. Mosby Co.
8. Hunt, R.H.: Use and abuse of H_2 receptor antagonists, J. Roy. Coll. Physicians Lond. **16**:33, 1982.
9. Ranitidine (Zantac), Med. Lett. **24**:111, Dec. 24, 1982.
10. Schlippert, W.: Cimetidine, H_2-receptor blockade in gastrointestinal disease, Arch. Intern. Med. **138**:1257, 1978.

Chapter 21

Serotonin and antiserotonins

Serotonin, or 5-hydroxytryptamine, occupies a surprisingly prominent position in the medical literature, considering the ignorance that surrounds its functions in the body. The reasons for this paradox are many. This endogenously produced amine is almost certainly one of the central neurotransmitters. It is also present in large quantities in the enterochromaffin system of the intestine and in platelets, where its functions are unknown. Moreover, studies on serotonin have contributed greatly to theories on biochemical mechanisms in disease states ranging from mental disease to migraine. The relationships between lysergic acid diethylamide (LSD) and serotonin and the release of the amine by reserpine provided potent stimuli for psychopharmacological research. The same can be said of the hallucinogenic properties of many serotonin derivatives.

In addition to serotonin, some of its therapeutically useful antagonists will be discussed in this chapter. Furthermore, the pharmacology of ergot alkaloids, lysergic acid derivatives that are generally serotonin antagonists, will also be considered at this point.

SEROTONIN

The discovery of serotonin (5-hydroxytryptamine; 5-HT) as a normally occurring amine resulted from independent studies on the vasoconstrictor substance in serum at the Cleveland Clinic and the active substance of intestinal enterochromaffin cells, named *enteramine* by investigators in Italy. The compound investigated by both groups was eventually shown to be 5-HT.

Occurrence and distribution

Serotonin is widely distributed in the animal and plant kingdom. Some fruits such as bananas contain a high concentration but represent no threat of causing serotonin poisoning because the amine is not well absorbed from the gastrointestinal tract and is rapidly metabolized. Ingestion of such fruits, however, may increase the urinary excretion of serotonin metabolites, giving false positive tests in the diagnosis of carcinoid tumor.

In mammals about 90% of the total serotonin is in the enterochromaffin cells of the intestine, about 8% in platelets, and 2% in the CNS, particularly in the pineal gland and the hypothalamus. In rats and mice serotonin is also present in mast cells along with histamine. Human mast cells probably do not contain serotonin, since in mastocytosis the excretion of the serotonin metabolite 5-hydroxyindoleacetic acid in the urine is not increased.

Serotonin is synthesized from tryptophan at the sites mentioned, except in the platelets, which actively concentrate the amine but do not make it.

Serotonin is made from tryptophan. Normally only a small fraction of the dietary tryptophan is used for serotonin synthesis. In patients with carcinoid tumors this fraction may increase so greatly that pellagra may result.

The various steps in the biosynthesis and biodegradation of serotonin are as follows:

Biosynthesis and metabolic degradation

Tryptophan → 5-Hydroxytryptophan → 5-Hydroxytryptamine → 5-Hydroxyindoleacetic acid

Tryptophan

5-Hydroxytryptophan

5-Hydroxytryptamine (serotonin)

5-Hydroxyindoleacetic acid

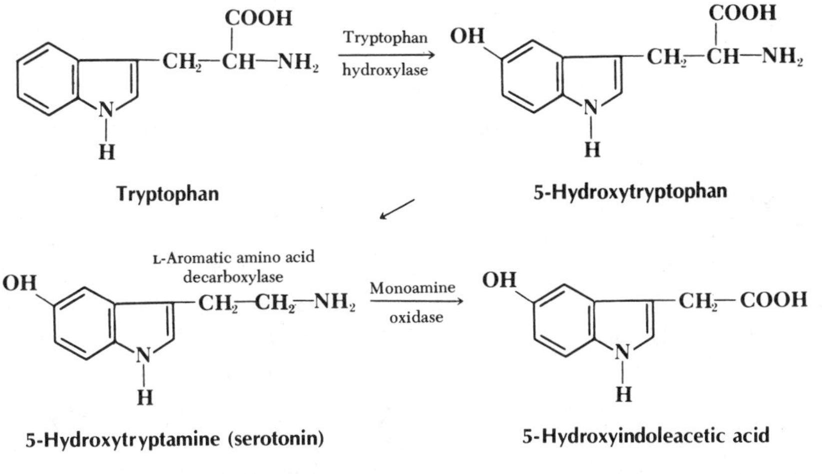

In addition, serotonin is converted in the pineal gland to *N*-acetyl serotonin and its *O*-methyl derivative, *melatonin*.

The biosynthesis of serotonin is blocked by *p-chlorophenylalanine*, which inhibits tryptophan hydroxylase, the rate-limiting enzyme. Degradation of serotonin is blocked by the MAO inhibitors. Turnover of serotonin is quite rapid in the CNS and also in the intestine. MAO inhibitors can double the serotonin content of brain in less than 1 hour.

The daily excretion of 5-hydroxyindoleacetic acid in the urine is 3 to 10 mg in a normal adult. It increases greatly in the presence of a carcinoid tumor and also with the ingestion of bananas and the administration of reserpine, which releases serotonin from its binding sites. Excretion of 5-hydroxyindoleacetic acid is decreased by MAO inhibitors.

The actions of serotonin are exerted on smooth muscles and on nerve elements including afferent nerve endings. The smooth muscle effects are prominent in the cardiovascular system and the gastrointestinal tract.

Intravenous injection of a few micrograms of serotonin as the creatinine sulfate complex produces a *triphasic* response: (1) a transient fall of blood pressure, (2) a brief period of hypertension, and (3) a more prolonged period of pressure lowering. The early depressor phase is probably caused by a reflex elicited by stimulation of chemoreceptors (Bezold-Jarisch effect). The blood pressure elevation is a consequence of constriction of blood vessels in many areas. Finally, the late depressor phase is attributed to the vasodilator action of serotonin in areas such as the skeletal muscle. Continuous intravenous infusion of serotonin produces only the prolonged lowering of peripheral resistance, with lowering of mean blood pressure.

In addition to its effect on the cardiovascular system, serotonin stimulates the gastrointestinal and bronchial smooth muscles. The gastrointestinal effects are both direct and also a consequence of excitation of ganglion cells. The direct effects are blocked by serotonin antagonists such as LSD; the ganglionic action is, interestingly, blocked by morphine. The bronchial stimulant action of the drug is probably unimportant in humans, although asthmatic individuals may be unduly responsive to it.

Serotonin can stimulate afferent nerve endings, ganglion cells, and adrenal medullary cells. It does not cross the blood-brain barrier but exerts striking effects when injected into the lateral ventricles of cats. Sleep, catatonia, and fever have been elicited by such injections.

The possible role of serotonin in mood and behavior and in mental disease comes from speculations based on several lines of evidence. First, the powerful psychotomimetic drug LSD was early found to inhibit the actions of serotonin on smooth muscles. The simple hypothesis based on these facts found little support, however, when it was shown that other antiserotonins, even the closely related D-2-bromolysergic acid diethylamide, were not psychotomimetic.

The final remaining speculation in regard to a link between serotonin and mental disease is the demonstrated hallucinogenic effect of a variety of compounds structurally related to the amine. For example, bufotenine is 5-hydroxy-dimethyltryptamine, and psilocin is 4-hydroxy-dimethyltryptamine. Bufotenine is present in some plants and in toads. Psilocin and its phosphoryl ester psilocybin are very potent LSD-like hallucinogens. Many other tryptamine derivatives have psychotomimetic effects, and it is intriguing to speculate on biochemical explanations of schizophrenia. A critical review of this problem concluded that all such speculations are interesting but up to then, at least, not convincing.

Serotonin probably plays a role in intestinal motility, since there is an abundance of this amine in the enterochromaffin cells that can be released by distention and other mechanical stimuli. Morphine blocks the effects of serotonin on intramural ganglion cells.

Serotonin probably plays a role in the causation of symptoms in the *carcinoid syndrome*. Flushing and increased intestinal motility have been attributed to serotonin release. However, the flush that occurs in carcinoid patients cannot be elicited by the injection of serotonin but will occur, on the other hand, after the administration of epinephrine or bradykinin. It has been shown that kinin-producing enzymes are released from the carcinoid tumor. In addition, in the gastric carcinoid syndrome histamine plays an important role. The ameliorating effects of *p*-chlorophenylalanine on intestinal motility of carcinoid patients suggests a role for serotonin in its causation.

The role of serotonin in platelets is completely unknown, although for years it was believed to play a role in hemostasis as the vasoconstrictor of serum. This hypothesis was put to a test when reserpine became available as a serotonin depletor. Reserpine was administered to patients in sufficient dosage to reduce serotonin levels to negligible amounts. This procedure had no effect on bleeding time or clotting time, a result that casts doubt on the role of serotonin in hemostasis.

Because of the effectiveness of several serotonin antagonists in the prevention of *migraine*, a role for the amine in the causation of vascular headaches has been suggested. The evidence for this is poor.

SEROTONIN ANTAGONISTS, OR ANTISEROTONINS

Serotonin antagonists include numerous *lysergic acid derivatives*, many of which are naturally occurring ergot alkaloids. Methysergide (Sansert) is a potent antiserotonin of clinical usefulness in the prevention of vascular headaches. Other lysergic acid derivatives that are potent antiserotonins include LSD and D-2-bromolysergic acid diethylamide. Many *antihistamines* have antiserotonin effects also. Among these, *cyproheptadine* (Periactin) is potent and has been discussed among the antihistamines (p. 222). *Chlorpromazine*, other *phenothiazines*, and *α-adrenergic blocking agents* such as *phenoxybenzamine* also block the effects of serotonin.

For practical purposes methysergide and cyproheptadine are the only two drugs available for antagonizing symptoms that might be attributed to serotonin clinically.

Methysergide maleate

Methysergide maleate (Sansert) is closely related to the ergot alkaloid methylergonovine, which is used as an oxytocic drug. It is 1-methyl-*d*-lysergic acid butanolamide and was introduced specifically as a prophylactic agent for migraine headaches. It is a potent serotonin antagonist, even more potent than ergotamine or LSD. The drug is useful only for the prevention and not for the treatment of migraine. Its mode of action is not well understood, since connections between migraine and serotonin are in the realm of speculation.

Methysergide

Adverse reactions to methysergide are many and include nausea, dizziness, insomnia, behavioral changes (reminiscent of mild LSD reactions), gastrointestinal disturbances, and others. A serious complication seen in several patients after long-term use of methysergide was retroperitoneal fibrosis and pleural pulmonary fibrosis. Retroperitoneal fibrosis may lead to urinary tract obstruction.

Contraindications to the use of methysergide are peripheral vascular disease, hypertension, peptic ulcer, coronary artery disease, and pregnancy.

Methysergide maleate (Sansert) is available in tablets containing 2 mg.

Cyproheptadine hydrochloride

Cyproheptadine hydrochloride (Periactin hydrochloride) is an antihistaminic drug that also has potent antiserotonin properties. It has been proposed for some indications that are different from those requiring the usual antihistamines. The drug is effective in the treatment of allergic rhinitis and for the relief of pruritus in a variety of skin disorders. In addition, it is claimed to be effective in promoting weight gain in children by mechanisms that are not understood.

The main untoward effect seen after the administration of cyproheptadine is drowsiness. Preparations of cyproheptadine hydrochloride (Periactin hydrochloride) include tablets, 4 mg, and syrup, 2 mg/5 ml.

Ergot alkaloids

Some of the ergot alkaloids are quite useful in treating vascular headaches, some are employed for stimulating the uterine smooth muscle, and still others have been tried as hypotensive agents. The work on LSD is an outgrowth of pharmacological studies on ergot alkaloids.

There is increasing interest in new semisynthetic ergot alkaloids such as bromocriptine, which act as dopaminergic agonists. Such drugs inhibit the release of prolactin from the pituitary gland and have been used successfully to suppress postpartum lactation and to treat galactorrhea and amenorrhea in patients with increased prolactin levels.

HISTORICAL ASPECTS OF PHARMACOLOGY

It has been known for centuries that ingestion of diseased rye can cause poisoning characterized by gangrene, abortion, and sometimes convulsions. The fungus that causes this disease of rye is *Claviceps purpurea*, often called *ergot*. It contains a large variety of potent pharmacological agents referred to as the ergot alkaloids, many of which are derivatives of lysergic acid. The structural formulas of lysergic acid and ergonovine, one of the ergot alkaloids, are shown below.

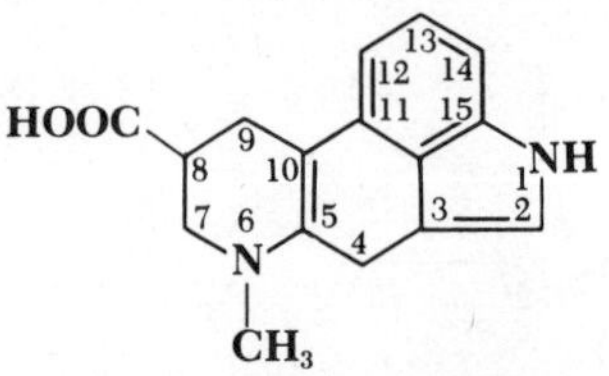

Lysergic acid

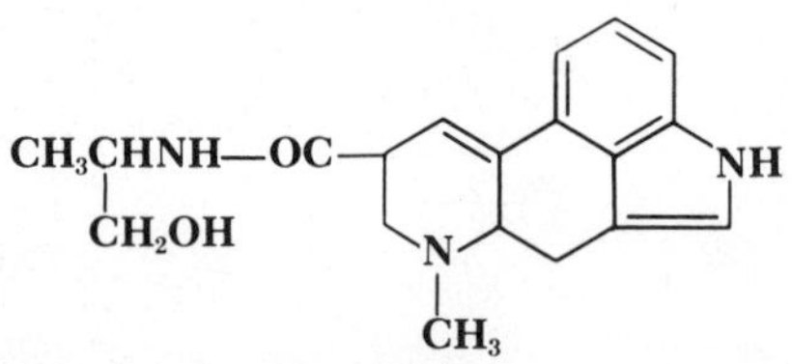

Ergonovine

The isolation of ergotamine and ergotoxine, a mixture of ergot alkaloids, led to the belief that most of the pharmacological properties of ergot resulted from these compounds. It was later shown, however, that crude ergot extracts had a greater effect on the uterus than did ergotamine or ergotoxine. Soon the alkaloid ergonovine was also isolated, and this unsuspected new compound served to explain the greater activity of the crude extracts.

CHEMISTRY

The important alkaloids of ergot are ergotamine, ergotoxine, and ergonovine. In addition, ergotoxine has been shown to be a mixture of three compounds: ergocristine, ergocryptine, and ergocornine.

From a chemical standpoint, ergonovine is the simplest compound. Its structural formula indicates that it is a combination of lysergic acid with *d*-2-aminopropranol.

In contrast to ergonovine, ergotamine and the ergotoxine group yield amino acids on hydrolysis and have a considerably higher molecular weight than ergonovine, although they also are lysergic acid derivatives.

PHARMACOLOGICAL EFFECTS

The ergot alkaloids have three major actions in the body: smooth muscle contraction, particularly evident on blood vessels and the uterus, adrenergic blocking effect, and CNS effects leading to hypotension. These actions are present to a varying extent in the different alkaloids. Ergonovine has powerful smooth muscle effects without the other properties characteristic of many of the other alkaloids. Ergotamine and the ergotoxine group have smooth muscle actions and can also block norepinephrine and epinephrine.

The two most commonly used ergot alkaloids in therapeutics are ergotamine (Gynergen) and ergonovine (Ergotrate). Ergotamine is extensively employed in the treatment of vascular headaches such as migraine, whereas ergonovine finds its greatest usefulness in obstetrics for its stimulant effect on the uterine smooth muscle.

ERGOTAMINE TARTRATE

Ergotamine tartrate (Gynergen) is used almost exclusively in the treatment of migraine and other vascular headaches, and its effects can be best illustrated by describing its actions when administered to a patient suffering from such headaches.

It is believed that during the early stages of the attack there is constriction of blood vessels, followed by their marked dilatation. The early visual disturbances are attributed to constriction of retinal vessels, whereas the headache itself may be related to dilatation and edema of the extracranial vessels.

Ergotamine tartrate is the drug of choice in the treatment of migraine and is believed to act by vasoconstriction. The drug may be given orally or injected subcutaneously or intramuscularly. Its effectiveness in relieving a headache is considered to be of diagnostic value.

Although the drug is very effective, it is not suitable for long-continued or prophylactic use because of serious adverse effects such as severe vasoconstriction and gangrene of the extremities. For prophylaxis of migraine, methysergide (discussed previously) is commonly used, but it also has many untoward effects and contraindications. Propranolol and other β blockers are the preferred agents for prophylaxis of migraine.

Adverse effects. Ergotamine tartrate may cause nausea, vomiting, diarrhea, vasoconstriction, and gangrene of the extremities. Because of its adverse effects the drug is contraindicated in pregnancy and all vascular diseases.

Preparations. Ergotamine tartrate (Gynergen) is available in 1 mg tablets and solution for injection, 0.5 mg/ml. Ergotamine tartrate is also available in sublingual tablets, 2 mg, and for inhalation in Medihalers, which dispense 0.36 mg of the drug in each inhalation.

ERGONOVINE MALEATE

Ergonovine maleate (Ergotrate maleate) and its derivative, methylergonovine (Methergine), are used exclusively in obstetrics. They are less effective than ergotamine in migraine.

Ergonovine maleate and methylergonovine maleate are powerful oxytocics and have significant vasoconstrictor effects, but they lack the adrenergic blocking action of ergotamine. They are well absorbed from the gastrointestinal tract, whereas the larger amino acid alkaloids are only partially absorbed. They may produce hypertension.

Ergonovine maleate and methylergonovine maleate are used in obstetrics in the third stage of labor, principally to decrease postpartum bleeding through their powerful effect on direct contraction of the uterine smooth muscle.

Although ergonovine maleate and methylergonovine maleate have powerful effects on the uterus, they do not promote normal uterine contractions as does oxytocin. For this reason they should not be employed for initiation of labor.

Adverse effects. Adverse effects of ergonovine maleate and methylergonovine maleate include nausea, vomiting, and elevations of blood pressure.

Preparations. Ergonovine maleate (Ergotrate maleate) is available in tablets containing 0.2 mg and in solution for injection, 0.2 mg/ml. Methylergonovine maleate (Methergine) is available in tablets, 0.2 mg, and solution for injection, 0.2 mg/ml.

DIHYDROERGOTOXINE MESYLATE

The dihydrogenated alkaloids of the ergotoxine group are available in sublingual tablets containing 0.167 mg each of dihydroergocornine, dihydroergocristine, and dihydroergokryptine as the mesylates. Dihydroergotoxine mesylate (Hydergine) is used in elderly patients in whom it may produce modest improvements in self-care and various symptoms commonly attributed to cerebral atherosclerosis, although without definitive evidence regarding cause. Dihydroergotoxine mesylate does not have vasoconstrictor properties and the sublingual tablets do not produce serious side effects.

From a pharmacological standpoint the dihydrogenated ergotoxine alkaloids are expected to produce some adrenergic blockade and an inhibitory effect on central sympathetic functions. Nevertheless, the effects of dihydroergotoxine mesylate sublingual tablets in elderly patients cannot be definitely attributed to a specific pharmacological action.

The synthetic ergot alkaloid, bromocriptine mesylate (Parlodel), is a dopaminergic agonist and may have numerous indications. It inhibits prolactin secretion, suppresses acromegaly, and postpartum lactation, and is useful in Parkinson's disease. The drug is claimed to decrease prolactin-producing adenomas. Adverse effects such as nausea, orthostatic hypotension, and many others are common, particularly at the beginning of therapy. Bromocriptine mesylate (Parlodel) is available in 2.5 and 5 mg tablets.

Bromocriptine mesylate

Poisoning with ergot alkaloids occasionally follows ingestion of bread prepared from ergot-contaminated rye. There were large epidemics in the past, and occasional outbreaks still occur in some parts of the world. Poisoning may also be produced when patients take ergot alkaloids in fairly large doses over a long period of time for migraine or for the purpose of inducing abortion.

ERGOT POISONING

The symptoms and signs of ergot poisoning depend on whether the poisoning is acute or chronic. In chronic poisoning the clinical picture is dominated by gangrene. In acute poisoning there may be vomiting, diarrhea, headache, vertigo, paresthesia, convulsions, and gangrene of the fingers, toes, nose, or ears. The skin may be cold and cyanotic. The pulse rate may slow, but more frequently it is rapid and weak. Treatment with vasodilators such as papaverine and sympathetic nerve block has been tried, but there is no consensus on its effectiveness. The most important preventive measure is avoidance of long-continued use of ergotamine tartrate for vascular headaches.

1. Maxson, S.W., and Hammond, C.B.: Clinical uses of bromocriptine, Hosp. Form. June 1981.
2. Surgical approaches and drug treatment in the carcinoid syndrome, Br. Med. J. 1(3):1572, 1978.
3. Symposium: Pharmacology of serotonin neurones in the central nervous system, Fed. Proc. **36**:2133, 1977.

REFERENCES

Chapter 22

Kinins and prostaglandins

In addition to various amines that act as neurotransmitters, there are numerous polypeptides and acidic lipids that exert powerful effects on various smooth muscles and glands. Since these compounds occur normally in the body, they probably perform important regulatory functions. The *kinins* are vasodilator polypeptides; among them the plasma kinins *bradykinin* and *kallidin* are of greatest interest. The *prostoglandins* are acidic lipids widely distributed in the body and having great pharmacological activity.

KININS
General concept

A variety of polypeptides have effects somewhat similar to those of histamine on vascular smooth muscle, capillary permeability, and bronchial and intestinal smooth muscle.

Bradykinin is a biologically active nonapeptide, a product of the enzyme *kallikrein* on its α_2-globulin substrate. It is a potent agent to which many functions have been attributed, such as the regulation of the microcirculation of exocrine glands, circulatory changes occurring after birth, and mediation of inflammatory processes.

Numerous related kinins occur widely distributed in nature, such as in wasp venom and in the skin of amphibia. What makes bradykinin of special interest, however, is the ease with which it may be made and destroyed in the body. It could have great importance in physiological and pathological processes, but its exact role is not likely to be defined until specific antagonists become available.

History and
nomenclature

The early studies on the kinins were carried out by two groups of investigators, one in Germany (Werle and co-workers) and the other in Brazil (Rocha e Silva and co-workers). Until recently the nomenclature on kinins was quite confusing because of the conflicting terms used by the various groups. The German group named their polypeptide *kallidin* and its plasma precursor *kallidinogen;* the enzyme that acted on kallidinogen was named *kallikrein*. The hypotensive substance was found in the urine and also in the pancreas, whose Greek name is *kallikreas* (although some Greeks disagree).

Independently the Brazilian group found that when snake venoms or trypsin acted on plasma globulin, a substance was produced that caused a slow contraction of the guinea pig ileum. The term *bradykinin* (from the Greek word *bradys*, meaning "slow") was coined to designate this substance.

Bradykinin is a polypeptide composed of a chain of nine amino acids (arginine-proline-proline-glycine-phenylalanine-serine-proline-phenylalanine-arginine). Kallidin is a decapeptide that contains an additional *N*-terminal lysine residue. The precursor of the kinins is called *kininogen*, sometimes referred to as bradykininogen or kallidinogen. The precursor of active *kallikrein* is *prekallikrein*. Enzymes that release kinins in general should be called *kininogenases*. Thus kallikrein and trypsin are kininogenases. The relationships between these factors are shown below:

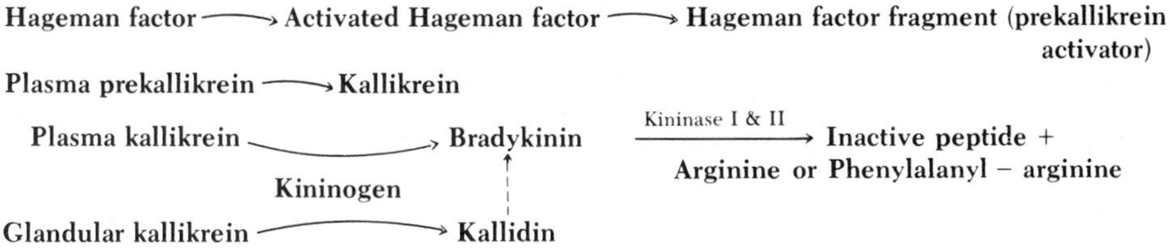

Hageman factor ⟶ Activated Hageman factor ⟶ Hageman factor fragment (prekallikrein activator)

Plasma prekallikrein ⟶ Kallikrein

Plasma kallikrein ⟶ Bradykinin $\xrightarrow{\text{Kininase I \& II}}$ Inactive peptide +
Kininogen ↑ Arginine or Phenylalanyl − arginine
Glandular kallikrein ⟶ Kallidin

Bradykinin is split by at least two enzymes. Kininase I is also known as carboxypeptidase N. Kininase II appears to be identical to the angiotensin I converting enzyme. Kininase I inactivates other biologically active peptides, for example, an anaphylatoxin derived from the activation of the complement system. Kininase I acts mostly in blood, whereas kininase II acts in various organs such as the lung.

The actual events are much more complex than indicated in the schema. Some of the kallidin released by glandular kallikrein may be converted to bradykinin. Kininogen may be acted on by trypsinlike proteases. There are activators in tissues that are not well characterized. Glandular tissues, such as salivary glands or pancreas and also urine, are among the richest sources of kallikrein. There are also numerous kallikrein inhibitors in tissues and in blood.

Kininogen has a role in blood clotting, and liberated plasma kallikrein activates factor XII (Hageman factor) by a positive feedback.

Kallikrein inhibitor. Aprotinin (Trasylol) is a peptide extracted from bovine lung. It inhibits kallikrein and many other proteases. It has been used clinically, particularly in Germany, in various types of shock, acute pancreatitis, and fibrinolytic states. It has not been approved for use by the Food and Drug Administration.

Roles of bradykinin. Some interesting relationships may exist between bradykinin and angiotensin (p. 192). Both are polypeptides split from plasma proteins. Angiotensin is a potent vasoconstrictor, whereas bradykinin has the opposite effect on vascular smooth muscle. The converting enzyme in the angiotensin system is a powerful inactivator of bradykinin.

Converting enzyme inhibitors are being tested at present both in treatment of hypertension and for their effect on the destruction of bradykinin. A nonapeptide (Pyr-Trp-Pro-Arg-Pro-Gln-Ile-Pro-Pro) blocks the conversion of angiotensin I to angiotensin II. It was found effective in the early phases of experimental renal hypertension if given intravenously. A newer inhibitor, captopril, is active orally. It is discussed in greater detail in connection with the antihypertensive drugs (p. 206).

The plasma kinins very likely play a role in inflammatory processes. They can reproduce the cardinal signs of inflammation such as vasodilatation, increased capillary permeability, and pain. Furthermore, they can be produced rather easily in the tissues following injury.

It is attractive to think of some types of inflammation as having two phases. In an early phase histamine and other mediators are released rather explosively. In a secondary phase kinins may be constantly produced and destroyed to perpetuate the inflammatory process. Interestingly, many of the kinins in fairly high concentration can cause histamine release from mast cells,[5] although their primary action in the body is probably not a consequence of histamine release.

Pharmacological effects

On a molar basis the plasma kinins are the most potent vasodilators known. They also cause increased capillary permeability and pain when applied to a denuded surface such as the base of a blister or after intraperitoneal injection. Pain produced by bradykinin is increased by prostaglandins.

Bradykinin also constricts the bronchial smooth muscle. Aspirin antagonizes the action of the peptide on guinea pig bronchi. This may be a result of an interaction between aspirin and prostaglandins released by the kinin.

Other smooth muscle effects. Bradykinin constricts the uterine smooth muscle and most gastrointestinal smooth muscles. The anomalous relaxing effect on the rat duodenum may be a consequence of catecholamine release. Bradykinin can cause the release of catecholamines from the adrenal medulla, histamine from mast cells,[5] and prostaglandin from the kidney.

Clinical significance of plasma kinins

In view of the ease with which plasma and tissue prekallikreins are activated and the availability of kininogen in the plasma, it is not surprising that numerous roles are being attributed to the kinins in health and disease. Plasma prekallikrein may be activated by the prior activation of the Hageman factor, antigen-antibody reactions, inflammation, trauma, trypsin, snake venoms, acid milieu, endotoxins, and heat. Similarly, tissue kallikreins may be activated and released by trauma, inflammation, toxins, and heat.

Some of the clinical conditions in which the kinins are believed to play a pathogenetic role are endotoxin shock, carcinoid syndrome (p. 229), hereditary angioneurotic edema with its deficiency of a kallikrein inhibitor, anaphylaxis, arthritis (particularly gout where urate crystals activate the Hageman factor), and acute pancreatitis. In addition, bradykinin may play a role in constricting the umbilical artery and the ductus arteriosus and in the transformation of the fetal to the neonatal circulation. An orthostatic syndrome, hyperbradykinemia, has recently been described.[9]

The significance of the kallikrein-bradykinin system may increase as a consequence of the observation indicating that some hypertensive patients excrete less kallikrein than normal controls. This is an old observation that has been confirmed recently.

In addition to bradykinin and kallidin, there are other peptides with somewhat similar properties. *Substance P* is present in the brain and in larger amounts in the intestine. *Eledoisin* is a powerful hypotensive peptide obtained from the salivary gland of the octopus.

Other hypotensive peptides

The prostaglandins, so named because they were first isolated from seminal fluid, represent a series of acidic lipids having powerful pharmacological activity. Their widespread occurrence in tissues (including those of the nervous system) suggests for these acidic compounds a regulatory function that may be exerted as a very basic control system related to adenyl cyclase. Great efforts are being made to develop this new class of agents into medically useful drugs. Preliminary indications are that they may find applications in the induction of labor, as abortifacients, and as nasal vasoconstrictors. All these uses and the many others that are being investigated must be considered as strictly experimental at present.

PROSTAGLANDINS

In 1930 two New York gynecologists reported that fresh human semen could cause contraction or relaxation of strips of human uterus. A few years later, Goldblatt in England and von Euler in Sweden studied the pharmacological effects of lipid extracts of seminal fluid. The name *prostaglandin* was coined by von Euler in 1935, and the structures of two were established by Sune Bergström at the Karolinska Institute. The Nobel prize was awarded to Sune Bergström, Bengt Samuelsson, and John Vane for their work concerning prostaglandins and related substances, such as the leukotrienes.

History and nomenclature

Prostaglandins are present in greatest amounts in human and sheep seminal plasma. In various species they occur also in the uterus, lung, brain, iris, thymus, pancreas, and kidney, and they are found in human menstrual blood. It is quite likely that the numerous acidic lipids with pharmacological activity isolated over the years from various tissues are actually prostaglandins.

As shown in the schema on p. 238, the prostaglandins are analogs of *prostanoic acid*, a C_{20} acid that contains a five-membered ring. Biosynthetically they originate from arachidonic acid or dihomo-γ-linolenic acid. The four major groups of prostaglandins are designated E, F, A, and B on the basis of their ring structure. The numeral in the subscript position indicates the degree of unsaturation in the side chains.

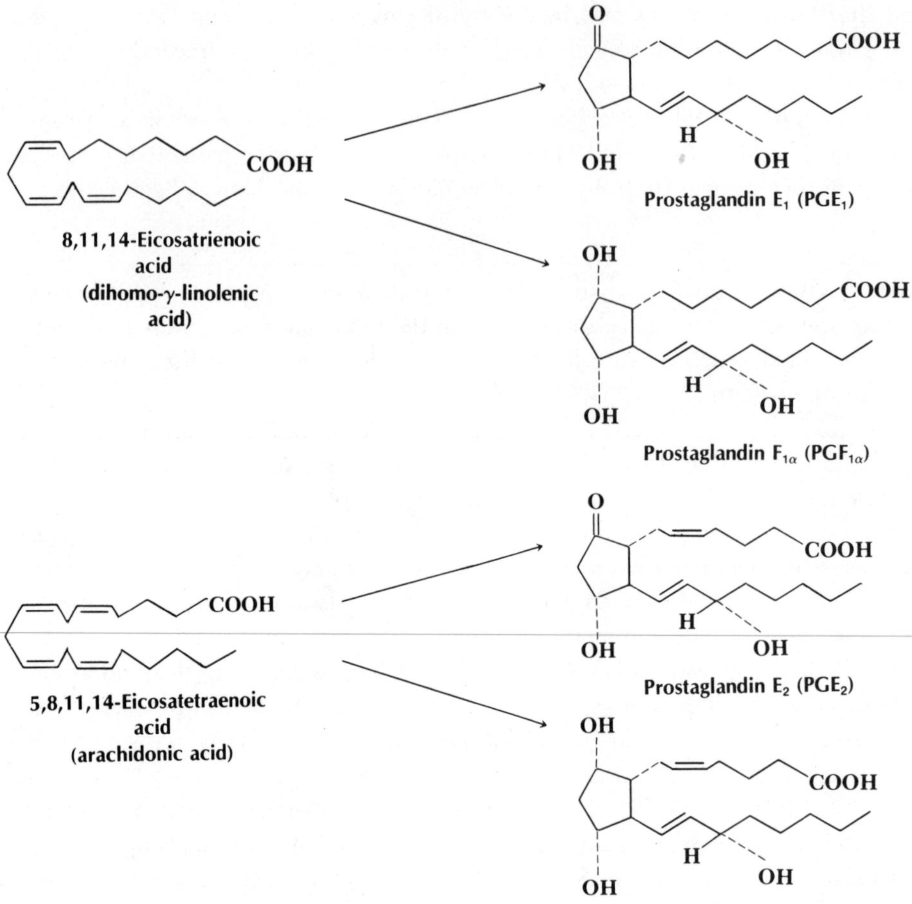

8,11,14-Eicosatrienoic
acid
(dihomo-γ-linolenic
acid)

Prostaglandin E_1 (PGE_1)

Prostaglandin $F_{1\alpha}$ ($PGF_{1\alpha}$)

5,8,11,14-Eicosatetraenoic
acid
(arachidonic acid)

Prostaglandin E_2 (PGE_2)

Prostaglandin $F_{2\alpha}$ ($PGF_{2\alpha}$)

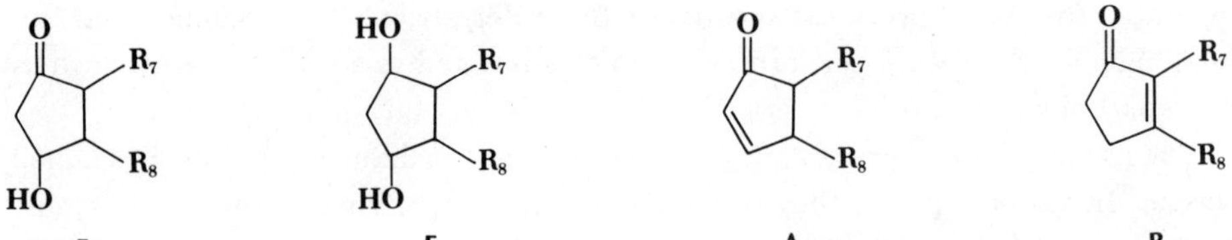

E   F   A   B

Biosynthesis   As shown in the formulas above, prostaglandins are made from dihomo-γ-linolenic acid and arachidonic acid. These fatty acids are probably released from phospholipids by phospholipases. According to current views, arachidonic acid is first converted by the enzyme prostaglandin synthetase to the cyclic endoperoxides, of very short half-life, also known as prostaglandin G_2 or H_2. This reaction is blocked by aspirin and indomethacin:

$$\text{Arachidonic acid} \xrightarrow[\overset{\text{Aspirin, indomethacin}}{}]{} \text{Prostaglandins } G_2, H_2 \text{ (cyclic endoperoxides)}$$

From the cyclic endoperoxides, the synthetic process may follow three different paths, forming several prostaglandins, thromboxanes, and prostacyclin.

$$\text{Cyclic endoperoxides} \begin{cases} \rightarrow \text{PGE}_2, \text{ PGF}_{2\alpha}, \text{ PGD}_2 \\ \rightarrow \text{Thromboxane } A_2 \rightarrow \text{thromboxane } B_2 \\ \rightarrow \text{Prostacyclin} \end{cases}$$

In addition to the cyclooxygenase pathway, which yields the endoperoxides, arachidonic acid may follow a lipoxygenase pathway, which produces hydroxy acids (HETE) and leukotrienes. One of these in combination with cysteine is SRS-A, which may play an important role in bronchial asthma.

The metabolic pathways of arachidonic acid are shown on pp. 240 and 241.*

Pharmacological effects

The mechanism of action of the prostaglandins may involve the stimulation of cyclic AMP production and calcium use by various cells. The synthesis of these compounds is inhibited by aspirin, indomethacin, and other nonsteroidal anti-inflammatory agents. Antagonists include the arachidonic acid analog eicosatetraynoic acid (ETYA) and polyphloretin phosphate.

The complex effects of the various prostaglandins may be summarized as follows: *cardiovascular*—PGE causes a decrease in blood pressure, PGF produces an increase in blood pressure; *kidney*—PGE but not PGF causes vasodilatation, natriuresis, diuresis, and renin release; *respiratory*—PGE is a bronchodilator, PGF is a bronchoconstrictor; *gastrointestinal*—PGE and PGF contract the smooth muscle and cause diarrhea, whereas PGE inhibits gastric secretion; *eye*—PGE and PGF cause miosis; and *reproductive system*—PGE relaxes the nonpregnant but contracts the pregnant uterus, whereas PGF contracts both the pregnant and nonpregnant uterus.

The possible role of the prostaglandins in inflammation and immune phenomena is of great interest. The intracutaneous injection of various prostaglandins has histamine-like effects. In addition, it has been shown that aspirin blocks the synthesis of prostaglandins by human platelets, guinea pig lungs, and some other tissues. On the basis of these findings it has been suggested that the action of aspirin and perhaps other nonsteroidal anti-inflammatory drugs may be attributed to inhibition of prostaglandin synthesis. The antithrombotic actions of aspirin are probably caused by this enzymatic effect.[10]

Although the prostaglandins do not produce much pain, there are reasons to believe that they may reinforce the pain-producing actions of bradykinin.

Precursors of prostaglandins, such as arachidonic acid, may have effects similar to the final product when injected. On the other hand, the *endoperoxide* interme-

---

*From Moncada, S., and Vane, J.R.: Pharmacology of endogenous roles of prostaglandin endoperoxides, thromboxane A_2 and prostacyclin, Pharmacol. Rev. **30**:293, 1979.

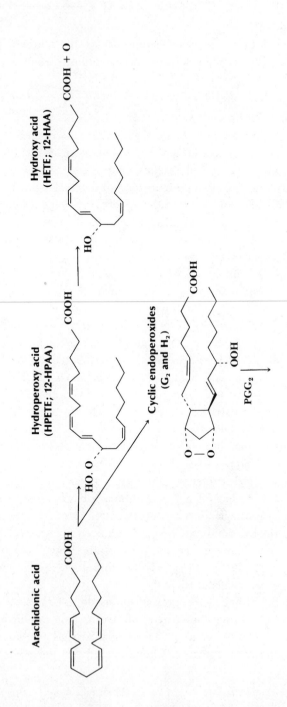

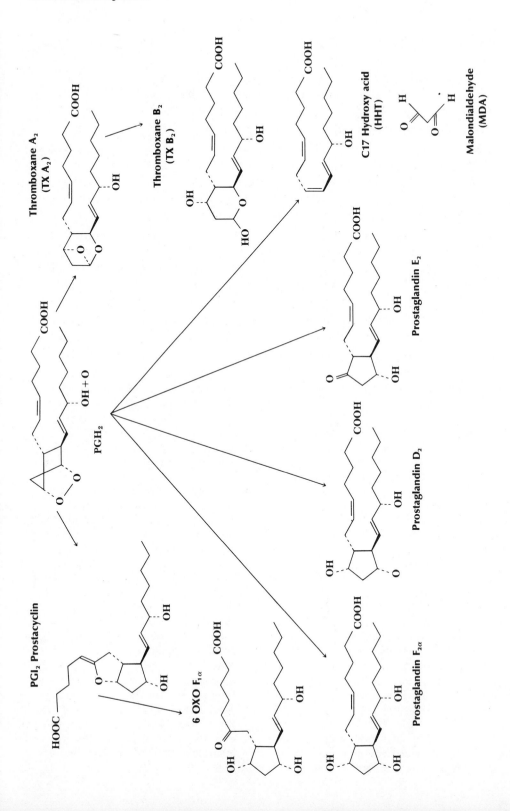

diates in the synthesis of the prostaglandins may have pharmacological effects of their own.

The thromboxanes are powerful but short-lived platelet aggregating agents. The newly discovered prostacyclin, or PGX, prevents platelet aggregation. It is postulated that the balance of these compounds, elaborated by the vascular endothelium, may play an important role in thrombosis and its prevention.

Diseases associated with excess production of prostaglandins

Various diseases may be associated with excessive prostaglandin production. The main evidence for such an association is based on the improvement that can be achieved by prostaglandin synthesis inhibitors. Some of these conditions are primary dysmenorrhea, Bartter's syndrome, threatened abortion, patent ductus arteriosus, pancreatic cholera, hypercalcemia of cancer, idiopathic orthostatic hypotension, and inflammation. The nonsteroidal anti-inflammatory drugs, such as aspirin, indomethacin, ibuprofen, and others, may owe their effectiveness to prostaglandin synthesis inhibition.

Possible therapeutic applications

Dinoprost tromethamine (Prostin F_2 Alpha) was introduced as an abortifacient in the second trimester of pregnancy. Synthetic analogs are being used investigationally in the treatment of peptic ulcer, hypertension, asthma, and hypercalcemia.[3] As an abortifacient, dinoprost tromethamine is administered intraamniotically. Adverse effects caused by the drug include nausea, vomiting, hypertension, allergic reactions, bronchospasm, hypotension, syncope, and uterine lacerations.

REFERENCES

1. Andersen, N.H., and Ramwell, P.W.: Biological aspects of prostaglandins, Arch. Intern. Med. **133:**30, 1974.
2. Bonta, I.L., and Parnham, M.J.: Prostaglandins and chronic inflammation, Biochem. Pharmacol. **27:**1611, 1978.
3. Clayman, C.B.: The prostaglandins, JAMA **233:**904, 1975.
4. Erdös, E.G.: Conversion of angiotensin I to angiotensin II, Am. J. Med. **60:**749, 1976.
5. Johnson, A.R., and Erdös, E.G.: Release of histamine from mast cells by vasoactive peptides, Proc. Soc. Esp. Biol. Med. **142:**1252, 1973.
6. Margolius, H.S., Geller, R.G., deJong, W., Pisano, J.J., and Sjoerdsma, A.: Urinary kallikrein excretion in hypertension, Circ. Res. **30:**11, 1972.
7. Moncada, S., and Vane, J.R.: Pharmacology of endogenous roles of prostaglandin endoperoxides, thromboxane A_2 and

prostacyclin, Pharmacol. Rev. **30:**293, 1979.
8. Samuelsson, B., Goldyne, M., Granstrom, E., Hamberg, M., Hammerstrom, S., and Malmsten, C.: Prostaglandins and thromboxanes, Ann. Rev. Biochem. **47:**997, 1978.
9. Streeten, D.H.P., Kerr, C.B., Kerr, L.P., Prior, J.C., and Dalakos, T.G.: Hyperbradykinism: a new orthostatic syndrome, Lancet **2:**1048, 1972.
10. Vane, J.K.: The mode of action of aspirin and similar compounds, J. Allergy Clin. Immunol. **58:**691, 1976.
11. Wilson, D.C.: Prostaglandins: their action on the gastrointestinal tract, Arch. Intern. Med. **133:**112, 1974.
12. Yang, H.Y.T., Erdös, E.G., and Levin, Y.: A dipeptidyl carboxypeptidase that converts angiotensin I and inactivates bradykinin, Biochim. Biophys. Acta **214:**374, 1970.

section three

Psychopharmacology

Chapter 23

General concepts of psychopharmacology

Before the 1950s there were no effective pharmacotherapeutic agents available for the treatment of the major mental diseases. Large doses of barbiturates were used to calm agitated psychotic patients, and amphetamine was sometimes used in an attempt to combat acute depression. In the early 1950s two drugs were introduced for the management of psychotic patients. These drugs, reserpine and chlorpromazine, proved to be agents that allowed a vast improvement in the medical management of psychotic persons and also provided the investigational tools for a major breakthrough in understanding the central transmitters and neuronal circuits involved in the antipsychotic actions of the drugs, as well as, possibly, in the etiology of the disease processes. At hand now are a large number of agents useful in the specific management of schizophrenia, depression, manic-depressive psychoses, and anxiety states.

Reserpine, the major active substance of *Rauwolfia serpentina* and related plants, provided the earliest insights into specific brain amines associated with mental disease. It was initially found that the drug depletes stores of serotonin (5-hydroxytryptamine) in the brain as well as peripheral organs and that only psychoactive alkaloids of *Rauwolfia* shared this action. It was later discovered that the drug also depletes stores of norepinephrine and epinephrine in the brain and periphery in a similar manner. Still later, after the identification of dopamine stores in the brain, it was found that reserpine and other psychoactive analogs also depleted the brain stores of this amine. Coupled with the observation that monoamine oxidase (MAO) inhibitors interfere with the metabolism of all of these brain amines and that the MAO inhibitors also altered the behavioral effects of reserpine in animals, it seemed apparent that one or more of the amines was involved in the central actions of reserpine.

The inability of the phenothiazine antipsychotic, chlorpromazine, to affect brain amine concentrations was at first an obstacle to further advances, but it was this drug that later allowed an important additional breakthrough when it was demonstrated

MONOAMINE BASIS OF PSYCHOPHARMACOLOGY
Antischizophrenic drugs

FIG. 23-1 *Metabolism of dopamine in the brain.*

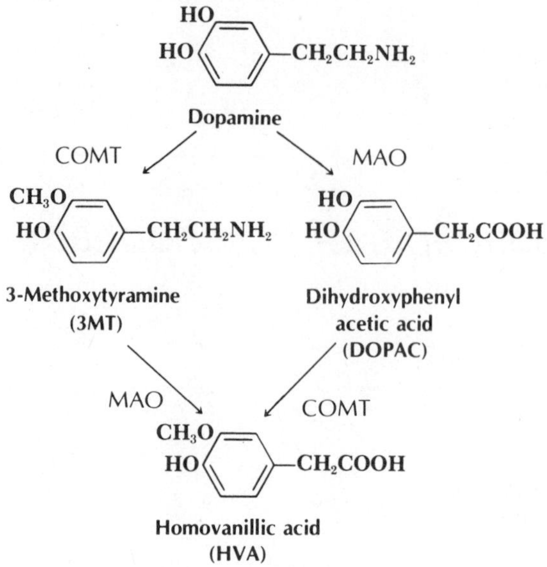

Dopamine

COMT   MAO

3-Methoxytyramine
(3MT)

Dihydroxyphenyl
acetic acid
(DOPAC)

MAO   COMT

Homovanillic acid
(HVA)

FIG. 23-2 *A, Antagonism by chlorpromazine (CPZ) of d-amphetamine (AMP)-induced slowing of dopaminergic cell activity in a nonanesthetized animal. AMP significantly decreased firing rate. After CPZ, cell firing resumed and increased. B, Effect of haloperidol on a dopaminergic cell in the nonanesthetized animal. Haloperidol increased basal activity. C, Effect of promethazine (PRO) on cell firing rate subsequent to d-amphetamine depression in an anesthetized animal. AMP markedly decreased unit activity. Promethazine failed to increase the rate usually seen with the antipsychotic phenothiazines. Perphenazine produced a rapid increase in rate to above baseline levels.*

From Bunney, B.S., et al.: J Pharmacol. Exp. Ther. **185:**560, 1973. Copyright 1973, The Williams & Wilkins Co., Baltimore.

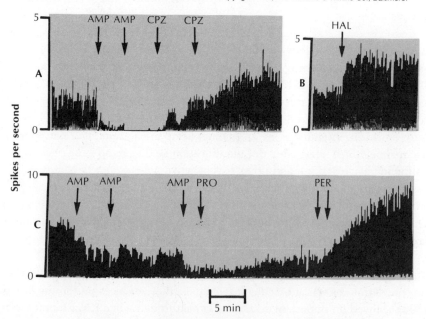

that chlorpromazine and related drugs are blockers of dopamine receptors in various brain areas.[1] With the further elucidation of central dopaminergic neuronal pathways, increasingly it appears that the major antipsychotic action of phenothiazine and related drugs is by blockade of dopamine receptors in mesolimbic or mesocortical brain areas, whereas the blockade of dopamine receptors in the corpus striatum is responsible for the major central side effects of these drugs.

Some of the major evidence for a role of dopamine in the therapeutic action of antischizophrenic drugs may be summarized as follows:

1. The potencies of antipsychotic drugs to stimulate dopamine turnover in general correlate well with their clinical potencies. This effect is seen in the elevation of the concentration of the dopamine metabolites, homovanillic acid (HVA) and dihydroxyphenylacetic acid in dopamine neuronal brain areas. Blockade of dopamine receptors causes a compensatory increase in the firing rate of dopamine neurons and in dopamine synthesis. The metabolic fate of dopamine in the brain is shown in Fig. 23-1.

2. Electrophysiological studies on dopamine neurons demonstrate again that there is a correlation between clinical antipsychotic potency and the ability of the drugs to alter dopamine neuronal firing rate. Some examples are given in Fig. 23-2.

3. Inhibition of tyrosine hydroxylase, the rate-limiting enzyme in the biosynthesis of catecholamines, in schizophrenic patients allows a major reduction in the dose of antipsychotic drug required to control their symptoms (Fig. 23-3).

4. Ligand-binding studies have shown a generally close association between clinical potency and affinity of binding of antipsychotic drugs to an apparent dopamine receptor on brain membrane fractions (Fig. 23-4).[2]

It is known that in certain neural tissues including dopaminergic brain areas there exists a dopamine-activated adenylate cyclase, which may be involved in dopamine receptor activation and coupling. This cyclase is inhibited by many antipsychotics in proportion to clinical potency. An excellent correlation appears in the case of phenothiazines, but haloperidol and other butyrophenones are relatively inactive.[3]

Recently it has been observed that antipsychotic drugs also bind to the calcium-dependent regulatory protein, calmodulin.[12] As this protein appears to be involved in adenylate cyclase activation and in phosphodiesterase activation, it may represent an appropriate target site for the action of antipsychotics. However, the correlation of binding affinity and clinical antipsychotic potency is limited.

It presently appears that there may be multiple receptors for dopamine, some linked to the adenylate cyclase and others not.[4] Such a dichotomy of receptor types may help clarify the overall interpretation of dopamine receptor–ligand-binding studies.

5. Administration of drugs such as amphetamines, known to release dopamine in the brain, can exacerbate schizophrenic symptoms or, in large, repeated doses, can initiate symptoms of paranoid schizophrenia. These effects are blocked by dopamine-blocking agents such as chlorpromazine.[9]

FIG. 23-3 *Social behavior* (solid lines) *and mental symptoms* (dashed lines) *in a patient with chronic schizophrenia. Patient had been receiving 1000 mg of chlorpromazine daily. The patient's condition worsened when this dose was reduced but improved when α-methyltyrosine was given with a small dose of chlorpromazine.*

From Carlsson, A., Persson, T., Roos, B.-E., and Walinder, J.: J. Neural Transm. **33**:83, 1972.

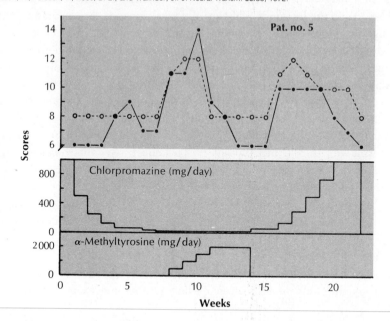

FIG. 23-4 *Concentration of various antipsychotic drugs required to produce a 50% inhibition of binding of haloperidol to a preparation of caudate nucleus are plotted against the average clinical dose in humans to control schizophrenic symptoms.*

From Seeman, P., Lee, T., Chau-Wong, M., and Wong, K. Reprinted by permission from Nature **261**:717. Copyright 1976, Macmillan Journals Ltd.

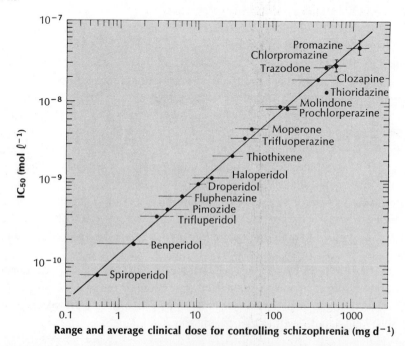

Although this brief summary for a role of dopamine is not a complete citation, it is an impressive array of evidence. It must be pointed out, however, that these findings do not, in themselves, constitute evidence for a role of dopamine neuronal abnormality in the *etiology* of schizophrenia. Furthermore, certain newer, experimental drugs thought to be useful in schizophrenia appear to have only subtle effects on dopamine receptors.

Of current interest are observations that certain dopamine agonists may act preferentially on dopamine neuronal presynaptic receptors to inhibit neuronal activity. It has been reported that low doses of the dopamine receptor agonist apomorphine lessen the symptoms of schizophrenia.[10] The possible development of more specific presynaptic dopamine agonists will be awaited with interest.

Endogenous psychotogenic substances

Based on the fact that ingestion of certain chemicals can result in abnormal mental function, for a number of years there have been suggestions that there might exist an endogenous substance capable of causing psychosis. The evidence for most such suggestions has proven inconclusive. A recent candidate for such a substance is phenylethylamine.[8] Small quantities have been reported in the brain, and injection can lead to amphetamine-like effects. It has been reported that higher than normal amounts are excreted in the urine of paranoid schizophrenics.[7] Interestingly, there is evidence that injected phenylethylamine may act through a dopaminergic mechanism.

Antidepressant drugs

Basic and clinical investigations have led to the development of drugs useful in the treatment of depression and to increased understanding of their basic actions. The first of these drugs, MAO inhibitors, were tried because they altered the unusual central depressant effects seen in animals given reserpine and because of an unusual stimulant effect seen in humans. The MAO inhibitors are thought to act through enhancement of free monoamines in central neuronal systems. These drugs have largely been replaced in clinical practice by the safer and more effective tricyclic antidepressants such as imipramine. Although the latter drugs are not MAO inhibitors, they inhibit the norepinephrine reuptake mechanism in adrenergic neurons. Serotonin uptake is also inhibited. Interestingly, the tricyclics have little effect on the dopamine uptake system in dopamine neurons.

It is currently thought that although uptake inhibition may be involved in the action of tricyclic antidepressants, this alone cannot explain their effects, since uptake inhibition occurs rapidly yet there is a delay of about 2 weeks for a clinical antidepressant effect. Recently it has been shown that with chronic administration of these drugs there occur slowly developing changes in the sensitivity of central adrenergic receptors, presynaptic[5] and postsynaptic,[11] or of serotonin receptors.[6] Chronic, but not acute, administration as well as electroconvulsive treatment, causes a decrease in the sensitivity of norepinephrine-stimulated adenylate cyclase in the brain.[11]

The actions and current view of the mechanisms of action of lithium and the antianxiety drugs are discussed in subsequent chapters.

REFERENCES

1. Carlsson, A.: Does dopamine have a role in schizophrenia? Biol. Psychiatry **13**:3, 1978.

2. Creese. I., Burt, D.R., and Snyder, S.H.: Dopamine receptor binding predicts clinical and pharmacological potencies of antischizophrenic drugs, Science **192**:481, 1976.

3. Iversen, L.L.: Dopamine receptors in the brain, Science **188**:1084, 1975.

4. Kehabian, J.M., and Calne, D.B.: Multiple receptors for dopamine, Nature **277**:93, 1979.

5. McMillen, B.A., Warnack, W., German, D.C., and Shore, P.A.: Effects of chronic desipramine treatment on rat brain noradrenergic responses to α-adrenergic drugs, Eur. J. Pharmacol. **61**:239, 1980.

6. Montigny, C. de, and Aghajanian, G.K.: Tricyclic antidepressants: long-term treatment increases responsivity of rat forebrain neurons to serotonin, Science **202**:1303, 1978.

7. Potkin, S.G., Karoum, F., Chuang, L.-W., Cannon-Spoor, H.E., Phillips, I., and Wyatt, R.J.: Phenylethylamine in paranoid chronic schizophrenia, Science **206**:471, 1979.

8. Sabelli, H.C., Borison, R.L., Diamond, B.I., Havdala, H.S., and Narasimhachari, N.: Phenylethylamine and brain function, Biochem. Pharmacol. **27**:1707, 1978.

9. Snyder, S.H., Banerjee, S.P., Yamamura, H.I., and Greenberg, D.: Drugs, transmitters, and schizophrenia, Science **184**:1243, 1974.

10. Tamminga, C.A., Schaeffer, M.H., Smith, R.C., and Davis, J.M.: Schizophrenic symptoms improve with apomorphine, Science **200**:567, 1978.

11. Vetulani, J., and Sulser, F.: Action of various antidepressant treatments reduces reactivity of noradrenergic cyclic AMP generating system in limbic forebrain, Nature **257**:495, 1975.

12. Weiss, B., and Levin, R.M.: Mechanism for selectively inhibiting the activation of cyclic nucleotide phosphodiesterase and adenylate cyclase by antipsychotic agents, Adv. Cyclic Nucleotide Res. **9**:285, 1978.

Chapter 24

Antipsychotic and antianxiety drugs

Antipsychotic and antianxiety drugs are the newer terms for major and minor tranquilizers, respectively. The antipsychotic drugs, represented by the *phenothiazines, thioxanthenes,* and *butyrophenones,* improve the mood and behavior of psychotic patients without excessive sedation and without causing drug dependence. Psychoses are not cured by antipsychotic agents, but the drugs do relieve signs and symptoms in a large percentage of affected individuals. The relapse rate for schizophrenics maintained on antipsychotic agents during remission is much lower than the rate for patients given placebo.

The antianxiety drugs include the *benzodiazepines, meprobamate,* and related drugs. Anxiety can be a disabling medical problem. Whether any drugs have selective anxiolytic properties is a matter of unresolved discussion, mainly because the label anxiety, like those of "mental stress" or "psychosomatic illness," is an amorphous, culture-laden diagnosis. Although controlled clinical trials may show one or more antianxiety agents to be superior to placebo, the differences are often small. Not infrequently, no differences emerge. Despite the difficulties in proving efficacy, prescribing patterns strongly suggest that a large percentage of physicians feel these drugs are useful. In general, antianxiety drugs have a spectrum of activity in humans and animals that resembles the spectra of barbiturates and ethanol[19]: they are sedatives, anticonvulsants, muscle relaxants, and potential inducers of drug dependency. The notable popularity of benzodiazepines derives from three differences between them and a barbiturate or meprobamate: they are less subject to tolerance and physical dependence; they are much safer when taken in accidental or intentional overdose; and the gap that separates doses that depress nonspecifically from doses that appear to be anxiolytic may be larger. On reflection, it would appear that these advantages may be as important to the prescriber of drugs as they are to recipients.

FIG. 24-1 *Brain nuclei and pathways especially relevant to the actions of antipsychotic drugs. The diagram depicts the base of the midbrain as viewed sagittally. Three cell bodies (unshaded) signify neurons of the three main pathways that synthesize dopamine (DA) and use it to communicate with target cells (shaded). Large arrows designate brain activities influenced by dopamine and altered by antipsychotic drugs.*

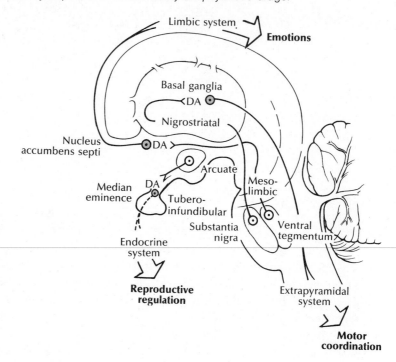

DEVELOPMENT   The field of tranquilizing agents was opened up by the almost simultaneous introduction of two powerful drugs, chlorpromazine and reserpine. Preparations of *Rauwolfia serpentina*, a wild shrub, have been used in India for centuries for the treatment of various illnesses. Reserpine, one of its alkaloids, was isolated in 1952.

A key feature of the central effects of reserpine is depletion of the stores of the brain monoamines—serotonin, norepinephrine, and dopamine.[16] For example, norepinephrine concentrations may be reduced by 90%. Reserpine disrupts binding sites for amines within the intraneuronal storage organelles, the small and medium diameter vesicles. Concurrently, there is loss of transmitter function, loss of formalin fluorescence in cells and terminal fields normally rich in amines, and degranulation of vesicles (fewer electron-dense cores) in autonomic terminals.

Chlorpromazine, the prototype phenothiazine tranquilizer, originated in France as a result of a search for new antihistamines having a phenothiazine structure. Chlorpromazine and drugs that act similarly block dopamine receptors (Fig. 24-1). Interference by phenothiazine derivatives in the regulation of endocrine and motor pathways normally mediated by dopamine is almost certainly responsible for many actions of the drugs, mostly undesirable. A hypothesis that blockade of dopamine receptors that lead into limbic pathways via the nucleus accumbens septi (Fig. 24-1) is responsible for the antipsychotic effects has generated much recent research but remains highly speculative.

At subhypnotic levels, reserpine and chlorpromazine exert striking calming effects on the behavior of wild animals and disturbed patients. The knowledge that these drugs could influence spontaneous and learned behavior in animals led to the development of extensive screening procedures for new tranquilizers. This research activity produced not only a variety of phenothiazine derivatives and reserpine-like compounds but also many antianxiety and antidepressant drugs. The list of compounds in each category continues to grow.

Once the unusually beneficial effect of chlorpromazine in psychotic patients was recognized, many related compounds were introduced. Considered as a group, these drugs calm psychotic persons without sedating them excessively, cause extrapyramidal effects, and lack the propensity of inducing drug dependence.[23] Most of these compounds have indications also as antiemetics, and some are antipruritic.

ANTIPSYCHOTIC DRUGS

From a chemical standpoint the antipsychotic drugs comprise the *phenothiazines, thioxanthenes, butyrophenones, dihydroindolones,* and *dibenzodiazepines.* The properties of these drugs are so similar that emphasis in this discussion will be placed primarily on the phenothiazines. Reserpine was at one time used as a "major tranquilizer" but has been essentially abandoned in psychiatric practice. Its use as an antihypertensive is discussed in Chapter 18.

The term *neuroleptic* is often used as a synonym for antipsychotic. A neuroleptic causes psychomotor slowing, emotional quieting, and, in higher doses, psychic indifference to the environment. It may or may not have a sedative effect but it is not hypnotic. The term is currently synonymous with *antipsychotic* because all antischizophrenic drugs used at the present time are neuroleptics. It is conceivable that at some time drugs will be developed that control the symptoms of schizophrenia without being neuroleptics.

Phenothiazine derivatives

Numerous phenothiazine derivatives are in current use. They resemble chlorpromazine in action but differ from it in potency, special clinical indications, and frequency of side effects.

The pharmacological effects of the phenothiazine tranquilizers are quite complex. In addition to their behavioral effects, these drugs are potent antiemetics and have important actions on the autonomic nervous system at various levels. They also produce significant toxic effects such as parkinsonism.

The phenothiazines are classified on the basis of their chemistry and pharmacology into three groups (Table 24-1).

The differences result mainly from substitutions on the nitrogen in the phenothiazine ring. Among the numerous *piperazines,* some of the most widely used are

TABLE 24-1   Classification of phenothiazines

Phenothiazine nucleus

	Substitution in (2)	Substitution in (10)	Average oral dose (mg)	Summary of effects by groups
Piperazine				
Prochlorperazine (Compazine)	C1	$CH_2-CH_2-CH_2-N\!\!\bigcirc\!\!N-CH_3$	5-10	Most potent antipsychotic and antiemetic. Highest incidence of extrapyramidal effects and catalepsy; least sedative
Trifluoperazine (Stelazine)	CF₃	$CH_2-CH_2-CH_2-N\!\!\bigcirc\!\!N-CH_3$	2-10	
Perphenazine (Trilafon)	C1	$CH_2-CH_2-CH_2-N\!\!\bigcirc\!\!N-CH_2-CH_2-OH$	4-8	
Fluphenazine (Prolixin; Permitil)	CF₃	$CH_2-CH_2-CH_2-N\!\!\bigcirc\!\!N-CH_2-CH_2-OH$	0.25-0.5	
Aliphatic				
Chlorpromazine (Thorazine)	C1	$CH_2-CH_2-CH_2-N-(CH_3)_2$	25-50	Intermediate antipsychotic and antiemetic potency; notable parkinsonian side effects, hypotension, sedation, and antihistamine activity
Promazine (Sparine)	—	$CH_2-CH_2-CH_2-N-(CH_3)_2$	25-50	
Triflupromazine (Vesprin)	CF₃	$CH_2-CH_2-CH_2-N-(CH_3)_2$	10-25	
Piperidine				
Mesoridazine (Serentil)	$SCH_3 \downarrow O$	$CH_2-CH_2-\bigcirc\!\!N-CH_3$	50-200	Least potent antiemetic and antipsychotic but lower incidence of extrapyramidal effects; most anticholinergic; most EKG changes
Thioridazine (Mellaril)	SCH₃	$CH_2-CH_2-\bigcirc\!\!N-CH_3$	25-100	

prochlorperazine (Compazine), trifluoperazine (Stelazine), perphenazine (Trilafon), fluphenazine (Prolixin; Permitil), and piperacetazine (Quide). The *aliphatic* compounds include chlorpromazine (Thorazine) and triflupromazine (Vespirin). The piperidines are represented by mesoridazine (Serentil) and thioridazine (Mellaril).

The *thioxanthene* group of antipsychotic drugs resembles in all respects the phenothiazines. The thioxanthenes include chlorprothixene (Taractan) and thiothixene (Navane). The *butyrophenone* haloperidol (Haldol) is similar pharmacologically to piperazine phenothiazines.

MAJOR DIFFERENCES AMONG DERIVATIVES

Phenothiazines differ from each other in their potencies, extrapyramidal effects, and sedative effects. Piperazines are more potent than other phenothiazines, cause significant extrapyramidal effects, and are not very sedative. The piperidines are least potent, cause fewer extrapyramidal effects, and produce sedation. The aliphatic compounds are between the piperazines and the piperidines as regards these properties.

Since extrapyramidal effects may be antagonized by anticholinergic drugs, it is possible that differences between phenothiazines in causing extrapyramidal side effects reflect differences in their intrinsic anticholinergic potency. Presumably, drugs with stronger antimuscarinic properties would be less likely to evoke motor disorders.

CHLORPROMAZINE

Chlorpromazine (Thorazine), an aliphatic or dimethylaminopropyl phenothiazine, is a sedative antipsychotic drug. In addition to its usefulness in agitated psychotic persons, the drug has other medical applications such as prevention of nausea and vomiting. It is used also for its ability to potentiate the actions of drugs such as anesthetics and analgesics.

The structural formulas of chlorpromazine (Thorazine) and the antihistaminic drug promethazine (Phenergan) are quite similar:

Promethazine hydrochloride   Chlorpromazine hydrochloride

Pharmacological effects. The pharmacological actions of chlorpromazine and other phenothiazines are antipsychotic, dyskinetic, anticholinergic, antiadrenergic, thermoregulatory, antiemetic, and endocrinological.

Antipsychotic effects. Phenothiazines produce emotional quieting, psychomotor slowing, and affective indifference. They tend to decrease paranoid ideation, fear, hostility, and agitation.[17] They make less intense the delusions and hallucinations of schizophrenia. In normal subjects phenothiazines produce dysphoria and impairment of intellectual functions.

Phenothiazines precipitate a surprising variety of motor disorders, presumably as a result of acute and chronic blockade of dopamine receptors in the basal ganglia.[5] Akathisia (restless pacing) and painful dystonic spasticities may occur very early in therapy, especially in young patients. Parkinsonian signs (tremor, rigidity, bradykinesia) are normally encountered after continuous administration of phenothiazines for several weeks or more. They can be a limiting factor in dose escalation. These "early" motor abnormalities are reversible, dose dependent (i.e., severity decreases if the daily phenothiazine intake is lowered), and at least partially controlled by antimuscarinic drugs used in true Parkinson's disease (benztropine, diphenhydramine, and so forth).

Tardive dyskinesia is increasingly recognized as a major medical problem in long-term use of antipsychotics.[15] It has been estimated that up to 50% of the patients receiving such drugs for 1 year or more develop some form of this syndrome, which is most often seen as grossly abnormal orofacial movements, although other body areas may be involved. Tardive dyskinesia is often "uncovered" when the dose of a phenothiazine is reduced or the drug is eliminated. However, dyskinetic signs can also "break through" during therapy.

Unlike the situation with other neuroleptic-induced parkinsonian symptoms, anticholinergic drugs are of no benefit in tardive dyskinesia, nor are compounds that may increase the availability of acetylcholine for synaptic transmission in the brain. Neuroleptics, which cause the syndrome, also tend to suppress the clinical signs, particularly if larger doses are administered. However, this approach to the problem is not recommended, because it seems probable that additional phenothiazine treatment would only add to the extent of the underlying damage. Dyskinetic responses may represent dopamine supersensitivity as a consequence of persistent receptor antagonism. Fig. 24-2 summarizes current perceptions on the complex relationships between transmitter activities and motor abnormalities in response to antipsychotic drugs and in true Parkinson's disease.

Anticholinergic and antiadrenergic effects. Chlorpromazine has atropine-like effects manifested by symptoms such as dry mouth, constipation, urinary retention, and paralysis of accommodation. On the other hand, dilatation of the pupil and tachycardia are unusual with phenothiazines.

Chlorpromazine can produce postural hypotension that has generally been attributed to an α-adrenergic blocking action. It appears, however, that this hypotensive action may be explained by an exaggeration of β-adrenergic vasodilatation, since chlorpromazine does not block the pressor action of norepinephrine. Marked hypotension may occur after parenteral administration of phenothiazines.

Temperature regulation. Although chlorpromazine is not an effective antipyretic, it does cause some lowering of body temperature and it prevents shivering. It is used sometimes when hypothermia is desired, such as in hypothermic anesthesia.

Antiemetic effects. Chlorpromazine blocks the emetic effect of apomorphine, which is exerted primarily on the chemoreceptor trigger zone (CTZ). The chemo-

Consequences of perturbations in the balance between dopamine and acetylcholine in   **FIG. 24-2**
the basal ganglia (neostriatum). Imbalances are depicted as results of aberrant amounts
of dopamine (DA) relative to unchanging cncentrations of acetylcholine (ACh).

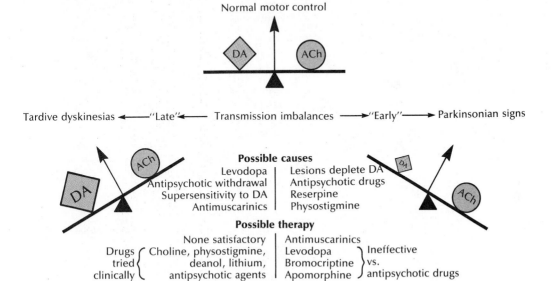

Normal motor control

Tardive dyskinesias ◄——"Late"◄—— Transmission imbalances ——►"Early"——► Parkinsonian signs

Possible causes

Levodopa	Lesions deplete DA
Antipsychotic withdrawal	Antipsychotic drugs
Supersensitivity to DA	Reserpine
Antimuscarinics	Physostigmine

Possible therapy

None satisfactory	Antimuscarinics
Drugs ⎰ Choline, physostigmine,	Levodopa ⎱ Ineffective
tried ⎰ deanol, lithium,	Bromocriptine ⎰ vs.
clinically ⎱ antipsychotic agents	Apomorphine ⎱ antipsychotic drugs

receptors are in the area postrema near the fourth cerebroventricle. The blood-brain barrier is weak in this region, and the chemoreceptors there normally respond to circulating toxins and emetic drugs by triggering a complex vomiting reflex. Trimethobenzamide, although structurally dissimilar to phenothiazines, has a similar antiemetic spectrum of activity and has extrapyramidal signs as a possible side effect. Phenothiazines are more effective in preventing vomiting by depressing the chemoreceptor trigger zone than they are in preventing motion sickness. In the latter, muscarinic receptor blockers and antihistamines that have strong atropine-like actions are more commonly used. Morphine and related analgesics, particularly on repeated administration, depress the vomiting "center," but these drugs are seldom used specifically for this purpose. Fig. 24-3 summarizes the sites of action of commonly prescribed antiemetics along the various avenues that provoke emesis.

Controlled clinical trials with domperidone (Motilium), which blocks enteric dopamine receptors but does not enter the brain, suggest that this drug may find use as an antiemetic. It proved more effective than placebo in controlling postoperative vomiting and the symptoms of chronic "dyspepsia."

The antiemetic properties of metoclopramide (Reglan) are thought to result from combined block of dopamine receptors in the CTZ and in the enteric nervous system. The drug is reported to be the most effective of several antiemetics evaluated against the nausea and vomiting of cisplatin, a chemotherapeutic agent and powerful emetic.

FIG. 24-3   Survey of mechanisms for emesis and the sites of action for several drugs or chemicals that initiate or control vomiting.

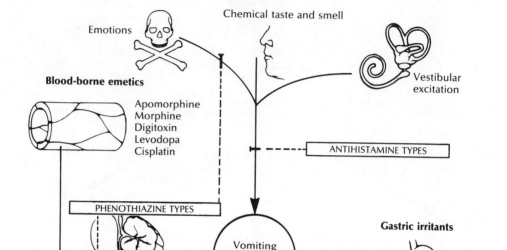

Phenothiazine-type antiemetics

Prochlorperazine (Compazine)
Promethazine (Phenergan)
Thiethylperazine (Torecan)
Trimethobenzamide (Tigan)

Antihistamine-type antiemetics

Benzquinamide (Emete-Con)
Cyclizine (Marzine)
Dimenhydrinate (Dramamine)
Meclizine (Bonine, Antivert)

Endocrine effects. Chlorpromazine may cause galactorrhea, delayed menstruation, amenorrhea, and weight gain. It is generally believed that these actions of the phenothiazine are exerted by disruption of hypothalamic control over the pituitary gland. For example, dopamine released into synapses in the tuberoinfundibular pathway (Fig. 24-1) normally inhibits prolactin production. Prolonged blockade of these receptors by chlorpromazine can lead to inappropriate lactation in women and gynecomastia in men.

Adverse effects and drug interactions. In addition to the extrapyramidal effects, chlorpromazine may cause numerous adverse reactions such as blood dyscrasias, cholestatic jaundice, increased responsiveness to barbiturates and other hypnotics, postural hypotension, electrocardiographic changes, skin reactions and photosensitivity, skin pigmentation, deposition of pigments in the cornea and lens, and the toxic consequences of its anticholinergic effect.

Drug interactions include intensification of the effects of alcohol, hypnotics, morphine-like analgesics, anesthetics, antihypertensives, and anticholinergics.

Chlorpromazine, the prototype phenothiazine, is absorbed somewhat erratically when given by mouth. Peak plasma levels occur in 2 to 4 hours, a plateau is maintained for several hours, and predose levels occur in 12 hours. Plasma half-lives are extremely variable, averaging 9 hours. Blood levels have not proved especially useful as guides to therapy. In a particular patient, the optimum dose is the one that relieves psychotic symptoms without causing intolerable side effects.

The distribution of chlorpromazine in various tissues is quite uneven.[17] The brain contains about four times as much as the plasma. Elimination takes place through the kidney and bile. The drug is also excreted in the milk. Chlorpromazine has numerous metabolites. The glucuronides and sulfoxides are excreted in the urine, whereas demethylated, nonpolar metabolites enter the bile and may undergo reabsorption, excretion in the feces, or storage in the tissue.

ANTIHISTAMINIC ACTIVITY

Some phenothiazines with powerful antihistaminic activity are used to relieve the itch of various skin diseases. Examples are **promethazine, trimeprazine tartrate** (Temaril), and **methdilazine** (Tacaryl). In general, these antihistaminic phenothiazines can cause drowsiness and all the toxic effects described previously. Precautions applicable to the other phenothiazines should be observed.

PREPARATIONS

The phenothiazines, as well as the thioxanthenes and butyrophenones, are available in a variety of dosage forms such as tablets, capsules, syrups, elixirs, injectables, and rectal suppositories. Fluphenazine, as the decanoate or enanthate ester, has an extended duration of action after intramuscular or subcutaneous injection. These dosage forms are useful for managing combative or noncompliant patients, since the effects of a single injection persist for 1 to 3 weeks.

Thioxanthene derivatives

The thioxanthene derivatives **chlorprothixene** (Taractan) and **thiothixene** (Navane) are similar chemically and pharmacologically to the phenothiazine derivatives. In the thioxanthene drugs a carbon is substituted for the nitrogen in the central ring of the phenothiazines.

Thiothixene is considerably more potent than chlorprothixene. The side chain on the carbon atom, which replaces the nitrogen of the phenothiazines, influences the activity in a similar way. Thiothixene has a piperazine side chain, whereas chlorprothixene is an alkylamine thioxanthene.

Thiothixene

Chlorprothixene

Chlorprothixene (Taractan) is effective in psychotic conditions in which agitation and anxiety are prominent symptoms.[20] The drug is available in tablets of 10, 25, 50, and 100 mg and in solutions for injection containing 12.5 mg/ml.

Thiothixene (Navane) is useful in the treatment of chronic schizophrenic patients who are apathetic. The drug is available in capsules containing 1, 2, 5, and 10 mg.

Substituted butyrophenones have been used increasingly as major tranquilizers, particularly in psychiatry and anesthesiology. **Haloperidol** (Haldol), the prototype of this series, has the following structure:

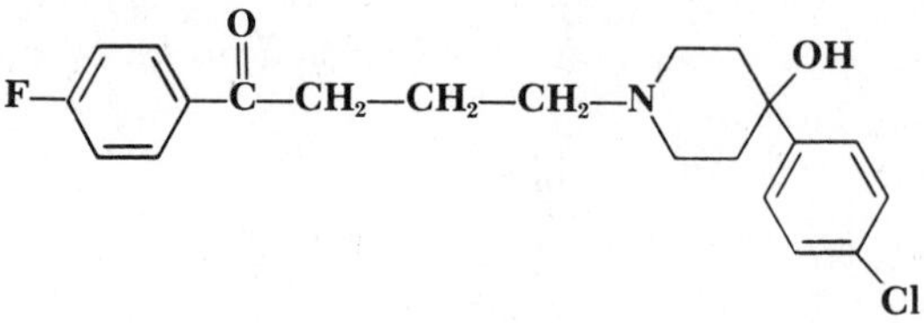

Haloperidol

Haloperidol is a potent antipsychotic and antiemetic.[14] Although there is no obvious chemical similarity, pharmacologically the drug resembles the piperazine phenothiazines in causing frequent extrapyramidal reactions. Haloperidol is often prescribed for depressed patients because it is less sedating than many other antipsychotics. It is also a first-line drug in the control of the neurological tics of Gilles de la Tourette's syndrome.

Many other butyrophenone-type drugs are currently being tested or are in use in other countries. It is likely that some of these will be introduced in the United States.

The tranquilizing butyrophenones are also used in anesthesiology in combination with a potent narcotic analgesic. The substituted butyrophenone droperidol, in combination with a meperidine-like analgesic (fentanyl), is employed in so-called neuroleptanesthesia. The fixed ratio combination is available under the trade name Innovar; however, droperidol and fentanyl can be administered separately.

Other antipsychotic drugs

Two recently introduced drugs are **loxapine** (Loxitane) and **molindone** (Moban). In general, their pharmacology resembles that of the other antipsychotic drugs, but their chemistry does not. They have antischizophrenic and antiemetic actions and cause extrapyramidal effects.

Choosing antipsychotic drugs

In a number of clinical trials it has been concluded that although the many antipsychotic drugs differ greatly in their potencies, side effects, and duration of action, there is little or no difference in efficacy when the drugs are used at optimal dosage regimens. Thus it is generally accepted that the best medical practice is to become familiar with a few of the drugs representative of the various types rather than to use a great number of drugs.

Lithium carbonate, a simple inorganic compound, lessens the intensiity of the manic phases of manic-depressive (bipolar) psychosis. In 1949 Cade[4] of Australia studied its effect on psychotic behavior following the observation that lithium carbonate caused lethargy in guinea pigs.

Lithium carbonate in manic psychosis

Patients in acute manic phases usually require doses as high as 600 mg three times a day, which should produce a serum lithium level of 0.5 to 1.5 mEq/L.[6] Continuous therapy for a week or more may be needed before the manic signs abate. As soon as a good response is achieved, the dosage should be reduced to 300 mg three times a day. Serum lithium levels should be monitored and should not be allowed to exceed 2 mEq/L. Diarrhea, vomiting, drowsiness, and ataxia are among the early signs of lithium intoxication. Thyroid involvement in the form of goiter may occur. Lithium is distributed in the total body water. Its renal clearance is proportional to its concentration in plasma. By interfering with sodium reabsorption, lithium may promote sodium depletion.[21,22]

The dose-related adverse effects of lithium carbonate administration may progress from *mild* symptoms such as nausea, vomiting, diarrhea, and muscle fasciculations to *moderately severe* symptoms that include hyperactive reflexes, epileptiform convulsions, and somnolence, leading finally to peripheral circulatory collapse, generalized convulsions, coma, and death. The very severe reactions are associated with serum lithium levels of 2.5 mEq/L or more. Excretion is hastened by forcing fluids while increasing the sodium intake.

The mechanisms of action of lithium carbonate in manic psychosis is not understood. Since there are many similarities in the biological actions of sodium and lithium and since sodium is required for a catecholamine uptake by the amine pump, current research is focusing on the possible effect of lithium on catecholamine uptake.[24] Lithium appears to accelerate the uptake of norepinephrine by isolated nerve-ending particles (synaptosomes).[6]

Lithium carbonate is available in capsules (Eskalith; Lithonate) and in tablets (Lithane; Lithobid), all containing 300 mg of the drug. A syrup (Cibalith-L) of lithium citrate is available that provides the equivalent of 300 mg of lithium carbonate in 5 ml.

Drugs for anxiety were once called "minor tranquilizers." This name is misleading, since it implies that these are simply less efficacious versions of phenothiazines. In fact, antipsychotic and antianxiety drugs differ with regard to their mechanisms of action, the beneficial and untoward effects they produce, and the indications for their use.[10,11,12]

ANTIANXIETY DRUGS

Anxiety in one form or another is a familiar emotion in an average day for most persons and is ordinarily a productive force. Anxiety merits medical attention only when it becomes so counterproductive that it is psychologically paralyzing. Administration of antianxiety drugs is the most common means for bringing levels of anxiety into a range where patients can cope, although other therapeutic approaches are possible. Anxieties that are prominent components of painful or paroxysmal organic diseases, such as angina pectoris or thyrotoxicosis, often vanish with treatment directed at the underlying condition. Injudicious overprescribing of antianxiety drugs has been a matter of justifiable concern. It appears to have decreased recently as physicians and patients have become increasingly aware of the perils of making nirvana a therapeutic goal.

Benzodiazepine derivatives currently dominate the field of antianxiety drugs. Compounds available in the United States and promoted mainly for this use are alprazolam (Xanax), chlorazepate (Tranxene), chlordiazepoxide (Librium), diazepam (Valium), halazepam (Paxipam), lorazepam (Ativan), oxazepam (Serax), and prazepam (Centrax). Their chemical structures are summarized below:

	R_1	R_2	R_3	R_4	R_5	R_6
Chlorazepate		Cl		(OH)$_2$	COOH	
Chlordiazepoxide		Cl		NHCH$_3$		→O
Clonazepam*	Cl	NO$_2$		O		
Diazepam		Cl	CH$_3$	O		
Flurazepam†	F	Cl	(CH$_2$)$_2$N(C$_2$H$_5$)$_2$			
Halazepam		Cl	CH$_2$CF$_3$	O		
Lorazepam	Cl	Cl		O	OH	
Oxazepam		Cl		O	OH	
Prazepam		Cl	CH$_2$—⊲	O		
Temazepam†		Cl	CH$_3$	O	OH	
Alprazolam		Cl				
Triazolam†	Cl	Cl				

*Main use as anticonvulsant.
†Main use as hypnotic.

Numerous nonbenzodiazepine antianxiety agents have been withdrawn by their manufacturers in recent years. Drugs in this category that remain available are meprobamate (Equanil; Miltown), chlormezanone (Trancopal), and hydroxyzine (Atarax; Vistaril). Chlormezanone and hydroxyzine cause less sedation than many other antianxiety agents. Hydroxyzine also has fairly strong antihistaminic and anticholinergic actions.

Benzodiazepine drugs

The clinical effects of biologically active benzodiazepines are qualitatively similar.[1] However, differences in the kinetics of their distribution and metabolism encourage marketing of certain benzodiazepines for purposes other than anxiety. For instance, flurazepam (Dalmane), temazepam (Restoril), and triazolam (Halcion) are promoted as hypnotics, whereas clonazepam (Clonopin) is offered as an anticonvulsant.

In animal models of epilepsy, convulsions produced by CNS stimulants such as strychnine, picrotoxinin, or pentylenetetrazol are antagonized by benzodiazepines. In this respect benzodiazepines are similar to phenobarbital but are quite different from phenothiazines or reserpine, which may lower seizure thresholds. Intravenous diazepam is a primary treatment for status epilepticus and seizures induced by drugs or toxins.[18] Diazepam, which relaxes skeletal muscle by depressing reflex pathways, is used to relieve spontaneous muscle spasms and those associated with procedures like endoscopy.[7]

Kinetics. Blood levels of benzodiazepines after oral administration peak between 1 and 4 hours. Absorption of diazepam is particularly rapid. Plasma protein binding ranges from 80% for alprazolam to 98% for diazepam. Chlorazepate is hydrolyzed in the stomach to N-desmethyldiazepam, an active, persistent metabolite. The rate of conversion is inversely proportional to gastric pH. Lorazepam and oxazepam, both short acting, are excreted as glucuronide conjugates. The rest are biotransformed by the hepatic microsomal system to one or more metabolites, some of them active and eliminated slowly. Doses and dosage forms are summarized in Table 24-2.

Adverse effects. Benzodiazepines cause drowsiness, ataxia, syncope, paradoxical excitement, rash, nausea, and altered libido.[9] Caution should be exercised in using them with other CNS depressants (barbiturates, ethanol, opiates, antihypertensives, anticonvulsants, and so forth). Diminished alertness from benzodiazepines in elderly patients may be mistaken for signs of senility. Apparently, with continued therapy, tolerance develops to the most common unwanted effect, drowsiness.

Anterograde amnesia from a benzodiazepine is not uncommon, especially after parenteral administration. This response can be beneficial, as well as adverse, and is one of the reasons for including a benzodiazepine in the presurgical regimen of balanced anesthesia.

Life-threatening reactions like agranulocytosis are very rare, and deaths from benzodiazepines alone seldom occur. Considering the extent to which benzodiazepines have been used worldwide for several decades, the incidence of true toxicity must be thought of as being very low indeed.

TABLE 24-2   Antianxiety benzodiazepines

Names and durations	Daily oral dose (mg)	Oral dosage† forms (mg)	Injectable forms (mg/ml)
Short acting (3-20 hr)*			
Alprazolam (Xanax)	1-4	T: 0.25, 0.5, 1.0	
Halazepam (Paxipam)	60-160	T: 20, 40	
Lorazepam (Ativan)	2-6	T: 0.5, 1.0, 2.0	2, 4
Oxazepam (Serax)	30-120	T: 15 C: 10, 15, 30	
Long acting (<24 hr)*			
Chlorazepate (Tranxene)	15-60	T: 11.25, 22.5 C: 3.75, 7.5, 15	
Chlordiazepoxide (Librium)	15-100	T: 5, 10, 25 C: 5, 10, 25	50
Diazepam (Valium)	4-40	T: 2, 5, 10	5
Prazepam (Centrax)	10-60	T: 10 C: 5, 10	

*$T_{1/2}$ of β phase of elimination from plasma at steady state.
†*T*, Tablet; *C*, capsule.

Physical and psychological dependence is a concern when benzodiazepines are taken for long periods of time. Abstinence signs such as tachycardia, tremor, and seizures have been reported, but the dependent individuals were taking larger than therapeutic doses continuously for several months or longer. The addictive liability for benzodiazepines seems to be lower than that of meprobamate or most barbiturates. Nevertheless, a prudent prescriber takes these precautions with benzodiazepines: (1) they are not normally given to persons with a history or drug or alcohol abuse; (2) the doses should be titrated for each patient's need so that daily intake is not needlessly large; and (3) an expected duration of treatment should be identified at the outset so that drug taking does not become prolonged through lack of planning.

Mechanism of action. The mode of action of benzodiazepines is unknown at the present time. Interesting interactions between benzodiazepines, picrotoxin, and the inhibitory neurotransmitter[13] γ-aminobutyric acid (GABA) have been observed at widespread receptors in the brain. Electrophysiological effects of GABA are enhanced in the presence of benzodiazepines. Furthermore, high-affinity binding sites for GABA and benzodiazepines have been demonstrated in vitro.

Some current ideas about how benzodiazepines act are shown in Fig. 24-4. The final common path at the GABA/benzodiazepine/picrotoxinin receptor complex appears to be the chloride channel. Influx of chloride from the extraneuronal to the

Hypothetical inhibitory synapse mediated by GABA. The postsynaptic receptor complex **FIG. 24-4**
consists of separate recognition sites for GABA, benzodiazepines, and picrotoxinin. Activation of GABA and benzodiazepine sites by appropriate agonists enhances the inward passage of chloride ions and tends to hyperpolarize the membrane. Ligands that activate the picrotoxinin site depress active inhibition by decreasing chloride conduction. An electric circuit equivalent of the chloride channel (ionophore) is shown at lower right: a resistor labeled $1/g_{Cl}$ (resistance is the reciprocal of conductance g) in series with a battery (E).

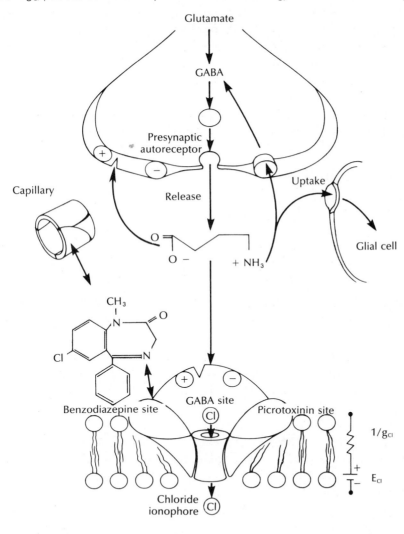

intraneuronal compartment initiates IPSPs (inhibitory postsynaptic potentials). Agonists or antagonists that bind to drug- or transmitter-recognition sites could induce steric changes in the membrane that alter the physical dimensions of the channel or the electrical charges within it.

The drug-binding sites in the receptor complex appear to be involved in the pharmacological actions of the drugs, since the ability of various benzodiazepines to displace labeled, bound diazepam parallels their clinical potency. At the present time efforts are being made to identify possible endogenous ligands for the benzodiazepine- and picrotoxin-binding sites. Several purines and β-carbolines normally present in the brain are of current research interest.

Meprobamate

Meprobamate (Miltown; Equanil) was developed as a result of studies on mephenesin-like drugs. Clinical trials of this central muscle relaxant indicated that compounds related to mephenesin have sedative and tranquilizing properties.

$$
\begin{array}{ll}
\text{Mephenesin} & \text{Meprobamate} \\
\\
\begin{array}{l}
\;\;\;\;\text{H} \\
\;\;\;\;| \\
\text{H--C--OH} \\
\;\;\;\;| \\
\text{H--C--OH} \\
\;\;\;\;| \\
\text{H--C--O--}\langle\text{ring}\rangle \\
\;\;\;\;| \\
\;\;\;\;\text{H}\;\;\;\;\;\text{CH}_3
\end{array}
&
\begin{array}{l}
\;\;\;\;\text{H} \\
\;\;\;\;| \\
\text{H--C--O--CONH}_2 \\
\;\;\;\;| \\
\text{C}_3\text{H}_7\text{--C--CH}_3 \\
\;\;\;\;| \\
\text{H--C--O--CONH}_2 \\
\;\;\;\;| \\
\;\;\;\;\text{H}
\end{array}
\end{array}
$$

Meprobamate (Miltown; Equanil) is available in 400 mg tablets. Oral administration of one of these tablets causes only very mild sedation. Larger doses tend to produce drowsiness and reduction of muscle spasm without interference with normal proprioceptive tone. In sufficiently large doses the drug causes ataxia.

The central muscle relaxant effect of meprobamate is illustrated by its reduction of experimental tremors induced by strychnine. The drug is also a fairly potent anticonvulsant and can protect mice against convulsions and death produced by pentylenetetrazol.

Mode of action. It is believed that meprobamate has a blocking action on spinal interneurons, since it has been shown that the drug has no effects on knee jerk, whereas flexor and crossed extensor reflexes are diminished by it. There are no interneurons interposed between the afferent and efferent reflex arcs in knee jerk. Thus the drug produces muscle relaxation without directly influencing transmission from motor nerve to skeletal muscle.

Muscle relaxant sedatives, although offered as tranquilizers, should be regarded as nonspecific sedatives similar in action to the barbiturates.[8] In addition to somnolence, addiction resembling that caused by barbiturates develops in patients who take large doses for a long time. Serious withdrawal symptoms characterized by muscle twitching and convulsions may result when these drugs are discontinued abruptly. It is very unlikely for these withdrawal symptoms to occur if the patient takes only two or three tablets a day. The drug should be withdrawn slowly.

Metabolism. Meprobamate is largely metabolized; only about 10% of the drug is excreted unchanged in the urine. Conjugation with glucuronic acid appears to be important in the metabolism of meprobamate, although it is first changed to hydroxymeprobamate.

Side effects and toxicity. Drowsiness occurs when fairly large doses of meprobamate are used. Skin rash, gastrointestinal disturbances, and purpura may rarely be caused by the drug. Severe hypotension associated with acute cardiac failure has been observed following the ingestion of large doses.[3]

REFERENCES

1. Bellantuono, C., Reggi, V., Tognoni, G., and Garattini, S.: Benzodiazepines: clinical pharmacology and therapeutic use, Drugs **19**:195, 1980.
2. Blackwell, B.: Rational drug use in the management of anxiety, Ration. Drug Ther. **9**:1, 1975.
3. Blumberg, A.G., Rosett, H.L., and Dobrow, A.: Severe hypotensive reactions following meprobamate overdosage, Ann. Intern. Med. **51**:607, 1959.
4. Cade, J.F.J.: Lithium salts in the treatment of psychotic excitement, Med. J Aust. **36**:349, 1949.
5. Creese, I., Burt, D.R., and Snyder, S.H.: Dopamine receptor binding predicts clinical and pharmacological potencies of antischizophrenic drugs, Science **192**:481, 1976.
6. Davis, J.M., and Fann, W.E.: Lithium, Annu. Rev. Pharmacol. **11**:285, 1971.
7. Diazepam as a muscle relaxant, Med. Letter **15**:1, 1973.
8. Domino, E.F.: Sites of action of some central nervous system depressants, Annu. Rev. Pharmacol. **2**:215, 1962.
9. Friend, D.G., and Cummins, J.F.: Use of chlorpromazine in the treatment of nausea and vomiting of uremia, N. Engl. J. Med. **250**:997, 1954.
10. Greenblatt, D.J., and Shader, R.I.: Benzodiazepines, N. Engl. J. Med. **291**:1011, 1974.
11. Greenblatt, D.J., and Shader, R.I.: Clinical use of benzodiazepines, Ration. Drug Ther. **15**(10):1, 1981.
12. Holister, L.E.: Mental disorders—antianxiety and antidepressant drugs, N. Engl. J. Med. **286**:1195, 1972.
13. Iversen, L.L.: GABA and benzodiazepine receptors, Nature **275**:477, 1978.
14. Jansen, P.A.J.: The pharmacology of haloperidol, Int. J. Neuropsychiatry **3**(suppl.):10, 1967.
15. Kobayashi, R.M.: Drug therapy of tardive dyskinesia, N. Engl. J. Med. **296**:257, 1977.
16. Murphy, D.L., Goodwin, F.K., and Bunney, W.E.: A reevaluation of biogenic amines in manic and depressive states, Hosp. Pract. Dec. 1972, p. 85.
17. Olsen, R.W.: Drug interactions at the GABA receptor-ionophore complex, Annu. Rev. Pharmacol. Toxicol. **22**:245, 1982.
18. Prensky, A.L., Raff, M.C., Moore, M.J., and Schwab, R.S.: Intravenous diazepam in the treatment of prolonged seizure activity, N. Engl. J. Med. **276**:779, 1967.
19. Randall, L.O., Scheckel, C.L., and Pool, W.: Pharmacology of medazepam and metabolites, Arch. Int. Pharmacodyn. Ther. **185**:135, 1970.
20. Scheckel, C.L.: Pharmacology and chemistry of thioxanthenes with special reference to chlorprothixene. In Freyhan,

F.A., Petrilowitsch, N., and Pichot, P., editors: Modern problems of pharmaco-psychiatry, vol. 2, The thioxanthenes, Basel, 1969, S. Karger, A.G.

21. Schildkraut, J.J.: Neuropsychopharmacology and the affective disorders, N. Engl. J. Med. **281:**197, 248, 302, 1969.

22. Schou, M.: Lithium in psychiatric therapy and prophylaxis, J. Psychiatry Res. **6:**67, 1968.

23. Shepherd, M., and Wing, L.: Pharmacological aspects of psychiatry, Adv. Pharmacol. **1:**229, 1962.

24. Singer, I., and Rotenberg, D.: Mechanisms of lithium action, N. Engl. J. Med. **298:**254, 1973.

Chapter 25

Antidepressant and psychotomimetic drugs

GENERAL
CONCEPT

Affective disorders (mental depression in its various forms) are the most frequent of the serious psychiatric illnesses. Most depressed persons are treated as outpatients by physicians who are not psychiatrists. The greatest danger to the patient is suicide, although the disease can cause severe physical and psychiatric debilitation.

A simple definition of depression is that it is sadness of duration and intensity that makes it incapacitating. Emotional complaints, which may not surface without probing, include apathy, guilt, self-reproach, disinterest in work or family, and preoccupation with tragedy or death. Physical complaints voiced frequently include abnormal eating and sleeping patterns, fatigue, headache, and vague gastrointestinal disturbances.

Four general types of depression are recognized. *Reactive* depressions are lingering reactions to some identified personal disaster or setback. *Endogenous* depressions occur without established cause. *Manic-depressive* illness is a separate subtype marked by abrupt mood swings between depression and hyperactivity (mania). The use of lithium in this condition is discussed in Chapter 24. *Psychotic* depression associated particularly with schizophrenia is just one of the numerous signs of psychosis. Antipsychotic tranquilizers, especially those that are least sedating, are the drugs of choice.

Some depressed individuals, especially those who have a reactive type, may respond to simple reassurance from family, friends, and physician. At the other extreme, profoundly depressed or suicidal individuals are often given a course of electroconvulsive therapy. Antidepressant drugs are indicated for many of the rest.[2]

Depressions tend to be cyclic, even without medical intervention. Moreover, clinical studies reveal positive placebo responses in as many as 30% of the patients. Some patients need therapy only during depressed episodes. Others benefit from more prolonged treatment that may increase the duration of remission.

Monoamine oxidase (MAO) inhibitors were introduced as the first antidepressants. *Iproniazid*, a chemical relative of a tuberculostatic drug and the first MAO inhibitor used clinically, has since been replaced by somewhat less toxic MAO inhibitors.

The *tricyclic antidepressant* imipramine (Tofranil) was discovered accidentally during clinical testing for antipsychotic drugs. It was soon followed by a series of related drugs, including two (desipramine and nortriptyline) that were identified as active metabolites of other tricyclics. *Central stimulants* such as dextroamphetamine (Dexedrine) and methylphenidate (Ritalin) are still used occasionally for depressions of short duration.

MAO INHIBITORS
Types and actions

On the basis of chemical structure, MAO inhibitors are categorized as hydrazines or nonhydrazines. Hydrazine types in current but limited use are **phenelzine** (Nardil) and **isocarboxazid** (Marplan). These drugs cause a variety of side effects including hepatotoxicity, overstimulation, postural hypotension, and hypertensive crises. The latter effects, which may be fatal, are generally associated with the ingestion of foods and drinks that have gone through a fermentation process so that they contain high levels of monoamines such as tyramine. Such foods and drinks include aged cheeses, some wines and beer, and others. Dietary monoamines are normally broken down by MAO in the intestine and liver. If this enzyme is blocked, amines may enter the circulation in sufficient concentration to release norepinephrine from adrenergic neurons already saturated with transmitter because of MAO inhibition. The beneficial action in depression is presumed to be inhibition of MAO type A in the mitochondria of the terminals of monoamine neurons. Enzyme inhibition increases the local concentration of amines and allows more transmitter to be released with each action potential.

Phenelzine

Isocarboxazid

Tranylcypromine (Parnate) is a potent *nonhydrazine* MAO inhibitor that also has a direct amphetamine-like stimulant action. Thus it is a *bimodal antidepressant*. The drug is closely related to amphetamine.

Tranylcypromine

Tranylcypromine's faster onset of action is advantageous, but like other MAO inhibitors it also causes postural hypotension. If the sense of euphoria produced by tranylcypromine progresses into unwanted mental excitement, the signs may be controlled with a phenothiazine.

Tranylcypromine, an extremely potent MAO inhibitor, can also cause hypertensive crises following ingestion of certain foods. This drug's use is restricted to hospitalized or closely supervised patients.

The MAO inhibitors are generally reserved for depressed patients not responding to other antidepressant therapy. Combined use of these drugs with the tricyclic antidepressants may cause a dangerous interaction resulting in hypertensive crisis, fever, and convulsions. At least a 1-week withdrawal period should be allowed for either the MAO inhibitor or the tricyclics before therapy with the other drug is initiated.

Drug interactions

Pargyline is discussed with the antihypertensive drugs in Chapter 18.

The tricyclic antidepressants have become the most widely used medications in the treatment of depression. Fig. 25-1 is a summary of the chemical structures of the drugs available in the United States: imipramine (Tofranil), amitriptyline (Amitid, Amitril; Elavil; Endep), desipramine (Pertofrane; Norpramin), nortriptyline (Aventyl; Pamelor), protriptyline (Vivactil), doxepin (Sinequan; Adapin), amoxapine (Asendin), and trimipramine (Surmontil). The latter pair are recent additions in this category.

TRICYCLIC ANTIDEPRES-SANTS

Structural formulas in the tricyclic antidepressant series.

FIG. 25-1

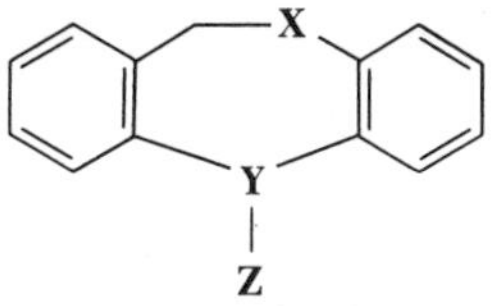

	X	Y	Z
Amitriptyline	C	C	$=CH(CH_2)_2N(CH_3)_2$
Desipramine	C	N	$(CH_2)_3NHCH_3$
Doxepin	O	C	$=CH(CH_2)_2N(CH_3)_2$
Imipramine	C	N	$(CH_2)_3N(CH_3)_2$
Nortriptyline	C	C	$=CH(CH_2)_2NHCH_3$
Protriptyline	$=C$	C	$(CH_2)_3NHCH_3$
Trimipramine	C	N	$CH_2CH_2CH_2NHCH_3$
			$\quad\quad\quad\mid$
			$\quad\quad\quad CH_3$

Amoxipine

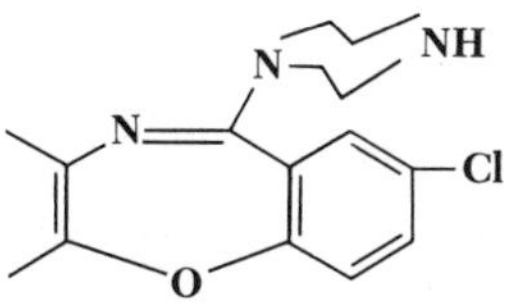

| *Pharmacological* | The major effects of the tricyclic antidepressants are their antidepressant and |
| *effects* | |

The major effects of the tricyclic antidepressants are their antidepressant and anticholinergic actions. Minor effects are related to sedation, antihistaminic action, and potentiation of the action of adrenergic drugs. They also have a quinidine-like effect on the heart.

ANTIDEPRESSANT
EFFECT

After a delay of several weeks, the tricyclic compounds elevate mood, increase alertness, and improve appetite in about 80% of depressed patients.

Current ideas about the mechanisms of action of tricyclic antidepressants may be found in Chapter 23. Fig. 25-2 summarizes the modes of action of several types of antidepressant drugs as these are commonly depicted in the monoamine hypothesis of affective disorders.

Other uses for tricyclic compounds are enuresis (bed wetting), motor hyperactivity in children, and chronic pain.

The anticholinergic action af the tricyclic compounds causes symptoms such as dry mouth, blurred vision, constipation, and urinary retention.[1] Disorientation and mental confusion may also be related to central anticholinergic (atropine-like) effects, since they can be counteracted with physostigmine.

Sedation may be considerable, and there is an increasing tendency for prescribing the tricyclic drugs in a single dose at bedtime. Most individuals become tolerant to the sedative effects after several weeks of continuous therapy. The antihistaminic action of these drugs is of no practical importance. The frequency of extrapyramidal side effects (mostly fine tremors) is much lower than with phenothiazines.

Cardiovascular side effects of the tricyclic antidepressants include orthostatic hypotension, tachycardia, arrhythmias, and prolongation of atrioventricular conduction time.

Tricyclic antidepressants prevent the antihypertensive actions of guanethidine by blocking the amine pump that transports guanethidine into the adrenergic fiber. Anticholinergic drugs and barbiturates should be used cautiously because of additive effects in patients who are taking one of the tricyclic antidepressants. MAO inhibitors are contraindicated in these same patients.

Dosage forms and some clinical comparisons of antidepressant drugs are summarized in Table 25-1.

Many new drugs for depression, known collectively as "second generation antidepressants," are now available or are in clinical trial. Compounds that have either been recently approved or may soon be released for use in the United States include trazodone (Desyrel), maprotiline (Ludiomil), viloxazine (Vivalan), nomifensine (Merital), bupropion (Wellbutrin), mianserin, and zimelidine.

The chemistry of these drugs is diverse. Maprotiline and mianserin are tetracyclics, zimelidine is bicyclic, and nomifensine is a tetrahydroisoquinoline. A considerable degree of selectivity is evident for block of uptake of one monoamine more than the others: bupropion is more effective against dopamine uptake; maprotiline

Synaptic effects of several types of antidepressant drugs as conceptualized in the biogenic   **FIG. 25-2**
amine hypothesis of mental illness. Four aminergic axon varicosities are in synaptic contact
with a target cell. Depicted is an association between intraneuronal and extraneuronal
transmitter (stippling) as governed by incorporation into vesicles (shading), release by
exocytosis, and uptake via the amine pump (arrows). Compared with the normal, drug-
free condition, the terminal altered by a tricyclic antidepressant has a much greater pro-
portion of transmitter in the synaptic cleft because of inhibition of uptake mechanisms.
The terminal subjected to an MAO inhibitor has a greater accumulation of transmitter
outside and inside the terminal as a result of decreased breakdown of the amine. Psy-
chomotor stimulants of the amphetamine type increase the amount of transmitter in the
cleft mainly by enhancing release mechanisms. Reuptake may be partially blocked. With
repeated administration of amphetamine, amine synthesis and vesicular incorporation may
not keep pace with release; therefore some vesicles are shown empty.

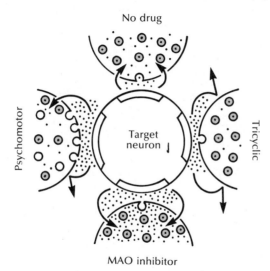

is more effective against norepinephrine; and trazodone and zimelidine are more effective against serotonin. Mianserin seems devoid of uptake blocker properties.

Information about "second generation" antidepressants is forcing a profound change in the monoamine hypothesis of mental illness.[4,5] The original postulate was that mental depression results from a deficiency of functional amines. A more recent idea is that depression arises from hyperfunctional amine pathways and that antidepressants "down regulate" (desensitize or inactivate) amine receptors.[6,7,8] In norepinephrine pathways, the drugs are thought to depress abnormally supersensitive receptors of the presynaptic α_2 and postsynaptic β types. Future refinements of the theories on the mode of action of antidepressants will need to account for seemingly selective actions of some drugs at synapses mediated by dopamine and serotonin.

TABLE 25-1   Antidepressants: synopsis of clinical responses and doses

Compound	Response onset (wk)	Adverse effects† Cardiovascular*	Anti-ACh	Sedative	Usual oral dose (mg/day)	Dosage‡ forms (mg)
MAO inhibitors						
Isocarboxazid	1	H	L	0	10-30	T: 10
Phenelzine	1	H	L	0	15-30	T: 15
Tranylcypromine	1	H	L	0	20-30	T: 10
Tricyclics						
Amitriptyline	2-3	H	H	H	75-200	T: 10,25,50,75,100,150 V: 100/10 ml
Amoxipine§	1	L	L	L	200-300	T: 25,50,100,150
Desipramine	2-3	H	L	±	100-200	C: 25,50 T: 25,50,75,100,150
Doxepin	2-3	L	H	H	75-150	C: 10,25,50,75,100,150 S: 10/ml
Imipramine	2-3	H	H	±	100-200	A: 25/2 ml T: 10,25,50
Nortriptyline	2-3	H	H	±	75-150	C: 10,25 S: 10/5 ml
Protriptyline	2-3	H	L	L	15-40	T: 5,10
Trimipramine§	2-3	H	H	H	50-150	C: 25,50

*Labile blood pressure and/or abnormal EKG.
†*H*, High; *L*, low; 0, none; ±, variable.
‡*A*, Ampule; *C*, capsule; *S*, oral solution; *T*, tablet; *V*, vial.
§Most recently introduced; clinical experience limited.

It seems unlikely that any of the newer compounds will displace the tricyclics because of remarkably greater efficacy or lower cost for a course of therapy. However, the tricyclics are vulnerable on the issue of safety, particularly their actions on cardiac rhythmicity and conduction. Estimates are that up to 20% of patients taking tricyclics develop EKG changes at therapeutic serum concentrations, although the changes may not cause overt symptoms. The relatively slow onset time for tricyclics is also a disadvantage in a population of patients prone to suicide.

Initial trials with the "second generation" drugs suggest that some may have less anticholinergic and quinidine-like effects. A few of these drugs may also have a faster onset of action. It remains to be seen if these claims will survive the scrutiny that comes with widespread clinical experience.

PSYCHOTO-MIMETIC DRUGS
Psychomotor stimulants

Amphetamine, particularly the more potent *dextro* form, has been used for years as a mood elevator in depressed patients. Its disadvantages are its cardiovascular effects and the letdown that follows the short period of stimulation. Other stimulants are also sometimes used in depressive states. These are pipradrol hydrochloride (Meratran) and methylphenidate hydrochloride (Ritalin).

Pipradrol hydrochloride   **Methylphenidate hydrochloride**

Pipradrol has been used as an antidepressant in depressive states, but its effectiveness is questionable. The related drug, methylphenidate hydrochloride, is more widely prescribed.

Methylphenidate resembles dextroamphetamine in its pharmacology except for its lower potency. The drug acts as a mild stimulant in depressive states but is not basically superior to dextroamphetamine. Its approved uses are in hyperkinetic children and in narcolepsy.

Although methylphenidate in the usual adult dose of 10 mg taken orally does not elevate the blood pressure, it should not be used in hypertensive persons or in any patients in whom sympathetic stimulation may be hazardous.

Preparations of methylphenidate hydrochloride (Ritalin hydrochloride) include tablets containing 5, 10, and 20 mg and powder for injection, 100 mg.

Psychomotor stimulants may be divided into two general types: amphetamine and nonamphetamine. Examples of the first are amphetamine and methamphetamine and, of the latter type, methylphenidate and cocaine. **TYPES AND ACTIONS**

This differentiation is not only on the basis of chemical structure, but also on mechanism of action. The central stimulant effect of amphetamine is dependent on a small, rapidly turning over pool of catecholamines. Thus its central actions are blocked by α-methyltyrosine, a catecholamine synthesis inhibitor. An important action of amphetamine is to promote release of monoamines from presynaptic terminals.

Nonamphetamines do not directly release dopamine. Rather, they block the dopamine neuronal uptake mechanism. The stimulant activity of the drugs parallels their potencies as dopamine uptake inhibitors. It has been proposed that such inhibition results in an intraneuronal translocation of stored dopamine so as to make more readily mobilized transmitter available for impulse-induced release.

Both types of stimulants can exacerbate or in high doses induce paranoid schizophrenic symptoms. These and other central actions of the drugs can be blocked by dopamine receptor–blocking agents such as chlorpromazine or haloperidol.

Certain chemicals produce toxic psychosis in small doses. Interest in these compounds has been great, partly because they have some usefulness in experimental psychiatry and partly because their actions suggest a chemical basis for mental illness. *Hallucinogens*

There is a significant difference between the central effects of the hallucinogens and the mental effects of high doses of the psychomotor stimulants such as amphetamine. In the case of the hallucinogens, human subjects generally retain insight into their experience, realizing that their reaction is drug induced. Thus their hallucinations might better be termed *pseudohallucinations*. Amphetamine and related drugs are more truly psychotomimetic and may cause symptoms of paranoid schizophrenia indistinguishable from the actual disease.

Some of the most interesting psychotomimetic agents are lysergic acid diethylamide, mescaline, and psilocybin.

Lysergic acid diethylamide (LSD; Delysid) is closely related to the ergot alkaloids. Discovery of its hallucinogenic properties was made by the chemist who synthesized the drug and noted these reactions in himself. Subjects who take a few micrograms of LSD develop auditory and visual hallucinations. The body may feel distorted, the arms, for example, appearing to be at a great distance. The subject may become fearful and irrational.

Lysergic acid diethylamide   Mescaline

In animal experiments, LSD may cause excitement and hyperthermia. With repeated administration, considerable tolerance develops.

LSD is a potent antagonist of the action of serotonin on smooth muscles. The association of antiserotonin activity with psychic effects has been the basis for speculations concerning the role of serotonin in behavior. Some evidence favors the idea that in the brain LSD may act as an agonist at serotonin receptors. Whether an interaction between LSD and serotonin has anything to do with hallucinations is an unresolved question. Brom-lysergic acid diethylamide, like LSD, has antiserotonin effects on smooth muscles, but no hallucinogenic properties.

Mescaline is obtained from the cactus known as peyote or mescal (*Lophophora williamsii*) that grows in the southwestern United States. This cactus is used by some Indians in religious ceremonies. Persons who have ingested dried peyote buttons report that they cause stupor with visual hallucinations. Colored lights, reported to be extremely beautiful, are the most striking feature of these hallucinations. Interestingly, some volunteers report that they have seen colors they did not know existed.

Mescaline, the active principle of peyote, is 3,4,5-trimethoxyphenethylamine, a structure resembling the sympathomimetic amines. It has been given in doses of 300 to 500 mg in experimental psychiatry. Trace amounts of β-phenethylamine are present in the normal human brain. Moreover, urinary concentrations of β-phenethylamine were much higher in paranoid schizophrenics than in other mental patients or in normal individuals.[3] The relationship of these observations to the actions of hallucinogens remains to be determined.

Psilocybin (*O*-phosphoryl-4-hydroxy-*N*, *N*-dimethyltryptamine) has been isolated from Mexican mushrooms that have hallucinogenic effects. Chemically it is closely related to serotonin.

It is of great interest that compounds related to the endogenously occurring amines have hallucinogenic properties. Further research is needed to explain why this should be so.

The abuse of psychotomimetic drugs is discussed in detail in Chapter 30.

REFERENCES

1. Burks, J.S., Walker, J.E., Rumack, B.H., and Ott, J.E.: Tricyclic antidepressant poisoning, JAMA **230**:1405, 1974.
2. King, D.J.: Drug management of depression, Irish Med. J. **76**:44, 1983.
3. Potkin, S.G., Karoum, F., Chuang, L.W., Cannon-Spoor, H.E., Phillips, I., and Wyatt, R.J.: Phenethylamine in paranoid chronic schizophrenia, Science **206**:470, 1979.
4. Shore, P.A., McMillen, B.A., Miller, H.H., Sanghera, M.K., Kiser, R.S., and German, D.C.: The dopamine neuronal storage system and nonamphetamine stimulants: a model for psychosis. In Catecholamines: basic and clinical frontiers, New York, 1979, Pergamon Press, Inc., p. 722.
5. Snyder, S.H., Banerjee, S.P., Yamamura, H.I., and Greenberg, D.: Drugs, transmitters and schizophrenia, Science **184**:1243, 1974.
6. Sulser, F., Vetulani, J., and Mobley, P.L.: On the mode of action of antidepressant drugs, Biochem. Pharmacol. **27**:257, 1978.
7. Sulser, F.: New perspectives on the mode of action of antidepressant drugs, Trends Pharmacol. Sci. **1**:92, 1979.
8. van Praag, H.M.: Depression, Lancet **2**:1259, 1982.
9. Vohra, J., Burrows, G.D., and Sloman, G.: Assessment of cardiovascular side effects of therapeutic doses of tricyclic antidepressant drugs, Aust. N.Z. J. Med. **5**:7, 1975.

section four

Depressants and stimulants of the central nervous system

Chapter 26

Hypnotic drugs and alcohol

By definition, hypnotic drugs are used to promote sleep. These drugs were previously called sedative-hypnotics because of their general sedating properties. For about 100 years drugs of this class (first the bromides and then after the turn of the century the barbiturates and chloral hydrate) were the only medications available to calm any agitated patient, from the anxious neurotic to the most disturbed psychotic. However, with the advent of modern psychopharmacology, following the discovery of the antipsychotic properties of chlorpromazine, many specific drugs have been developed for the sedation, as well as the overall pharmacologic treatment, of patients with different psychiatric disorders (e.g., neuroleptics for the manic or schizophrenic patient). Thus hypnotics are now used strictly in the adjunctive treatment of patients with the complaint of insomnia.

Until a few years ago barbiturates, such as secobarbital and pentobarbital, and nonbarbiturates, including glutethimide, methyprylon, ethchlorvynol, and methaqualone, dominated among the drugs used as hypnotics.[28] However, tolerance develops fairly rapidly to these drugs,[24] often leading to the use of higher doses. This in turn increases the likelihood that an abstinence syndrome will occur following abrupt drug withdrawal and thus creates a greater potential for drug dependence and addiction.[18,20,25,29] Another concern with these drugs has been their rather narrow margin of safety.[17]

Currently the most commonly used hypnotics belong to the benzodiazepine drug class, with the first benzodiazepine hypnotic, flurazepam, introduced in 1970. The benzodiazepines are safer drugs and have a relatively low dependence liability. Nevertheless, barbiturates and a few nonbarbiturate nonbenzodiazepine drugs such as chloral hydrate and paraldehyde are still being used as hypnotics, albeit to a much lesser extent.

At the present time there are three benzodiazepine hypnotics available in this country, each with different elimination half-lives: flurazepam (long), temazepam (intermediate), and triazolam (short). After discussing the chemical structure, pharmacokinetics, and mechanisms of action of benzodiazepines in general, the efficacy, side effects, and the potential for withdrawal difficulties will be discussed in relation to each of these three drugs.

Flurazepam   **Temazepam**   **Triazolam**

Benzodiazepines with a rapid rate of absorption have a fast onset of action.[1,7] Diazepam is the most rapidly absorbed benzodiazepine; flurazepam is intermediate in its rate of absorption, followed by triazolam, while the U.S. formulation of temazepam has a very slow rate. The clinical correlation of these data is strong, since diazepam, flurazepam, and triazolam are all effective for inducing sleep, whereas temazepam has been shown to have little or no efficacy for sleep induction when taken at bedtime or only shortly before bedtime.[8,11]

Lipid solubility is a major determinant of the rate at which a specific benzodiazepine enters the CNS.[1,7] Diazepam has high lipophilicity and thus a rapid onset for its CNS effects. The duration of action of a given benzodiazepine is in part related to the rate and extent of redistribution of the drug and its metabolites to peripheral tissues from the CNS. Thus a more rapid and extensive redistribution leads to a shorter duration of activity.

Drug clearance of the benzodiazepines is dependent almost exclusively on the liver's ability to metabolize them. Hepatic biotransformation, which is achieved through the microsomal drug-metabolizing enzyme systems of the liver, may be accomplished by several metabolic pathways: oxidation, conjugation, and nitroreduction. Thus chronic liver disease seriously impairs the liver's ability to metabolize benzodiazepines, although not all drugs are equally affected.

An important characteristic of benzodiazepine metabolism is the formation of active metabolites.[1,2,4] Diazepam is metabolized to several compounds with CNS effects that contribute to the efficacy of the parent drug. Desmethyldiazepam, the major active metabolite of diazepam, has an elimination half-life of about 50 hours. Similarly, the hypnotic benzodiazepine flurazepam is biotransformed to two ultra-rapidly eliminated metabolites (hydroxyethyl flurazepam and flurazepam aldehyde) and one slowly eliminated metabolite (desalkylflurazepam with a half-life of 50 to

TABLE 26-1   Benzodiazepines: elimination half-life and clinical data

Generic name	Trade name	Elimination half-life* (hr)	Clinical use	Dosage (mg)
Chlordiazepoxide	Librium	7-28	Anxiolytic	5-20
Diazepam	Valium	20-90	Anxiolytic	2-10
Flunitrazepam	Rohypnol†	10-20	Hypnotic	1-2
Flurazepam	Dalmane	50-100	Hypnotic	15-30
Lorazepam	Ativan	10-20	Anxiolytic	2-4
Nitrazepam	Mogadon†	18-34	Hypnotic	5-10
Oxazepam	Serax	3-21	Anxiolytic	10-15
Prazepam	Verstran	24-200	Anxiolytic	10-20
Temazepam	Restoril	10-20	Hypnotic	10-30
Triazolam	Halcion	2.7-4.5	Hypnotic	0.25-0.5

*Pertains to parent compound and active metabolites if any.
†Commercially available only in Europe.

100 hours).[1,2] Certain benzodiazepine anxiolytics such as oxazepam and lorazepam, as well as the hypnotic triazolam, are metabolized directly to inactive substances and thus have much shorter elimination half-lives. The half-lives of these drugs range from 2.5 to 4.5 hours for triazolam and up to 10 to 20 hours for lorazepam (Table 26-1).

Mechanisms of action

The ratio between anxiolytic and sedative effects for benzodiazepines is greater than for barbiturates. Benzodiazepines have been found to have calming and taming effects in animals similar to those of barbiturates; however, contrary to the barbiturates, these effects occur at doses markedly lower than those that produce decreased activity or result in sleepiness. Benzodiazepines consistently attenuate the effects of punishment or lack of reward on animal behavior; again, sedation is not a necessary component for the anxiolytic or antipunishment effects of the drug. In general, benzodiazepines also reduce both evoked and spontaneous hostility and aggressive behavior, but the disinhibitory effects of these drugs may produce paradoxical increases in aggression. Muscle relaxation is another property of the benzodiazepines; it is possible that this effect may also contribute to the relief of anxiety. Finally, by raising the seizure threshold benzodiazepines have anticonvulsant effects.

Recently the presence of high-affinity binding sites (receptors) for the benzodiazepines was demonstrated in various brain regions, including the cerebral cortex, midbrain, and hippocampus.[3,5,7] Although the physiological meaning of some high-density areas for benzodiazepine receptors is not well understood, there appears to be a relationship between certain high-density areas and the pharmacological effects of these drugs. Anxiolytic effects of the benzodiazepines may relate to the presence of high concentrations of these receptors in parts of the limbic system (amygdala, hippocampus, and olfactory bulb) and frontal cortex. Also, high concentrations of receptors in the cerebral cortex, hippocampus, and amygdala may account for anticonvulsant effects, and receptors in the reticular formation and other structures of the pons and medulla oblongata are more likely related to the sedative effects of benzodiazepines.

The benzodiazepine receptors appear to be located in close proximity to GABA receptor sites. GABA's role on its own receptor sites is to inhibit neuronal activity.[7] The interaction of benzodiazepines with these specific receptors enhances the inhibitory action of GABA and potentiates its effect. The effect of the interaction between benzodiazepines and GABA receptors, however, may be to produce secondary changes in other neurotransmitters such as catecholamines, serotonin, or acetylcholine.

Abrupt withdrawal of benzodiazepine drugs with a relatively rapid elimination rate results in intense rebound insomnia and rebound anxiety (marked increases in wakefulness and daytime anxiety, respectively, compared with baseline levels), presumably because of a lag in the production and replacement of endogenous benzodiazepine-like compounds.[11,12,14] However, when benzodiazepines with long elimination half-lives are withdrawn, effects on the benzodiazepine receptors are less abrupt because the endogenous benzodiazepine-like compounds may be partially restored before the active metabolites of the exogenously administered drugs are completely eliminated. Thus following withdrawal of benzodiazepines with a short elimination half-life, rebound insomnia and rebound anxiety usually occur and are of an intense degree; with benzodiazepines with an intermediate half-life, they frequently occur and are of a moderate degree; and with benzodiazepines with a long half-life, they may infrequently occur and be of a lesser degree.

Rebound insomnia and rebound anxiety both appear to be related to the relatively rapid rates of elimination of certain benzodiazepines and the rate of change in occupancy of benzodiazepine receptors.[14] Moreover, an interrelationship between rebound insomnia and rebound anxiety is highly likely on the clinical level. Patients experiencing rebound insomnia at night caused by withdrawal of a short-acting benzodiazepine hypnotic may also experience rebound anxiety during the day. Part of patients' rebound anxiety may be resulting from the drug's pharmacokinetics and receptor interaction; another part may be caused by psychological reactions to the sleep disturbance itself. Conversely, patients experiencing rebound anxiety following withdrawal of a benzodiazepine anxiolytic with a rapid elimination rate may also experience rebound insomnia at night.

Flurazepam   Flurazepam (Dalmane), the first benzodiazepine hypnotic to be introduced commercially in the United States (1970), has been studied more extensively than any other hypnotic agent.[11] With short-term administration of 30 mg of flurazepam, studies show a marked improvement in sleep, both in terms of sleep induction and sleep maintenance.[10,11,24] Although sleep is markedly and significantly improved on

Comparison of effectiveness of temazepam, triazolam, and flurazepam. The percentage   FIG. 26-1
of change in total wake time from baseline is illustrated for each of the three drugs (tem-
azepam [clear bar], triazolam [diagonally hatched bar], and flurazepam [stippled bar]
during short- (STD), intermediate- (ITD), and long-term (LTD) drug use. Data for triazolam
with long-term use were not included in the figure, since the drug was not studied beyond
2 weeks of continuous nightly usage. Statistically significant reductions in total wake time
were obtained with flurazepam on STD, ITD, and LTD and with triazolam on STD.

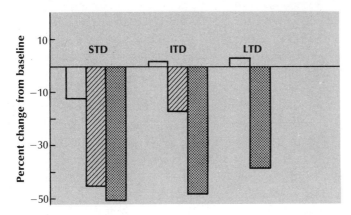

the first night of drug administration, peak effectiveness of the drug occurs on the second and third consecutive drug nights. These data indicate that the ultrashort elimination half-life metabolites of the drug, hydroxyethyl flurazepam and flurazepam aldehyde, account for much of the drug's efficacy, since the long half-life metabolite desalkylflurazepam is not available on the first night of use to affect sleep induction and is available only to a limited extent to affect sleep maintenance.[1,2,8,11]

An important consideration is that flurazepam's effectiveness, in contrast to that of most nonbenzodiazepine hypnotics and the more rapidly eliminated benzodiazepine hypnotics, is maintained with consecutive nightly administration of the drug over a 2-week period.[11,24] Even with long-term use of the drug (1 month), sleep is still markedly and significantly improved; there is only a slight loss of efficacy over this lengthy period of drug administration[10] (Fig. 26-1).

During the first 2 to 3 nights following withdrawal of flurazepam, there is clear-cut evidence of carry-over effectiveness; that is, levels of total wake time remain somewhat below the baseline values.[10,11] The carry-over effect for flurazepam is an advantage not only in terms of enhancing effectiveness but in facilitating withdrawal. Rebound insomnia has not been demonstrated following flurazepam's withdrawal; sleep disturbances observed have been mild in intensity and delayed in appearance.

The incidence of adverse effects with flurazepam administration is generally low. Because of the drug's carry-over, however, daytime sedation and performance decrements have been found to be greater with flurazepam than with the more rapidly eliminated benzodiapines.[9] Daytime sedation and performance decrement generally peak following the first several nights of drug administration and decrease as drug administration continues.[8] Short-term efficacy, effectiveness with continued use, and an absence of rebound phenomena following withdrawal have also been demonstrated with the 15 mg dose of flurazepam.[11] Since daytime sedation and performance decrement are much less frequent with the 15 mg dose, therapy should be initiated with this dose in the majority of patients, particularly the elderly.

Temazepam

Temazepam's (Restoril) usefulness is severely restricted by the drug's ineffectiveness for inducing sleep, since difficulty falling asleep is the most frequent complaint of insomniac subjects.[8,11] In the hard gelatin capsule formulation available in the United States, temazepam has a slow rate of absorption from the gastrointestinal tract; peak concentrations are reached an average of 2.5 hours after oral ingestion. Thus the drug's lack of efficacy for inducing sleep is not surprising and has been demonstrated both in sleep laboratory studies and clinical trials of hospitalized patients awaiting surgery. For sleep maintenance, the drug is moderately effective. However, because of the drug's lack of efficacy for inducing sleep, its effect on reducing total wake time is limited (Fig. 26-1).

Since it takes several hours for the drug to reach peak blood concentrations and the drug has an intermediate elimination half-life, there may be a significant carryover the next morning, resulting in excessive drowsiness.[11] The U.S. formulation of temazepam should produce a greater degree of morning drowsiness and possible performance decrements than the European preparation, since the latter is absorbed more quickly and lower doses are often used.

Since temazepam has an intermediate half-life, sleep disturbances following its withdrawal occur often, are moderate in intensity, and may be somewhat delayed in appearance.[11] In several studies rebound insomnia has been noted following the withdrawal of temazepam; increases in total wake time of greater than 50% over baseline levels have been reported.

Triazolam

Triazolam (Halcion) is rapidly eliminated; it has an ultrashort elimination half-life of approximately 2.7 to 4.5 hours.[1,7,8] The major advantage of the drug therefore is that there is little drug accumulation and less likelihood of daytime drowsiness and performance decrements than with drugs that are eliminated more slowly. However, the drug has a number of disadvantages, including a rapid development of tolerance, a strong potential for producing sleep disturbances both during drug administration and following drug withdrawal, and the occurrence of serious behavioral side effects, particularly at higher doses.[11]

With short-term use, triazolam is effective both for inducing and maintaining sleep.[11] Studies, however, have not demonstrated efficacy for the drug with continued drug administration. Data for some studies in which efficacy is claimed actually show that total sleep time increases by only 5 to 15 minutes a night, a rather small and clinically insignificant degree of change. Also, triazolam administration, particularly

Efficacy and withdrawal effects of triazolam, 0.5 mg. Changes in total wake time with drug   FIG. 26-2
administration and following drug withdrawal of triazolam, 0.5 mg. The ± standard error
of the minutes of total wake time is represented by the vertical bars. Values are plotted
for the following conditions: baseline (nights 2-4), initial (nights 5-7), and continued (nights
16-18) drug administration and drug withdrawal (nights 19-21). The baseline mean is
indicated by the broken line. The mean degree of worsening of sleep following drug
withdrawal is considerably greater than even the maximum degree of improvement of
sleep with drug administration.

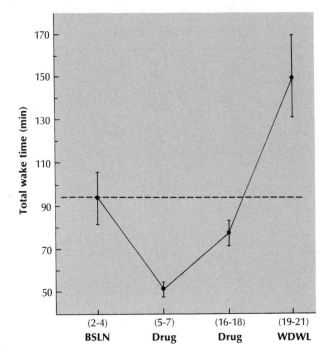

when tolerance has developed, can produce both significant increases in wakefulness during the final hours of drug nights (early morning insomnia[13]) and increases in levels of daytime anxiety or tension the next day.[13,15]

Since triazolam is rapidly eliminated, its withdrawal is usually accompanied by an immediate and intense degree of rebound insomnia.[11,12,14] Total wake time may increase by two to three times over the levels of the predrug baseline nights. Early morning insomnia, daytime anxiety, and rebound insomnia are all factors that may reinforce drug-taking behavior and thus contribute to the development of drug dependence (Fig. 26-2).

Memory impairment and even cases of prolonged anterograde amnesia have been reported during administration of 0.5 mg of triazolam.[11] A report from the Netherlands on the occurrence of serious behavioral side effects during triazolam administration (confusional states, depersonalization, severe anxiety, or hallucinations) has been minimized by some as being a result of patients using doses higher than those clinically recommended. However, these doses are only two to four times the 0.5 dose of the drug, and it is quite possible that the ultrashort half-life of triazolam, its high potency, and the occurrence of amnesia, early morning insomnia, daytime anxiety, and rebound insomnia all contribute to the development of adverse behavioral effects in susceptible persons.[11,14]

BARBITURATES
Chemistry and
pharmacokinetics

Barbituric acid, the parent compound of the barbiturate series, is synthesized through the combination of urea and malonic acid.[16,19]

Urea   Malonic acid   Barbituric acid

The parent compound, barbituric acid, has no hypnotic properties. Most of the clinically useful barbiturates are synthesized through replacing the two hydrogens in position 5 of the molecule with alkyl or aryl groups. The resulting substances are weak acids and tend to be un-ionized at physiologic pH. Pharmacokinetic variables such as absorption, distribution, protein-binding, metabolism, duration of action, and excretion of the barbiturates are influenced strongly by the degree of ionization and lipid solubility of these compounds. The ultrashort-acting barbiturates used as anesthetics are highly lipid-soluble and penetrate the brain very rapidly, whereas the long-acting barbiturates are less lipid-soluble and more ionized, and thus are distributed to and penetrate the brain more slowly. In Table 26-2 the barbiturates are classified as ultrashort- , intermediate- , and long-acting drugs.

After rapid entry into the CNS, the ultrashort-acting barbiturates are quickly redistributed to other parts of the body. The general CNS depression caused by barbiturates depends primarily on the general level of barbiturate in the brain, since barbiturates do not selectively concentrate in specific brain areas. For the short-acting barbiturates, the rate of redistribution is more important in determining the duration of action than is the rate of metabolism.

The barbiturates in general are metabolized in the liver to more water-soluble compounds that then can be more effectively excreted in the urine. The microsomal drug-metabolizing enzyme system of the liver has the critical role in this process. The long-acting barbiturate phenobarbital is metabolized slowly, and as a consequence a significant amount is excreted unchanged in the urine. Excretion of phenobarbital is enhanced by an alkaline pH, a fact that is important in the management of cases of overdose with this drug. Because of the roles of the liver and kidney in

TABLE 26-2	Barbiturates: elimination half-life and clinical data				
Generic name	Trade name	Elimination half-life (hr)	Clinical use	Dosage (mg)	Route of administration
Long acting					
Barbital	Veronal		Hypnotic	300-500	Oral
Butabarbital	Butisol	34-42	Hypnotic	100-200	Oral
Phenobarbital	Luminal	24-140	Hypnotic	100-200	Oral
Intermediate acting					
Amobarbital	Amytal	8-42	Hypnotic	100-200	Oral
Pentobarbital	Nembutal	15-48	Hypnotic	100	Oral
Secobarbital	Seconal	19-34	Hypnotic	100	Oral
Ultrashort acting					
Thiopental	Pentothal	3-6	Anesthetic	2.5%*; 0.3%†	Intravenous
Thiamylal	Surital		Anesthetic	2.5%*; 0.3%†	Intravenous
Methohexital	Brevital	1-2	Anesthetic	1.0%*; 0.2%†	Intravenous

*Concentration of intravenous solution for induction of anesthesia.
†Concentration of a continuous intravenous drip when used as a sole anesthetic.

the metabolism and excretion of barbiturates, diseases of these organs may significantly prolong the effects of these drugs.

Sites and mechanism of action

Barbiturates depress the activity of all brain cells; however, they selectively depress the diffuse pathways in the brain stem known as the reticular activating system.[19,21] Barbiturates can also selectively depress neuronal activity in the posterior hypothalamus, the amygdaloid complex, and certain limbic structures such as the septal region and the hippocampus. Neurochemical studies have shown that barbiturates reduce stress-induced turnover of norepinephrine and serotonin in rat brain, particularly in cell bodies of the raphe nuclei. Low doses of the drugs appear to enhance the effects of GABA or have GABA-like activity.[23] In anesthetic doses, the barbiturates may lead to reduced sensitivity of the postsynaptic membranes to excitatory neurotransmitters.

Clinical effects HYPNOTIC AND ANESTHETIC EFFECTS

The ultrashort-acting barbiturates are used almost exclusively in anesthesia for induction as well as for supplementation of inhalation agents. Their main advantage is their rapid redistribution in the body, which allows a minute-to-minute adjustment of their effects. Short- to intermediate-acting barbiturates have been extensively used as hypnotics and have been shown in both sleep laboratory and clinical trials to be effective initially and over short-term periods for inducing and maintaining sleep. However, there is a rapid development of tolerance with the barbiturates, since most of their effectiveness is lost with continued administration over a 2-week period.[24,26]

This rapid development of tolerance explains the common clinical finding of patients taking multiple doses of the drug; the patients become drug dependent and experience an abstinence syndrome when attempting to withdraw from the drug.[18,20,25,29]

In certain individuals, these drugs may produce paradoxical restlessness, excitement, and delirium. Elderly people are generally more prone to hangover effects; they are more likely to develop confusion and agitation. The most serious shortcoming of using barbiturates as hypnotics relates to their narrow margin of safety; only 10 times the therapeutic dose may be a lethal dose.[17] For example, in 1976 barbiturates were implicated in 14.5% of all drug-related deaths in the Drug Abuse Warning Network (DAWN). In contrast, there have been few well-documented cases in which benzodiazepines have been the sole factor causally associated with death. Since insomnia may be a symptom of depression with serious suicidal potential, safety is an important issue in prescribing barbiturates as hypnotics.

OTHER EFFECTS   Most of the barbiturates are capable of inhibiting the development of epileptic activity in the CNS. Barbiturates such as phenobarbital and metharbital are particularly effective in the treatment of grand mal seizures and jacksonian epilepsy. These drugs can abolish convulsions secondary to tetanus and eclampsia and can be used as antidotes for convulsant drugs.

Although barbiturates are not primarily analgesics, they may modify the reaction to pain. Large doses of barbiturates lead to depression of the respiratory center and a decrease of its responsiveness to carbon dioxide. The low blood pressure in barbiturate poisoning may be in part caused by impaired gaseous exchange or it may be a result of the direct action of barbiturates on central and peripheral elements of the autonomic nervous system. Such effects on respiration and circulation are commonly the cause of death from barbiturate overdosage.

DRUG INTERACTIONS   Whenever other drugs are administered in combination with barbiturates, possible drug interactions should be carefully considered, since the effects of these drugs may be additive to those of the barbiturates, thereby creating potential clinical hazards. Alcohol, reserpine, and phenothiazine neuroleptics, as well as sedative-hypnotics belonging to other drug classes, may enhance the action of the barbiturates. Such drug interactions may lead to serious impairment of daytime performance or even to respiratory depression with lower than expected doses of barbiturates.

The most significant drug interactions encountered with the barbiturates are based on the fact that these drugs induce hepatic microsomal enzymes. Thus chronic administration of barbiturates stimulates the metabolism of other drugs such as the MAO inhibitors, tricyclic antidepressants, phenytoin, and the coumarin anticoagulants. Moreover, discontinuation of the barbiturates may result in an exaggerated clinical response of the drugs whose metabolism had previously been stimulated by the microsomal enzymes induced by the barbiturates.

Barbiturates can produce both psychological and physiological depen- **ADDICTION**
dence.[18,20,25,29] Abrupt withdrawal from barbiturates following physical addiction produces a condition that is characterized by anxiety, irritability, insomnia, restlessness,
tremors, and even convulsions. Most barbiturate addicts have an underlying personality disorder that predisposes them to chronic barbiturate abuse. They may suffer
from anxiety or affective disorders, although most often they have antisocial person-
alities. Many narcotic addicts and alcoholics may also use barbiturates, either in
combination or as a substitute, if their preferred drug is unavailable. Since barbiturate
addicts may develop decreased intellectual capacity and impaired judgment, many
are unable to work or even care for themselves. They may also become hostile,
paranoid, or suicidal and in general manifest a loss of emotional control.

Withdrawal from chronic use of high doses of barbiturates and any other sedative-
hypnotic should be done only on an inpatient basis. Close medical supervision and
continuous monitoring of the patient are necessary because of the serious and potentially life-threatening consequences of barbiturate withdrawal. The basic strategies
of treatment are slow withdrawal of the addicting drug or substitution with a long-
acting barbiturate (phenobarbital) and subsequent gradual withdrawal of the substitute agent. When substitution with phenobarbital is employed, one sedative dose
of phenobarbital (30 mg) is substituted for each hypnotic dose (100 mg) of the shorter
acting barbiturate. The long-acting drug produces very slight fluctuations in blood
levels, allowing for safe use of smaller doses. If during phenobarbital withdrawal
symptoms of CNS hyperexcitability occur, the daily dosage of phenobarbital is temporarily increased by 25%. If, on the contrary, signs of phenobarbital intoxication
appear (nystagmus, slurred speech, staggering gait), the daily dosage should be
reduced by 25% before phenobarbital withdrawal proceeds further.

Before the development of the benzodiazepine hypnotics, which currently dom- **NONBARBITURATE**
inate among prescribed sleeping pills, various agents were used as hypnotics besides **NONBENZODIAZ-**
the barbiturates. The most commonly used drugs in this category were chloral hy- **EPINE HYPNOTICS**
drate, paraldehyde, ethchlorvynol, glutethimide, methyprylon, and methaqualone.
Chloral hydrate and paraldehyde, although the oldest, are the safest among these
compounds. Ethchlorvynol, a tertiary alcohol with a β-chlorovinyl group, is a short-
acting drug, which may lead to the development of physical dependence, although
it is less effective than most of the commonly used hypnotics. Glutethimide and
methyprylon, both piperidinedione derivatives (i.e., chemically similar to barbiturates), are intermediate-acting drugs with some hypnotic efficacy but with many
shortcomings, including a considerable potential for tolerance and addiction. An
important consideration is that overdose with glutethimide presents a special hazard
because the drug is highly lipid soluble and the use of dialysis is not effective. Finally,
methaqualone, a 2,3-disubstituted quinazolone, is a fast-acting hypnotic, which in
spite of its short duration of action can produce morning hangover. It may also cause
dizziness, urticaria, and paresthesias and frequently has been a drug of abuse.

Except for chloral hydrate and paraldehyde, the nonbarbiturate nonbenzodiaze-pine hypnotics appear to have at least as great a potential for tolerance and addiction as the barbiturates. Since their hypnotic efficacy is quite limited,[24] these compounds are currently underprescribed or have been withdrawn from the market in some countries, as is the case with methaqualone.

Chloral hydrate   Chloral hydrate is a crystalline material, water and lipid soluble, which is rapidly reduced in vivo to trichloroethanol, CCl_3CH_2OH, the active form of the drug.

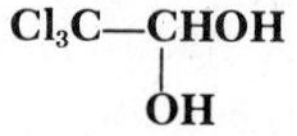

$$Cl_3C-\underset{\underset{OH}{|}}{CHOH}$$

Chloral hydrate

Chloral hydrate was introduced in 1869 and is still an occasionally used hypnotic. It is a short-acting drug especially useful in pediatric and geriatric patients, since in these individuals it produces a lower incidence of paradoxical excitation than the barbiturates. The usual dosage of chloral hydrate is 1 g. Development of tolerance to its hypnotic effect occurs after about 2 weeks of continued use. In its concentrated form, chloral hydrate causes some gastric irritation. The drug is also available in tablet form (chloral betaine), and this formulation may be less likely to cause gastric irritation.

The toxicity of chloral hydrate is generally low. The lethal dose of the drug is variable, that is, between 3 and 30 g. Although usual hypnotic doses have no de-tectable effect on the heart, overdosage may adversely affect the cardiac muscle. Thus chloral hydrate should be avoided in patients suffering from heart disease. Finally, administration of chloral hydrate can cause acute potentiation of other pro-tein-bound drugs such as warfarin, phenytoin, or tolbutamide, since chloral hydrate is metabolized to trichloroacetic acid, which is tightly bound to serum albumin and displaces the other drugs from their binding sites.

Paraldehyde   Paraldehyde is a cyclic ether, a polymer of acetaldehyde. On exposure to light and oxygen it decomposes to acetaldehyde, whereas in vitro and in vivo it is oxidized to acetic acid.

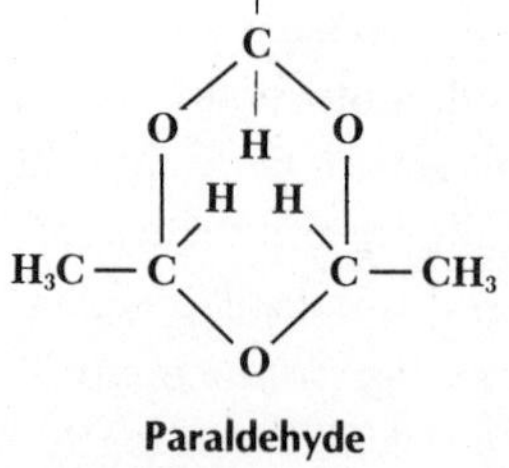

Paraldehyde

The drug, which is available in liquid form, has a strong odor and a characteristic disagreeable taste. Thus it is usually administered in a cold beverage to disguise its taste. An effective hypnotic dose is 4 to 8 ml at bedtime. Currently, paraldehyde is almost exclusively used in the management of hospitalized patients undergoing alcohol withdrawal or in patients with convulsive states such as eclampsia or tetanus. It is also used for patients with renal shutdown, since about one third of the total amount of the drug administered is eliminated through the pulmonary route and the remainder is metabolized to such simple chemicals as carbon dioxide and water.

Because of its causing gastric irritation, paraldehyde should not be administered orally to patients suffering from inflammatory conditions or ulcers in the esophageal, gastric, or duodenal areas. Similarly, rectal administration should be avoided in patients with inflammatory conditions of the anus and rectum.

Over-the-counter hypnotics

The ingredients of most nonprescription sleep medications include one or two antihistamines and occasionally salicylamide. The manufacturers' intent is to use the sedative side effects of the antihistamines to facilitate sleep. The widespread availability of over-the-counter (OTC) medications can be justified if they were indeed effective in relieving the symptoms of insomnia. As with many prescription drugs, however, claims of efficacy of the OTC preparations in inducing and/or maintaining sleep have not been verified. When the effectiveness of a standard OTC sleep preparation (Sominex) was evaluated in the sleep laboratory, it was shown that its recommended clinical dose did not produce any favorable changes either for inducing or maintaining sleep.[27] Similarly, sodium salicylamide, an ingredient of other OTC preparations, was shown to be almost completely devoid of any hypnotic efficacy.

Many insomniacs, fearing addiction to prescription hypnotics, may turn to these nonprescription medications in the belief that they are safer. However, clinical disturbances have been reported with varying dosages of these drugs. Even the recommended doses for these drugs may precipitate acute glaucoma, especially in elderly patients who have a narrow corneal-iris angle. Two to three times the recommended dosage may result in transient disorientation and hallucinations, especially in emotionally unstable individuals. With a marked overdose of these drugs (15 to 30 tablets), a stuporous state, confusion, extreme psychiatric disturbance, coma, and even death have been reported.

TREATMENT OF INSOMNIA

Hypnotics are only an adjunctive part of the overall treatment of insomnia.[30,31] Effective evaluation and treatment of this condition is dependent on a thorough knowledge of its multifaceted nature. Insomnia is by far the most prevalent sleep disorder; over 40% of the population has had a current or past problem with insomnia. The complaint of insomnia is more frequent with increasing age, in women, and in persons with high levels of psychological distress.

Transient sleep disturbances are extremely prevalent and may relate to situational problems at home, at work, or involving finances. Jet travel or changes in work shift may disrupt circadian rhythms and result in sleep disturbance. Medical conditions with significant pain, physical discomfort, anxiety, or depression are likely to produce complaints of insomnia.

Pharmacological agents themselves can disrupt sleep.[30,31] Insomnia can result from stimulant drugs, steroids, energizing antidepressants, or β-adrenergic blockers, particularly when these drugs are taken close to bedtime. Coffee or cola taken close to bedtime, as well as cigarette smoking, may similarly cause sleep difficulty, mostly in terms of delayed sleep induction, whereas alcohol consumption can lead to difficulty staying asleep, mainly in the form of early morning awakenings. Abrupt withdrawal of high doses of nonbenzodiazepine or benzodiazepine hypnotics may cause an abstinence syndrome that may include both insomnia and nightmares, whereas withdrawal of relatively low doses of benzodiazepines with short to intermediate elimination half-lives may produce rebound insomnia. Benzodiazepines with a rapid elimination rate may also produce early morning insomnia.

Aging is also a factor contributing to disturbed sleep; the elderly obtain less total sleep time and have very little of the "deeper" stages 3 and 4 sleep. Although medical conditions and aging may often contribute to the problem of chronic insomnia, psychopathology is by far the most predominant etiological factor.[30,31] Personality patterns of most patients with chronic insomnia are characterized by an internalization of emotions. Retrospective studies suggest that chronic insomnia develops at a time when life-stress factors are prevalent, in individuals who are predisposed by having inadequate coping mechanisms.

A thorough evaluation of patients with chronic insomnia includes taking a sleep history, drug history, and psychiatric history. Taking a sleep history includes defining the specific sleep problem, assessing the clinical course, ruling out other sleep disorders, evaluating sleep/wakefulness patterns, questioning the bed partner, and evaluating the impact of the sleep problem on the patient's life.

A drug history includes information on the current use of any prescribed and nonprescribed medication, as well as the timing of administration of the drug, particularly in relation to bedtime. In terms of past drug use, the history focuses on dosage and length of administration of any sedative-hypnotics recently discontinued. Also included is a review of current or past use of other substances such as alcohol, caffeine, and nicotine.

Since transient insomnia usually develops in reaction to some immediate stress, it can be expected to subside when the individual adapts through his or her own coping mechanisms. If the stress-generating situation cannot be eliminated, the physician is best able to help by identifying adaptive coping mechanisms and by aiding the patient in strengthening them.

The treatment of chronic insomnia is more complex, since chronic insomnia is multifaceted; any approach that is directed to only one of the factors involved will usually be inadequate or unsuccessful.[30,31] In general, the most effective treatment for the patient with chronic insomnia combines the following elements: (1) non-pharmacological treatment, including the use of general measures (regularizing schedules including time for bed, gradually increasing levels of physical exercise during the day, restricting the use of caffeinated beverages, and avoiding the use of alcohol as a sedative), supportive counseling, behavioral therapy, and psychotherapy; and (2) pharmacological treatment consisting of the adjunctive use of hypnotic medication or the use of antidepressant medication.

ALCOHOL*

As a therapeutic agent, alcohol is only of moderate importance. Alcohol has great toxicological interest, however, and chronic alcoholism is one of the great social problems of humankind.

Pharmacological effects

The main action of alcohol is exerted on the CNS. It may be looked on as an unusual hypnotic and anesthetic. There is general agreement that the apparent stimulant action of the drug is a consequence of primary depression of the higher centers, resulting in uninhibited behavior.

In addition to its action on behavior and consciousness, alcohol influences cardiovascular, gastrointestinal, and renal functions.

Cutaneous vasodilatation and a feeling of warmth are generally observed following the ingestion of an alcoholic beverage. This vasodilatation is not a direct effect of the drug on blood vessels but is a consequence of its CNS actions. There is a popular impression that alcohol dilates the coronary vessels, but it has been shown that alcohol does not prevent the electrocardiographic evidences of coronary insufficiency following exercise tolerance. Alcohol may lessen precordial pain, but this action is likely to be exerted on the brain rather than on the coronary vessels. Adverse myocardial responses to alcohol have been demonstrated in animal experiments.

The ingestion of alcohol promotes the secretion of acid gastric juice. It has been postulated that this action may be mediated through the release of histamine or gastrin in the stomach wall.

The diuresis observed in persons who drink alcoholic beverages is partly caused by the ingestion of water. Inhibition of the release of antidiuretic hormone from the posterior pituitary lobe by alcohol has also been demonstrated.

Metabolism

Ingested alcohol is absorbed rapidly from the stomach and the small intestine. The rate of absorption is influenced by the concentration of the alcohol ingested and most importantly by the presence of food in the stomach. On an empty stomach the drinking of an alcoholic beverage produces peak blood levels in less than 1 hour. There may be considerable delay if the stomach is filled with food.

---

*Sections on alcohol contributed by Dr. Andres Goth.

TABLE 26-3	Relative concentration of alcohol in various body fluids, tissues, and alveolar air (concentration in blood is 1.0)
Serum	1.15
Urine	1.3
Saliva	1.3
Spinal fluid	1.15
Brain or liver	0.85 to 0.90
Kidney	0.83
Alveolar air	0.0005 of blood concentration

Once absorbed, alcohol is distributed in total body water. The concentration of alcohol in different tissues and body fluids correlates well with the concentration of water at these sites. If the concentration of alcohol in blood is assigned the value of 1.0, the relative values given in Table 26-3 may be expected in the various body fluids, tissues, and alveolar air.

The concentration of alcohol in the blood has great medicolegal importance, since it is generally accepted that a blood level of alcohol of 100 mg/100 ml may be taken as evidence that the person is drunk. It is of some importance to know also the relationship between the quantities of alcohol ingested and the blood levels that may be expected. The concentration of alcohol in the blood will depend on the following factors: (1) quantity of alcohol ingested and rate at which it is drunk, (2) speed of absorption, (3) body weight and the percentage of total body water, and (4) rate of metabolism of alcohol.

The blood levels of alcohol that may be expected following the ingestion of various alcoholic beverages may be calculated. Since intoxication occurs when a blood level of 100 mg of alcohol/100 ml of blood is reached (0.100%) it can be calculated that this will occur if approximately 6 fluid ounces of a distilled spirit containing 45% alcohol is drunk rapidly. If a distilled spirit is drunk over a period of several hours, the number of ounces required for producing a blood level of 0.15% may be calculated by the following formula: 8 + H = Number of ounces of distilled spirits required to cause intoxication, where H is the number of hours during which the beverage is drunk.

The corresponding formula for fortified wine (containing 20% alcohol) is 18 + 2H; for ordinary wine (containing 10% alcohol) it is 36 + 4H; for beer (containing 4.5% alcohol) the figure would be 80 + 10H.

The relationships between the ingestion of various beverages, blood levels of alcohol, and prognosis in terms of ability in driving an automobile are shown in Fig. 26-3.

Level of alcohol in blood of an automobile driver relative to his being "under the influence."   FIG. 26-3

From Harger, R.N. In Economos, J.P., and Kreml, F.M., editors: Judge and prosecutor in traffic court, Chicago, 1951, American Bar Association and The Traffic Institute, Northwestern University.

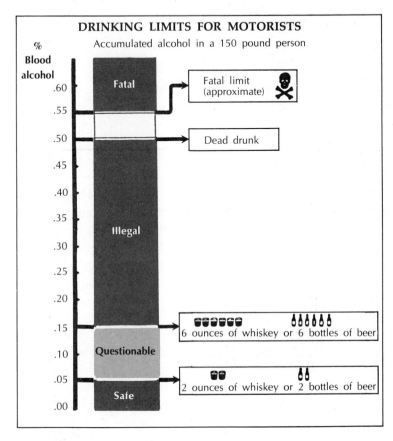

Elimination

The quantity of alcohol excreted in the urine, exhaled through the lungs, or lost in the perspiration ordinarily represents less than 10% of the total ingested. The remainder is metabolized; the end products are carbon dioxide and water.

The steps in the metabolism of alcohol appear to be as shown on p. 298.

The liver plays an important role in the metabolic transformation of alcohol. The first step occurs almost entirely in the liver.

The average person metabolizes 6 to 8 g (7.5 to 10 ml) of alcohol per hour. This figure is fairly constant for a given individual and is independent of the quantity present in the body. Habitual drinkers may metabolize alcohol slightly more rapidly than abstainers.

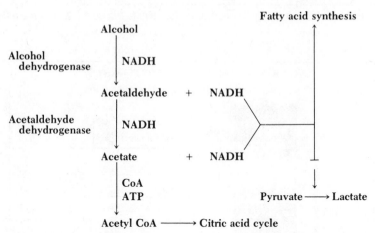

It has been claimed that the administation of glucose and insulin, various vitamins, dinitrophenol, and muscular exercise accelerate the metabolism. However, most of these claims have been denied.

The metabolism of 1 g of alcohol yields 7 calories. Since the maximal amount that can be metabolized in 24 hours is approximately 170 g, it may be calculated that alcohol can contribute up to 1200 calories per day to the metabolic requirements of an individual.

Metabolic effects   The influence of alcohol on carbohydrate and lipid metabolism has received much attention in recent years. Hypoglycemia can be induced in humans by the ingestion of 35 to 50 ml of ethanol after a 2-day fast. Such individuals must have low liver glycogen because they do not respond to glucagon with the characteristic increase in blood glucose. Animal studies indicate that alcohol can inhibit glycogen synthesis, probably by interfering with glyconeogenesis from amino acids.

It is quite likely that acute hyperlipemia following alcohol ingestion and the hyperlipemia of the chronic alcoholic have different mechanisms. The acute hyperlipemia is probably mediated through sympathetic activation, norepinephrine release, and lipolysis from fat depots. This effect of norepinephrine can be prevented by β-adrenergic blocking agents. Conversely, hyperlipemia in the chronic alcoholic may depend largely on deficient removal of lipid from the blood. Evidence for decreased lipoprotein lipase activity in alcoholic patients has been presented.

Fatty livers are commonly observed in alcoholic patients. The most likely explanations would appear to be (1) increased mobilization from fat deposits, (2) increased esterification to triglycerides rather than to phospholipids and cholesterol esters, and (3) decreased triglyceride release from the liver.

Tolerance and   It is commonly known that the experienced drinker shows fewer and less marked
addiction   effects from moderate amounts of alcohol than does the abstainer. This moderate tolerance cannot be explained on the basis of what is known about absorption, distribution, and metabolism in the chronic alcoholic. It is concluded therefore that

the experienced drinker has learned to behave and to perform habitual tasks at blood alcohol levels that would seriously disturb the unaccustomed individual. This apparent tolerance probably does not extend to the lethal effects of alcohol, and blood levels exceeding 550 mg/100 ml may produce death in the chronic alcoholic.

The severely intoxicated patient represents a medical emergency and should be managed according to the following recommendations[34]:

1. Respiratory support should be given if necessary.
2. Aspiration of vomitus should be prevented by placing the patient in semi-lateral decubitus position with head forward and mouth down.
3. Fluid needs should be assessed. The patient may be fluid overloaded or may have fluid deficits.
4. Gastric lavage can be helpful.
5. Hypoglycemia is suspected on the basis of unusual neurological findings, such as convulsions or coma. Intravenous glucose and intramuscular thiamine are recommended.
6. Metabolic acidosis, if severe, may require the use of sodium bicarbonate.
7. Hemodialysis may be useful in patients with excessive blood levels of alcohol.
8. Fructose and other measures that supposedly increase the rate of metabolism of alcohol are not recommended.

In alcohol withdrawal, magnesium replacement is often indicated. Intramuscular magnesium sulfate in 2 ml doses of a 50% solution may be given three times a day for 2 days. The benzodiazepines—chlordiazepoxide and diazepam—are commonly used, but their prolonged use can lead to a secondary abstinence syndrome.[34] Propranolol has a favorable effect on alcoholic tremor, but its usefulness in alcohol withdrawal has not been established.

The blood alcohol levels that may be lethal are usually in excess of 0.5% or 500 mg/100 ml. If the person has taken some other CNS depressant such as a barbiturate, even lower blood alcohol levels may result in a lethal outcome.

Chronic alcoholism

A variety of pathological changes occur in the alcoholic with much greater frequency than in the general population. Chronic gastritis, cirrhosis of the liver, and the neuropsychiatric condition known as Korsakoff's syndrome have received considerable attention. The mechanism of production of these abnormalities is difficult to state because the chronic alcoholic often suffers from nutritional deficiencies also. When benefited by psychiatric treatment or the organization known as Alcoholics Anonymous, about 50% of chronic alcoholics may be able to abstain from drinking.

Another approach to the problem has been the administration of drugs that will make the effects of alcohol extremely unpleasant or even dangerous. The best known of these is disulfiram.

DISULFIRAM

The development of the disulfiram (Antabuse) approach to chronic alcoholism was the consequence of a chance observation. While testing certain new drugs as potential anthelmintics, it was observed that following ingestion of tetraethylthiuram disulfide even a few bottles of beer caused very unpleasant side effects. Careful study of this unusual occurrence led to the discovery of the probable mechanism involved and to the eventual introduction of disulfiram into therapeutics.

From a chemical standpoint, disulfiram is tetraethylthiuram disulfide. Certain other disulfides have similar properties with respect to alcohol intolerance.

If alcohol is ingested several hours after taking disulfiram in doses of 1 to 2 g,

$$C_2H_5 \qquad\quad S \qquad\qquad S \qquad\quad C_2H_5$$
$$\diagdown \qquad\quad \| \qquad\qquad \| \qquad\quad \diagup$$
$$N\!-\!C\!-\!S\!-\!S\!-\!C\!-\!N$$
$$\diagup \qquad\qquad\qquad\qquad\qquad\quad \diagdown$$
$$C_2H_5 \qquad\qquad\qquad\qquad\qquad\quad C_2H_5$$

Disulfiram

the individual develops the typical reaction characterized by nausea, vomiting, flushing, palpitation, and headache. There may be lowering of the blood pressure, even to shock levels. These symptoms are so unpleasant that the patient simply cannot drink alcohol while on a maintenance dose of 0.25 to 0.5 g of disulfiram. Even when the drug administration is stopped, it may take a week before the alcohol intolerance disappears. Disulfiram by itself can cause some effects. Dizziness, metallic taste, reduced sexual potency, electroencephalographic changes, and skin reactions have occurred following its use.

It seems reasonable to assume that disulfiram interferes with the metabolism of alcohol, resulting in the accumulation of some toxic intermediate. Indeed, it has been demonstrated that acetaldehyde accumulates in the blood when the patient ingests alcohol while taking disulfiram. Blood acetaldehyde levels under these conditions may be of the order of 1 mg/100 ml. It has also been demonstrated that the intravenous infusion of acetaldehyde, which would produce comparable blood levels, reproduces the manifestations of the "Antabuse reaction." It has also been demonstrated in experimental animals that the administration of disulfiram delays the metabolism of administered acetaldehyde.

On the basis of these facts it may be concluded that disulfiram inhibits the second step in alcohol metabolism: the further utilization of acetaldehyde. This intermediate is a very potent pharmacological agent with vasopressor and vasodepressor properties.

Acetaldehyde apparently can cause the release of catecholamines from the tissues and thus behaves as an indirect-acting sympathomimetic drug. It is quite likely that it releases other amines also, which may account for the symptoms of the "Antabuse reaction."

Disulfiram is usually administered in a dosage of 1 to 2 g the first day, the quantity administered being gradually decreased in 4 days to about 0.5 g, but it may be even further reduced to 0.25 g as a maintenance dose.

Other drugs that create intolerance to alcohol and may elicit an "Antabuse reaction" include the hypoglycemic sulfonylureas, such as **tolbutamide** (Orinase) and **chlorpropamide** (Diabinese); and the antimicrobials, such as **chloramphenicol, furazolidone** (Furoxone), **griseofulvin** (Fulvicin), **isoniazid, metronidazole** (Flagyl), and **quinacrine** (Atabrine).

The aliphatic alcohols other than ethyl alcohol are of interest in medicine largely because they are sometimes involved in cases of poisoning. **OTHER ALCOHOLS**

Generally the toxicity of the alcohols increases with the chain length. An exception to this statement is methyl alcohol, which is unique in producing marked acidosis and blindness in primates but not in lower animals. As little as 30 ml of methanol has caused serious poisoning, and even death has been attributed to this quantity or even less. In addition to the acidosis, methanol intoxication involves the CNS, with the production of headache, dizziness, delirium, and coma. Blindness, which is a common accompaniment of these effects, may be total or partial. *Methanol*

Although methanol is metabolized in part to formaldehyde and formic acid, the amount of the latter is not sufficient to explain the profound metabolic acidosis that may result from ingestion of relatively small quantities of the alcohol. Blindness is probably a consequence of the toxic effects of formaldehyde on the retina. Interference with adenosine triphosphate generation by uncoupling oxidative phosphorylation has been postulated.

Metabolism of methyl alcohol in the body is much slower than that of ethyl alcohol, a fact that further complicates the management of methanol poisoning. The treatment of methanol poisoning is based largely on the correction of the acidotic state with appropriate intravenous fluids. Another approach is based on the observation that ethanol delays the metabolic transformation of methanol. Although some investigators favor the use of ethanol in treating methanol poisoning, it must be kept in mind that correction of the acidotic state with sodium bicarbonate given orally or intravenously (500 ml of a 5% solution) is the most important therapeutic procedure.

Isopropyl alcohol has some toxicological interest also. It is metabolized to acetone in the body. Severe renal damage is found in patients who have recovered from ingestion of a few ounces of isopropyl alcohol. The fatal dose is estimated as 120 to 240 ml. *Isopropyl alcohol*

REFERENCES

Benzodiazepines: general pharmacology

1. Greenblatt, D.J., Abernethy, D.R., Divoll, M., Harmatz, J.S., and Shader, R.I.: Pharmacokinetic properties of benzodiazepine hypnotics, J. Clin. Psychopharmacol. 3:129, 1983.
2. Kaplan, S.A., de Silva, A.F., Jack, M.L., Alexander, K., Strojny, N., Weinfeld, R.E., Puglisi, C.V., and Weissman, L.: Blood level profile in man following chronic oral administration of flurazepam hydrochloride, J. Pharm. Sci. 62:1932, 1973.
3. Mohler, H., and Okada, T.: Benzodiazepine receptor: demonstration in the central nervous system, Science 198:849, 1977.
4. Randall, L.O., and Kappell, B.: Pharmacological activity of some benzodiazepines and their metabolites. In Garattini, S., Mussini, E., and Randall, L.O., editors: Benzodiazepines, New York, 1973, Raven Press.
5. Squires, R.F., and Braestrup, C.: Benzodiazepine receptors in rat brain, Nature 266:732, 1977.

6. Sternbach, L.H., Randall, L.O., Banziger, R., and Lehr, H.: Structure-activity relationship in the 1,4-benzodiazepine series. In Burger, A., editor: Drugs affecting the central nervous system, New York, 1968, Marcel Dekker, Inc.

7. Usdin, E., Skolnick, P., Tallman, J.F., Jr., Greenblatt, D., and Paul, S.M., editors: Pharmacology of benzodiazepines, London and Basingstoke, 1982, Macmillan Press, Ltd.

Benzodiazepines: clinical use

8. Greenblatt, D.J., Divoll, M., Abernethy, D.R., and Shader, R.I.: Benzodiazepine hypnotics: kinetic and therapeutic options, Sleep 5:S18, 1982.

9. Johnson, L.C., and Chernik, D.A.: Sedative-hypnotics and human performance, Psychopharmacology 76:101, 1982.

10. Kales, A., Bixler, E.O., Soldatos, C.R., Vela-Bueno, A., Jacoby, J., and Kales, J.D.: Quazepam and flurazepam: long-term use and extended withdrawal, Clin. Pharmacol. Ther. 32:781, 1982.

11. Kales, A., and Kales, J.D.: Sleep laboratory studies of hypnotic drugs: efficacy and withdrawal effects, J. Clin. Psychopharmacol. 3:140, 1983.

12. Kales, A., Scharf, M.B., and Kales, J.D.: Rebound insomnia: a new clinical syndrome, Science 201:1039, 1978.

13. Kales, A., Soldatos, C.R., Bixler, E.O., and Kales, J.D.: Early morning insomnia with rapidly eliminated benzodiazepines, Science 220:95, 1983.

14. Kales, A., Soldatos, C.R., Bixler, E.O., and Kales, J.D.: Rebound insomnia and rebound anxiety: a review, Pharmacology 26:121, 1983.

15. Morgan, K., and Oswald, I.: Anxiety caused by a short-life hypnotic, Br. Med. J. 284:942, 1982.

Barbiturates: general pharmacology

16. Bush, M.T.: Sedatives and hypnotics. In Root, W.S., and Hofmann, F.G., editors: Physiological pharmacology, vol. 1, New York, 1963, Academic Press, Inc.

17. Cooper, J.R., editor: Sedative-hypnotic drugs: risks and benefits, National Institute on Drug Abuse Report, U.S. Department of Health, Education, and Welfare Pub. No. (ADM) 79-592, Washington, D.C., 1977, U.S. Government Printing Office.

18. Essig, C.F.: Addiction to nonbarbiturate sedative and tranquilizing drugs, Clin. Pharmacol. Ther. 5:334, 1964.

19. Harvey, S.C.: Hypnotics and sedatives: the barbiturates. In Goodman, L.S., and Gilman, A., editors: The pharmacological basis of therapeutics, ed. 5, New York, 1975, Macmillan Publishing Co., Inc.

20. Isbell, H., and Fraser, H.F.: Addiction to analgesics and barbiturates, Pharmacol. Rev. 2:355, 1950.

21. Magoun, H.W.: The waking brain, Springfield, Ill., 1958, Charles C Thomas, Publisher.

22. Mark, L.C.: Archaic classification of barbiturates: commentary, Clin. Pharmacol. Ther. 10:287, 1969.

23. Nicoll, R.A.: Pentobarbital: differential postsynaptic actions on sympathetic ganglion cells, Science 199:451, 1978.

Barbiturates and nonbarbiturates: clinical use

24. Kales, A., Bixler, E.O., Kales, J.D., and Scharf, M.B.: Comparative effectiveness of nine hypnotic drugs: sleep laboratory studies, J. Clin. Pharmacol. 17:207, 1977.

25. Kales, A., Bixler, E.O., Tan, T.L., Scharf, M.B., and Kales, J.D.: Chronic hypnotic-drug use: ineffectiveness, drug-withdrawal insomnia, and dependence, J.A.M.A. 227:513, 1974.

26. Kales, A., Hauri, P., Bixler, E.O., and Silberfarb, P.: Effectiveness of intermediate-term use of secobarbital, Clin. Pharmacol. Ther. 20:541, 1976.

27. Kales, J.D., Tan, T.L., Swearingen, C., and Kales, A.: Are over-the-counter sleep medications effective? All-night EEG studies, Curr. Ther. Res. 13:143, 1971.

28. Koch-Weser, J., and Greenblatt, D.J.: The archaic barbiturate hypnotics, N. Engl. J. Med. 291:790, 1974.

29. Oswald, I., and Priest, R.G.: Five weeks to escape the sleeping-pill habit, Br. J. Med. **ii:**1093-1095, 1965.

Insomnia

30. Kales, A., Kales, J.D., and Soldatos, C.R.: Insomnia and other sleep disorders, Med. Clin. North Am. **66:**971, 1982.
31. Soldatos, C.R., Kales, A., and Kales, J.D.: Management of insomnia, Ann. Rev. Med. **30:**301, 1979.

Alcohol

32. Becker, C.E., and Scott, R.: The treatment of alcoholism, Ration. Drug. Ther. **6:**1, 1972.
33. Bueno, F., and Mezey, E.: Management of alcoholism, Ration. Drug. Ther. **10:**1, 1976.
34. Redetzki, H.M.: Treatment of ethanol intoxication, Hosp. Formulary, Oct, 1979, p. 934.
35. Seller, E.M., and Kalant, H.: Alcohol intoxication and withdrawal. N. Engl. J. Med. **294:**757, 1976.

Chapter 27

Central nervous system stimulants of the convulsant type

GENERAL CONCEPT	*Analeptic* drugs have two main actions: they promote generalized arousal, and they increase the rate and depth of respiration. The sites of action for these potentially useful effects are the reticular activating system and the vital centers in the medulla. Unfortunately, analeptics also work in corticospinal pathways to raise levels of reflex excitability, which can lead to convulsions.[3,5] Many analeptics, once important in *materia medica*, are now mainly of toxicological interest or are tools for basic research on neurotransmission. A few are still used as respiratory stimulants. Analeptics of note are strychnine, picrotoxin, bicuculline, pentylenetetrazol, nikethamide, doxapram, and the methylxanthines.
MECHANISMS OF CONVULSANT ACTION	Stimulants may excite neurons directly (doxapram), block presynaptic inhibition (picrotoxin), or block postsynaptic inhibition (strychnine). The antagonism between strychnine and glycine on spinal motoneurons is discussed in Chapter 10.
CNS STIMULANTS	The older analeptics such as pentylenetetrazol (Metrazol), picrotoxin, and nikethamide (Coramine) have a low margin of safety between their analeptic and convulsant doses. Newer analeptics such as doxapram (Dopram) have replaced older ones because of a more favorable therapeutic index.
Pentylenetetrazol	There is much experience with the convulsant action of pentylenetetrazol in humans because the drug has been used extensively in shock treatment for mental disease. When approximately 5 ml of 10% solution of pentylenetetrazol is injected rapidly by the intravenous route, the individual becomes apprehensive and in a few seconds convulses and becomes unconscious. The major convulsive movements are tonic at first but rapidly become clonic. The convulsive phase may last only a minute, then is followed by exhaustion and sleep.

Sites of action of several neuronal stimulants and depressants as hypothesized for the   FIG. 27-1
GABA receptor/chloride ionophore. The complex is depicted as it might appear on the
outer surface of a membrane. With the exception of GABA, endogenous ligands (italics)
are identified only tentatively, and the effects of their binding on cellular responsiveness
are unknown. Drugs that tend to close the chloride channel (presumably by inducing
allosteric changes) are stimulants and convulsants. Stimulant drugs can bind at the ben-
zodiazepine (BZD) and picrotoxinin (PICRO) sites, as well as at the GABA receptor itself.

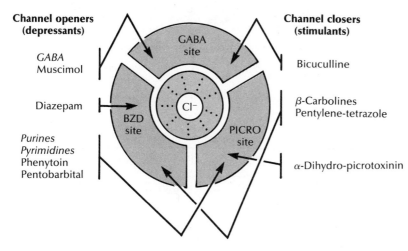

Channel openers
(depressants)

GABA
Muscimol

Diazepam

Purines
Pyrimidines
Phenytoin
Pentobarbital

GABA
site

BZD
site

Cl⁻

PICRO
site

Channel closers
(stimulants)

Bicuculline

β-Carbolines
Pentylene-tetrazole

α-Dihydro-picrotoxinin

$$H_2C-CH_2-CH_2-N-N$$
$$H_2C-CH_2-C{=\!=}N-N$$

Pentylenetetrazol

Muscular contractions may be so powerful that fractures of vertebrae and other bones may occur. For this reason, it was customary to administer muscle relaxants such as succinylcholine before the convulsant.

This drug is now largely obsolete both as an analeptic and for convulsive therapy.

Picrotoxin is a mixture of nonnitrogenous substances obtained from an East Indian   *Picrotoxin*
shrub. The more active component is picrotoxinin. It is available in injectable solution containing 3 mg/ml.

It is a typical convulsant of the pentylenetetrazol rather than the strychnine type. In normal animals it stimulates respiration only in doses close to the convulsant dose. Barbiturate-anesthetized animals may show significant respiratory stimulation without a convulsant action because the barbiturates antagonize the convulsive tendency.

Picrotoxin, once recommended for barbiturate poisoning, is seldom used today and is largely obsolete as a clinical drug. It has been an important research tool in the recent elucidation in vitro of GABA receptor mechanisms.[2] The scenario of convulsant drug activities clustered around the chloride channel (Fig. 27-1) may prove eventually to be too simplistic, since some of these drugs have properties in vivo inconsistent with the model. Nevertheless, the scheme has the virtue of focusing attention on the interrelationships of drugs, a specific transmitter, and ionic events in neural membranes.

Nikethamide   Nikethamide (Coramine) is closely related to nicotinamide and is converted to the vitamin in the body. The structural relationships are as follows:

Nicotinamide   Nikethamide

Nikethamide (Coramine) is available in ampules containing 0.4 g/1.5 ml or 1.25 g/5 ml. The drug is not a cardiac stimulant, and as an analeptic it is seldom used today.

Doxapram   Doxapram (Dopram) is a powerful respiratory stimulant. It increases respiratory volume more than rate. Its therapeutic index, expressed as convulsant dose$_{50}$/respiratory stimulant dose$_{50}$, is higher than that of the older analeptics, as determined in animals. This ratio may be as high as 25. The drug is administered intravenously in doses of 1 to 1.5 mg/kg of body weight.

Doxapram has a short duration of activity (3 or 4 minutes). It is used as a post-anesthetic respiratory stimulant. It has sympathomimetic side effects like hypertension and may be considered a very short-acting sympathomimetic stimulant.

Doxapram

Strychnine   Strychnine is a complex alkaloid obtained from the seeds of the plant *Strychnos nux vomica*.

Strychnine probably affects all levels of the neuraxis, but actions in the spinal cord seem to predominate. Strychnine lowers the threshold of excitability of various neurons. More recent studies indicate that it opposes the inhibitory influence of Renshaw cells on the motoneurons, probably by blocking glycine receptors. At some synapses the drug may act presynaptically to prevent transmitter release. Strychnine convulsions differ from pentylenetetrazol seizures in humans by the predominance of the tonic extensor phase, opisthotonos being characteristic of both this type of poisoning and of tetanus. The individual becomes highly susceptible to various stimuli, so that sudden stimuli such as noise or light precipitate a tonic extensor seizure.

Strychnine

Toxicological interest arises from uses of strychnine as a rodenticide and a contaminant in "street drugs."

Death by strychnine poisoning probably results from asphyxia or exhaustion after a prolonged series of seizures. Barbiturates are effective antagonists against the convulsant and lethal actions of strychnine. The muscle relaxants such as mephenesin (Tolserol) are also capable of protecting animals against strychnine poisoning.

Treatment of strychnine poisoning is based on the prompt uses of intravenous barbiturates. The stomach may be lavaged with a dilute potassium permanganate solution to remove and alter the poison at the early stages of intoxication.

Caffeine

Caffeine (1,3,7-trimethylxanthine) is one of the most widely used stimulants by the lay public, and it also has some medical uses. Coffee contains approximately 1.3% caffeine. A cup of coffee may contain from 100 to 150 mg of the alkaloid, which approximates a clinical dose for adults. It has been estimated that the annual consumption of caffeine in the United States in the form of coffee is about 7,000,000 kg.

The main pharmacological actions of caffeine are exerted on the CNS and the cardiovascular system. In addition, the drug is a diuretic and stimulates gastric secretion (Table 27-1).

Caffeine stimulates the cerebral cortex and medullary centers. In ordinary doses it causes wakefulness, restlessness, and mental alertness. These actions of caffeine are considered pleasant by most persons. It is not surprising that wherever a caffeine-containing plant grows, the inhabitants of the region have usually learned to utilize the drug. Some habituation to the use of caffeine occurs, but the drug is not truly addictive. Many "look alike" drugs that counterfeit the physical appearance of controlled substance dosage forms contain caffeine.

In larger doses, caffeine stimulates respiration and can also precipitate clonic convulsions in animals.

Caffeine stimulates the myocardium and can increase cardiac output.[4] Increased coronary blood flow is probably a consequence of increased myocardial work. Systemic blood pressure is not changed by ordinary doses of caffeine, although the drug directly dilates some blood vessels. The cerebral vessels are constricted by caffeine.

TABLE 27-1 Chemical structures and relative activities of methylxanthines

Xanthine

Alkaloid	Source	Methyl	Analepsis and gastric secretion	Cardiac stimulation, bronchodilatation, and diuresis
Caffeine	Coffee, tea, cocoa, cola	1,3,7	+ + +*	+
Theophylline	Tea	1,3	+ +	+ + +
Theobromine	Cocoa	3,7	+	+ +

*+, Least potent; + + +, most potent.

The end product of caffeine metabolism in the body appears to be 1-methyluric acid and other methyl derivatives of uric acid. It is quite certain that caffeine does not increase the miscible pool or urinary excretion of uric acid itself and is not contraindicated in gout.

For therapeutic use, caffeine is available as caffeine sodium benzoate in ampules of 0.25 and 0.5 g in 2 ml for intramuscular injection. For oral administration, citrated caffeine is available in 60 and 120 mg tablets. In addition, caffeine is often added to headache remedies containing salicylates and acetophenetidin and to ergotamine (Cafergot) for the treatment of migraine.

Visceral smooth muscle relaxation such as bronchodilatation is accomplished better with theophylline or aminophylline. The latter is a soluble physical complex of theophylline and ethylenediamine. Methylxanthines inhibit the enzyme phosphodiesterase which inactivates cyclic adenosine-3′,5′-phosphate. Since catecholamines promote the formation of the cyclic nucleotide whereas the methylxanthines inhibit its destruction, a very interesting hypothesis could be constructed for explaining similarities of pharmacological action at many sites such as the heart and the bronchial smooth muscle. The action of methylxanthines and epinephrine on cyclic adenylic acid metabolism is discussed further in Chapters 15 and 40.

1. Graham, D.M.: Caffeine—its identity, dietary sources, intake and biological effects, Nutr. Rev. **36**:97, 1978.

2. Olsen, R.W.: Drug interactions at the GABA receptor-ionophore complex, Ann. Rev. Pharmacol. Toxicol. **22**:245, 1982.

3. Smythies, J.R.: Relations between chemical structure and biological activity of convulsants, Ann. Rev. Pharmacol. **14**:9, 1974.

4. Stimulants and other drugs for treatment of mental symptoms in the elderly, Med. Letter **20**:75, 1978.

5. Wang, S.C., and Ward, J.W.: Analeptics, Pharmacol. Ther. **3**(**B**):123, 1977.

REFERENCES

Chapter 28

Antiepileptic drugs

GENERAL
CONCEPT

Convulsions are involuntary, general paroxysms of muscular contractions. Unconsciousness may occur, but this is not a necessary component. Convulsions can arise from pathological processes within or outside the brain and from various toxins, drugs, and xenobiotics. A frequent etiology for convulsions is the assortment of neuronal defects grouped under the collective term *epilepsy*.

A focal area is an essential feature in the origin of epileptic seizures. The focus may be functional (arising from proximity to a tumor, hypoxic tissue, a cyst) or cryptogenic (a biochemical lesion or abnormal synaptic connections). Within the focal area, neurons discharge rapidly in bursts that coincide with periodic waves of depolarization.

An epileptic fit arises when discharges from focal neurons invade extrafocal regions, recruiting neurons there into a synchronously discharging aggregate of excited cells.[5] Numerous reasons for spread of the excitation have been identified in individual patients, including changes in blood sugar, plasma pH, osmotic pressure, electrolytes, and circulating hormones. Fatigue, physical or mental stress, and nutritional deficiencies also trigger spread in certain individuals.

If spread is sufficiently extensive, focal or generalized seizures ensue. As part of the excitation process, certain neurons feedback inhibitory information to the neuronal aggregate (Fig. 28-1). Inhibitory synaptic potentials summate with time, gradually hyperpolarizing and desynchronizing the aggregate. This latter process terminates the motor or sensory manifestations (ictus) and may be partially responsible for the usual period of postictal lethargy.

Epilepsies are categorized for purposes of therapeutic management, but it should be borne in mind that epilepsy is a symptom much more than it is a specific disease. Diagnosis is based mainly on the clinical patterns of the seizure.[6] Electroencephalography can be helpful. For instance, monotonous three per second spike-wave complexes are characteristic in petit mal. A brief, annotated classification of the epilepsies follows:

A. *Generalized seizures* (abrupt bilateral spread from focus into both hemispheres)
  1. *Grand mal* (unconsciousness; tonic-clonic convulsions)
  2. *Petit mal* (staring or absence reaction; no motor signs; prepubertal age)
  3. *Myoclonic attacks* (rhythmic body jerks without loss of consciousness; infants; may respond to ACTH or antiinflammatory steroids if usual anticonvulsants fail)
B. *Focal or partial seizures* (spread contained within limits)
  1. *Simple motor* (jacksonian types)
  2. *Temporal-limbic* (psychomotor types)
    a. Simple sensory (visual; auditory; olfactory; autonomic)
    b. Complex (automatisms; intense emotions; psychic experience)
C. *Focal becoming generalized* (prodromal sensation or aura; focal EEG discharge before generalized seizure occurs; focal behavioral events before or after grand mal attack)

Bromides were the earliest antiepileptic drugs, followed by phenobarbital in 1912 and phenytoin in 1938. Significant newer developments include primidone, carbamazepine, benzodiazepines such as diazepam and clonazepam, valproic acid, and drugs for absence attacks such as trimethadione and ethosuximide.

Diagram of neuronal connections thought to be important in the genesis of major motor (tonic-clonic) convulsions. Excitation spreads from focal neuron (asterisk) through excitatory synapses (e) to form an aggregate of excited cells (shaded). Involvement of motor pathways leads to skeletal muscle contractions. Some neurons (unshaded), when activated feed back inhibitory signals through synapses (i) on focal and other neurons in the chain to terminate the seizure episode. Intracellular recordings depicted are typical for cells in a focal area during interictal periods: bursts of action potentials on waves of depolarization. Such bursts are often coincident with spikes in electroencephalographic spike/wave combinations (three combinations are shown). A paroxysm of exaggerated amplitude, slow (3 to 5/sec) waves appears in the EEG during spread. These paroxysms can occur in the absence of clinical convulsions if spread is not extensive. The time calibration is 200 msec for the intracellular record and 1 sec for the electroencephalograms. FIG. 28-1

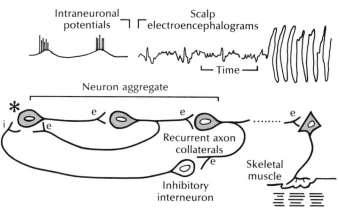

MODE OF ACTION   The modes of action of antiepileptic drugs are unknown. Targeted effects on just the focal neurons would be desirable; however, none of the useful drugs have this degree of specificity. At the neurophysiological level, the spread of seizure discharge is decreased by phenytoin, phenobarbital, and primidone. Convulsive threshold, as measured by electroshock or pentylenetetrazol convulsions, is elevated by most drugs in this class.

Working hypotheses for the effects of anticonvulsants on threshold and spread stem from the idea of membrane stabilization. Events thought to enhance stability include altering the activity of (Na/K) ATPase, shifting the production of cyclic nucleotides, and interfering with protein phosphorylation. Interest has also centered on drug-induced changes in permeability to specific ions because ion flux governs excitability. Phenytoin and phenobarbital may depress sodium influx into axons and somata and calcium influx into dendrites. These actions would tend to stabilize membranes. Trimethadione and ethosuximide, drugs effective in petit mal, may alter potassium permeability.

Interest in "active inhibition" has emerged with recent descriptions of binding of anticonvulsants within the GABA receptor complex. The ion in this instance is chloride, which hyperpolarizes membranes as it enters cells. GABA inhibits certain cells by virtue of promoting inward chloride conductance. Receptors for drugs are located in the vicinity of chloride channels. See Fig. 24-4 for a stylized version of a GABA receptor complex.

Some anticonvulsants may bind to drug receptors in the complex in such a way as to enhance GABA-mediated inhibition. Phenytoin and phenobarbital seem to act as ligands at what has been called the picrotoxin site. Benzodiazepine anticonvulsants (diazepam, clonazepam) have a separate binding site in the complex. Valproic acid has several actions at GABA synapses, including inhibition of GABA catabolism and presynaptic uptake, and agonist effects at the GABA receptor itself. The overall contribution of these actions to the anticonvulsant properties of valproic acid is still unclear.

CLASSES   From a chemical standpoint the various drugs used in epilepsy may be categorized as follows:

Barbiturates and related drugs
  Phenobarbital (Luminal)
  Mephobarbital (Mebaral)
  Metharbital (Gemonil)
  Primidone (Mysoline)
Hydantoins
  Phenylethylhydantoin (Nirvanol)
  Mephenytoin (Mesantoin)
  Phenytoin (Dilantin)
Oxazolidinediones
  Trimethadione (Tridione)
  Paramethadione (Paradione)

Succinimides
  Phensuximide (Milontin)
  Methsuximide (Celontin)
  Ethosuximide (Zarontin)
Miscellaneous anticonvulsants
  Phenacemide (Phenurone)
  Acetazolamide (Diamox)
  Clonazepam (Clonopin)
  Diazepam (Valium)
  Carbamazepine (Tegretol)
  Valproic acid (Depakene)

The structural formulas of barbiturates, hydantoins, oxazolidines, and succinimides have certain similarities.

Whereas barbituric acid is malonylurea, hydantoins have five-membered rings formed by condensation of acetic acid and urea. In the oxazolidine series, the nitrogen in the hydantoin ring is replaced by oxygen. Succinimides obviously resemble the oxazolidines.

Phenobarbital (Luminal), one of the oldest and least expensive antiepileptic drugs, is administered orally in a total daily dose of 0.1 to 0.2 g. Blood and brain levels peak at 10 to 12 hours. Phenobarbital differs from most hypnotic barbiturates in possessing significant antiepileptic effects at dose levels that do not cause excessive sedation. When phenobarbital is used, care must be taken never to withdraw it suddenly, because this procedure can precipitate a grand mal attack.

Barbiturates and related drugs

The major usefulness of phenobarbital is in the management of grand mal and focal epilepsy. It has little effect on petit mal but may be combined with trimethadione in patients who have mixed types of generalized epilepsy. Phenobarbital has a long half-life of 50 to 150 hours. Therapeutic blood levels are 10 to 30 μg/ml. Drowsiness and irritability are the main side effects of phenobarbital, but most patients become tolerant to the sedative effects with the passage of time. In children, hyperactivity and interference with learning ability are distinct disadvantages. However, phenobarbital is frequently prescribed in the prophylaxis of febrile convulsions.

Mephobarbital (Mebaral) is *N*-methylphenobarbital. Its indications and uses are similar to those of phenobarbital. In fact, the compound is demethylated to a significant extent to phenobarbital in the body. As a consequence, the antiepileptic effects of mephobarbital are due at least in part to phenobarbital. The dosage of mephobarbital (Mebaral) is 300 to 600 mg/day.

Metharbital (Gemonil) is *N*-methylbarbital and is probably demethylated in the body to barbital. Its dosage is 100 mg two or three times a day.

Primidone (Mysoline), although not a true barbiturate, is similar in structure to phenobarbital. Because sedation and vertigo can be pronounced, it should be started in small doses, about 50 mg, with a gradual increase to as much as 250 mg three times a day. Primidone is converted into two active metabolites: phenobarbital and phenylethylmalonamide. Therapeutic blood levels are 5 to 10 μg/ml when the drug is used for generalized tonic-clonic seizures.

Phenobarbital   **Primidone**

Phenylethylhydantoin   Mephenytoin   Phenytoin

Phenylethylhydantoin (Nirvanol) was withdrawn as a sedative because it produced an extraordinarily high incidence of drug fever, skin sensitization, and eosinophilia. Interestingly, replacement of the ethyl radical by a phenyl group yielded the highly useful anticonvulsant phenytoin.

On the other hand, **mephenytoin** (Mesantoin), which is the *N*-methyl derivative of phenylethylhydantoin, is demethylated in the body to this highly toxic and sensitizing drug. It is not surprising therefore that a high incidence of drug reactions has been reported for mephenytoin. Some of these are skin rashes and fever, granulocytopenia, and aplastic anemia. Clearly the drug should be used only if other compounds are ineffective.

Phenytoin (Dilantin), introduced in 1938, is still one of the most valuable antiepileptic drugs. It is administered in capsules containing 0.1 g of the drug as its sodium salt. The daily dose in adults varies from 0.2 to 0.6 g.

The main advantage of phenytoin in the management of grand mal and focal epilepsy is that it exerts little sedative action at effective dose levels. It may be given intravenously in status epilepticus. Fifty milligrams per minute is administered up to a total dose of 1 g for adults.

Adverse effects of phenytoin. The unwanted effects of phenytoin are of three categories. It has *toxic effects,* true *side effects,* and *idiosyncratic reactions.* Intoxication is characterized by sedation, ataxia, nystagmus, and a paradoxical increase in seizures. These manifestations are dose related and appear at plasma levels of 20 to 40 μg/ml. Severe and prolonged intoxication may lead to degeneration of cerebellar Purkinje cells.

Side effects include osteomalacia and hypocalcemia caused probably by interference with vitamin D metabolism. Long-term use of phenytoin may lead to lowered serum folic acid levels, resulting in megaloblastic anemia.

A frequent side effect of phenytoin is hypertrophy of the gums. It occurs in 20% of patients and is generally attributed to a disorder of fibroblastic activity.

Increased risk of teratogenesis is associated with the use of phenytoin during pregnancy. A "hydantoin syndrome" consisting of cleft lip, heart defects, and slow mental and physical maturation has been described. Other antiepileptic drugs, and perhaps epilepsy itself, may contribute to the teratogenesis. Current thinking is that seizures during pregnancy pose a greater risk to the developing fetus than do anticonvulsant drugs.[4]

Drugs of the hydantoin group may produce blood dyscrasias and rarely a clinical picture resembling malignant lymphoma. Phenytoin's use as an antiarrhythmic drug is dicussed in Chapter 35.

Pharmacokinetics of phenytoin. Phenytoin is absorbed rapidly from the gastrointestinal tract, and the drug is about 90% protein bound. The half-life of phenytoin is 24 to 30 hours; thus steady state concentrations are achieved in 4 to 5 days. The therapeutic blood level range is 10 to 24 μg/ml. Phenytoin shows some unusual pharmacokinetic features. Once plasma concentrations of 10 μg/ml are reached, further increases in dosage produce greater than expected plasma levels. It appears that metabolic pathways for the elimination of the drug, mainly hepatic parahydroxylation, become saturated. As a consequence the half-life of the drug increases as plasma concentrations rise. Monitoring of plasma concentrations is quite important, since minor increases in dosage can result in markedly elevated plasma concentrations. High blood levels lead to toxic manifestations and even paradoxical seizures.

Trimethadione   Paramethadione

Trimethadione (Tridione) and **paramethadione** (Paradione) are useful in the management of petit mal. They are available in capsules containing 0.3 g. The daily dose varies from 1 to 2 g.

Oxazolidinediones

Toxic effects of oxazolidines include drowsiness, ataxia, photophobia, and white halos around objects in the visual field. Bone marrow depression and kidney damage have also been described after prolonged use of the oxazolidines. Skin rashes and alopecia also have been reported. Trimethadione is used mainly in patients hypersensitive or refractory to ethosuximide.

Succinimides such as **phensuximide** (Milontin), **methsuximide** (Celontin), and **ethosuximide** (Zarontin) are useful in the management of petit mal. They may be less toxic than the oxazolidones, although dizziness or skin rashes may occur following their use. Rare cases of neutropenia and other blood dyscrasias have also been reported. The mechanism of action of succinimides is obscure.

Succinimides

Usual dosages of these drugs are phensuximide (Milontin), 0.5 to 1 g three times a day; methsuximide (Celontin), 0.3 to 0.6 g three times a day; and ethosuximide (Zarontin), 0.5 g two to four times a day. Ethosuximide is now considered the drug of choice in the treatment of petit mal. It has a mean half-life of about 48 hours. Therapeutic blood concentrations are thought to be between 40 and 100 μg/ml. Monthly blood counts are recommended.

Phensuximide   Ethosuximide

Phenacemide (Phenurone), a very potent but quite toxic anticonvulsant, should be used only after all other measures fail. Given in doses of 0.5 g three times a day, it may cause severe bone marrow depression, hepatocellular damage, and toxic psychoses.

Bromides were used extensively at one time but are now obsolete. Their use is associated with mental depression, toxic psychoses, and skin rashes.

Acetazolamide (Diamox), a carbonic anhydrase inhibitor, is used adjunctively as an anticonvulsant. Metabolic acidosis induced by a ketogenic diet was at one time used in epilepsy. The carbonic anhydrase inhibitors, which produce metabolic acidosis, have been found useful in all types of epilepsy. There is a possibility that their effectiveness is not caused by systemic acidosis but rather by inhibition of carbonic anhydrase in the CNS. The activity of the enzyme is high in the choroid plexus, which regulates the composition of cerebrospinal fluid. Acetazolamide (Diamox) is given in doses of 250 to 500 mg two or three times a day.

Carbamazepine (Tegretol) is an iminostilbene derivative related structurally to the tricyclic antidepressants. The drug is useful in the treatment of generalized tonic-clonic seizures and focal seizures, in the prophylaxis of childhood febrile seizures, and in trigeminal neuralgia. Carbamazepine's beneficial actions in psychomotor types of epilepsy are particularly important because this rather common form of epilepsy is most refractory to drug therapy.

The drug is absorbed slowly from the gastrointestinal tract and is 75% protein bound. Its half-life is 12 hours; therefore it must be given in divided daily doses. Adverse effects of carbamazepine include ataxia, dizziness, drowsiness, diplopia, and rarely hepatic damage, cardiotoxicity, and bone marrow depression. The drug is available in 200 mg tablets.

Clonazepam (Clonopin) and **diazepam** (Valium) are the two benzodiazepines used as antiepileptic drugs. Clonazepam is useful in the treatment of drug-resistant absence seizures and progressive myoclonic epilepsy. Diazepam, administered intravenously, is indicated for status epilepticus.[3]

Therapeutic blood concentrations of clonazepam are from 20 to 80 ng/ml. The drug has a half-life of elimination of about 18 hours. Adverse side effects produced by the drug include drowsiness, ataxia, and, in children, personality changes. The drug is available in tablets containing 0.5, 1, or 2 mg. Diazepam (Valium) for intravenous use is available in ampules containing 10 mg/2 ml.

Valproic acid (Depakene) is dipropylacetic acid and is one of the more recently introduced antiepileptics. The drug may act by increasing the effectiveness of γ-aminobutyric acid in the brain. It is absorbed rapidly from the gastrointestinal tract and has a short half-life of 6 to 13 hours. Thus it must be administered three or four times daily.

Valproic acid is useful in the treatment of generalized seizures, both tonic-clonic and absence, and is indicated also in myoclonic seizures. Thus the drug has a remarkably wide range of applications.[2]

Adverse effects of valproic acid include drowsiness, gastrointestinal discomfort, transient hair loss, weight gain, and rarely hepatotoxicity. Valproic acid interacts with other antiepileptic drugs. It inhibits the metabolism of phenobarbital, and it lowers phenytoin plasma concentrations by competition for protein binding.

Valproic acid (Depakene) is available in 250 mg capsules and as a syrup containing 250 mg/5 ml as the sodium salt. The recommended dose is 30 mg/kg with therapeutic blood concentrations of 50 to 100 µg/ml.

The usefulness of the antiepleptic drugs in various types of seizures is indicated below:

CLINICAL PHARMACOLOGY

Generalized tonic-clonic and focal seizures	Absence seizures	Status epilepticus
Phenytoin	Ethosuximide	Diazepam
Phenobarbital	Clonazepam	Clonazepam
Primidone	Valproic acid	Phenytoin
Carbamazepine		
Valproic acid		

The general incidence of side effects is less if anticonvulsant doses are low initially, then built up slowly. Complete seizure control is a desirable goal but may not be attainable because of intervening side effects.[1] Patient compliance is a major problem. More often than not "nonresponders" are either not taking their medication at all or are not taking it as prescribed. Some patients are candidates for cautious drug withdrawal to determine if anticonvulsants are still needed. Usual criteria for slowly decreasing the dose are no seizures in the previous 3 to 4 years, no overt neurological deficits, and normal electroencephalograms.

The adverse effects of antiepileptic drugs tend to be gastrointestinal, neurological, cutaneous, mental, hematopoietic, and renal. Gastrointestinal side effects, usually seen at the initiation of treatment, respond to a reduction in dosage. Drowsiness and ataxia are common side effects. Ataxia is common with hydantoins and barbiturates. Skin eruptions are produced by many of the antiepileptic drugs. Rarely, they can become major medical problems.

ADVERSE EFFECTS AND DRUG INTERACTIONS

Personality, mood, and mental changes in patients treated with the antiepileptic drugs are not uncommon. Megaloblastic anemias that respond to folic acid may occur with hydantoins, barbiturates, and primidone. Lymphadenopathies resembling malignant lymphomas have been reported in association with phenytoin, mephenytoin, paramethadione, and trimethadione. Nephropathies have been reported for trimethadione and paramethadione.

Among the miscellaneous adverse effects, gingival hyperplasia during therapy with phenytoin has been commented on before. Congenital abnormalities have been reported following ingestions of trimethadione and paramethadione by pregnant women. If primidone is used during pregnancy, an injectable vitamin K should be given before delivery. Maternal and neonatal hemorrhagic problems have been ascribed to primidone.

Drug interactions are numerous in connection with the antiepileptic drugs. Phenobarbital speeds up the metabolism of phenytoin, although this interaction seldom creates a serious problem. The metabolism of the coumarin anticoagulants is also increased by phenobarbital. On the other hand, dicumarol inhibits the metabolism of phenytoin.

Isoniazid, aminosalicylic acid, chloramphenicol, and disulfiram potentiate the actions of phenytoin by inhibiting its metabolism. Reserpine may oppose the actions of anticonvulsants by lowering convulsive thresholds.

REFERENCES

1. Browne, T.R.: Clinical pharmacology of antiepileptic drugs, Am. J. Hosp. Pharm. **35**:1048, 1978.
2. Bruni, J., and Wilder, B.J.: Valproic acid: review of a new antiepileptic drug, Arch. Neurol. **36**:393, 1979.
3. Delgado-Escueta, A.V., and Bajorek, J.G.: Status epilepticus: mechanisms of brain damage and rational management, Epilepsia **23**(suppl. 1):S29, 1982.
4. Montouris, G.D., Fenichel, G.M., and McLain, L.W.: The pregnant epileptic, Arch. Neurol. **36**:601, 1979.
5. Schwartzkroin, P.A., and Wyler, A.R.: Mechanisms underlying epileptiform burst discharge, Ann. Neurol. **7**:95, 1980.
6. Spero, L.: Epilepsy, Lancet **2**:1319, 1982.

Chapter 29

Narcotic analgesic drugs

Suffering and disability caused by unrelieved pain lower the quality of life for vast numbers of individuals. Relief of pain is one of the great objectives in medicine. Drugs with a predominant pain-relieving action are called *analgesics* and are commonly classified as *narcotic* and *nonnarcotic*. Although our knowledge about analgesia is far from complete, improper application of the information we now have is a recognized problem. Narcotic analgesics include the alkaloids of opium and their semisynthetic derivatives (opiates) and synthetic compounds (opioids) that resemble opium alkaloids in their pharmacology if not their chemistry. However, opioids and opiates are only part of a larger picture of approaches to pain management (Fig. 29-1). The use of opiates and opioids in most instances is regulated by the Federal Controlled Substances Act of 1970.

The opiate analgesics and related compounds produce physical dependence characterized by withdrawal symptoms. Tolerance develops to some of their effects. The recent characterization of the opiate receptor and discovery of endogenous opioid peptides, the endorphins and enkephalins, give an entirely new perspective to the topics of pain and analgesia.

Morphine, the prototype opiate, has been available for 200 years, but opium, a crude botanical product, has been used for thousands of years. Opiate antagonists were introduced in 1941.

It has been suspected for some time that there are specific opiate receptors in the brain. First of all, some opiates are extremely potent, etorphine being 10,000 times as potent as morphine. In addition, the actions of opiates are stereospecific, the levo isomers representing the active form. Finally, there are pure opiate antagonists, such as naloxone, which exert no analgesia but block the effect of the opiates.

The concept of specific opiate receptors was greatly strengthened by the demonstration that opiate agonists and antagonists bind stereospecifically in vitro to membranes of pinched-off nerve terminals. The potencies of these drugs in competing for binding sites parallel closely their clinical potencies.

THE OPIATE RECEPTOR

319

FIG. 29-1 *Correlation of neural projections and chemical mediators in pain perception with some of the different types of drugs that alleviate pain.*

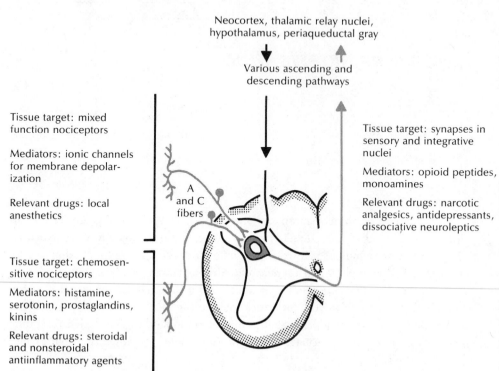

Neocortex, thalamic relay nuclei,
hypothalamus, periaqueductal gray

Various ascending and
descending pathways

Tissue target: mixed
function nociceptors

Mediators: ionic channels
for membrane depolar-
ization

Relevant drugs: local
anesthetics

A
and C
fibers

Tissue target: synapses in
sensory and integrative
nuclei

Mediators: opioid peptides,
monoamines

Relevant drugs: narcotic
analgesics, antidepressants,
dissociative neuroleptics

Tissue target: chemosen-
sitive nociceptors

Mediators: histamine,
serotonin, prostaglandins,
kinins

Relevant drugs: steroidal
and nonsteroidal
antiinflammatory agents

Opiate receptors in the brain are concentrated in the limbic system, spinoreticular tracts (especially the periaqueductal gray), medial thalamic nuclei, hypothalamus, and other regions involved in pain perception. Opiate receptors are also found in the *substantia gelatinosa* of the spinal cord and spinal trigeminal nucleus, the *nucleus tractus solitarii*, and related nuclei concerned with vagal reflexes. High receptor densities in these latter areas suggest participation in the cough reflex, gastric secretion, and orthostatic hypotension. The amygdala is highest in receptor binding, followed by the periaqueductal gray, hypothalamus, and medial thalamus. Several subtypes of opiate receptors may exist. The type most responsible for the analgesic properties of drugs such as morphine has been designated the μ receptor.

Endogenous opioid
peptides
ENKEPHALINS AND
ENDORPHINS

Presumably, most drug receptors in the body exist for the purpose of binding some ligand produced endogenously. Thus the demonstration of specific receptors for opiates suggested the existence of endogenous morphine-like compounds.[2,6] Pentapeptides with opiate-like activity such as methionine enkephalin (H-tyrosine-glycine-glycine-phenylalanine-methionine-OH) and leucine enkephalin (H-tyrosine-glycine-glycine-phenylalanine-leucine-OH) have been isolated from brain tissue and appear to act as neurotransmitters or neuromodulators.

Other peptides that are opiate-like from the standpoint of competing for the receptor have also been isolated. β-Lipotropin, isolated from the pituitary some years ago, contains the amino acid sequence of methionine enkephalin in residues 61 to 65. The function of β-endorphin is not clear. The enkephalins and endorphins are further discussed in Chapter 30. The probability seems reasonably high that in the future peptides will be introduced as analgesics. The challenge will be to design analogs of endogenous peptides that are reasonably resistant to catabolism, that can cross the blood-brain barrier, and that provide pain relief without problems of tolerance or drug dependence. Unless the last goal is achieved, we will have succeeded only in rediscovering another morphine.

Quantitative studies on analgesics are difficult because the pain experience in humans depends not only on the perception of the painful stimulus but also on psychological factors.

Two types of experimental approaches are commonly used for evaluation of analgesic action. In one, the threshold for pain is determined in humans or animals by the application of painful stimuli of graded intensity. Analgesics are evaluated by elevations in threshold. In the other method, analgesics are administered to postoperative patients, and pain-relieving efficacy is compared with that of a placebo. Positive placebo responses are often in the vicinity of 30% of patients tested in acute situations.

METHODS OF STUDY OF ANALGESIC ACTION

Narcotic analgesics and antagonists can be divided into several categories:

CHEMISTRY AND CLASSIFICATION

Naturally occurring alkaloids and semisynthetic opiates
  Morphine
  Codeine (methylmorphine)
  Oxymorphone (Numorphan)
  Hydromorphone (Dilaudid)
  Methyldihydromorphinone (Metopon)
  Hydrocodone (Dicodid)
  Nalbuphine (Nubain)
  Heroin (diacetylmorphine)
Benzomorphans (agonists and partial antagonists)
  Phenazocine (Prinadol)
  Pentazocine (Talwin)
Morphinan derivatives
  Levorphanol (levo-Dromoran)
  Butorphanol (Stadol)
  Dextromethorphan

Meperidine and related phenyl-piperidines
  Meperidine (Demerol)
  Alphaprodine (Nisentil)
  Anileridine (Leritine)
  Piminodine (Alvodine)
  Diphenoxylate (in Lomotil)
Methadone and related drugs
  Methadone (Dolophine)
  Propoxyphene (Darvon)
Narcotic antagonists (allyl substituted compounds)
  Nalorphine (Nalline)
  Levallorphan (Lorfan)
  Naloxone (Narcan)

Pharmacological studies indicate a basic similarity among the more potent narcotic analgesics. They all obtund severe pain, can be substituted for each other in the addict (although tolerance develops to them), and are antagonized by drugs such as nalorphine.[1] It could be anticipated from these facts that some basic chemical similarity must exist in this series, and in fact examination of the formulas of all of these drugs reveals the presence of a common moiety, γ-phenyl-*N*-methyl-piperidine. The "chair" form of piperidine is thought to be the more realistic representation, with heavy lines indicating projection outward from the plane of the paper. Substituent R is often quite bulky.

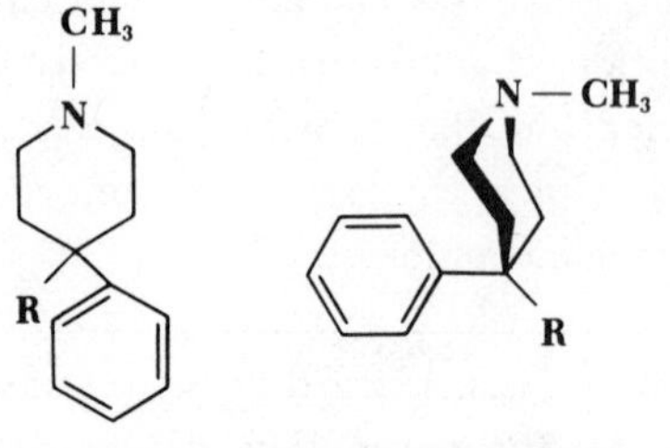

Disubstituted *N*-methylpiperidine

<table>
<tr><td>

NATURAL OPIATES AND SEMISYNTHETIC DERIVATIVES

Morphine
CHEMISTRY

</td><td>

Morphine, which has been used extensively for many years, remains the most important narcotic analgesic. It is obtained from opium, the dried juice of the poppy plant *Papaver somniferum*. Alkaloids in opium are of two types: phenanthrene and benzylisoquinoline. Of the latter, papaverine and noscapine have medical importance. Papaverine is an antispasmodic and vasodilator, whereas noscapine is used for cough. Neither has analgesic properties.

</td></tr>
</table>

Morphine and codeine are the important narcotics in the phenanthrene group. Opium contains 10% morphine and 0.5% codeine. Much of the codeine in clinical use is made commercially from morphine.

Morphine, the first alkaloid ever obtained in pure form, was isolated in 1803 by Sertürner. Its total synthesis in 1952 confirmed a structure proposed by Gulland and Robinson in 1925.

Two hydroxyl groups, one phenolic and the other alcoholic, are of importance because some morphine derivatives are simple modifications of one or both groups. For example, codeine is methylmorphine, the substitution being in the phenolic hydroxyl. Heroin is diacetylmorphine. In dihydromorphinone the alcoholic hydroxyl is replaced by a ketonic oxygen and the double bond adjacent to it is removed. Although many useful semisynthetic alkaloids are prepared by substitutions in the hydroxyl groups, the antidotal (narcotic antagonist) compounds, nalorphine and naloxone, are prepared by replacing the CH_3 group on the nitrogen with an allyl radical—$CH_2CH = CH_2$.

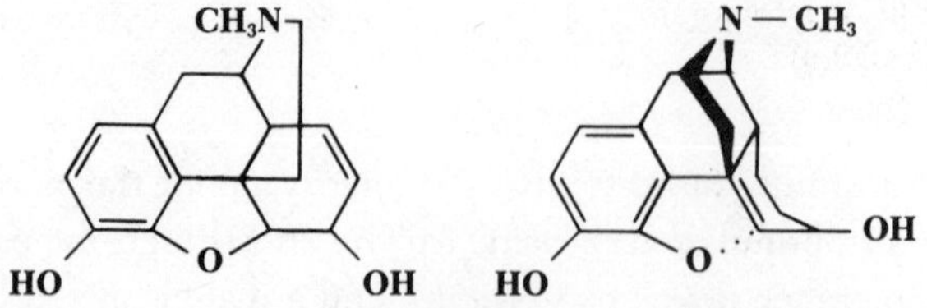

Morphine

Morphine sulfate is the most commonly employed salt. It is available in ampules of 1 ml or in tablets of various sizes for preparing the injectable solution. It is also available in ampules of larger sizes. An ampule is not a dose. The subcutaneous dose range is 8 to 15 mg.

When morphine is administered by the subcutaneous route to normal persons in the amount of 10 to 15 mg, it produces drowsiness and euphoria in some, but more commonly it causes anxiety and nausea. The individual may sleep, the respiration slows, and the pupils constrict. Dysphoria is less frequent in patients with pain.

ANALGESIC AND OTHER CNS EFFECTS

There are at least two factors involved in the pain relief afforded by morphine. The drug elevates the pain threshold, and it alters the reaction of the individual to the painful experience.[3]

Ten milligrams of morphine gives relief of moderate postoperative pain to at least 90% of patients. This is reduced to 70% in severe postoperative pain. A dose of 15 mg may raise this to 80%. Interestingly, a placebo can provide relief to 30%, whereas morphine by the oral route may benefit just 40%.

The respiratory center is markedly depressed by morphine, and cessation of respiration is the usual cause of death in morphine poisoning. Therapeutic doses of morphine moderately lower respiratory minute volume and lessen the response to carbon dioxide inhalation without affecting respiratory rate. Larger doses also depress the rate of respiration. Carbon dioxide retention becomes severe. The onset of respiratory depression after morphine depends on the method of administration. Maximal depression occurs within 5 minutes of an intravenous injection, whereas it may be delayed for 60 minutes or longer if the drug is injected by the intramuscular route. As tolerance develops to the analgesic and euphoric actions of morphine, the respiratory center becomes tolerant also. For this reason an addict may tolerate otherwise lethal doses of morphine.

RESPIRATION

Carbon dioxide retention is probably responsible for the cerebral vasodilation and increased intracranial pressure that follow the administration of morphine.

Morphine is not a uniform depressant of neural structures. It does not oppose the action of stimulants such as strychnine or picrotoxin. Indeed, it may be synergistic with such drugs. Also, morphine may enhance monosynaptic reflexes, whereas it depresses multineuronal reflexes. Thus knee and ankle jerks in the cat with spinal cord section are enhanced or unaffected by the drug, whereas the flexor and crossed extensor reflexes are depressed.

Morphine may actually be excitatory in susceptible persons. Some patients become nauseated and may vomit following a morphine injection. Others may become delirious. Cats and horses are consistently stimulated by morphine. The violent excitement of cats caused by morphine is still present after decortication, requiring lesions in the hypothalamus for its prevention.

EXCITATION

EMESIS   The emetic effect of morphine is exerted on the chemoreceptor trigger zone in the medulla. Apomorphine, which is obtained from morphine, is used as a potent stimulant of the chemoreceptor trigger zone in some types of poisoning.

MISCELLANEOUS   *Effect on pupils.* The pupils are constricted by morphine, and this action is an-
EFFECTS   tagonized by atropine. The response is a consequence of stimulation of pupillocon-strictor centers in the brain. Addicts do not develop tolerance to the pinpoint pupils, but during withdrawal their pupils become widely dilated. Animals excited by mor-phine show pupillary dilatation.

Gastrointestinal effects. Morphine has a marked constipating effect, and opiates are time-honored remedies in the management of diarrhea.

In general, morphine tends to increase the tone of intestinal smooth muscle and decrease propulsive peristalsis. Morphine delays gastric emptying through decreased gastric motility and contraction of the pylorus and perhaps of the duodenum as well. Atropine tends to partially oppose this spasmogenic action of morphine.

The constipating effect of morphine may result from several factors. The most important ones are (1) increased tone and decreased propulsive activity throughout the gastrointestinal tract and (2) failure to perceive sensory stimuli that would other-wise elicit the defecation reflex. It seems likely that the antidiarrheal effects of morphine may represent actions on opioid receptors in the enteric nervous system.

Effect on biliary tract. Morphine increases intrabiliary pressure as a consequence of contracting the smooth muscles of the biliary tract. Pain relief in biliary colic is probably caused by a central analgesic action. Atropine may not be effective in relieving spasm of the biliary tract induced by morphine.

Cardiovascular effects. Morphine reduces arterial resistance and venous tone. These effects are beneficial in reducing ventricular work, pulmonary congestion, and edema. The hemodynamic effects may become excessive, leading to postural hy-potension. The depressor response to intravenous morphine is decreased but not abolished by atropine.

In some species, histamine released by intravenous morphine administration may contribute to the hypotensive reactions. The hemodynamic effects of morphine are unfavorable in hemorrhagic shock.

Effect on bronchial smooth muscle. Contraction of bronchial smooth muscle by morphine tends to decrease the diameter of the airway. Many investigators have attributed deaths in asthmatic patients to the bronchconstrictor action of morphine. It is quite possible, however, that mortality in asthmatics may be caused by depression of the stimulant effects of carbon dioxide on the respiratory center. According to this view, carbon dioxide narcosis, rather than bronchial constriction, may be the cause of death; however, the question is not settled.

Effect on genitourinary tract. Opiates contract the smooth muscle of the ureter and the detrusor muscle of the bladder to increase the tone of the vesicle sphincter. Atropine tends to relieve the ureteral spasm induced by morphine. Despite its spasmogenic actions, morphine is often used in the relief of ureteral colic, where its effectiveness must be a result of its analgesic action.

The urinary retention that may follow administration of morphine results from difficulty in micturition and decreased perception of the stimulus for micturition. Morphine is also antidiuretic. It releases the antidiuretic hormone, and its hemo-dynamic actions also contribute to an antidiuretic effect.

Uterine contractions during labor are not significantly affected by a therapeutic dose of morphine, although they may be slowed somewhat.

Metabolic effects. Morphine lowers total oxygen consumption, probably because of decreased muscle tone. Hyperglycemia after the injection of morphine is probably a consequence of increased sympathetic activity, since total sympathectomy will prevent the rise in blood sugar.

Morphine is absorbed readily after subcutaneous or intramuscular injection. It is estimated that about 60% of subcutaneously injected morphine is absorbed in the first 30 minutes. Absorption is strongly influenced by cutaneous circulation. Because absorption from the gastrointestinal tract is erratic and because first-pass hepatic inactivation is significant, the parenteral route is preferred.   METABOLISM

Morphine partitions from blood into most tissues. The half-life in humans is about 3 hours, and the period of effective analgesia is 4 to 5 hours.

About 90% of an administered dose can be recovered from the urine in a con-jugated form, and a small percentage can be recovered from the feces. Biliary ex-cretion may account for the presence of morphine in the feces. A small percentage of a dose of morphine is *N*-demethylated in the liver to normorphine.

A striking feature of the pharmacology of morphine and related drugs is the gradual tolerance that develops to some of its effects.   TOLERANCE

If a patient in chronic pain is given 10 to 15 mg of morphine sulfate by the subcutaneous route twice a day, it is often observed that after a week or so he will not receive as much pain relief as was received at the beginning. The dose must be gradually increased. On the other hand, no tolerance develops to the gastrointestinal or pupillary constrictor actions of morphine or to the excitatory effects of the drug. Tolerance to the analgesic effects may occur more rapidly than tolerance to respiratory depression. Thus tolerance is often a limiting factor in the use of morphine for chronic pain.

If the administration of morphine is prolonged, both patients and addicts will require progressively larger doses of morphine to obtain the same subjective effects. Tolerance may reach incredible proportions. Addicts have been known to take as much as 4 g of the drug in 24 hours. This quantity is far greater than the lethal dose in a nontolerant person. The duration of tolerance is 1 to 2 weeks, and following this period of abstinence the individual again responds to a small dose of the drug. Addicts may die as a consequence of taking their usual large dose of an opiate after a period of abstinence during which they have lost their tolerance.

PROBLEM 29-1. Could tolerance to morphine be a consequence of altered absorption, increased rate of metabolism, and excretion? Obviously not, because the tolerant addict can administer doses of morphine intravenously that would depress the respiratory center of a nonaddict permanently. There must be a true cellular tolerance of some nervous elements. In agreement with this view, there is no difference in the metabolism of morphine in tolerant and nontolerant dogs.

Many factors influence the development of tolerance. Regular frequent administration of the drug is more likely to produce tolerance than widely spaced, irregular modes of administration. The administration of the narcotic antagonists nalorphine or naloxone produces acute withdrawal symptoms in individuals who are tolerant to large doses of morphine.

The mechanisms of tolerance may become understandable as a consequence of the discovery of the enkephalins. If the enkephalins are neurotransmitters or neuromodulators, the continued presence of morphine at the opiate receptor could turn off peptide production or release (Fig. 29-2). Thus larger doses of morphine would be required in the face of steadily decreasing peptide availability. If the supply of morphine is withdrawn abruptly, the insufficient concentrations of analgesic compounds (endogenous plus exogenous) may cause abstinence signs.

FIG. 29-2 *Possible servomechanisms in morphine tolerance and abstinence. Opioid peptides are assumed to act as neurotransmitters or neuromodulators. Peptide binding to μ receptors initiates effects on target neurons compatible with normal function. Synthesis and release of peptide commensurate with need is under feedback control. Morphine competes with the peptide either directly or indirectly. Continuously available morphine is responsible for persistent feedback signals to decrease peptide production. With time, higher concentrations of morphine are required to maintain a specified level of responsiveness in the target neuron (tolerance). If morphine is withdrawn or blocked abruptly with naloxone, the available level of "analgesia" (opioid plus morphine) is grossly inadequate to meet need. In response to the deficit, target cells enter into activities that lead to withdrawal signs. The abstinence syndrome subsides as peptide stores are replenished.*

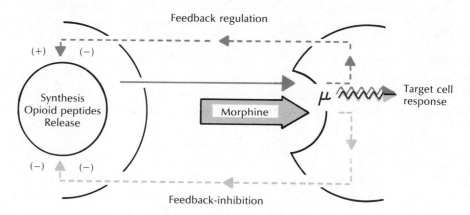

In *acute* morphine poisoning the individual is comatose and cyanotic, the respirations are slow, and the pupils are of pinpoint size.

The management of a patient in acute morphine poisoning is quite different from that of the barbiturate-poisoned patient. Central stimulant drugs such as picrotoxin or pentylenetetrazol (Metrazol) should not be used, since there is little evidence they have antidotal value. Morphine, in contrast to the barbiturates, has many excitatory actions and may be synergistic with the convulsants.

The major development in the treatment of acute morphine poisoning has been the discovery of specific antidotes. Naloxone is the antagonist of choice, since it has few deleterious effects of its own. Intravenous injection of naloxone or nalorphine improves respiration and circulation promptly in acutely poisoned individuals. Opiate antagonists are of no use in overdoses with barbiturates or general anesthetics. Naloxone is so specific that if a course of therapy does not dramatically reverse respiratory depression, the initial diagnosis must be questioned. In narcotic-dependent individuals, whether abusers or patients in chronic pain, naloxone will precipitate a severe abstinence syndrome.

Codeine, or methylmorphine, is a very important analgesic and antitussive drug. In therapeutic doses it is less sedative and analgesic than morphine. Tolerance to codeine develops more slowly, and it is less addictive than morphine. It has less effect also on the gastrointestinal and urinary tracts and on the pupil, and it causes less nausea and constipation than morphine. It is the opiate most frequently prescribed.

Codeine administered orally is not as effective an analgesic as when it is injected subcutaneously. In one study performed on postoperative patients, 60 mg of codeine administered by mouth produced relief in 40% of the patients, whereas a placebo was effective in 33%. On the other hand, administered subcutaneously, the drug was effective in 60% of the patients, whereas 10 mg of morphine provided relief in 71%. Although effective, codeine is not quite as effective an analgesic as morphine, even when its dosage is six times higher.

Codeine phosphate is widely used in oral doses of 15 to 64 mg for moderately severe pain, often in dosage forms combined with acetylsalicylic acid or acetaminophen. Codeine is injected subcutaneously for severe pain.

Codeine is partly demethylated to morphine in the body and is partly changed to norcodeine. The conjugated forms of these compounds are excreted in the urine.

Oxymorphone (Numorphan) is a more potent analgesic than morphine, but it causes more side effects.

Hydromorphone (Dilaudid) is five to ten times more potent than morphine in producing analgesia. Its respiratory depressant effect is correspondingly greater, although it may be less nauseating and constipating. It may have a more rapid onset and shorter duration of action than morphine.

Hydrocodone (Dicodid) resembles codeine but may be a more effective antitussive compound and is also more addictive. The recommended oral dose for adults is 5 to 15 mg, which may be given three to four times a day.

Methyldihydromorphinone, or metopon, is more potent than morphine, but it has no significant advantages over the latter, except that it is effective by oral administration.

Heroin, or diacetylmorphine, is a highly euphoriant and analgesic drug. It is much preferred by the addict, who usually takes it by the intravenous route in order to obtain a peculiar orgastic sensation. Apparently, a significant amount of the drug enters the brain during the first circulatory pass. Because of its great addictive liability, heroin may not be legally manufactured in or imported into the United States, although it is used elsewhere clinically for its analgesic properties.

Pantopium (Pantopon) contains the alkaloids of opium in the same proportion as they exist naturally. Since it contains about 50% morphine, its dosage is correspondingly higher than morphine alone. It has no significant advantages over morphine.

Nalbuphine hydrochloride (Nubain) is a phenanthrene with both agonist and antagonist properties. As an agonist, it is equivalent to morphine in potency. As a narcotic antagonist, it has one fourth the potency of nalorphine. Although abrupt discontinuation after prolonged use causes withdrawal signs, the drug is said to have a much lower potential for abuse than morphine and perhaps less than codeine. Nalbuphine hydrochloride (Nubain) is available as a solution containing 10 mg/ml for intravenous, intramuscular, or subcutaneous injection.

MEPERIDINE AND RELATED COMPOUNDS

Meperidine (pethidine; isonipecaine; Demerol; Dolantin) was introduced originally as an antispasmodic of the atropine type. It is probably the most frequently prescribed of the opioids.

The analgesic potency of meperidine is such that 50 mg is equivalent to 8 mg of morphine or 100 mg is equivalent to 12 mg of morphine. Analgesia lasts only about two hours at therapeutic doses.

Despite early claims, it appears that meperidine is just as depressant to respiration as is morphine when the two drugs are compared in equianalgesic doses. It lacks antitussive activity and may cause mydriasis and tachycardia by reason of its erratic atropine-like properties.

Meperidine

The drug may be slightly less sedative than morphine, but there is no basis for the belief that it has a significantly different action on the gastrointestinal or biliary tract or on bronchial smooth muscle. Intravenous injection of meperidine may be followed by severe hypotension, caused at least in part by histamine release. Meperidine is definitely addictive.

The liver plays an important role in the metabolism of meperidine; therefore usual doses of the drug may be toxic to persons with liver disease. Ordinary doses of meperidine have caused severe untoward reactions and death in patients who had been taking MAO inhibitors.

Alphaprodine (Nisentil) is a piperidine derivative resembling meperidine. Its analgesic action is prompt and of short duration, but its superiority to meperidine remains to be demonstrated.

Anileridine (Leritine) is related to meperidine but is slightly more potent. It is well absorbed from the gastrointestinal tract; the oral dose in adults is 25 to 50 mg. It may be given intramuscularly in 40 mg dosage for severe pain.

Piminodine (Alvodine) and **diphenoxylate** (with atropine, as Lomotil) are related chemically to meperidine. Piminodine is used primarily as an analgesic, either orally or by injection. Diphenoxylate has been recommended for the control of diarrhea in doses of 5 mg three times a day by mouth. Atropine is added to discourage overzealous self-medication.

Loperamide hydrochloride (Imodium), recently introduced as an antidiarrheal drug, is similar to diphenoxylate, but it is not combined with atropine. It is available in 2 mg capsules. Chemically, it is a derivative of meperidine and haloperidol. Thus it has a potential for acting at enteric receptors for monoamines and endogenous opioids.

Methadone (Amidone; Dolophine) was developed in Germany during World War II as a substitute for morphine. The two-dimensional structural formula of methadone does not resemble that of meperidine; however a disubstituted *pseudo*piperidine ring is evident in three-dimensional representation. Methadone's analgesic potency and some other effects, including antagonism by nalorphine, are quite similar to those of morphine. The analgesic actions of *dl*-methadone reside mainly in the levo isomer.

Methadone

The analgesic potency of methadone is about as great as that of morphine, but methadone has a longer duration. As a consequence, it is administered in doses of 10 mg and is quite effective following oral administration. It causes considerable respiratory depression, but its emetic and constipating actions are less than those of morphine. Tolerance and addiction to methadone occur, but abstinence signs are less severe than those of morphine.

Methadone is employed as an analgesic, especially in severe chronic pain. Sedation and euphoria are slight. The unique applications of methadone in the withdrawal or maintenance of opiate addicts are discussed in Chapter 30. Acetylmethadol (LAAM) is in clinical trial as a methadone substitute. An oral dose has a duration of action of 2 to 3 days.

Propoxyphene is one of the most widely used drugs in medicine despite serious reservations about its efficacy. Results from carefully controlled double-blind studies cast doubt on the claim that propoxyphene and codeine have similar analgesic potency. However, the undesirable side effects of codeine (lethargy, nausea, constipation) are less frequent with propoxyphene when the drugs are used in ordinary doses for pain relief.

Propoxyphene

Propoxyphene is dispensed alone as the hydrochloride (Darvon; numerous generics) or the napsylate (Darvon-N). Combination proprietary products contain one of the propoxyphene salts plus aspirin, acetaminophen, or the APC combination (aspirin, phenacetin, and caffeine). These mixtures (Darvon Compound, Darvon ASA, Darvocet-N, and so forth) usually rate higher than propoxyphene alone in tests for pain relief. Because of its antiinflammatory activities, aspirin confers analgesic properties that propoxyphene alone does not possess.

The overall bioavailabilities of the two propoxyphene salts are comparable. The apparent half-life in plasma is 6 to 12 hours; thus steady state levels are achieved in about 2 days of oral dosing at 6-hour intervals. Occasional doses for pain probably have placebo value only. The dextro isomer of propoxyphene is used for analgesia. The levo isomer has been introduced as an antitussive.

Propoxyphene overdoses are responsible for hundreds of deaths each year in the United States, partly because the drug is so readily available. The signs of serious overdose resemble those of morphine: respiratory depression, stupor, and pinpoint pupils. Convulsions are not uncommon. Respiratory depression responds to naloxone. The presence of aspirin or other drugs in excess quantities complicates management of toxicity. It may be necessary to restore acid-base balance. Concomitant ingestion of alcohol and other depressants also accentuates the toxicity.

When its widespread use is taken into consideration, the number of persons addicted to propoxyphene is low, although tolerance and dependence are known to occur. Apparently propoxyphene will not substitute for heroin or morphine in withdrawal situations. The prudent physician, however, exercises caution in prescribing propoxyphene for persons with a history of substance abuse.

Phenazocine (Prinadol) is a synthetic addictive analgesic that is about four times as active as morphine but is without other significant advantages.

BENZOMORPHANS

Pentazocine (Talwin) is an *N*-allyl derivative of phenazocine. It is actually a weak narcotic antagonist with a significant analgesic effect of its own. Its potency is moderate and of short duration, but its low addiction liability makes it useful in chronic illnesses in which the more addictive drugs would constitute a hazard. It will precipitate an abstinence syndrome in patients dependent on narcotics. Administered in 20 to 40 mg doses by the subcutaneous or intramuscular route, pentazocine may be as effective as 10 mg of morphine. Larger doses do not increase its analgesic power. Pentazocine (Talwin) is also available in tablet form (50 mg) for oral administration, although it is not well absorbed across the gastric mucosa. Its analgesic potency by the oral route is thought to be roughly equivalent to 60 mg of codeine. Pentazocine is more likely to precipitate hallucinations than other analgesics.

Pentazocine

Levorphanol

Levorphanol (Levo-Dromoran) is a synthetic phenanthrene related chemically to morphine.

Morphinan derivatives

The levo isomer is about five times as analgesic as morphine and consequently is administered in dosages of 2 mg. Its duration of action is somewhat longer than that of morphine. Respiratory depression and addiction liability are marked, but emetic and constipating actions are only moderate.

Butorphanol tartrate (Stadol), a substituted morphinan, has five times the potency of morphine as an analgesic and 30 times the potency of pentazocine as an antagonist. Its clinical applications and abuse potential appear to be roughly comparable to those of pentazocine. Butorphanol tartrate (Stadol) is available in injectable solutions of 1 or 2 mg/ml.

Dextromethorphan (Romilar), the methyl ether of dextrorphan, has about the same antitussive potency as codeine, with no analgesic or respiratory-depressant properties. It is widely used as a cough suppressant, an action that is clearly unrelated to any narcotic analgesic property. It is a CNS depressant in high doses.

NARCOTIC
ANTAGONISTS

An allyl substitution on the nitrogen atom of morphine or levorphanol yields compounds that antagonize narcotic responses, especially respiratory depression. Nalorphine and levallorphan are important narcotic antagonists. Pentazocine is a weak antagonist and is much more useful as an analgesic of low addiction liability.

Subclassification of
opiate receptors

Differences in the actions of agonist-antagonists and morphine-type drugs have led to a subclassification of their receptors. At the μ receptor, morphine acts as an agonist and nalorphine as a competitive antagonist. At the κ receptor, nalorphine acts as an agonist and morphine is weak or inactive. Finally, the σ receptor may mediate the dysphoric and psychotomimetic effects of drugs such as pentazocine.

According to this hypothesis, pentazocine is a weak competitive antagonist at the μ receptor, a strong agonist at the κ receptor, and is also a σ receptor agonist. Naloxone is a competitive antagonist at all three receptor sites. Butorphanol and nalbuphine may act like pentazocine but cause less euphoria and psychotomimetic effects.

Nalorphine (Nalline) is *N*-allylnormorphine. Although there was evidence in the literature for many years that *N*-allyl derivatives of opiates antagonized respiratory depression produced in animals by narcotics, it was not until 1950 that nalorphine received clinical recognition.

Nalorphine antagonizes practically all the effects of morphine and other narcotics, including meperidine and methadone. It is still used as an antidote in cases of poisoning from these drugs and can also precipitate acute withdrawal symptoms in an addicted person. The "Nalline test" is sometimes used to determine if a person in a heroin withdrawal program has remained "clean."

Interestingly, in the normal person nalorphine behaves only as a weak opiate. It has been suggested that the antidotal action of the drug may be caused by competitive inhibition with replacement of potent drugs by a less efficacious compound having higher affinity for μ receptors.

Nalorphine (Nalline) is administered in doses of 5 to 10 mg, usually by the intravenous route in cases of poisoning. The dosage should not exceed 40 mg.

Nalorphine hydrochloride

Levallorphan tartrate

Levallorphan tartrate (Lorfan) is a morphine antagonist very similar in indications to nalorphine. From the pharmacological standpoint, it has the same relationship to levorphanol as nalorphine has to morphine. Levallorphan (Lorfan) is used in doses of 0.3 to 1.2 mg by injection.

Naloxone hydrochloride (Narcan), the *N*-allyl derivative of oxymorphone hydrochloride (Numorphan), is an important and specific narcotic antagonist. The usual adult dose is 0.4 mg, intravenous route, repeated at 3-minute intervals two or three times. Naloxone has a duration of action of about an hour, whereas some agonists such as methadone depress respiration for a day or two. Therefore repeated administrations of naloxone may be necessary.

Naloxone reverses the respiratory-depressant action of the narcotics such as morphine, meperidine, methadone, and pentazocine. It differs from the other narcotic antagonists in several important respects. By itself, naloxone does not cause respiratory depression, pupillary constriction, sedation, or analgesia. Although naloxone does not antagonize the depressant effects of hypnotics and anesthetics, neither does it add to the hypoxic burden. As with other narcotic antagonists, naloxone precipitates an abstinence syndrome when administered to patients addicted to opiate-like drugs.[4]

The following medical conditions are generally considered to be contraindications to the use of morphine and related drugs:

 Head injuries and following craniotomy
 Bronchial asthma and other hypoxic states
 Acute alcohol intoxication
 Convulsive disorders
 Undiagnosed acute abdominal conditions

CONTRA-INDICATIONS TO THE USE OF MORPHINE AND RELATED AGENTS

The important problem of physical dependence to narcotics is discussed in detail in Chapter 30. Pain associated with terminal illnesses may require the use of gradually escalated doses of narcotics, although this is not a universal rule. The aim should always be to provide pain relief. Tolerance may or may not become a problem in management, but drug dependence per se is inconsequential in such instances.[5]

Of considerable interest is a recent finding that opiate withdrawal symptoms are inhibited by clonidine. Clonidine may depress central noradrenergic neurons by an action on presynaptic α receptors that mediate firing rates of locus ceruleus neurons. Inhibitory receptors in the locus ceruleus may become tolerant to opiates, thus allowing excessive neuronal activity following opiate withdrawal.

PHYSICAL DEPENDENCE

Coughing is normally considered a defense mechanism for clearing the respiratory tract. However, some coughs signal cardiac dyspnea, pleurisy, hiatal hernia, or other conditions not directly related to tracheobronchial irritation. In many instances coughs should not be restrained lest their prevention lead to pneumonia or other infections. Medical intervention is indicated if a cough is serving no useful purpose and is interfering with sleep or other normal activities.

CLINICAL PHARMACOLOGY OF ANTITUSSIVE DRUGS

From a pharmacological standpoint, antitussives may suppress the neural component of the cough reflex or may influence the quantity or viscosity of respiratory tract fluid. Drugs that act on the neural component may act in the CNS or on sensory endings in the mucous membranes of the respiratory tract. The specific effectiveness of antitussives is difficult to determine because nonspecific sedation and placebos can be of benefit. Furthermore, in many cough mixtures, the demulcent action of vehicles may play a significant part in the effects claimed.

There is little doubt that morphine and synthetic opiate-like drugs are potent cough suppressants. Those with significant addiction liability are not ordinarily used for this purpose. Codeine is the traditional cough suppressant, and all nonaddictive antitussives should be compared with codeine in controlled clinical trials. Too often claims for effectiveness are based on impressions from uncontrolled clinical trials.

Codeine is the standard narcotic antitussive. It is highly effective, and its addiction liability is not nearly as great as that of stronger narcotics. Nausea, constipation, and drowsiness are among the common side effects of codeine. In contrast with morphine, excessive doses of codeine may cause convulsions, especially in children. These convulsions are attributed to disinhibitory effects of codeine on spinal neurons. The usual adult dose of codeine phosphate USP is 8 to 15 mg three or four times daily. For antitussive applications, the drug is usually dispensed in a demulcent syrup (elixir of terpin hydrate is a time-honored vehicle) or suspension. Polypharmacy mixtures of codeine with an assortment of antihistamines, antipyretics, and other drugs are common; however, these would seem to have little advantage over codeine alone.

Hydrocodone bitartrate (Dicodid) is a more potent antitussive than codeine, but its addiction liability is greater. It is available in 5 mg tablets.

Dextromethorphan (Romilar) is a substituted dextro isomer of the narcotic levorphan (Dromoran). It is not analgesic and is not addictive. It is claimed that it approaches codeine in antitussive potency. The usual dose is 10 to 20 mg by mouth.

Noscapine (Nectadon) is the isoquinoline alkaloid narcotine found in opium. The drug is not addictive or analgesic but is claimed to be antitussive. The dose is 15 to 30 mg by mouth three times a day.

Benzonatate (Tessalon) is a local anesthetic related to tetracaine. It is used as an antitussive in doses of 100 mg. It is thought to influence the cough reflex both at stretch receptors in the lungs and within the CNS. It does not depress respiration.

Antihistaminics are also claimed to be of benefit as antitussives. Although there may be some rationale for their use in asthmatic bronchitis of allergic etiology, their mode of action in other types of cough is not understood and according to some investigators is not well documented. Drugs of this type include carbetapentane (Toclase), dimethoxanate (Cothera, a phenothiazine), and numerous other antihistaminic drugs.

Levopropoxyphene (Novrad), in contrast to its dextro form (Darvon), is said to have antitussive properties without being an analgesic. The drug is claimed to be as effective as codeine.

In addition to depressing the cough reflex, drugs could be beneficial in the treatment of respiratory illnesses by reducing the viscosity of thick mucus.

Glyceryl guaiacolate (Guaifenesin) is a component of many cough mixtures. It is thought to have expectorant properties, that is, to increase the volume and decrease the viscosity of bronchial secretions. Its dose is 100 to 200 mg by mouth, which may be repeated in 2 to 4 hours. Its efficacy is in doubt.

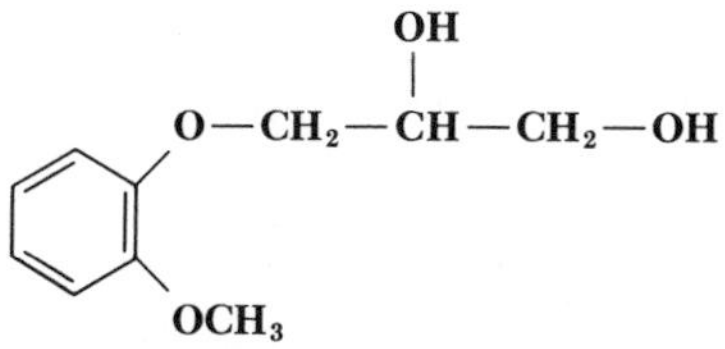

Glyceryl guaiacolate

Iodides such as potassium iodide are sometimes employed in bronchial asthma. The mode of action of these drugs is not known with certainty, but they may dilute bronchial mucus by reflex stimulation of secretory cells in the mucosa.

Ipecac and **ammonium chloride** are believed to cause thinning of bronchial mucus, perhaps by some reflex mechanism.

As a general statement, the antitussive drugs may be valuable in reducing a useless cough. They are purely symptomatic medications, and their use should not obviate the necessity of determining the cause of the cough. Claims made for the many nonaddictive antitussives should be examined critically.

REFERENCES

1. Foley, K.M.: The practical use of narcotic analgesics, Med. Clin. North Am. **66**(5):1091, 1982.
2. Goldstein, A.: Opioid peptides (endorphins) in pituitary and brain, Science **193**:1081, 1976.
3. Lewis, J.W., and Rance, M.J. : Opioids in the management of pain, Pharmaceut. J. **221**:395, 1978-1979.
4. Martin, W.R.: History and development of mixed opioid agonists, partial agonists, and antagonists, Br. J. Clin. Pharmacol. **7**(suppl. 3): 273, 1979.
5. Newburger, P.E., and Sallan, S.E.: Chronic pain: principles of management, J. Pediatr. **98**:180, 1981.
6. Pert, A.: Mechanisms of opiate analgesia and the role of endorphins in pain suppression, Adv. Neurol. **33**:107, 1982.

Chapter 30

Contemporary drug abuse

The term *abuse* implies that a particular application of a drug is more destructive than constructive for society or the individual. Needless to say, it is sometimes difficult to decide whether an application is preponderantly destructive or constructive. Some observers assert that the connotation of "drug abuse" represents solely a cultural value judgment, a biased accusation; it is nevertheless obvious that some drug usage would be considered abusive from almost any cultural frame of reference. Prolonged dependence on amphetamines in high doses, for example, invariably invokes a progressive organic brain syndrome.

It is important to distinguish between *drug abuse* and *drug dependence;* the two concepts are not synonymous. Drug abuse may exist without drug dependence, drug dependence without drug abuse, or both may coexist. A single administration of a hazardous drug may represent abuse without dependence, whereas the maintenance of a diabetic person on insulin represents dependence without abuse. The concept of abuse also depends in part on cultural values, unlike the concept of dependence.

Most abused drugs are drugs with a primary action on the CNS. The reason is obvious: drug users wish to modify their mental state. Abuse of drugs without primary CNS activity is mostly a matter of misuse by medical or paramedical personnel, such as the indiscriminate prescription of penicillin and the "treatment" of obesity with digitalis, thyroid hormone, and diuretics.

Drug dependence has traditionally been conceptualized in terms of a rigid duality: psychological dependence and physical dependence. This duality probably originates in the ancient distinction between mind and body. The dual concepts are still used today and are incorporated into the discussions of individual drugs in this chapter. If a physiologically disruptive withdrawal illness follows the abrupt discontinuation of a drug taken over a prolonged period of time, the drug is said to be physically addicting. Physically addicting drugs include the opiates, barbiturates, antianxiety agents, ethanol, and some nonbarbiturate sedatives. Psychological drug dependence, on the other hand, has been described as a craving for a drug producing a desired effect and to which one has become accustomed by habit; the habit has become a crutch and may assume enormous importance to the individual. It is said that psychological dependence, not physical dependence, drives opiate addicts back to their drug after months or years of successful abstinence.

Bridging the gap between psychological and physical dependence now seems feasible. Central mediation of reward perception appears to occur in association with modification of neurotransmitter actions at limbic synapses; the nature of the modification seems to differ with different drugs. A tighter linkage of behavior with neural substrate will help bridge the gap between psychological and physical dependence, because both may be reducible to physicochemical changes at central synapses.

OPIATES AND OPIATE-LIKE DRUGS

In some state statutes the legal category "narcotics" embraces the opiates, opiate-like drugs, marijuana, and cocaine. Medically defined, however, the term *narcotic* refers only to drugs having both a sedative and an analgesic action and is essentially restricted to the opiates and opiate-like drugs. These drugs are classified on p. 321.

Physical dependence and tolerance

Marked physical dependence develops rapidly during continued administration of any of the narcotic drugs. A striking tolerance also develops to all but the miotic action; the addict continues to have constricted pupils, even after low doses. A high degree of cross-tolerance exists among all the opiates and opiate-like drugs in spite of chemical dissimilarities.

Characteristics of abuse

Heroin is generally the opiate most preferred by the drug user, except for physician addicts, who use meperidine more than any other. Many users consider heroin more euphorigenic than any other opiate. In regions of the United States where good-quality heroin is hard to obtain, however, the addict may prefer "drugstore dope" (usually morphine or hydromorphone stolen from drugstores). Until recently narcotic addiction in the United States had been mostly confined to the lower socioeconomic classes of the larger cities and to members of the medical profession; it is now spreading alarmingly to youth from all socioeconomic levels.

The veteran heroin addict seeks two principal desired effects from the drug: avoidance of the withdrawal illness and a feeling described most commonly as "relief." These effects are usually more important to the addict than the transitory "kick" or "rush" felt immediately after intravenous injection. The opiates tend to leave the user in a state of drive satiation; everything is "as it should be." Accordingly, sexual drive is usually diminished.

There is no evidence that the opiates produce organic CNS damage or other organ pathology, even after years of continuous use. An 84-year-old physician morphine addict was found to exhibit no evidence of mental or physical deterioration after continuous use for 62 years.[4] Complications of parenteral administration, however, are legion and include viral hepatitis, bacterial and fungal endocarditis, nephropathy with massive proteinuria, systemic and pulmonary mycoses, lung abscess, pulmonary fibrosis or granulomatosis, pneumonia, chronic liver disease (of obscure type), transverse myelitis, osteomyelitis (frequently *Pseudomonas*), acute and chronic

TABLE 30-1   Comparison of commonly abused centrally acting drugs

Drug category	Physical dependence*	Tolerance	Psychotogenic in high doses
Opiates	X	X	
Marijuana		X	X
Ethanol	X	X	
Barbiturates	X	X	
Amphetamines		X	X
Cocaine		X	X
Psychotomimetics		X	X
Phenothiazines			
Antianxiety agents	X		
Inhalants†		?	X

*An abstinence syndrome results from abrupt discontinuation of any drug producing physical dependence.
†See text for details.

polyneuropathy, acute and chronic myopathy, acute rhabdomyolysis with myoglobinuria, tetanus, tuberculosis (including tuberculous vertebral osteomyelitis), malaria (now rare in the United States), thrombophlebitis, cellulitis, local abscesses, and sclerosis and occlusion of veins. In addition, there is a constant risk of overdose and death from an unexpectedly concentrated sample of heroin; the triad of coma (or stupor), respiratory depression, and pinpoint pupils strongly suggests opiate overdose. Death from overdose may be a result of respiratory depression or acute pulmonary edema or both; the mechanism of production of pulmonary edema is obscure. Still another ever present hazard is the masking of pain, which may delay awareness of a serious medical condition; cigarette burns between the fingers of opiate addicts are a common finding. Since 1955 most cases of tetanus in New York City have occurred in heroin addicts.

Additional dangers arise from foreign substances intentionally added to the sample by the supplier. Heroin is commonly "cut" with lactose or quinine; other adulterants include barbiturates, procaine, mannitol, aminopyrine, methapyrilene, and baking soda.

Social consequence of narcotic addiction include crime, interruption of employment, and personal and family neglect. Criminal activity is usually restricted to property offenses and peddling, which may become necessary in the absence of employment in order to support the habit. Some addicts become functionally disabled, spending much of the 24-hour period "nodding" (remaining inactive in a semistuporous state) or suffering withdrawal symptoms; other addicts who have an uninterrupted drug supply and are careful with dosage may lead a seemingly normal life at work and at home. The concept of the opiate addict as a dangerous "dope fiend" is not justified; in contrast to alcohol, the opiates tend to quell aggressive drives. When an addict's supply of drugs is exhausted, however, violence may be resorted to in order to obtain a continuing supply. Another incentive for assaultive behavior is fear of police detection. A fellow addict suspected of collaborating with the police may be silenced permanently by an overdose of drug, either arranged by a supplier who provides an unusually concentrated sample of heroin to the victim or accomplished more directly by assault and enforced injection. The apparent cause of death in either case is accidental overdose.

Pentazocine, a synthetic opiate with both agonist and weak antagonist properties, has become increasingly popular as a street drug since its introduction as an analgesic of low addiction liability in 1967. The combination of pentazocine with the antihistamine tripelennamine, called "Ts and blues," is currently widely abused in the United States, and serious medical complications have resulted. Seizures and acute psychotic episodes are being seen with increasing frequency in emergency rooms. In addition, severe skin ulcerations, subcutaneous abscesses, and muscle necrosis have followed parenteral administration of the combination.

Symptoms first appear about 8 hours after the last dose, reaching peak intensity between 36 and 72 hours. Lacrimation, rhinorrhea, yawning, and diaphoresis appear between 8 and 12 hours. Shortly thereafter, at about 13 hours, a restless sleep (the "yen") may intervene. At about 20 hours, gooseflesh, dilated pupils, agitation, and tremors may appear. During the second and third day, when the illness is at its peak, symptoms and signs include weakness, insomnia, chills, intestinal cramps, nausea, vomiting, diarrhea, violent yawning, muscle aches in the legs, severe low back pain, elevation of blood pressure and pulse rate, diaphoresis, and waves of gooseflesh. The skin may have the appearance of a cold plucked turkey, hence the expression "cold turkey," denoting abrupt withdrawal. Fluid depletion during the withdrawal period has at times resulted in cardiovascular collapse and death. At any point during the course of withdrawal, administration of an opiate in adequate dosage will dramatically eliminate the symptoms and restore a state of apparent normalcy. The duration of the syndrome is roughly 7 to 10 days.

Abstinence syndromes
MORPHINE OR HEROIN

Most narcotic abstinence syndromes are similar to that of morphine or heroin. Narcotics with a shorter duration of action tend to produce a shorter and more severe abstinence syndrome; those with a longer duration of action or slower rate of elimination, such as methadone, usually produce a milder and more prolonged syndrome.

OTHER NARCOTIC DRUGS

Withdrawal from an opiate may be accomplished simply by administering smaller and smaller doses of the same opiate over a period of days. Rehabilitation of the opiate addict, however, is another matter. The craving for the drug long after withdrawal is one factor in the very low success rate. In 1964 Drs. Vincent P. Dole and Marie E. Nyswander reported that if heroin addicts were maintained on oral methadone they could give up heroin and engage in an active rehabilitation program.[1] Methadone, a synthetic opiate-like drug, substitutes well for most other opiates and

Methadone maintenance

is well absorbed from the gastrointestinal tract, unlike morphine or heroin; parenteral administration is thereby avoided. In addition, methadone has a longer duration of action than other opiates, permitting administration only once or twice in a 24-hour period. The total period of drug administration is shortened, since methadone remains in the body for 36 to 72 hours after the last dose.

In the early 1970s methadone maintenance was attempted with federal support on a nationwide scale. It was found to be less effective on a large scale than on the small personal scale initiated by Dole and Nyswander, but more effective than any other known approach. One-year retention rates were found to be about 50% at best. After a period of 12 to 36 months of methadone maintenance, withdrawal of methadone ("methadone detoxification") is attempted. One study has shown a 58% return to narcotic use 6 years after methadone detoxification.[18] The highest recidivism rates appear to be associated with premature detoxification from methadone maintenance.

A synthetic congener of methadone, l-α-acetylmethadol hydrochloride (methadylacetate), can prevent withdrawal symptoms for more than 72 hours. Because of this relative advantage, methadylacetate is currently being evaluated as a substitute for methadone. It appears that the two drugs are equivalent in rehabilitative efficacy, but that one or the other may be more effective with different subsets of the addict population.[9,15]

Clonidine, a centrally acting antihypertensive drug, is remarkably effective in reducing the severity of opiate withdrawal. Like opiates, clonidine produces sedation, analgesia, and respiratory depression, but it is not an opiate itself and is not antagonized by naloxone. The discovery that clonidine, like opiates, decreases the excitability of noradrenergic locus ceruleus neurons suggested that it might be effective in opiate withdrawal. It was subsequently found that clonidine and opiates both depress preganglionic sympathetic activity; the effectiveness of clonidine in opiate withdrawal may be related in part to this action on nonopiate receptors.[5] Clonidine has been found to be a safe and effective nonopiate method of opiate detoxification.[6,19]

Narcotic antagonists	A search is under way for the "ideal" narcotic antagonist, namely, a pharmacological agent that blocks the effects of opiates, has few or no side effects of its own, requires relatively infrequent administration, and is not prohibitively expensive to produce. No drug has yet met these criteria but some have come close. Naloxone, for example, abolishes the euphoria, respiratory depression, nausea, and gastrointestinal disturbances produced by opiates and produces virtually no side effects; it is expensive, however, and its limited duration of action requires more than one dose per day for the treatment or prevention of addiction. A new experimental drug, naltrexone, has come closer than any other substance to fulfilling the criteria of an ideal narcotic antagonist.

The earliest known narcotic antagonists were nalorphine (Nalline) and levallorphan (Lorfan). Administration of a narcotic antagonist precipitates a telltale abstinence syndrome if physical dependence on an opiate has become established. A severe abstinence syndrome may be precipitated that cannot be suppressed during the period of action of the antagonists, and some antagonists may further embarrass respiration that has been compromised by alcohol, barbiturates, or other nonnarcotic depressants.

This exciting new area of neuropharmacology began with the finding in 1971 that opiates bind to receptors on the cell membrane of some neurons of the CNS. The neurons are distributed in brain regions corresponding to anatomical structures and pathways involved in pain perception. Receptor binding has been demonstrated in many vertebrate species, from fish to primates. The natural question arose: Why should receptors exist in vertebrates for the alkaloids of the poppy? The logical answer was that there may be *endogenous* opiate-like compounds that are recognized by the receptors and serve some purpose in brain function.

Opiate receptors and endogenous opiates

Many drugs after all turn out to be mimics of endogenous substances. An accident of molecular shape allows them to fit into our receptors, either activating or blocking them.

The receptor theory of opiate action is supported by several lines of evidence. First, all natural and some synthetic opiate agonists have basic similarities of structure, suggesting the possibility of common recognition by an opiate receptor. Second, the extraordinary potency of some synthetic opiate agonists can be explained only by considering a highly selective receptor site. Etorphine, for example, is 5000 to 10,000 times more potent than morphine and produces euphoria and analgesia in doses as small as 0.0001 g, making it even more potent than LSD. Third, usually only levorotatory opiate isomers are active, suggesting stereospecific receptor function. Finally, opiate antagonists can be synthesized by effecting very slight molecular modifications of opiates, and the rapid action of these antagonists in reversing the effects of opiates suggests receptor site blockade.

The receptor theory of opiate action provoked a search for endogenous opiate-like compounds. This search has been successful; since 1975 two groups of brain peptides have been found with opiate-like activity: pentapeptides, called *enkephalins*, which appear to be neurotransmitters or neuromodulators with a distribution paralleling that of opiate receptors, and larger peptides, called *endorphins*, isolated from the hypothalamus and anterior pituitary gland.

The enkephalins and endorphins are indistinguishable from morphine in opiate-binding bioassays. When administered in vivo to laboratory animals, the enkephalins display weak analgesic action, and the endorphins evoke a host of variable effects: α-endorphin produces apparent tranquilization, analgesia of face and neck, and hypothermia; γ-endorphin produces agitation, hyperthermia, and no analgesia; and β-endorphin also produces hypothermia and profound analgesia of the whole body. β-Endorphin also produces prolonged muscular rigidity and immobility similar to a catatonic state. In every case the effects are abolished rapidly by the administration of a narcotic antagonist. The profound behavioral effects of the endorphins have led to speculation that opiate receptors may have functions other than modulating pain sensation. Just as exogenous opiates induce a state of euphoria and emotional detachment from the experience of suffering, endogenous opiates may play some central role in affective and behavioral homeostasis.

Avram Goldstein has asked the following questions: Do opiate addicts suppress or damage their endogenous opioid systems? Are some people more vulnerable to opiate addiction because of a relative deficiency of endogenous opioids?[7]

New dimensions in pain relief have emerged with the exciting discovery that animals can learn to activate their endogenous opiate systems to inhibit pain.[20]

ALCOHOL

It is often forgotten that alcoholism is still the most serious form of drug abuse in western society. It is estimated that over 9 million Americans are alcoholics and that over 50% of crimes and over 50% of highway accidents in the United States are alcohol-related.

Physical dependence and tolerance

A marked degree of physical dependence and a moderate degree of tolerance develop to alcohol when ingested regularly and in large amounts. Tolerance may be explained in part by induced hypertrophy of hepatic smooth endoplasmic reticulum with stimulation of alcohol metabolism.

Characteristics of abuse

Alcohol is a primary and continuous depressant of the CNS. Even a small amount decreases mental acuity and impairs motor coordination; at times, however, this deficit may be more than compensated for by the improved performance accompanying the induced state of euphoria and release from inhibitory attitudes.

In chronic alcoholism one may observe organ pathology and clinical syndromes not usually associated with other types of drug abuse, including fatty metamorphosis and cirrhosis of the liver, peripheral polyneuropathy, alcoholic gastritis, Korsakoff's psychosis, Wernicke's encephalopathy, and the complications of portal hypertension. Some of these changes are thought to be the result of nutritional deficiency rather than the direct action of alcohol; unlike other commonly abused drugs, alcohol supplies calories, depressing the appetite and encouraging a dietary deficit in the face of a deceptive maintenance of body weight. It is believed that alcohol is directly incriminated, however, in the pathogenesis of alcoholic fatty liver.

Chronic alcohol consumption leads to hypertrophy of hepatic smooth endoplasmic reticulum, with consequent stimulation of drug metabolism. This finding may explain in part the tolerance of alcoholics, *when sober*, to drugs such as barbiturates. *When inebriated*, alcoholics display a *heightened* sensitivity to barbiturates, not only because of the synergistic action of the two drugs but perhaps also because hepatic metabolism of other drugs is temporarily slowed during the active metabolism of alcohol.

A study of blood pressure in relation to drinking habits of over 80,000 men and women of three races strongly suggests that regular use of three or more drinks per day is a significant risk factor predisposing to hypertension.

In the history of many opiate addicts there occurs a turning from alcohol to opiates. The addict recalls that he was frequently "getting into fights" while under the influence of alcohol and that such poorly controlled behavior diminished or disappeared entirely "behind heroin."

Alcoholism appears to be a genetically influenced disorder. This conclusion is strongly suggested by familial incidence, twin studies, genetic marker studies, and adoption studies.[8,12] A higher incidence of elevated blood acetaldehyde levels after an ethanol test dose has also been shown to occur in families of alcoholics.

After prolonged, heavy intake of alcohol, withdrawal symptoms may appear within a few hours after the last dose; these include tremulousness, weakness, anxiety, intestinal cramps, and hyperreflexia. Between 12 and 24 hours the stage of "acute alcoholic hallucinosis" may appear, in which visual hallucinations are reported, at first only with the eyes closed. By 48 hours an acute brain syndrome may become apparent, with confusion, disorientation, and delusional thinking. When this syndrome is accompanied by gross tremulousness, it is called "delirium tremens." Major convulsive seizures ("rum fits") may occur but are less common than in barbiturate withdrawal. The chronic alcoholic may be in too poor a condition to withstand the stress of withdrawal; if death is not the price, recovery occurs by the fifth to the seventh day.

Abstinence syndrome

MARIJUANA

SLANG EQUIVALENTS:

Grass, weed, pot, dope, hemp
  Marijuana cigarette = joint, "j," number, reefer, root
  Cigarette butt = roach

Marijuana is inadequately described by any one drug category, as it possesses properties of a sedative, euphoriant, and hallucinogen.

The source of marijuana is the Indian hemp plant *Cannabis sativa*, an herbaceous annual growing wild in temperate climates all over the world. The plant is dioecious; that is, male and female flowers are borne on separate plants. The active compounds are most concentrated in the resinous exudate of the female flower clusters.

In the United States the term *marijuana* refer to any part or extract of the plant. The smoking mixture termed "bhang" consists only of the cut tops of uncultivated female plants. The most concentrated natural supply of cannabinols is found in the preparations called "hashish" and "charas," which consist largely of the actual resin from the flower clusters of cultivated female plants. The potency of any marijuana preparation varies from the plant strain and the growth conditions.

The principal psychoactive compound in marijuana appears to be l-Δ^9-transtetrahydrocannabinol (hereafter referred to as Δ^9THC; Δ^1THC and Δ^9THC represent different systems of nomenclature for the same compound). A varying, usually small, amount of $\Delta^{8(9)}$THC may also be present.

Black-market samples labeled "THC" virtually never contain THC but are comprised of any number of other psychotomimetic agents.

Δ⁹THC   Δ⁸⁽⁹⁾THC (Δ¹⁽⁶⁾THC)

| Physical dependence and tolerance | Physical dependence is not known to develop, and tolerance has been observed in most species tested. One study has demonstrated a dose-related cross-tolerance between Δ^9THC and ethanol, and the cross-tolerance is symmetric (either drug inducing cross-tolerance to the other). |

| Characteristics of intoxication ANECDOTAL REPORTS | Most users report that marijuana induces a dreamy, euphoric state of altered consciousness, with feelings of detachment, gaiety, and jocularity and preoccupation with simple and familiar things. In the company of others there is a tendency toward laughter and loquaciousness. Perceptual distortion of space and time is regularly reported; distances may be judged inaccurately, and things may seem to be happening very slowly or very rapidly. |

Dissociative phenomena such as partial amnesia or a feeling of being outside of oneself looking on are frequently reported. Libido is variably affected; since sexual desire may be enhanced, marijuana has gained a reputation as an aphrodisiac. There may be an unusually vivid remembrance or reliving of experiences or mood states of the past. The continuity of a story or movie may be lost, to be replaced by an intense experiencing of individual segments or scenes. Users are sometimes recognized by the characteristic hiliarity of their mutual laughter, which may become prolonged and uncontrolled. Appetite and appreciation of the flavor of food are usually enhanced, and weight gain may accompany regular smoking.

A paranoid state is sometimes reported, in which the smoker is keenly sensitive of others watching him; some forsake marijuana for this reason. Antisocial behavior under the influence of marijuana appears to be rare; users ordinarily withdraw from company that they find unpleasant.

Adverse reactions to unadulterated preparations of marijuana are relatively rare, but they may be serious when they do occur. Such reactions include acute paranoid states, dissociative states, and, less commonly, acute psychotic reactions. Adverse reactions to marijuana appear to be dose related (they are more frequent with hashish) and highly individualized (some users regularly have adverse reactions and some never do). The evaluation of reports of adverse reactions is complicated by the fact that marijuana is frequently adulterated with other drugs; some reports have failed to take this possibility into consideration.

Regular use of marijuana may result in a pervasive feeling of apathy, the so-called amotivational syndrome. The user discovers that "things just don't seem important to me any more." This development may be especially damaging to the psychological maturation of the adolescent. Such a syndrome is undoubtedly multidetermined, but in many adolescents undergoing psychotherapy, its development has been observed to coincide temporally with regular use of marijuana.

CLINICAL STUDIES

A study of marijuana-induced temporal disintegration was conducted at the Stanford University School of Medicine,[10,11] using doses of 20, 40, and 60 mg of THC (the higher two doses were admittedly larger than the dose to be expected from ordinary social smoking). All three doses significantly impaired serial operations in performing a task requiring sequential cognitive functions. Progressively more errors were made with increasing dose. The subjects reported a feeling of timelessness and uncertainty of how much time had elapsed; the time line extending from past to future seemed discontinuous, and past and future seemed unrelated to the present. One individual stated: ". . . I can't stay on the same subject. . . . I can't remember what I just said or what I want to say . . . because there are just so many thoughts that are broken in time, one chunk there and one chunk here." Impairment of short-term memory with emergence of loose associations was noted, and the latter was considered to have its probable origin in the former. The serious implications of such an effect over a prolonged period of time are clear.

Apparent overestimation of the passage of time was also reported in chimpanzees to whom Δ^9THC was administered orally. Temporally spaced responses of the chimps came to be made closer and closer together as the dose of THC was increased, suggesting that the chimps perceived shorter and shorter intervals of time as being of the original familiar duration.

In a study of aggression in mice, rats, and squirrel monkeys, THC was shown to decrease species-specific attack behavior. Comparatively low doses of THC were administered and did not appear to induce a general depression or incapacitation; other social interactions, such as allogrooming, actually increased in frequency.

It appears that a serious hazard of marijuana smoking is enhancement of a paranoid thought disorder and exacerbation of psychosis in schizophrenic patients.

In contrast to anecdotal reports that marijuana smoking increases interpersonal communication, studies have demonstrated an overall decrease in affective exchange and interpersonal skills during marijuana use.

Studies of marijuana and driving skills suggest that marijuana has a detrimental effect on driving ability. This effect is dose related and not uniform for all persons. Marijuana and alcohol are commonly used together; driving performance deteriorates rapidly with simultaneous use of both.

A report of 31 American soldiers who were heavy hashish smokers suggests that respiratory tract irritation may be a prominent feature of hashish smoking. Bronchitis, asthma, rhinopharyngitis, and sinusitis were common findings, with a mild obstructive pulmonary dysfunction in five who underwent pulmonary function studies. It was noted that the uvula becomes swollen and edematous while hashish is smoked and remains so for 12 to 24 hours afterward.

A 3-year study of 720 hashish smokers in an American Army population revealed a marked difference in the effects of light versus heavy hashish smoking. Occasional smoking in small, intermittent doses caused only minor respiratory ailments with no adverse mental effects. Heavier smoking, several times a day, resulted in a chronic intoxicated state with frequent acute adverse effects, such as disorientation, panic reaction, or acute psychotic reaction. Many chronic users become psychotic for long periods of time and were unresponsive to treatment with antipsychotic agents. Symptoms of chronic intoxication were similar to those of long-term dependence on depressant-hypnotic drugs and included apathy, dullness, and lethargy with mild to severe impairment of judgment, concentration, and memory. The heavy user, dubbed a "hashaholic" in Army jargon, appeared dull and maintained poor hygiene. He rarely resorted to violence or overt criminal behavior. His consumption of hashish reached 500 to 600 g per month, the equivalent of several thousand American marijuana cigarettes. The frequent practice of abusing ethanol and hashish simultaneously was reported to greatly increase the likelihood of adverse reaction and long-term morbidity.

Studies of the acute pulmonary physiological effects of marijuana show that both smoked marijuana and orally administered Δ^9THC produce significant bronchodilatation of relatively long duration (6 hours for the 20 mg dose). Another pulmonary function study suggests that occasional social smoking of marijuana does not result in functional respiratory impairment in healthy young men, but that heavy marijuana use for 6 to 8 weeks produces mild but definite *narrowing* of large, medium, and small airways, in spite of the acute bronchodilator action of THC.

The neoplastic potential of marijuana smoking has been inadequately researched. No reliable data are available on the incidence of carcinoma of the lung and upper respiratory passages in cannabis users. Studies have suggested, however, that marijuana smoke may prove carcinogenic and that a combination of marijuana and tobacco smoking may have greater carcinogenicity than either alone.

Long-term marijuana use may impair the expression of cell-mediated immunity, rendering the host more susceptible to infectious diseases and cancer. An in vitro study demonstrated that blastogenic responses to phytohemagglutinin and allogeneic lymphocytes were depressed in lymphocytes of long-term marijuana smokers; these responses were comparable to those of patients with uremia and patients undergoing immunosuppressive therapy. Other in vitro studies have also suggested that natural cannabinoids inhibit nucleic acid synthesis. Other studies, however, have failed to demonstrate impaired immune response in long-term marijuana smokers. Although this is currently an area of dispute, it appears that immunological suppression does occur in conjunction with marijuana smoking in some instances.

In various studies THC has been shown to impair spermatogenesis, inhibit the synthesis of testosterone, and, in the female, decrease serum levels of follicle-stimulating hormone (FSH), luteinizing hormone (LH), and prolactin. Oral administration of cannabinoids to female mice late in pregnancy and during early lactation produces a permanent alteration in body weight regulation, pituitary-gonadal function, and adult copulatory activity in male offspring. Clearly the cannabinoids exert profound effects on reproductive function, the mechanisms of which are unknown. Dose-related fetal resorptions are produced by administering cannabinoids to rats and mice; the mechanism may involve disruption of placental function.

In several species of animals THC induces hypothermia at room temperature. In human subjects marijuana smoking results in little or no change in body temperature in a cool environment but in a hot environment produces inhibition of sweating and hyperthermia. THC thus interferes with thermoregulation, although the mechanism is unknown.

[^{14}C] Δ^9THC administered to rats was shown to accumulate in tenfold greater concentrations in fat than in other tissues; 11-hydroxy THC, an active metabolite of Δ^9THC, showed a similar distribution, with highest concentration in body fat. The importance of fat localization of drugs in prolonging pharmacological activity is well known; it is conceivable that slow release from fat stores may help explain the phenomenon of "reverse tolerance," in which regular users of marijuana achieve a "high" more quickly and easily than sporadic users.

Plasma levels of THC fall rapidly to a low value, which remains for days, suggesting penetration into and release from storage sites. One study has demonstrated a half-life in tissues of 7 days; after 5 days, 15% of the THC is found as metabolites excreted by the kidney and 40% to 50% is excreted by the intestines.

Although it is too early to predict, THC and related compounds may become useful drugs. THC reduces intraocular pressure, has a bronchodilator action, may be an effective antiemetic, and has properties of a sedative and an antianxiety agent. Its toxicity in laboratory animals and in humans is low, as is its respiratory-depressant activity.

FURTHER CONSIDERATIONS

Marijuana is sometimes said to "lead to other drugs." Many drug users experiment first with marijuana, and in this sense marijuana may serve as a "stepping-stone" to the more potent agents. Most drug users believe strongly, however, that they would have eventually tried other drugs whether they had first smoked marijuana.

The potency of street marijuana in the United States has tended to increase so that there is less difference now between marijuana and hashish than formerly. Recent evidence suggests that the THC content of hashish is only twice that of strong marijuana.

Marijuana is often compared with alcohol. Unlike alcohol, marijuana is not known to be physically addicting and tolerance does not develop to the effects of ordinary marijuana preparations. When inebriated, the alcoholic usually suffers a greater temporary loss of judgment and control than the marijuana user, whose "highs" are usually characterized by mild alterations in perception and mood without marked loss of behavioral control. Hostility and aggression are commonly released by alcohol but rarely by marijuana. The appetite is stimulated by marijuana, whereas calories are provided by alcohol; nutritional deficiency commonly complicates the syndrome of chronic alcoholism. Psychological dependence on either drug may develop, and both drugs may impair the physical performance essential to safe automobile driving. Acute paranoid states, dissociative reactions, and near-psychotic reactions are occasionally seen with marijuana use; moderate drinking rarely if ever induces such reactions. There is strong suggestive evidence that chronic marijuana use interferes with motivational and goal-directed thinking; chronic alcoholism may do the same and ultimately result in brain damage and general physical deterioration.

In summary, in the light of our present incomplete knowledge, the principal medical risks in the use of marijuana appear to be (1) the occasional adverse reaction, characterized by paranoid thinking and extreme anxiety, sometimes with an acute psychotic reaction; (2) enhancement of preexisting paranoid thought disorders and exacerbation of psychosis in schizophrenic patients; (3) alteration of time and space perception, with loosening of associations and impairment of driving skills; (4) impairment of learning and short-term memory; (5) loss of motivation and drive, associated with regular and frequent use; (6) probable impairment of vascular reflex responses; (7) possible impairment of immune response; (8) disturbance of hypothalamopituitary function with impairment of reproductive functions; and (9) interference with temperature regulation.

For a more detailed analysis of current research findings, the student should consult the Institute of Medicine's report, *Marijuana and Health* (National Academy Press, Washington, D.C., 1982).

AMPHETAMINES

SLANG EQUIVALENTS:

Dextroamphetamine (Dexedrine) = dexies, copilots, oranges
Amphetamine (Benzedrine) = bennies, splash, peaches
Methamphetamine (Methedrine; Desoxyn) = meth, speed, crystal, crank, white cross (tablets)
Dextroamphetamine + amphetamine (Diphetamine; Biphetamine) = footballs

It appears that little if any physical dependence develops to the amphetamines. A change in sleep pattern on abrupt withdrawal has been reported in association with minimal EEG changes, but there is no physiologically disruptive abstinence syndrome. Abrupt withdrawal is physiologically safe and is characterized by the onset of lethargy, somnolence, and often a precipitous depressive reaction; the possibility of suicide should be kept in mind. Some consider the period of lethargy and somnolence an abstinence syndrome in itself.

Tolerance to amphetamines develops slowly and becomes marked. At any level of tolerance the margin between euphoria and toxic psychosis remains narrow.

Characteristics of abuse

The amphetamines are direct CNS stimulants and in ordinary therapeutic doses produce the following effects: euphoria, with increased sense of well-being; heightened mental acuity, until fatigue sets in from lack of sleep; nervousness, with insomnia; and anorexia. Amphetamines are useful in circumstances demanding optimal endurance and mental acuity; they have been prescribed for airmen in the military and for astronauts during difficult maneuvers. They are commonly abused by students, housewives, truck drivers, and all-night workers who self-administer the drugs for extended periods of time. Liberal dispensing by physicians of amphetamines for dietary management has contributed significantly to the abuse of these agents.

Undesirable and potentially hazardous effects accompany the prolonged use of amphetamines. As many a student has learned the hard way, fatigue eventually sets in and blocks coherent thought at inopportune times, such as during an examination. In addition, brief lapses of alertness, with sudden drooping of the head ("nodding"), may occur without warning as fatigue "breaks through"; this phenomenon, like the seizure of the epileptic individual, may result in a catastrophic loss of control in dangerous circumstances.

High doses of amphetamines reduce mental acuity and impair performance of complex acts, even in the absence of fatigue. Behavior may become irrational. A peculiar phenomenon observed among amphetamine users is a condition described as being "hung up." The user may get stuck in a repetitious behavioral sequence, repeating an act ritually for hours; the perseverative behavior may become progressively more irrational.

The "amphetamine psychosis" may develop during long-term or short-term abuse of amphetamines and is characterized by visual and auditory hallucinations and paranoid delusions in the setting of a clear sensorium and full orientation. The psychosis clears within a few days after the drug is discontinued. It has been compared with a severe paranoid state closely resembling paranoid schizophrenia, with fixed, systematized delusions aggravated by attempts at intervention.

The expressions "meth is death" and "speed kills" reflect the belief, widespread among drug users, that brain damage may result from administration of methamphetamine in large doses. In most cases a prolonged acute brain syndrome follows withdrawal.

Tolerance develops to such a degree that the habitual user may come to inject several hundred milligrams of an amphetamine every few hours. A total 24-hour dose of methamphetamine estimated at over 10 g has been reported. Some users report that the subjective effects of intravenous amphetamines are similar to the effects of intravenous cocaine except for the longer duration of action of the amphetamines.

The mechanism behind the "paradoxical" calming effect of amphetamines and methylphenidate in hyperkinetic children remains unknown. A recent study with possible relevance demonstrated that amphetamine administration to preweanling rats appeared to enhance the normal tendency to approach and maintain contact with conspecifics. In contrast, adult rats responded to amphetamines with marked increase in random, nondirected locomotor activity.

Physiological effects of high doses of amphetamines include mydriasis, elevation of blood pressure, hyperreflexia, and hyperthermia. Hypertensive crisis wtih intracranial hemorrhage has been reported following oral and intravenous administration of methamphetamine. It is important to recall that amphetamine is an indirectly acting adrenergic drug, promoting the release of dopamine in the CNS (p. 247).

Amphetamines have sometimes been used, and abused, for the relief of pain. It appears that they may have some effectiveness, at least in combination with an analgesic agent. When morphine was administered with 10 mg of dextroamphetamine, it was found to be twice as potent as morphine alone; the combination with 5 mg was one and one-half times as potent as morphine.

Other sympathomimetic agents that are chemically related to the amphetamines and commonly abused include ephedrine, phenmetrazine (Preludin), mephentermine (Wyamine and Dristan inhalers), and methylphenidate (Ritalin). These drugs all produce central stimulation much like the amphetamines, but generally less marked. As with the amphetamines, physical dependence is not known to develop.

COCAINE

SLANG EQUIVALENTS:

Coke, snow, toot, happy dust, white girl

Cocaine is a local anesthetic and vasoconstrictor agent and powerful CNS stimulant. It occurs naturally in the leaves of the coca plant *Erythroxylon coca* and in other species of *Erythroxylon*, which are indigenous to Peru and Bolivia. Coca chewing has been a way of life for centuries for the Inca Indians living in the Andean highlands. Cocaine use by intranasal application has become popular with many who can afford the high price of the drug.

Physical dependence and tolerance

Neither physical dependence nor tolerance is known to develop to the prolonged use of cocaine. It is possible that heightened responsiveness actually develops in some cases.

Characteristics of abuse

Euphoric excitement, often of orgastic proportions, is rapidly produced even when cocaine is sniffed ("snorted" or "horned"). Grandiose feelings of great mental and physical prowess may cause the user to overestimate his capabilities. Strong sexual desire is often aroused. After intravenous injection, spontaneous ejaculation in the absence of genital stimulation has been reported; some users joke about letting the drug "replace" a sexual partner.

Acute toxicity from intranasal absorption is characterized by agitation, dizziness, blurred vision, and tremors. With prolonged use, cardiac arrhythmias, convulsions, and respiratory arrest may ensue.

With intravenous injection the effects are short lived, in contrast to the longer duration of action of intravenous amphetamines. To recapture the fleeting "high," the user repeats the dose at short intervals of 5 to 15 minutes, often leaving the needle in place. Users have been known to lock themselves in a room and enjoy 48 hours of uninterrupted cocaine euphoria, sharing a large supply until it is exhausted.

Symptoms of cocaine toxicity include visual, auditory, and tactile hallucinations and paranoid delusions. Delusions may be compelling and may provoke assault. The agitated paranoid state is similar to that of amphetamine psychosis except that it is more short lived in cases of parenteral injection. Experienced users may inject an opiate to "come down" from a toxic state.

It has long been assumed that orally administered cocaine is hydrolyzed in the gastrointestinal tract and rendered ineffective. A study in human subjects demonstrated that cocaine is well absorbed from the gastrointestinal tract, with peak plasma levels occurring 50 to 90 minutes after ingestion.

Smoking of cocaine alkaloid ("free base") is becoming more widespread and appears to be frequently associated with cocaine toxicity.

One complication among cocaine sniffers is perforation of the nasal septum, occurring as a result of ischemic necrosis in the wake of the intense and prolonged vasoconstriction induced by the drug. Plasma concentrations reach a peak between 15 and 60 minutes after intranasal application, and cocaine persists in the plasma for 4 to 6 hours. The long plasma life may result from continuous absorption secondary to the vasoconstrictor action of cocaine and brings about a far more enduring toxic state than does parenteral injection. Cocaine remains on the nasal mucosa for 3 hours after application.

Physiological disturbances from high doses of cocaine include pyrexia, dilated pupils, tachycardia, irregular respiration, abdominal pain, vomiting, and major convulsive seizures. Central stimulation is followed by depression; the higher centers are the first to become depressed, making this transition while the lower centers are still excited. Death results from medullary paralysis and respiratory failure. Acute poisoning may pursue a rapid course. In one survey of deaths from recreational cocaine use, respiratory collapse occurred rapidly after intravenous injection, but occurred suddenly as late as 1 hour after oral or nasal administration.

Street cocaine is often adulterated with a variety of substances, including amphetamines, procaine, mannitol, and lactose. The sky-high price of cocaine has resulted in the appearance of substitutes advertised as being "like the real thing;" these substitutes contain caffeine, ephedrine, nicotine, and menthol. Cases of acute intoxication from these substitutes have been reported.

SLANG EQUIVALENTS: *BARBITURATES*

Barbiturates in general = goofballs, fool pills
  Short acting: secobarbital (Seconal) = red birds, red devils, reds; pentobarbital
    (Nembutal) = yellow jackets
  Intermediate acting: amobarbital (Amytal) = blue heavens
  Long acting: phenobarbital (Luminal) = purple hearts
  Combinations: secobarbital + amobarbital (Tuinal) = tooies, Christmas trees,
    rainbows

A marked degree of both physical dependence and tolerance develops to all the barbiturates. There is a sharp upper border to the tolerance, so that a slight increase in dosage may precipitate toxic symptoms. *Physical dependence and tolerance*

Characteristics of abuse

The effects of ordinary doses of barbiturates include sedation (without analgesia), decreased mental acuity, slowed speech, and emotional lability. Toxic symptoms resulting from overdose include ataxia, diplopia, nystagmus, difficulty in accommodation, vertigo, and a positive Romberg sign. There is risk of overdose as a result of the delayed onset of action of the longer acting barbiturates and also as a result of perceptual time distortion, which induces users to ingest more than they intended in a short period of time. Death from overdose, as with the opiates, results from respiratory depression; the respiratory depression of barbiturate overdose, however, is not antagonized by nalorphine or levallorphan.

In contrast to opiate addiction, the direct harm to the individual and society stems more from the toxic effects of the drug than from the difficulty of maintaining a continuing supply.

The barbiturates are rapidly becoming archaic drugs in modern medicine because of their disadvantages and hazards. REM rebound commonly follows use for insomnia; toxicity and respiratory-depressant action are great risks of higher doses; and induction of hepatic microsomal enzymes by barbiturates accelerates the biotransformation of many other drugs.

Abstinence syndrome

The barbiturate abstinence syndrome is one of the most dangerous drug withdrawal syndromes. Symptoms progress from weakness, restlessness, tremulousness, and insomnia to abdominal cramps, nausea, vomiting, hyperthermia, blepharoclonus (clonic blink reflex), orthostatic hypotension, confusion, disorientation, and eventually major convulsive seizures. The syndrome is sometimes mistaken for the "delirium tremens" of alcohol withdrawal. The seizures may become prolonged, as in status epilepticus. Agitation and hyperthermia may lead to exhaustion and cardiovascular collapse. With the short-acting barbiturates, convulsions are most likely to appear during the second or third day of abstinence; with the longer acting barbiturates, convulsions are less likely to occur and usually appear between the third and the eighth day.

The barbiturate type of abstinence syndrome is occasionally observed in an addict being withdrawn from heroin who insists that he or she has used no other drug. In such cases one should suspect that the lot of heroin last used by the patient had been "cut" (diluted) with barbiturates, a practice that is known to exist. A barbiturate withdrawal regimen is then instituted immediately.

Withdrawal from barbiturates

Hospitalization is advisable for the duration of the withdrawal period. Instead of accepting the addict's word for the level of barbiturate to which he has become addicted, an objective test is made to determine the level of tolerance to barbiturates. An ordinary therapeutic dose of pentobarbital is administered, and the patient is observed for clinical signs of drug effect. If the sedative action of the drug is not soon apparent, it is concluded that the patient's level of tolerance is higher and that he or she has become accustomed to higher individual doses. Additional increments of pentobarbital are administered until drug effect is evident; at this point the total dose of drug administered is considered the baseline from which subsequent doses are tapered over the ensuing 7 to 14 days. The long withdrawal period is advisable to minimize the likelihood of convulsions.

NONBARBITURATE
SEDATIVES

Methaqualone (Quaalude; Sopor; Parest): Nicknamed "quaas" and "ludes," methaqualone has become one of the leading drugs of abuse in the United States after marijuana and alcohol.[21] In contrast to barbiturate overdose, overdose may result in restlessness, hypertonia, and convulsive seizures. Pulmonary edema has been reported with large overdoses. Death may occur from respiratory arrest, pulmonary edema, or other causes. Physical dependence may develop after prolonged use in high doses. "Street" methaqualone may be adulterated with or may consist entirely of diazepam, PCP, or virtually any other agent, often in very large doses.

Glutethimide (Doriden): Marked physical dependence develops. resulting in a severe abstinence syndrome characterized by nausea, vomiting, abdominal cramps, tachycardia, pyrexia, hyperesthesia, dysphagia, and major convulsive seizures.

Chloral hydrate (Noctec; Somnos): Moderate physical dependence develops, as manifested by a "chloral delirium" on abrupt withdrawal, characterized by agitation, confusion, disorientation, and hallucinations. Slight to moderate tolerance develops; a "break in tolerance" may result from abrupt impairment of the mechanism of hepatic detoxification, with resulting overdose and death.

Methyprylon (Noludar): Abrupt withdrawal has resulted in confusion, agitation, hallucinations, and generalized convulsions.

Paraldehyde: Moderate physical dependence develops, as seen by the withdrawal symptoms of tremulousness, visual and auditory hallucinations, and a state of agitation and disorientation similar to delirium tremens.

Bromides: Physical dependence has not been demonstrated. In low doses bromides act as sedatives; in toxic doses they produce a so-called bromide psychosis characterized by confusion, disorientation, vivid hallucinations, and eventually coma. The slow elimination of bromide from the body may lead to chronic accumulation when it is administered over a period of time, with the subtle onset of the toxic syndrome.

Antianxiety agents

Drugs in this category, unlike the antipsychotic agents, characteristically produce a marked physical dependence of the barbiturate type, as evidenced by the common occurrence of major convulsive seizures after abrupt withdrawal. Barbiturates may, in fact, be substituted for any of the following drugs for purposes of controlled withdrawal.

Diazepam (Valium): Major convulsive seizures have been reported during the withdrawal illness. One study suggests that ethanol ingested simultaneously with diazepam accelerates diazepam absorption; plasma diazepam levels from 30 to 240 minutes after ingestion were significantly higher after administration with ethanol than with water alone.

Chlordiazepoxide (Librium): Withdrawal symptoms are reported to progress from agitation and insomnia to major convulsive seizures. Because of slow elimination of the drug, seizures may be delayed as long as 1 week after the last dose.

Meprobamate (Equanil; Miltown; Meprospan): Withdrawal symptoms may progress from insomnia, tremors, ataxia, and vomiting to an acute psychotic reaction, major convulsive seizures, coma, and death. Seizures occur between 24 and 48 hours after the last dose.

Ethchlorvynol (Placidyl): Abrupt withdrawal may result in agitation, hallucinations, and generalized convulsions.

Antipsychotic agents

It is remarkable that no significant physical dependence develops during long-term administration of the antipsychotic drugs in high doses. One author has described a syndrome characterized by anxiety, insomnia, and gastrointestinal disturbances following the abrupt discontinuation of phenothiazines,[2] but, as in the case of amphetamine withdrawal, there is no gross physiological disturbance. The issue of whether to call this an "abstinence syndrome" is largely a matter of semantics.

Moderate tolerance develops to the sedative effects of the phenothiazines; it is not known whether a true tolerance develops to the antipsychotic effects.

The antipsychotic drugs have low abuse potential for drug users, since they do not produce a "high" or pleasurable emotional state.

PSYCHOTO-MIMETIC DRUGS

Considered in this category are psychotogenic (hallucinogenic) drugs taken primarily for their psychotomimetic effects. Many other drugs such as the amphetamines and cocaine are also psychotogenic in high doses.

Phencyclidine

SLANG EQUIVALENTS:

PCP, angel dust, DOA, peace pill, hog

Phencyclidine hydrochloride (Sernylan, Sernyl)[16,17] 1-phenylcyclohexyl piperidine, a veterinary anesthetic agent, has become increasingly popular since the late 1970s as a psychotomimetic drug, in part because it is easily synthesized from readily available precursors. It is administered by ingestion, inhalation (sprinkled on smoking preparations or inhaled directly), and injection.

In low doses, from 1 to 5 mg, phencyclidine may induce euphoria and disinhibition, with release from social inhibitory attitudes and increased emotional lability. Many use the drug for this effect alone. In higher doses a variable clinical picture is produced, with excitement, somatic perceptual distortions, impairment of pain and touch perception, confusion, disorientation, and difficulty speaking. The user may appear agitated or quiet and withdrawn. The clinical syndrome may resemble schizophrenia in many respects and may persist for days or weeks. Posturing, catatonic states, and mutism have been reported. Attack behavior, directed or chaotic, has also been observed with large doses.

Phencyclidine produces both sympathomimetic effects (tachycardia, hypertension) and cholinergic effects (flushing, diaphoresis, drooling, miosis). Increased deep tendon reflexes, clonic movements, nystagmus, ataxia, and dysarthria are common effects. Paresthesias and analgesia may occur. At higher doses major convulsions, status epilepticus, hypertensive crisis, and cardiac or respiratory arrest may occur. Atypical coma may be the presenting clinical picture, mimicking head injury.

Treatment measures include emesis (if early after ingestion), control of hypertension, ventilatory support, and control of behavioral disturbance.

It is obvious that phencyclidine is one of the most dangerous drugs ever to appear on the street. Like most other street drugs, it is commonly misrepresented by sellers as THC, mescaline, peyote, or other drugs. It appears in powder form or in tablets or capsules, and the color is variable. It is inexpensive to produce and may bring great profits (1 pound may cost $100 to produce and bring $20,000), so its spread across North America and Europe is not surprising.

At least five PCP analogues have been widely distributed in the United States and marketed as PCP. Their structure varies from a piperidine to a phenylcyclohexylamine.

LSD

SLANG EQUIVALENT:

Acid; many different local names. The term *mikes* refers to micrograms, *clinical mikes* to actual micrograms, *street mikes* to a fictional microgram one-third to one-fourth as potent.

LSD (LSD-25; D-lysergic acid diethylamide tartrate) was first synthesized from the alkaloids of ergot *(Claviceps purpurea)* a fungus that parasitizes rye and other grains in Europe and North America. The ergot alkaloids, which include ergotamine and ergonovine, are active oxytocics and vasoconstrictors. The chance synthesis of LSD was accomplished in 1938 by a research chemist working for Sandoz, Ltd., who attached a diethylamide radical to lysergic acid, the skeletal structure common to all the ergot alkaloids. The sample was set aside until 1943, when it was first tested by the researcher and found to have strange and potent central effects.

Physical dependence and tolerance

Physical dependence is not known to develop. Tolerance, however, develops rapidly and is lost as rapidly after discontinuance of LSD. The usual initial dose of 200 to 400 μg is often raised to several thousand micrograms after a few days of continuous use. Cross-tolerance between LSD, mescaline, and psilocybin has been shown; it appears that cross-tolerance between LSD and DMT (dimethyltryptamine) and between LSD and Δ^9THC does not develop.

Characteristics of abuse

The nature of the "trip" taken with LSD is not predictable in advance but is influenced to some degree by the state of mind, mood, and expectations at the time the drug is taken. This is also true of one's response to marijuana, which may act as a stimulant, aphrodisiac, or sedative, depending largely on the environment and the state of mind. The usual trip wih LSD is characterized by exhilarating feelings of strangeness and newness of experience, vividly colored and changing hallucinations, reveries, "free thinking," and "new insight." Colors become alive and may seem to glow; the space between objects may take on greater subjective importance as a thing in itself; and there is dazed wonderment at the beauty in common things. The introspective experience may be intense and sobering; it has been described as an intellectual earthquake in which conditioned attitudes and feelings are reevaluated and values are reshuffled. To some degree there appears to be a regression to primary process thinking.

Unpleasant experiences with LSD are relatively frequent and may involve an uncontrollable drift into confusion, dissociative reactions, acute panic reactions, a reliving of earlier traumatic experiences, or an acute psychotic hospitalization. Prolonged nonpsychotic reactions have included dissociative reactions, time and space distortion, body image changes, and a residue of fear or depression stemming from morbid or terrifying experiences under the drug.

Catastrophic reactions to LSD are better understood when one conceptualizes the disruption by the drug of psychological defense mechanisms such as repression and denial in an individual precariously defended against confrontation of conflict material. With the failure of the usual defenses, the onslaught of repressed material overwhelms the integrative capacity of the ego, and a psychotic reaction results. It appears that this disruption of long-established patterns of adapting may be a lasting or semipermanent effect of the drug.

It also appears that LSD removes the usual intrinsic restraints on the intensity of affective response. It is well known to LSD users that a specific emotional response, whether it be fear, dread, delight, or sadness, may become rapidly more intense under the influence of the drug until it reaches overwhelming proportions. The users are then virtually in the grip of the reaction; they may indeed derive insight from the introspective experience, as most users report, but they may become so disturbed as to engage in behavior that endangers their own life. Deaths while under the influence of LSD have occurred by drowning, falling from a window, and walking into the path of a car. The meaningless question has been asked: "Was it an accident or suicide?" An instance of homicide by a 22-year-old student during an LSD-induced psychotic reaction has been reported; the student, not previously psychotic except for one other experience with LSD, killed a stranger with a knife in response to persecutory delusions. During 4 years of observation after the episode, the student was not again psychotic.[14]

Disturbing implications are inherent in the finding of many "acid heads" that after 25 to 50 trips the frequency of taking LSD may be reduced progressively without sacrificing the desired state of mind. Users may discover that between trips they begin to feel as they did while under the influence of the drug, until they eventually find themselves on a continuous trip with no further ingestion of the drug. They state that their thinking has become different, and they no longer "need" the drug.

Indeed, their changed behavior is apparent to others; with no further drug ingestion, they remain preoccupied with any trivial thing at hand, feel "at one" with all living things, and act as they often did while under the influence of the drug. The ultimate duration of these changes as well as their significance remains unknown.

Symptoms occurring during an LSD trip may recur unpredictably days, weeks, or months after a single dose. Strangest of drug effects, these "flashback" reactions may occur at intervals following the administration of many drugs with CNS activity, but they most commonly follow an LSD reaction. Flashback symptoms vary from gentle mood states to severely disruptive changes in thought and feeling and may occur with or without further administration of the drug. The reaction may be initiated voluntarily in some cases. The mechanism remains unknown, but the existence of the phenomenon suggests a residual impairment of psychological defense mechanisms, with periodic emergence of repressed feelings. Flashback reactions may also be "triggered" by strong affective states or by administration of a drug with CNS activity.

The physiological effects of LSD are few and include mydriasis, hyperreflexia, and muscular incoordination. Grand mal seizures have been observed following ingestion of LSD.

It has been demonstrated that injections of LSD in rats decrease the turnover rate of serotonin (5-hydroxytryptamine). Some investigators suggest that this may in part explain the psychotomimetic effects of LSD.

Numerous studies suggest that LSD may induce mutations, damage chromosomes, or have teratogenic effects. The studies are complicated, however, by many etiological variables, such as exposure to other drugs during pregnancy. The question of reproductive hazard remains unanswered though suspected.

Because it is water soluble, odorless, colorless, and tasteless and because by weight it is one of the most potent drugs known, LSD is easily administered to the unwary. At a party it will not be detected in the punch until its effects are evident.

LSD is usually taken by mouth. It is occasionally "mainlined," however, alone or in combination with other drugs. It is also absorbed through the lungs when marijuana soaked in an LSD solution is smoked.

It was once believed that a transient "model psychosis" resembling schizophrenia could be experimentally induced with LSD. It was soon recognized, however, that the psychotic reaction from LSD differs substantially from most types of schizophrenic reactions. In schizophrenia one usually finds a disordered thought pattern characterized by subtle or flagrant delusions that are systematized and integrated into the personality structure of the individual. The LSD psychosis, on the contrary, is characterized by a chaotic and unpredictable thought disturbance with little or no organization or integration. It resembles an acute brain syndrome more closely than it does most types of schizophrenic reaction, although it differs somewhat from a brain syndrome in the wide range of affective disturbance and in the complex nature of the hallucinatory experiences.

In the opinion of some investigators, LSD may become useful as a psychotherapeutic agent when administered under strictly controlled conditions in the course of psychotherapy. Two studies, however, failed to demonstrate superiority of LSD in the treatment of alcoholism.

Phenothiazines and barbiturates, singly or in combination, have sometimes been found effective in treating the acutely intoxicated state. The regular LSD user knows this well and may keep a supply of chlorpromazine on hand.

Other psychotomimetic agents

p-**Chlorophenylalanine** ("PCPA") has been found to induce long-lasting sexual excitation in male rats. Nicknamed "steam" by drug users, it has gained a reputation as a dangerous drug capable of inducing a prolonged psychotic reaction when taken in high doses. Drug users warn each other that "steam burns."

Dimethyltryptamine (DMT), **Diethyltryptamine** (DET), and **Dipropyltryptamine** (DPT) are commonly abused for their psychotomimetic effects. All three tryptamine derivatives produce a syndrome resembling an LSD reaction but differing in the following ways: the onset is more rapid, increasing the likelihood of panic reaction; the duration of action is only 1 to 2 hours (the experience has been dubbed a "businessman's trip"); and the autonomic effects consisting of pupillodilatation and elevation of blood pressure are more marked than with LSD. DMT is present in several South American snuffs, including cohoba snuff.

The labels "**STP**" and "**DOM**" have been given to the hallucinogenic drug 2,5-dimethoxy-4-methyl amphetamine. It is said to induce an LSD-like reaction lasting 72 hours or longer. Many who have tried the drug dislike the long "come-down" period of 1 to 3 days; perhaps for this reason, among others, it is generally less popular than LSD.

Another psychotomimetic agent related to the amphetamines is "MDA," or the "love pill" (3-methoxy-4,5-methylenedioxy amphetamine), which is said to induce a relatively mild LSD-like reaction lasting 6 to 10 hours. An amphetamine-like effect is also produced and tends to persist longer than the psychotomimetic effect, so that the period of "crashing" or "coming down" may be characterized by euphoria instead of the psychic depression that frequently concludes an LSD trip.

Morning glory seeds

VARIETIES:

1. *Rivea corymbosa:* ololiuqui, Mexican morning glory, Heavenly Blue (used in ceremony by Aztec Indians of Mexico)
2. *Ipomoea versicolor* (alternate names: *I. violacea, I. tricolor*): Pearly Gates

Morning glory seeds, readily purchasable in stores, contain compounds similar to LSD—D-lysergic acid amide among others. Up to several hundred seeds are ingested at a time to produce effects; less commonly an extract is injected intravenously.

Symptoms incude drowsiness, perceptual distortion, confusion, lability of affect, and hallucinations; giddiness and euphoria may alternate with intense anxiety. Common side effects of oral ingestion include nausea, vomiting, and diarrhea.

An instance of suicide apparently related to a morning glory seed flashback re-action has been described. A 24-year-old college student ingested 300 Heavenly Blue seeds and developed an acute psychotic reaction. Three weeks later the symptoms recurred for no apparent reason, and the student expressed a fear of losing his mind. The symptoms persisted and one morning he awoke, communicated his distress to others, and drove his car at an estimated 90 to 100 miles per hour down a hill to his death.[3]

Mescaline

The dumpling (peyote) cactus, *Lophophora williamsii*, is indigenous to the Rio Grande Valley. Protuberances atop the plant are cut off and dried in the sun to form the peyote or mescal buttons; these contain the active drug, mescaline (peyote; peyotl; 3,4,5-trimethoxyphenethylamine). The buttons are prepared into cakes, tablets, or powder; the powder is water soluble and may be administered orally or parenterally. Peyote is used in ceremonies by the Indians of northern Mexico and by the Navahos, Apaches, Comanches, and other tribes of the southwestern United States.

Mescaline produces effects similar to those of LSD, but it is less potent. Vivid and colorful hallucinations are reported. Flagrant psychotic reactions are far less common than with LSD.

Mescaline has been found in smaller quantities in another North American cactus, *Pelecyphora aselliformis*, and is known also to occur in some species of South American cacti.

Psilocybin and psilocin

The hallucinogenic agents psilocybin and psilocin, available in powder and lquid form, are extracted from the mushrooms *Stropharia* spp. and *Psilocybe* spp., which occur principally in Mexico.

A native religious cult in which these mushrooms are consumed as a sacrament has deep roots in Mexican tradition. Psilocybin is now popular with drug users in the United States and produces an effect similar to mescaline.

Anticholinergics

Commonly abused anticholinergic agents include atropine, scopolamine, syn-thetic atropine substitutes, and preparations or plants containing these agents (such as the over-the-counter preparation Asthmador and the plants jimsonweed and angel's trumpet [*Datura* spp.]). In high doses these agents produce a central anticholinergic syndrome characterized by fever, agitation, veridical hallucinations (bugs, spiders, etc.), and confusion. Severe intoxication may result in convulsions, flaccid paralysis, coma, and death. Other signs of anticholinergic intoxication are present, such as mydriasis, tachycardia, decreased salivary secretion, anhidrosis, urinary retention, and warm, flushed skin. Anticholinergic agents abused for their psychotomimetic effects are sometimes falsely marketed as LSD.

Nutmeg

Nutmeg (*Myristica*), a spice used throughout the world, is the powdered seed kernel of the East Indian tree *Myristica fragrans*. Unknown to many, it contains a hallucinogen thought to be myristicin. Ingestion of large amounts of nutmeg produces euphoria, hallucinations, and an acute psychotic reaction. Side effects, which may be confused with atropine poisoning, include flushing of the skin, tachycardia, and decreased salivary secretion. Unlike atropine, nutmeg may produce early pupillary constriction.

INHALANTS

The term *inhalant*, as used here, includes gases and highly volatile organic compounds and excludes liquids sprayed into the nasopharynx (droplet transport required) and substances that must be ignited before inhalation (such as marijuana).

This category of drug abuse attracts the youngest customers. Not infrequently one learns of elementary schoolchildren who have experimented dangerously with inhalants for weeks or months before being discovered.

Among the currently most popular inhalants are the volatile nitrites, principally amyl nitrite and isobutyl nitrite. They are nicknamed "poppers" and "snappers" because of the sound produced by breaking open the thin glass ampule in which amyl nitrite is marketed. Isobutyl nitrite has been marketed in various containers with trade names such as "Bolt," "Heart-On," "Rush," and "Locker Room." The effects of inhalation of the volatile nitrites are immediate and fleeting and may consist of light-headedness, euphoria (variable), headache, and enhancement of sexual orgasm. The latter effect accounts for the most common usage of the drugs. The basic pharmacological action is relaxation of vascular smooth muscle; complaints of users include a prolonged pulsatile headache and symptoms of orthostatic hypotension, glaucoma, recent head injury, or intracranial hemorrhage. If inhalation is prolonged or practiced regularly, hemoglobin may be converted to methemoglobin; this should be kept in mind in the evaluation of the regular user.

Other popular inhalants include model airplane glues, plastic cements, gasoline, brake and lighter fluids, paint and lacquer thinners, varnish remover, cleaning fluid (spot remover), and nail polish remover. These household agents contain a variety of volatile aliphatic and aromatic hydrocarbons, including benzene, toluene, xylene, carbon tetrachloride, chloroform, acetone, amyl acetate, trichloroethane, naphtha, ethyl alcohol, and isopropyl alcohol. Some of these compounds are depressants of the CNS and may produce anesthesia and death in high concentrations. Some have known toxic effects. Chloroform and carbon tetrachloride, for example, are toxic to the myocardium, liver, and kidney and may produce hepatic or renal failure or cardiac arrhythmias with severe hypotension; mild poisoning with either agent may produce a reversible oliguria of a few days' duration. Exposure to high concentrations of toluene may result in renal tubular acidosis, acute hepatic failure, bone marrow suppression, and permanent encephalopathy. Lead poisoning has resulted from gasoline sniffing.

A case of fatal aplastic anemia secondary to glue sniffing has been reported.[6] A drug user habituated to one inhalant may resort to using another when the first inhalant is unavailable; a gasoline sniffer substituted carbon tetrachloride with near-fatal results. Chronic toluene abuse has resulted in severe brain damage characterized by cognitive impairment, defective modulation of affect, scanning speech, tremors, and ataxia.

Symptoms produced by inhalation of the agents just listed are essentially similar for all. A sense of exhilaration and light-headedness are usually reported, progressing to hallucinations. Judgment and reality perception are impaired. Transient ataxia, slurred speech, diplopia, and vomiting have been reported in cases of glue sniffing. If inhalation is not interrupted, coma and death may result.

The development of a definite tolerance has been reported. Physical dependence is not known to develop.

Anesthetic agents such as nitrous oxide ("laughing gas"), diethyl ether, cyclopropane, trichloroethylene (Trilene), and halothane (Fluothane) are also subject to abuse. Nitrous oxide, currently a very popular inhalant, represents an exception to the general rule that inhalants are organic compounds.

"Sudden sniffing death" is a new phenomenon associated with inhalant abuse. In the usual reported case a young person inhales a volatile hydrocarbon deeply and gets the urge to run; after sprinting a short distance he falls to the ground dead. The cause of death is assumed to be a cardiac arrhythmia induced by the inhaled agent and intensified by exercise and hypercapnia. Most reported cases have followed inhalation of fluoroalkane gases such as the pressurized propellants of many aerosol sprays. Once called "inert," fluoroalkane gases have been found to sensitize the hearts of mice to asphyxia-induced sinus bradycardia, atrioventricular block, and ventricular T-wave depression. Inhalation of airplane glue or toluene has likewise been shown to sensitize the heart of mice to asphyxia-induced atrioventricular block. Some reported deaths have occurred while running just after sniffing vapors; in one case inhalation of vapors was incidental to siphoning only. Fatal cardiac arrhythmias have been produced in dogs by inhalation of fluorinated hydrocarbons (trichloromonofluoromethane and dichlorodifluoromethane) in the absence of hypoxia, with careful maintenance of normal arterial oxygen tension, carbon dioxide tension, pH, serum carbon dioxide level, and base excess.

MISCELLANEOUS DRUGS

Propoxyphene

There is no evidence that significant physical dependence or tolerance develops when propoxyphene (Darvon) is administered in ordinary therapeutic doses. In very large doses, however, both physical dependence and tolerance have been observed to develop. The withdrawal syndrome is characterized by chills, diaphoresis, rhinitis, yawning, muscle aches, irritability, abdominal cramping, and diarrhea. Evidence suggesting that propoxyphene is pharmacologically related to the opiates is provided by the finding that it can suppress the morphine abstinence syndrome to a slight degree. Perhaps the most convincing evidence of such a relationship is the finding that the toxic effects of an overdose of propoxyphene (muscular fasciculations, respiratory depression, and convulsive seizures) are antagonized by the narcotic antagonists nalorphine and levallorphan.

In a study at the Addiction Research Center in Lexington, Kentucky, comparison of propoxyphene with codeine was made on the basis of the occurrence of an abstinence syndrome following abrupt withdrawal, suppression of morphine abstinence syndrome, and precipitation of an abstinence syndrome on administration of nalorphine. It was concluded that propoxyphene induces considerably less physical dependence than codeine and has substantially less addiction liability than codeine. The same investigators also found that a toxic psychosis was induced by single doses of propoxyphene in excess of 900 mg. Propoxyphene overdosage may be rapidly fatal. Respiratory depression, convulsions, and pulmonary edema are common terminal events.

Propoxyphene has become a major drug of abuse in the United States. In some cities it is associated with more deaths than either heroin or morphine, and it ranks near the top in drugs mentioned in emergency room visits.

Nicotine

Nicotine is extracted from the tobacco plant *Nicotiana tabacum*, which has been cultivated from remote antiquity and in every country of the world where the climate has permitted. It has never been found as a wild plant and fails to survive outside of cultivation. Nicotine is one of the most toxic of all drugs; the dosage encountered in cigarettes is extremely small. Physiological effects of nicotine include elevation of blood pressure, increased bowel activity, and an antidiuretic action. Apparently a moderate tolerance and a mild to moderate physical dependence develop.

Caffeine

Caffeine occurs naturally in the coffee bean (seeds of *Coffea arabica* and related species), the leaves of the tea plant *(Thea sinensis)*, and the seeds of the chocolate tree *(Theobroma cacoa)*. Caffeine is added to many soft beverages and over-the-counter medications. It stimulates the CNS at all levels, beginning with the cortex; a more rapid and clear flow of thought is produced and a sense of fatigue is diminished. Physical dependence on caffeine has not been demonstrated. It appears that a mild degree of tolerance develops during continued use.

Caffeine is probably the most widely consumed psychoactive drug in the world. It has recently been shown that caffeine elevates plasma catecholamine concentration when ingested in doses encountered in beverages; hyperadrenergic syndrome has been reported from overdose of caffeine, from either coffee or caffeine tablets, and is characterized by agitation, psychosis, hyperventilation, tachycardia, and dilated, reactive pupils. Metabolic acidosis may also result from generation of lactate. Caffeine poisoning should be considered along with salicylate poisoning and diabetes in the differential diagnosis of metabolic acidosis, hyperglycemia, and hyperventilation.

Cantharidin

Cantharidin (Spanish fly) is erroneously reputed to have a specific aphrodisiac effect, presumably because priapism may result from irritation of the male urethra when the drug is excreted in the urine. Ingestion of cantharidin may be followed by stomatitis, abdominal cramps, vomiting, bloody diarrhea, urinary urgency, dysuria, hematuria, and priapism. Cantharidin is directly toxic to the kidneys; deaths from renal damage and cardiorespiratory collapse have been reported.

The dried leaves of the catnip plant *(Nepeta Cataria)* are smoked like marijuana *Catnip* or the extract is sprayed over ordinary tobacco. Effects are said to be euphoria and enhanced appreciation of sensory experiences. No definite pharmacological activity has yet been demonstrated. One wonders to what extent the alleged effects of catnip, like those of banana peels, are the result of placebo effect and hyperventilation.

Drug users are aware that the combination of two or more centrally active drugs *DRUG MIXING* may provide a novel dimension of feeling unobtainable with a single drug alone. A second drug may be taken to enhance the effects of the first drug, to prevent undesired effects of the first drug, or to reduce the discomfort of discontinuing the first drug. Adulteration is virtually the rule with black-market drug samples.

When drugs of abuse are classified as they are in this chapter and in Appendix *CLINICAL* B (p. 761), it is often forgotten that a large percentage of drugs taken by people *EVALUATION OF* today are black-market samples and that three unknowns are thereby introduced: *THE DRUG USER* dose, actual identity, and purity. Any one of these three unknowns constitutes a serious danger in itself, and all three are present in any black-market sample.

Fundamental to the diagnostic evaluation of the suspected drug user is an attempt to place the apparent drug-related symptoms into one or more of four categories: symptoms occurring during intoxication; symptoms of withdrawal; "flashback" symptoms; and the "masking" of symptoms of illness or injury by a drug.

The lack of symptom specificity in cases of intoxication makes the evaluation tricky even for an experienced observer; manic excitement, panic reaction, dissociative reaction, paranoid reaction, and overt psychotic reactions may occur during a "bad trip" with most of the drugs discussed. An etiological diagnosis is best reached through laboratory analysis of drug sample, gastric aspirate, blood, or urine; even laboratory identification may be difficult, however, because of introduction of new chemical agents in an evolving drug scene. To make matters more complicated, a patient may be simultaneously in withdrawal from one drug and intoxicated with another.

Contrary to earlier thinking, it is now apparent that discontinuing almost any drug after heavy use is likely to result in serious abstinence symptoms. It may be unrealistic to describe the phenomenon of "crashing" (discontinuing a drug after heavy use or a large dose) in either physiological or psychological terms; it is clearly neither the one nor the other alone.

Symptoms of coincident illness or injury may not be reported by intoxicated drug users because of the analgesic action of the drug or because of a mental state in which they are only vaguely aware of the symptoms (or lack of the incentive to report them). Heart attack or head injury may thereby escape detection. Systemic infection, metabolic disturbance (especially diabetic crisis), and head injury may contribute to the moribund state of patients who have taken a depressant drug.

It is important to remember that a patient under the influence of, or in withdrawal from, almost any drug may show no obvious symptoms or signs referable to recent drug use.

A syndrome of necrotizing angiitis associated with drug abuse has been described. It appears to be pathologically indistinguishable from periarteritis nodosa and is manifest clinically by few or no symptoms in some patients and multiple-system involvement, with pulmonary edema, hypertension, pancreatitis, and renal failure, in others. Although the etiology is unclear, a frequent associated finding has been the intravenous injection of methamphetamine. The actual existence of this syndrome as a new drug-related phenomenon is challenged by some observers.

Injection of oral drug preparations may release a shower of vascular emboli in the form of tablet filler material, which becomes deposited in capillary beds of the retina, lung, endocardium, liver, spleen, and kidney. Pulmonary angiothrombotic granulomatosis has been reported, with consequent pulmonary hypertension and fatal cor pulmonale, as a result of deposition of talc (magnesium trisilicate) in the pulmonary vessels. Ophthalmological examination may reveal crystals of talc and cornstarch clustered in the macular region. Retinopathy and retinal detachment have resulted. The list of tablet filler materials is endless and includes lactose, colloidal silica, microcrystalline cellulose, magnesium stearate, and dibasic calcium phosphate. The list may be almost as long as that of contaminants added to black-market drugs.

Gangrene of an extremity is a common end result of inadvertent arterial injection of a drug. The mechanism of vascular injury is not known, but chemical damage to the intima by the concentrated drug may play an important role. Tissue ischemia after intraarterial injection of *oral* drug preparations appears to be more severe than that after injection of parenteral preparations, perhaps because of the presence of the many additives of the filler.

A drug habit carries a proportionately greater risk if (1) black-market drugs are used, (2) the higher risk drugs such as LSD, amphetamines, or heroin are used, and (3) the route of administration is intravenous. The intravenous route introduces a number of risks of its own, including greater likelihood of adverse reaction or lethal overdose, viral hepatitis, bacterial endocarditis, serious sequelae of injecting filler from oral drug preparations, and development of a "needle habit" (craving for injection of anything by needle).

REFERENCES

1. Ausubel, D.P.: The Dole-Nyswander treatment of heroin addiction, JAMA **195**:949, 1966.
2. Brooks, G.W.: Withdrawal from neuroleptic drugs, Am. J. Psychiatry **115**:931, 1959.
3. Cohen, S.: Suicide following morning glory seed ingestion, Am. J. Psychiatry **120**:1024, 1964.
4. Cutting, W.C.: Morphine addiction for 62 years: a case report, Stanford Med. Bull. **1**:39, 1942.
5. Franz, D.N., Hare, B.D., and McCloskey, K.L.: Spinal sympathetic neurons: possible sites of opiate-withdrawal suppression by clonidine, Science **215**: 1643, 1982.
6. Gold, M.S., Pottash, A.C., Sweeney,

D.R., and Kleber, H.D.: Opiate withdrawal using clonidine, JAMA **243:**343, 1980.

7. Goldstein, A.: Endorphins: physiology and clinical implications. In Recent developments in chemotherapy of narcotic addiction, vol. 311, New York, 1978, Ann. N.Y. Acad. Sci.

8. Goodwin, D.W.: Alcoholism and heredity, Arch. Gen. Psychiatry **36:**57, 1979.

9. Marcovici, M., O'Brien, C.P., McClellan, A.T., and Kacian, J.: A clinical, controlled study of l-α-acetylmethadol in the treatment of narcotic addiction, Am. J. Psychiatry **138:**234, 1981.

10. Melges, F.T., Tinklenberg, J.R., Hollister, L.E., and Gillespie, H.K.: Marihuana and temporal disintegration, Science **168:**1118, 1970.

11. Melges, F.T., Tinklenberg, J.R., Hollister, L.E., and Gillespie, H.K.: Marihuana and the temporal span of awareness, Arch. Gen. Psychiatry **24:**564, 1971.

12. Mendelson, J.H., and Mello, N.K.: Biologic concomitants of alcoholism, N. Engl. J. Med. **301:**912, 1979.

13. Powars, D.: Aplastic anemia secondary to glue sniffing, N. Engl. J. Med. **273:**700, 1965.

14. Reich, P., and Hepps, R.B.: Homicide during a psychosis induced by LSD, JAMA **219:**869, 1972.

15. Senay, E.C., Dorus, W., and Renault, P.F.: Methadyl acetate and methadone, JAMA **237:**138, 1977.

16. Showalter, C.V., and Thornton, W.E.: Clinical pharmacology of phencyclidine toxicity, Am. J. Psychiatry **134:**1234, 1977.

17. Snyder, S.H.: Phencyclidine, Nature **285:**355, 1980.

18. Stimmel, B., Goldberg, J., Rotkopf, E., and Cohen, M.: Ability to remain abstinent after methadone detoxification, JAMA **237:**1216, 1977.

19. Washton, A.M., and Resnick, R.B.: Clonidine for opiate detoxification: outpatient clinical trials, Am. J. Psychiatry **137:**1121, 1980.

20. Watkins, L.R., and Mayer, D.J.: Organization of endogenous opiate and nonopiate pain control systems, Science **216:**1185, 1982.

21. Wetli, C.V.: Changing patterns of methaqualone abuse, JAMA **249:**621, 1983.

Chapter 31

Nonsteroidal antiinflammatory antipyretic analgesics

GENERAL CONCEPTS

A group of chemically unrelated drugs classified as nonsteroidal antiinflammatory antipyretic analgesics (NSAIA) produce similar pharmacological effects by inhibiting the synthesis and release of prostaglandins. These pharmacological effects include reducing (1) the symptoms of inflammation (antiinflammatory), (2) the elevation in body temperature during fever (antipyretic), (3) the experience of pain without loss of consciousness (analgesia), and (4) platelet aggregation. Drugs in this class include salicylates, arylalkanoic acid derivatives (ibuprofen; naproxen; fenoprofen), tolmetin, zomepirac, mefenamic acid, and derivatives of pyrazolone (phenylbutazone; oxyphenbutazone), indoles (indomethacin; sulindac) and *p*-aminophenol (acetaminophen; phenacetin) (Fig. 31-1). Many of these compounds are used to reduce the

FIG. 31-1 *Chemical structures.*

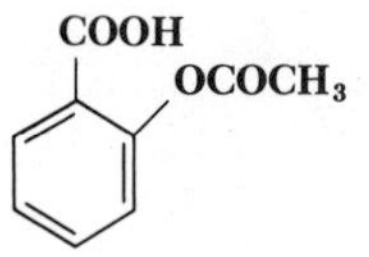

Aspirin
(salicylate)

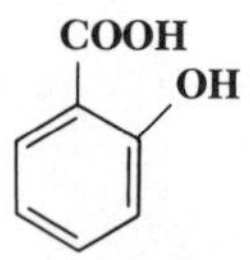

Salicylic acid
(salicylate)

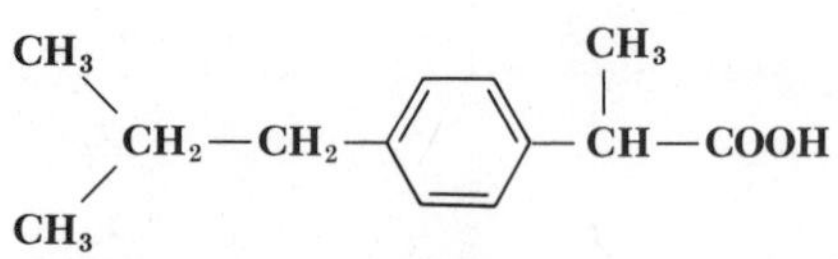

Ibuprofen
(arylalkanoic acid derivative)

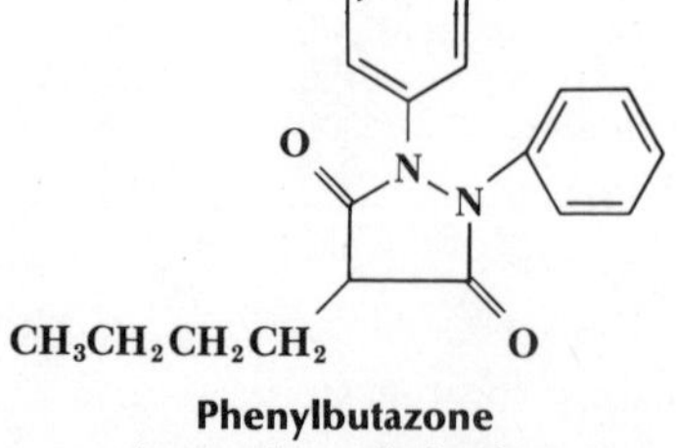

Phenylbutazone
(pyrazolone derivative)

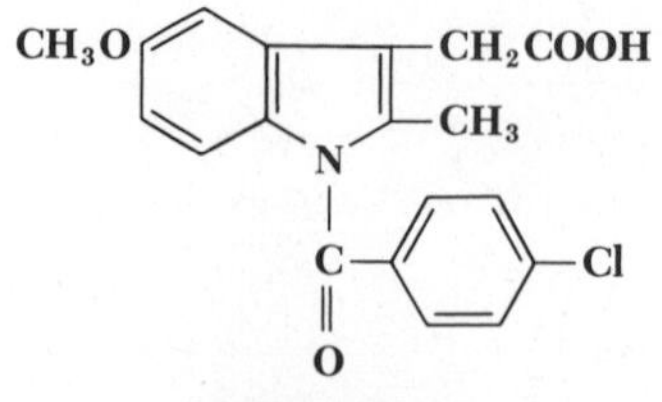

Indomethacin
(indole derivative)

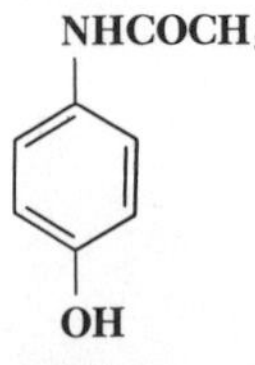

Acetaminophen
(*p*-aminophenol)

inflammation and pain associated with arthritic diseases. Frequently, irritation of the gastrointestinal tract limits the use of these compounds as antiinflammatory agents. The salicylates and many of the salicylate-like antiinflammatory drugs displace oral anticoagulants, sulfonylureas, hydantoins, and sulfonamides from binding proteins in plasma and increase their toxicity. The NSAIAs should not be used in pregnant women or patients with bleeding disorders, gastrointestinal ulcers, renal disease, or an intolerance to aspirin.

The NSAIAs are classified according to their therapeutic uses (Fig. 31-1).

DRUG CLASSIFICATION

Salicylates—antiinflammatory antipyretic analgesics
  Acetylsalicylic acid (aspirin)
  Salts of salicylic acid
  Sodium and magnesium salicylate
  Choline magnesium trisalicylate
  Never ingest
  Salicylic acid—topical use for wart and corn removal
  Methylsalicylate (oil of wintergreen)—used as a counterirritant in ointments
Salicylate-like antiinflammatory agents
  Arylalkanoic acid derivatives
    Ibuprofen
    Naproxen
    Fenoprofen
  Tolmetin
  Pyrazolone derivatives
    Phenylbutazone
    Oxyphenbutazone
  Indole derivatives
    Indomethacin
    Sulindac
Salicylate-like antipyretic analgesics
  p-Aminophenol derivatives
    Acetaminophen
    Phenacetin
  Mefenamic acid
  Zomepirac sodium
Analgesic combination and mixtures
  Narcotic and antipyretic analgesics (codeine and aspirin or acetaminophen)
  Antipyretic analgesic mixtures (aspirin and acetaminophen)
  Caffeine and antipyretic analgesics (APC-aspirin phenacetin and caffeine)
  Sedatives and antipyretic analgesics (phenobarbital or promazine and aspirin)

NSAIAs produce their antiinflammatory, antipyretic, analgesic and antiplatelet effects by inhibiting the synthesis and release of prostaglandins.[10,11,35,38] These drugs inhibit the enzyme cyclooxygenase, which catalyzes the synthesis of cyclic endoperoxides important in the formation of prostaglandins[24,26] (Fig. 31-2). All mammalian cells studied thus far contain microsomal enzymes necessary for the synthesis of prostaglandins. In contrast to the ubiquitous distribution of prostaglandin synthetase,

PHARMACO-DYNAMICS
Mechanism and sites of action

FIG. 31-2   Biosynthesis of prostaglandins.

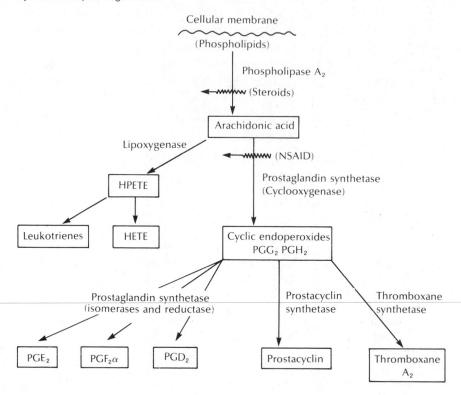

enzymes required for the production of both prostacyclin (prostacyclin synthetase) and thromboxane A_2 (TXA$_2$; thromboxane synthetase) are selectively present in certain tissues. The NSAIAs inhibit cyclooxygenase activity without selectively altering either prostacyclin synthetase or thromboxane synthetase. Neither do these drugs act as direct receptor antagonists of prostaglandins. Since prostaglandins are not stored in the cell, their release during inflammation is dependent on their de novo synthesis. Thus inhibition of cyclooxygenase activity by NSAIA drugs reduces the influence of prostaglandins at the site of inflammation. Since prostaglandins produce symptoms of inflammation (erythema; edema) and potentiate the effect of bradykinin on receptors mediating pain, a reduction of prostaglandins at the sight of inflammation results in the therapeutic response, for example, antiinflammatory action and analgesia.

The antipyretic action of NSAIAs is also mediated by inhibition of cyclooxygenase activity. The site at which cyclooxygenase activity is inhibited to produce antipyresis is presumed to be in neurons of the hypothalamus. Fever results from a resetting of the temperature set–point (thermostat) by the action of endogenous pyrogen on neurons of the thermoregulatory center in the preoptic region of the

Fever production.   FIG. 31-3

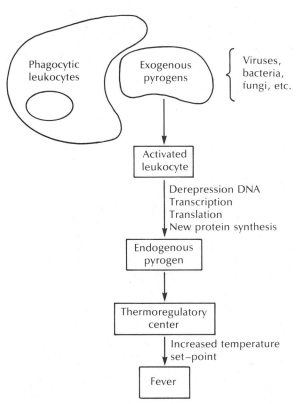

hypothalamus[8] (Fig. 31-3). NSAIAs reduce elevated body temperature associated with fever but do not alter normal basal body temperature.[11,16] Neither do these drugs reduce an elevated body temperature associated with hyperthermia produced by exercise (heat stroke; heat exhaustion), drugs (atropine; inhalation anesthetics; muscle relaxants), hypothalamic lesions, disturbances in monoamine metabolism in the CNS, or metabolic disorders.[36] Salicylates and salicylate-like compounds are useful as antipyretics only when the elevated body temperature results from a change in the temperature set–point in the thermoregulatory center of the hypothalamus. Hyperthermia does not involve a change in the "thermostat" but rather results from heat production in excess of heat dissipation. Whole-body cooling procedures are effective in treating hyperthermia, whereas salicylates, acetaminophen, or indomethacin are used as antipyretics in the treatment of fever. Since the physiological importance of fever in combating infection is not well understood, antipyretic agents should be utilized only when the body temperature is dangerously high or when significant relief is experienced by the patient when the temperature is lowered.

FIG. 31-4 *Thromboxane A₂ and prostacyclin effects on platelet aggregation.*

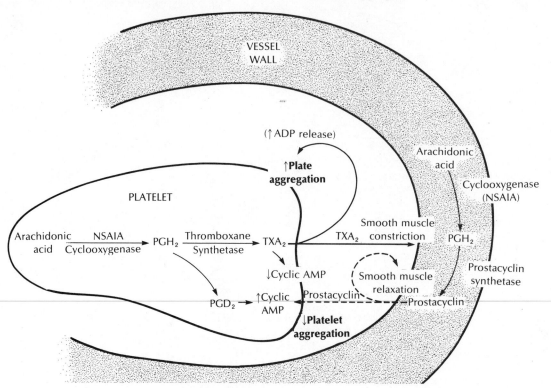

The antiplatelet action of salicylates and other NSAIAs is also mediated by inhibition of cyclooxygenase activity. In addition to cyclooxygenase, the platelet contains thromboxane synthetase, which catalyzes the formation of TXA_2 from the cyclic endoperoxides.[17] The opposing effects on platelet homeostasis of TXA_2 formed in the platelet and prostacyclin synthesized in the vessel wall are illustrated in Fig. 31-4. TXA_2 promotes platelet aggregation and vasoconstriction, whereas prostacyclin does the reverse, that is, inhibits platelet aggregation and promotes vasodilatation. The antiplatelet effect of NSAIAs indicates the relative importance of inhibiting the formation of TXA_2 on platelet function. Because of the antiplatelet action of these drugs, NSAIAs should not be used in patients either with blood-clotting problems or who are taking oral anticoagulants. NSAIAs are currently being evaluated for their effectiveness in treating or preventing diseases associated with reduced platelet life and increased thrombi formation such as atherosclerosis,[15,33] myocardial infarction, pulmonary emboli, thrombi associated with mitral stenosis and prosthetic valve replacement, transient ischemic attacks, and stroke.[15]

NSAIAs also have a uricosuric effect, resulting from inhibition of uric acid reabsorption from the proximal tubule of the nephron. Many of these drugs are organic acids and are transported by the same systems mediating both secretion and reabsorption of organic acids such as uric acid in the proximal tubule. For this reason the effect of NSAIAs on uric acid excretion is dose related and varies from producing no change to increased or decreased secretion.[39] Sulfinpyrazone, a pyrazolone derivative similar to phenylbutazone, is used to promote uric acid excretion in patients with gout (see Chapter 48).

Side effects and toxicity associated with NSAIAs affect four organ systems consistently: hematopoetic, renal, hepatic, and gastrointestinal.[11,37] Blood dyscrasias and injury to the kidney and gastrointestinal tract are associated primarily with salicylates and salicylate-like antiinflammatory compounds used in the treatment of arthritis. NSAIAs are nonselective in reducing the symptoms of inflammation; that is, frequently they produce hemorrhage, irritation, and gastric ulcers after prolonged use at therapeutic doses. These drugs are contraindicated in patients with a history of gastrointestinal ulcers and should not be used concurrently with other drugs known to promote ulcer formation, such as alcohol.

Side effects

Liver damage is not typically associated with salicylates but occurs predictably following overdose of acetaminophen. Liver necrosis is distinctly localized to hepatocytes in the centrolobular region of the liver. These cells contain the highest activity of the cytochrome P-450 mixed-function oxidase system. At recommended doses acetaminophen is metabolized largely by conjugation to glucuronide and sulfate.[4,5,12] A small fraction ($\leq 4\%$) is converted by oxidation via cytochrome P-450 to a highly reactive and toxic metabolite (Fig. 31-5). This metabolite, suggested to be either a semiquinone or quinoneimine, is conjugated with glutathione and excreted as mercapturic acid or cysteine conjugates.[23,31] However, when the dose of acetaminophen is increased and enzymes catalyzing glucuronide and sulfate conjugation are saturated, a larger proportion of the drug is metabolized by the cytochrome P-450 system to the reactive metabolite(s). Hepatic damage will not result as long as glutathione stores are sufficient to allow conjugation of the reactive metabolite. Factors affecting hepatic necrosis after overdose of acetaminophen include the (1) amount of acetaminophen consumed, (2) blood levels of drug attained, (3) activity of the cytochrome P-450 mixed-function oxidase system, (4) clearance of toxic and nontoxic metabolites, and (5) glutathione stores.[31] Hepatic necrosis is predicted if the half-life of acetaminophen in plasma is greater than 4 hours or if the concentration of drug in plasma exceeds 120 µg/ml and 50 µg/ml at 4 hours and 12 hours after ingestion, respectively.[4,31] Treatment of acetaminophen overdose includes (1) gastric lavage and (2) administration of a substance that donates sulfhydryl groups, such as N-acetylcysteine, 140 mg/kg by mouth as a loading dose followed by 70 mg/kg by mouth every 4 hours for 17 doses or until the plasma concentration of acetaminophen falls 25% below the nomogram.[4]

FIG. 31-5   *Metabolism of acetaminophen.*

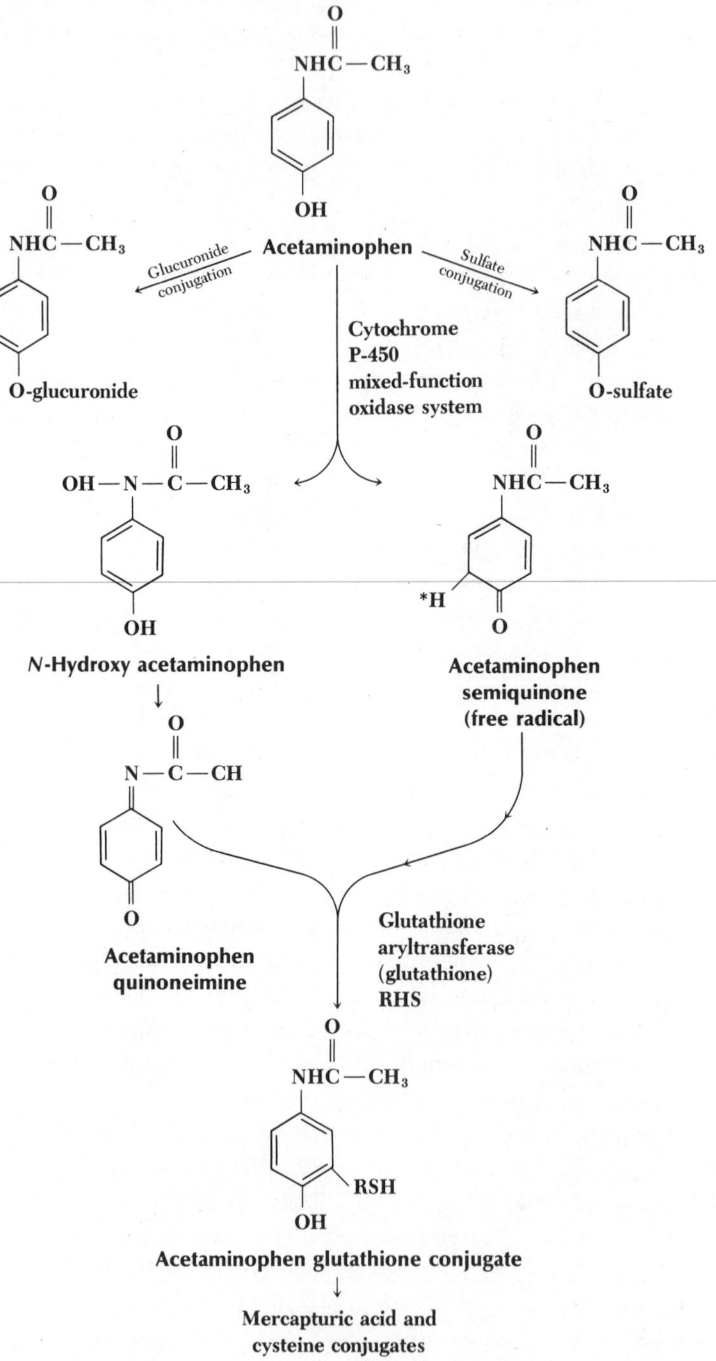

Renal toxicity is associated with the use of salicylates and salicylate-like antiinflammatory compounds following prolonged use in high doses for the treatment of arthritis. Although drugs in this class are regarded as nonaddicting, some people become chronic users of combination analgesics. In particular, combinations of aspirin, phenacetin, and caffeine (APC tablets) have been abused. Renal toxicity, which begins as papillary necrosis followed by chronic interstitial nephritis, frequently leads to renal failure in chronic users of combination analgesics.[29] Initially it was believed that phenacetin was the drug mediating the renal damage, since phenacetin was the one drug found in all combinations eliciting the toxicity. However, when administered itself even in very high doses, phenacetin does not produce renal damage characteristic of analgesic nephropathy. When renal damage results from the use of combination analgesics, the prognosis is good if none of the NSAIAs are used, rather than restricting only the use of phenacetin.[29] Kidney damage appears to result from both a reduction in prostaglandin influence on renal function and a direct toxic action of the drug on the tubular cell. Dehydration resulting in increased concentration of the interstitial fluid in the papilla augments renal damage from NSAIAs.

Blood dyscrasias resulting from drug-induced injury to the hematopoetic system include thrombocytopenia, leukocytopenia, and agranulocytosis, which is frequently fatal. NSAIAs with a higher risk of producing blood dyscrasias are mefenamic acid, phenylbutazone, and indomethacin.[11,37] Mefenamic acid is recommended for continuous use for no longer than 7 days, and probably for this reason should not be used at all. Other NSAIAs are as effective as analgesics with less risk of toxicity. Phenylbutazone and its hydroxylated metabolite oxyphenbutazone are more toxic than other NSAIAs, an effect that appears to be increased in older patients.[11] When these drugs are used in the treatment of arthritis, particularly in the elderly, frequent blood tests should be required for early detection of blood dyscrasias. Indomethacin also results in a higher incidence of blood dyscrasias than other salicylates or salicylate-like antiinflammatory drugs.

Hypersensitivity to aspirin develops in approximately 0.9% of the population. Although only a relatively small number of people are affected, the hypersensitivity to aspirin is frequently fatal.[1] Hypersensitivity or "aspirin intolerance" is defined as "acute urticaria-angioedema, bronchospasm, severe rhinitis, or shock occurring within 3 hours of aspirin ingestion."[34] The hypersensitivity response to aspirin is manifested by two distinctive symptomologies: bronchospasm and urticaria-angioedema.[34] Patients intolerant to aspirin who also experience chronic asthma, chronic urticaria, or chronic rhinitis (with or without nasal polyps) have their symptoms exacerbated by aspirin.[1,34] The use of NSAIAs in these patients should be avoided. The exact mechanism by which individuals become hypersensitive to aspirin is unknown. Since no specific antibodies for aspirin have been found in the serum of hypersensitive patients, it has been suggested that aspirin directly releases autacoids itself.[1] Perhaps a shift in the metabolism of arachidonic acid to the synthesis of a leukotriene(s) identified as the slow-reacting substance of anaphylaxis contributes to the mechanism of aspirin hypersensitivity.[32] Patients hypersensitive to aspirin frequently show a cross-reaction to other NSAIAs and to chloro-tarquin, a yellow dye used in many pharmaceutical preparations. For this reason, *no NSAIAs* should be used in patients allergic to aspirin.

Duration of Action	The duration of action of NSAIAs is variable as determined by both the pharmacokinetic properties of the drug and the endogenous turnover of cyclooxygenase. A majority of drugs in this class produce a competitive irreversible inhibition of cyclooxygenase activity.[10] Aspirin directly acetylates the enzyme, resulting in irreversible inhibition. This becomes of clinical significance when cyclooxygenase cannot be resynthesized as in the platelet. The antiplatelet action of aspirin is therefore prolonged until new platelets can be formed (8 to 12 days). For this reason aspirin use should be discontinued at least 1 week before surgery.

Drug interactions	Many salicylates and salicylate-like agents displace oral anticoagulants and other drugs such as hydantoins, sulfonylureas, and sulfonamides from plasma-binding proteins and thus increase their toxicity. The risk of gastrointestinal ulceration is increased when salicylates are administered with steroids, phenylbutazone, or alcohol. Salicylates antagonize the uricosuric effects of probenecid and sulfinpyrazone, as well as reduce the clearance and increase the toxicity of methotrexate.

PHARMACO- **KINETICS** **Aspirin** **ABSORPTION**	Aspirin, a weak acid with a pKa of 3.5, is rapidly and completely absorbed from the upper gastrointestinal tract. Factors affecting the absorption of aspirin include (1) dosage form, (2) intragastric pH, and (3) the rate of gastric emptying.[19] Dosage form is an important determinant of the rate of aspirin absorption, since only the dissolved drug is available for passive diffusion into the cell. A tablet of aspirin must first disintegrate into smaller particles, which then dissolve in the gastric juice (Fig. 31-6). The rate of dissolution is the rate-limiting step in absorption. Dosage forms of aspirin in which the drug is already dissolved (e.g., effervescent preparations [Alka Seltzer] and solutions of sodium salicylate) result in higher concentrations of salicylate in plasma as compared with those attained at similar times after ingestion of a tablet. Increasing the pH in the microenvironment surrounding the disintegrated particles promotes dissolution. This is the rationale for buffered preparations. However, buffered aspirin tablets neither prevent gastric irritation nor differ therapeutically from unbuffered preparations.[3]

Once aspirin is dissolved, the un-ionized fraction penetrates the cellular membrane of the mucosal cell by passive diffusion. The rate of absorption is then dependent on the lipid solubility of the un-ionized fraction (HA) and its concentration at the site of absorption. The pH of the gastric juice and the pKa of the drug determines the fraction of un-ionized drug available for absorption according to the Henderson-Hasselbalch equation. As illustrated in Fig. 31-6, a larger proportion of aspirin is in the un-ionized state when the pH is low as in the gastric juice. Once inside the cell this equilibrium is shifted in favor of the ionized moiety, resulting in

Absorption of aspirin.   *FIG. 31-6*

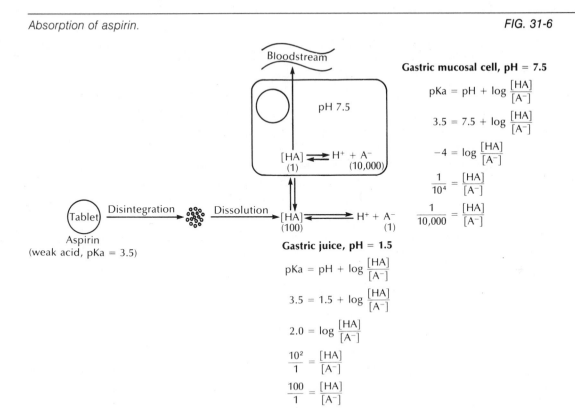

a large intracellular concentration of drug. Although some aspirin is absorbed in the stomach, more of the drug is absorbed in the duodenum and upper small intestine because of the increased surface area. Although the pH is higher in the intestine, which increases the fraction of ionized salicylate, this effect is more than compensated for by the increased surface area for absorption. Thus an increased rate of gastric emptying augments absorption of aspirin. Rectal absorption of the drug is slow and incomplete in contrast to the rapid absorption of methylsalicylate and salicylic acid from the skin. Enteric-coated aspirin is erratically absorbed, and the sustained-release preparations do not result in a prolongation of the therapeutic action.

DISTRIBUTION

Approximately 80% to 90% of aspirin in plasma is bound to protein, primarily to albumin. The unbound fraction of drug distributes rapidly throughout all body tissues by passive, pH-dependent processes.[14] Aspirin and its active metabolite salicylate are found in cerebrospinal fluid, saliva, and peritoneal and synovial fluids. Salicylate crosses the placental barrier and reaches the developing fetus. Aspirin distributes in effective concentrations to sites at which inhibition of cyclooxygenase activity results in antiinflammatory (synovium; arthritis), antipyretic (CNS), and analgesic (sites of inflammation; CNS) actions.

METABOLISM   Aspirin, or acetylsalicylic acid, is rapidly deacylated to form salicylic acid, a pharmacologically active metabolite. The half-life of acetylsalicylic acid in plasma is short, only 15 to 20 min. Salicylic acid is further metabolized, primarily in the liver, by oxidation to gentisic acid and by conjugation with both glycine to form salicyluric acid and glucuronide to form the ester and ether conjugates[7] (Fig. 31-7). The fastest rate of metabolism is via conjugation with glycine, resulting in approximately 75% of salicylate excreted as salicyluric acid.[7,14,20,21] Approximately 5% to 10% of the dose is excreted as glucuronide conjugates, and ≤1% as gentisic and gentisuric acids. The half-life of salicylate in plasma ranges from 3 to 6 hours at lower doses, reaching 15 to 30 hours after prolonged administration of high doses necessary for the treatment of arthritis.[14,20,21] This increased time for excretion of salicylate results from the saturation of enzymes required for conjugation of salicylate with both glycine and glucuronide (ether formation). Since glycine conjugation is the fastest route for me-

FIG. 31-7   *Metabolism of aspirin.*

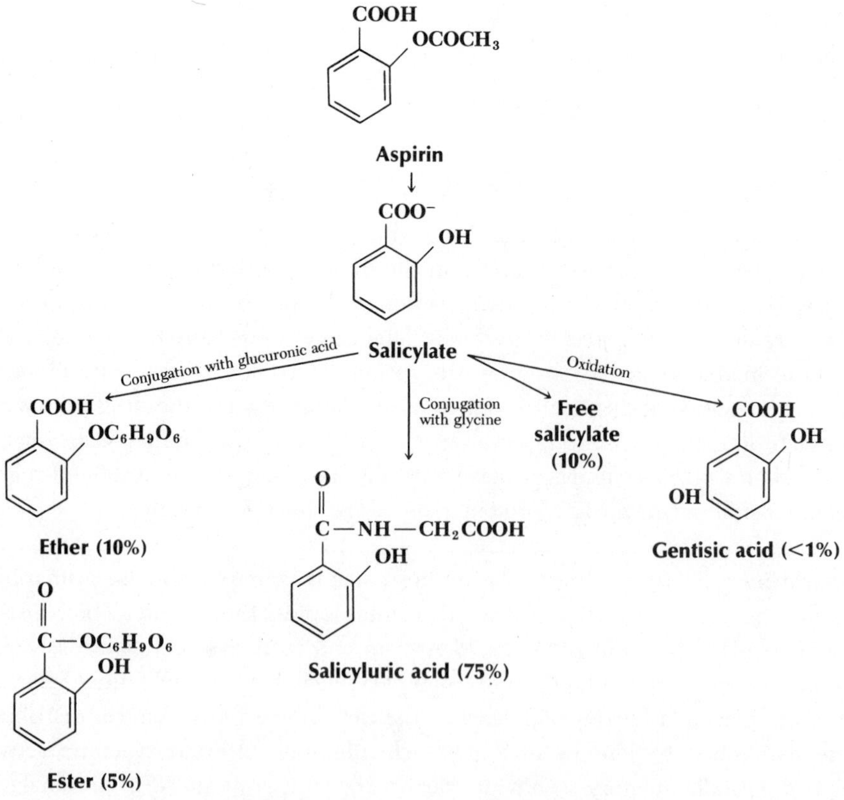

tabolism when this system becomes saturated (≥650 mg aspirin), the rate of aspirin elimination no longer follows first-order kinetics but becomes zero order.[7,21] After ingestion of ≥1 g of drug, the phenolic conjugation of glucuronide to salicylate also becomes saturated. Saturation of these metabolic pathways results in a prolongation of the half-life of free salicylate in plasma. The rate of metabolism is no longer determined by the concentration of salicylate but depends on the constant rate of enzyme(s) action. Frequently, these metabolic changes become of clinical significance when therapeutic misuse results in aspirin toxicity.

Salicylates are excreted mainly by the kidney. Salicylic and salicyluric acids are filtered at the glomerulus, then reabsorbed by passive pH-dependent processes.[11] The clearance of salicylate is increased approximately fourfold when the pH of urine is ≥8.0. At this pH, both acids are highly ionized and therefore cannot be reabsorbed from the tubular fluid. A high rate of urine flow decreases, whereas oliguria increases, reabsorption of salicylate from the renal tubule. The glucuronide conjugates of salicylic acid and gentisic acid derivatives are water-soluble organic acids and thus do not readily back-diffuse across the renal tubular cells. These metabolites are not excreted by pH-dependent processes but are filtered at the glomerulus and secreted by the organic acid transport system.

EXCRETION

Arthritis is a term meaning "inflammation of a joint." The five most common arthritic diseases are rheumatoid arthritis, osteoarthritis, ankylosing spondylitis, systemic lupus erythematosus, and gout. The NSAIAs used to reduce inflammation associated with these diseases are the salicylates and salicylate-like antiinflammatory drugs (see Chapter 48 for drugs used in the treatment of gout). NSAIAs reduce the symptoms of inflammation but do not alter the progression of the disease. There is considerable individual variability in drug responsiveness. Frequently, because of the nonselectivity of NSAIAs used to treat inflammation, side effects limit the drug's usefulness. For these reasons, treatment of patients with rheumatoid arthritis is individualized. Aspirin, 5 to 8 g/day, should be tried first, since it is the "drug of choice" in the treatment of rheumatoid arthritis. If aspirin is ineffective or not tolerated, usually tolmetin, sulindac,[6] or one of the arylalkanoic acid derivatives, is recommended. When necessary, indomethacin or phenylbutazone is used. A majority of patients with rheumatoid arthritis are responsive to one of the NSAIAs. However, some individuals require treatment with more toxic drugs such as gold salts, immunosuppressive agents, penicillamine, adrenocorticosteroids, or hydroxychloroquine. Two patient populations are exceptions to these guidelines: children and pregnant women. Only drugs such as aspirin, indomethacin or ibuprofen, which have been tested extensively in children, should be prescribed. Low doses of aspirin are probably the safest to use in pregnant women. However, aspirin should be discontinued before parturition to avoid complications to both the mother and neonate.[28,30]

CLINICAL USES
Arthritis

Pain   Salicylates and salicylate-like antipyretic analgesics are most effective in alleviating pain of mild to moderate intensity. Aspirin, acetaminophen, ibuprofen, and mefenamic acid are NSAIAs used as analgesics. Zomepirac sodium, an effective salicylate-like analgesic,[25] was recently removed from the market because of fatal hypersensitivity reactions. NSAIAs may be more effective than narcotic analgesics in alleviating pain associated with prostaglandin-stimulated smooth muscle contractions. The salicylate and salicylate-like antipyretic analgesics do not bind to opiate receptors nor are they addicting with chronic use. These drugs are less toxic and have a lower maximum effect, or efficacy, than narcotic analgesics.

Fever   Salicylates and salicylate-like antipyretic analgesics are used to lower elevated body temperature associated with fever. Aspirin and acetaminophen are NSAIAS used clinically for their antipyretic actions. Only one other NSAIA is used to treat febrile states. Indomethacin is recommended to lower the fever of Hodgkins' disease that is uncontrolled by other salicylate-like drugs.

Thromboembolism and atherosclerotic disease   A thrombus is a blood clot resulting from a pathological disturbance in blood flow or hemostasis. Thrombi formed in arterial vessels, termed *white thrombi*, are formed by platelet aggregation. Venous thrombi, or *red thrombi*, resemble a blood clot formed in vitro and are composed of a network of fibrin "enmeshed with red blood cells and platelets."[27] Arterial thrombi cause disease by local tissue ischemia, whereas the "tail" of venous thrombi frequently become dislodged, resulting in ischemic tissue damage at distant sites. Atherosclerosis is the deposition of fatty substances into the inner layer of the arteries. Atherosclerotic plaque formation is believed to result from injury to the endothelial cell, which stimulates platelet adhesion and aggregation, release of platelet constituents, migration of smooth muscle into the intima of the vessel, formation of a connective tissue matrix, and extracellular lipid accumulation.[33]

NSAIAs are used for their platelet-inhibitory action in the treatment of arterial and venous thromboembolic diseases including cerebrovascular disease (transient ischemic attacks; stroke), coronary artery disease (myocardial reinfarction), valvular heart disease (mitral valve disease; prosthetic heart valves), and pulmonary emboli.[15,33] Salicylates are currently being evaluated for prevention and/or treatment of atherosclerosis, particularly of the coronary arteries.[15,33] Although the role of platelet aggregation in atherogenesis remains controversial, inhibition of prostaglandin formation and release by NSAIAs may provide a beneficial antiplatelet action in the treatment of this disease.[15,18,33] Salicylates have been shown effective in the treatment of cerebrovascular disease and prevention of thromboembolism in patients with mechanical heart valves.[15] Aspirin, 1.3 g/day, reduces the risk of recurrent transient ischemic attacks, stroke, and death in men.[15] Women, however, do not benefit from this therapy. The secondary prevention of myocardial infarction has been evaluated in several prospective, randomized, and double-blind trials. Although favorable trends have been associated with aspirin (300 to 1500 mg/day), no significant differences have been observed.[15] The incidence of thromboembolism in patients with mechanical prosthetic heart valves has been significantly reduced by combination of oral anticoagulants and aspirin. Current recommended therapy for patients with prosthetic heart valves is first to try anticoagulants with dipyridamole. If the patient can not tolerate either drug, then an anticoagulant with aspirin (325 mg/day) or dipyridamole plus aspirin (1.3 g/day) is recommended.[15] Aspirin (1.2 to 1.5 g/day) reduces postoperative complications from venous thromboemboli and pulmonary embolism. However, it should be emphasized that secondary prophylactic treatment of pulmonary embolism and venous thrombi requires heparin and oral anticoagulants (see Chapter 37).

Dysmenorrhea

Primary dysmenorrhea (painful menstruation) results from an excess production of prostaglandins by the uterus. The prostaglandins formed stimulate smooth muscle contractions in the uterus and gastrointestinal tract, resulting in cramps, diarrhea, and vomiting.[22] Oral contraceptives, which prevent ovulation, are the recommended therapy for treatment of primary dysmenorrhea. However, ibuprofen, acetaminophen, and aspirin have been shown effective.[2,9] Although mefenamic acid also provides relief from dysmenorrhea, its use cannot be recommended because of its toxicity. Treatment with NSAIAs beginning a few days before menstruation may be most effective; however, these drugs should be administered only after menstrual flow has begun, to avoid exposure of a developing fetus to the drug. Dysmenorrhea resulting secondarily from endometriosis, intrauterine devices, pelvic inflammation, or adhesions is also relieved by NSAIAs.

Patent ductus arteriosus

The ductus arteriosus is the distal segment of the sixth aortic arch, which connects the pulmonary artery with the descending aorta, allowing blood to bypass the lungs in the developing fetus. The ductus arteriosus normally constricts during the first day of life, resulting in functional closure.[13] In some neonates, particularly in premature infants of low body weight, the ductus arteriosus does not close but remains patent after birth. Although surgical closure of the patent ductus is the preferred therapy, NSAIAs are also effective. Buffered aspirin and indomethacin promote closure of the patent ductus arteriosus and alleviate the associated symptoms of cardiac failure in the neonate. Drug-induced renal toxicity, however, restricts the use of these drugs to individuals at high risk for surgery. Early diagnosis and treatment of the patent ductus is important, since the sensitivity to closure by NSAIAs decreases with time after birth. The patency and closure of the ductus arteriosus is believed to be mediated by prostaglandins. Salicylates and salicylate-like compounds therefore most likely promote closure by inhibiting cyclooxygenase activity.

Other proposed clinical uses

Salicylates and salicylate-like compounds have also been shown effective in treating ocular inflammation, acute and chronic glomerulonephritis, Bartter's syndrome, and traveler's diarrhea. Aspirin is recommended as prophylaxic therapy in the treatment of migraine.

REFERENCES

1. Abrishami, M.A., and Thomas, J.: Aspirin intolerance—a review, Ann. Allergy 39:28, 1977.

2. Anderson, A.B.M., Fraser, I.S., Haynes, P.J., and Turnbull, A.C.: Trial of prostaglandin-synthetase inhibitors in primary dysmenorrhea, Lancet 1:345, 1978.

3. Aspirin Products, Med. Lett. Drugs Ther. 23:65, 1981.

4. Black, M.: Acetaminophen hepatotoxicity, Gastroenterology 78:382, 1980.

5. Brodie, B.B., and Axelrod, J.: The fate of acetophenetidin (phenacetin) in man and methods for the estimation of acetophenetidin and its metabolites in biological material, J. Pharmacol. Exp. Ther. 97:58, 1949.

6. Brogden, R.N., Heel, R.C., Speight, T.M., and Avery, G.S.: Sulindac: a review of its pharmacological properties and therapeutic efficacy in rheumatic diseases, Drugs 16:97, 1978.

7. Davison, C.: Salicylate metabolism in man, Ann. N.Y. Acad. Sci. 179:249, 1971.

8. Dinarello, C.A.: Production of endogenous pyrogen, Fed. Proc. 38:52, 1979.

9. Drugs for dysmenorrhea, Med. Lett. Drugs Ther. 21:81, 1979.

10. Flower, R.J.: Drugs which inhibit prostaglandin synthetase, Pharmacol. Rev. 26:33, 1974.

11. Flower, R.J., Moncada, S., and Vane, J.R.: Analgesic-antipyretics and anti-inflammatory agents: drugs employed in the treatment of gout. In Gilman, A.G., Goodman, L.S., and Gilman, A., editors: The pharmacological basis of therapeutics, New York, 1980, Macmillan Publishing Co., Inc., p. 682.

12. Forrest, J.A.H., Clements, J.A., and Prescott, L.F.: Clinical pharmacokinetics of paracetamol, Clin. Pharmacokinet. 7:93, 1982.

13. Friedman, W.F., Fitzpatrick, K.M., Merritt, T.A., and Feldman, B.H.: The patent ductus arteriosus, Clin. Perinatol. 5:411, 1978.

14. Furst, D.E., Tozer, T.N., and Melmon, K.L.: Salicylate clearance, the resultant of protein binding and metabolism, Clin. Pharmacol. Ther. 26:380, 1979.

15. Fuster, V., and Chesebro, J.H.: Antithrombotic therapy: role of platelet inhibitor drugs. III. Management of arterial thromboembolic and atherosclerotic disease, Mayo Clin. Proc. 56:265, 1981.

16. Gander, G.W., Chaffee, J., and Goodale, F.: Studies on the antipyretic action of salicylates, Proc. Soc. Exp. Biol. Med. 126:205, 1967.

17. Gorman, R.R.: Modulation of human platelet function by prostacyclin and thromboxane A_2, Fed. Proc. 38:83, 1979.

18. Haft, J.I.: Role of blood platelets in coronary artery disease, Am. J. Cardiol. 43:1197, 1979.

19. Levy, G., Gumtow, R.H., and Rutowski, J.M.: The effect of dosage form upon the gastrointestinal absorption rate of salicylates, Can. Med. Assoc. J. 85:414, 1961.

20. Levy, G.: Pharmacokinetics of salicylate elimination in man, J. Pharm. Sci. 54:959, 1965.

21. Levy, G., Vogel, A.W., and Amsel, L.P.: Capacity-limited salicylurate formation during prolonged administration of aspirin to healthy human subjects, J. Pharm. Sci. 58:503, 1969.

22. Lundstrom, V., and Green, K.: Endogenous levels of prostaglandin $F_{2\alpha}$ and its main metabolite in plasma and the endometrium of normal and dysmenorrheic women, Am. J. Obstet. Gynecol. 130:640, 1978.

23. Michell, J.R., Thorgeirsson, S.S., Potter, W.Z., Jollow, D.J., and Keiser, H.: Acetaminophen-induced hepatic injury: protective role of glutathione in man and rationale for therapy, Clin. Pharmacol. Ther. 16:676, 1974.

24. Moncada, S., and Vane, J.R.: Mode of action of aspirin-like drugs, Adv. Intern. Med. 24:1, 1979.

25. Morley, P.A., Brogden, R.N., Carmine, A.A., Heel, R.C., Speight, T.M., and Avery, G.S.: Zomepirac: A review of its pharmacological properties and analgesics efficacy, Drugs 23:250, 1982.

26. Nickander, R., McMahon, F.G., and Ridolfo, A.S.: Nonsteroidal anti-inflammatory agents, Ann. Rev. Pharmacol. Toxicol. **19**:469, 1979.

27. O'Reilly, R.A.: Anticoagulant, antithrombotic, and thrombolytic drugs. In Gilman, A.G., Goodman, L.S., and Gilman, A., editors: The pharmacological basis of therapeutics, New York, 1980, Macmillan Publishing Co., Inc., p. 1347.

28. PG-synthetase inhibitors in obstetrics and after, Lancet **2**:185, 1980.

29. Prescott, L.F.: Analgesic nephropathy: a reassessment of the role of phenacetin and other analgesics, Drugs **23**:75, 1982.

30. Rudolph, A.M.: Effects of aspirin and acetaminophen in pregnancy and in the newborn, Arch. Intern. Med. **141**:358, 1981.

31. Ruffalo, R.L., and Thompson, J.F.: Cimetidine and acetylcysteine as antidote for acetaminophen overdose, South. Med. J. **75**:954, 1982.

32. Samuelsson, B.: Prostaglandins, thromboxanes, and leukotrienes: formation and biological roles, The Harvey Lectures, Series 75, New York, 1981, Academic Press, Inc., p. 1.

33. Saunders, R.N.: Evaluation of platelet-inhibiting drugs in models of atherosclerosis, Ann. Rev. Pharmacol. Toxicol. **22**:279, 1982.

34. Settipane, G.A.: Adverse reactions to aspirin and related drugs, Arch. Intern. Med. **141**:328, 1981.

35. Smith, J.B., and Willis, A.L.: Aspirin selectively inhibits prostaglandin production in human platelets, Nature (New Biol.) **231**:235, 1971.

36. Stitt, J.T.: Fever versus hyperthermia, Fed. Proc. **38**:39, 1979.

37. Toxicity of nonsteroidal anti-inflammatory drugs, Med. Lett. Drugs Ther. **24**:15, 1983.

38. Vane, J.R.: Inhibition of prostaglandin synthesis as a mechanism of action of aspirin-like drugs, Nature **231**:232, 1971.

39. Yu, T.F., and Gutman, A.B.: Study of the paradoxical effects of salicylate in low, intermediate, and high dosage on the renal mechanisms for excretion of urate in man, J. Clin. Invest. **38**:1298, 1959.

section five

Anesthetics

Chapter 32

Pharmacology of general anesthesia

GENERAL
CONCEPT

The scope of anesthesiology touches nearly every specialty of medicine. Drugs that allow painless, controlled surgical, obstetrical, and diagnostic procedures constitute one of the cornerstones of modern-day pharmacological therapy. It is estimated that 20 million anesthetics are administered annually in the United States alone.

The hallmark of anesthetic drugs is *controllability*. For this reason, most of the potent anesthetics are gases or vapors. Such drugs can be administered at required dosages via the lungs with consequent rapid uptake into the systemic circulation. Elimination of these drugs is also primarily by the pulmonary route. Unlike "fixed" or nonvolatile drugs, elimination and pharmacological termination of action therefore do not depend on intrinsic hepatic biotransformation or renal excretion; rather they depend on a pulmonary process, which can be actively controlled by the anesthesiologist. The lungs possess a large surface area, which can be utilized for precise dosage administration or elimination.

Anesthetics are nonspecific; that is, they do not function by means of interaction with specific receptors. As a corollary to this general action, there are no specific antagonists to anesthetics. Inhalation anesthetics should produce all of the following characteristics, although there may be quantitative differences among various drugs: (1) hypnosis, (2) analgesia (freedom from pain), (3) skeletal muscle relaxant properties, and (4) reduction of certain autonomic reflexes. When combined, these four attributes constitute the definition of general anesthesia.

Selection of a particular anesthetic or combination of anesthetics is predicated on the patient's pathophysiological state and the nature of the anticipated surgical procedure. Anesthetics differ in degrees of depression of various organ systems, in potency, in speed of induction and awakening, in degree of skeletal muscle relaxation, and in other effects. Thus one anesthetic may be superior to another, depending on the clinical circumstances. Final selection of an anesthetic or anesthetic sequence is based on three factors in order: (1) those drugs and anesthesia techniques judged to be safest for the patient, (2) drugs and techniques facilitating performance of the

TABLE 32-1 Distribution of inhalation anesthetic concentrations in various biophases following partial pressure equilibrium

| | Biophase | | |
Anesthetic	Blood	Lean tissue	Fat
Concentration at equilibrium	3 mM ⇌	6 mM ⇌	660 mM
Partial pressure at equilibrium	8 mm Hg ⇌	8 mm Hg ⇌	8 mm Hg

surgical procedure, and (3) techniques most acceptable to the patient. The last factor is generally a judgment between general and regional (e.g., spinal) anesthesia.

Popular potent organohalogen inhalation anesthetics include enflurane, isoflurane, and halothane. Isoflurane is the newest halogenated anesthetic in clinical practice. Nitrous oxide, a weak gaseous anesthetic, is frequently used in combination with these volatile compounds or with intermittent dosages of fixed intravenous drugs such as barbiturates (for hypnosis), narcotics (for analgesia), and neuromuscular blockers (for skeletal muscle relaxation). Use of nitrous oxide in this latter circumstance is termed *balanced anesthesia*. The older anesthetics cyclopropane and diethyl ether are used infrequently because of flammability. This feature is inconsistent with modern operating suites loaded with cautery and electronic monitoring gear.

The intravenous anesthetics are used for specific purposes or to supplement inhalation anesthetics but lack controllability and other salutary features of the inhalation anesthetics. Thiobarbiturates (e.g., thiopental) are still highly preferred induction agents, as they rapidly and pleasantly produce hypnosis. Lack of analgesic and muscle relaxant properties and slow elimination limit both dose and usefulness. Narcotics such as morphine and the more rapidly eliminated fentanyl are frequently used to supplement nitrous oxide anesthesia. Combinations of narcotics and tranquilizers, such as fentanyl plus droperidol (Innovar), are employed commonly with nitrous oxide. The sobriquet "dissociative anesthesia" has been given to the effect of certain phencyclidine drugs such as ketamine. Such drugs have limited scope, however, as they do not allow for other than superficial procedures and often have prolonged effects including abnormal psychic reactions.

POTENCY AND EFFICACY

Because volatile and gaseous anesthetics distribute and reach equilibrium in the body by virtue of partial pressure, it is convenient to establish potency in terms of this physical characteristic rather than the more conventional ED_{50}. The minimal anesthetic concentration (MAC) is defined as *that concentration of anesthetic (in v/v percent or mm Hg) measured in end-tidal gas, which prevents response to a standard painful stimulus in 50% of humans or test animals*. In the clinical situation anesthetics are usually given in multiples of MAC (1.5 to 2.5 × MAC). Several factors change MAC. These include circadian rhythm, body temperature (direct proportional

Schematic illustrating derivation of blood-gas solubility coefficient (λ). Gas or vapor is inhaled into lungs perfused with pulmonary arterial blood. Anesthetic partial pressure in lungs is high initially and absent in blood. Anesthetic molecules diffuse into blood and reach partial pressure equilibrium. Because of solubility coefficient, partial pressure equilibrium results in concentration differences in anesthetic. Anesthetic of low blood-gas coefficient will have fewer molecules in blood than in gas phase; high coefficient produces fewer molecules in gas than in blood at equilibrium.   **FIG. 32-1**

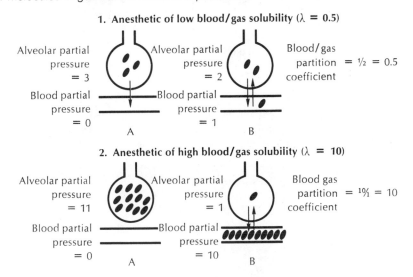

decrease), age (direct proportional decrease), other drugs (sedative, hypnotic, anesthetics, and other CNS depressants decrease MAC). Factors that do not influence MAC include sex, species, state of oxygenation, acid-base changes, and arterial blood pressure changes.

SOLUBILITY

Anesthetic gases and vapors are soluble in blood, tissue fluids, and tissues. Anesthetics in general are quite lipophilic. Since various tissues and fluids differ in lipid content, any particular gas or vapor will distribute to an eventual equilibrium with different concentrations in biophases, depending on solubility of the anesthetic. Table 32-1 illustrates this effect with a hypothetical inhalation anesthetic at equilibrium. Note that although the partial pressure of the anesthetic in all phases is the same, the concentration of those tissues varies several hundredfold. This is caused by the difference in solubility of the drug in various tissues. Table 32-1 illustrates the large fat-storage capacity of an anesthetic due to its high lipophilic nature.

There are three solubility coefficients germane to anesthetic distribution. All are based on Henry's law and are temperature dependent. For clinical purposes these coefficients are measured at 37° C.

1. *Blood-gas partition coefficient (λ).* This is the most important solubility parameter for understanding uptake of inhaled gases and vapors. Fig. 32-1 illustrates

FIG. 32-2   *Flow of anesthetic gases and vapors from anesthesia machine to peripheral tissues.*

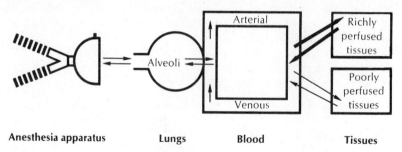

Anesthesia apparatus   **Lungs**   **Blood**   **Tissues**

FIG. 32-3   *Equilibrium curve for two anesthetics. Note that anesthetic with lower blood-gas solubility approaches equilibrium much faster than anesthetic with higher solubility. Anesthetic with lower solubility will achieve state of anesthesia more rapidly.*

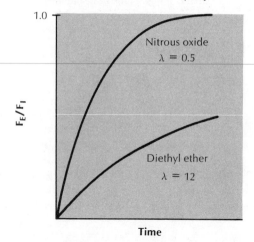

how this coefficient is derived. It will be noted from this figure that when equilibrium is reached, the end-tidal concentration of the anesthetic in the alveoli (*upward-directed arrows*) is proportional to the pulmonary blood concentration. Thus end-tidal concentration or partial pressure (abbreviated F_E) can be used as a measure of degree of equilibrium steady-state. The partial pressure of anesthetics being administered to the lungs for uptake by the blood is inspired alveolar partial pressure (F_I). Thus when $F_E/F_I = 1$, blood-gas equilibrium has been reached.

2. *Tissue solubility.* Anesthetics enter the lungs, are picked up by pulmonary arterial blood, and then are distributed to peripheral tissues. Obviously, those organs with the highest degree of blood flow per unit time will receive more anesthetic molecules than organs with lower flow. Richly perfused organs include brain, heart, liver, and kidney; skeletal muscle perfusion is intermediate; lowest perfusion goes

TABLE 32-2   MAC, blood-gas, and oil-gas partition coefficients for six general anesthetics

Anesthetic	MAC in humans (v/v%)	Blood-gas (λ)	Oil-gas
Halothane $CF_3CHBrCl$	0.78	2.3	224
Enflurane CF_2HOCF_2CFClH	1.7	1.8	98
Diethyl ether $(C_2H_5)_2O$	2.0	12.1	65
Isoflurane $CF_3CClHOCF_2H$	1.3	1.4	99
Nitrous oxide N_2O	188*	0.4	1.4
Methoxyflurane $CCl_2HCF_2OCH_3$	0.16	12.0	970

*Extrapolated data.

to bone, ligaments, and fat. The blood and tissue partition coefficient is usually between 1 and 2 for most anesthetics. Fat solubility is much higher, however. At times it exceeds blood solubility several hundredfold. As a result of the combination of low flow and high solubility, it is apparent that body fat requires a long time to achieve complete equilibrium. In Fig. 32-2 transfer of anesthetics from the anesthesia machine to peripheral tissues is demonstrated.

3. *Oil-gas partition coefficient.* This partition coefficient is an artificial one in certain respects because the oil commonly used, olive oil, is not a biological constituent of the body. However, olive oil has certain solubility characteristics similar to body fat and correlates with it. Lipid solubility of anesthetics is proportional to potency. This is the basis of the Meyer-Overton correlation of directly proportional fat solubility to anesthetic potency. Thus a high oil-gas partition coefficient indicates a potent anesthetic (e.g., one with low MAC and low partial pressure required for anesthesia). This correlation does nothing to define mechanism of anesthesia but can be used to predict MAC. In fact, the correlation between MAC and the oil-gas partition of inhalation anesthetics is essentially linear.

Importance of blood-gas partition coefficient in speed of induction. A low blood-gas partition coefficient of an anesthetic gas dictates that uptake of the anesthetic will occur rapidly, and consequently induction will be rapid (e.g., FE/FI = 1 will be attained rapidly). Because such a gas or vapor is relatively insoluble, equilibrium with blood is quickly attained. Thus clinical induction of anesthesia is rapid with such an agent. On the other hand, a high blood-gas solubility mandates a long time interval before blood-gas equilibrium is attained. This implies a slow induction. Due to the higher solubility, it takes a longer time for the blood to become equilibrated with molecules of anesthetic. Therefore attainment of final partial pressure required for anesthesia is delayed. The difference between the speed of eventual equilibrium of an inhalation anesthetic of low blood-gas partition coefficient compared with one of high blood-gas partition coefficient is seen in Fig. 32-3. Table 32-2 lists MAC, blood-gas, and oil-gas partition coefficients for six commonly employed inhalation anesthetics.

UPTAKE OF AN ANESTHETIC

Ventilation with an inhaled anesthetic causes a rapid rise in alveolar anesthetic partial pressure or concentration (F_I). The rise in F_I is antagonized by uptake into arterial pulmonary blood, removing the gas or vapor from the lungs. Arterial blood containing anesthetic then distributes the anesthetic to peripheral tissues. Uptake of the anesthetic by any tissue is a function of solubility, blood flow to the tissues, and the arterial to tissue anesthetic partial pressure difference. The partial pressure difference acts as the driving force. When the partial pressure difference is zero, no uptake occurs.

Uptake from the lungs (as from any tissue) is directly related to three variables: (1) blood-gas partition coefficient of the anesthetic, (2) cardiac output ($\dot{Q}$), and (3) alveolar to venous anesthetic partial pressure difference. As described before, when equilibrium at one partial pressure particular is attained, uptake falls to zero. The time to such equilibrium depends on the peripheral tissue capacity, which is related to the particular volume and capacity of the tissue concerned. In summary:

$$\text{Uptake} = \lambda \cdot \dot{Q} \cdot (P_A - P_V)/BP$$

where

$$
\begin{aligned}
(P_A - P_V) &= (\text{Alveolar} - \text{Venous partial pressure of anesthetic}) \\
\dot{Q} &= \text{Cardiac output} \\
\lambda &= \text{Blood-gas partition coefficient} \\
BP &= \text{Barometric pressure}
\end{aligned}
$$

An increase in any of these factors will increase uptake. It is worthwhile noting that if uptake of an anesthetic is plotted graphically, the resulting curve is reciprocal of the equilibrium curve.

Factors that prevent zero uptake

There are several variables that prevent or slow the equilibrium curve from reaching the $F_E/F_I = 1$ state. Because of these, equilibrium is slowed.

1. *Fat solubility*. Because of the poor perfusion and large storage solubility characteristics of general anesthetics, body fat may take hours or even days to achieve total equilibrium with alveolar anesthetic partial pressure.

2. *Biotransformation of anesthetics*. Inhalation anesthetics interact with microsomal enzyme systems and are metabolized. Actually, the degree of metabolism is small compared with the overabundance of drug molecules given during the course of an anesthetic. Obviously, metabolism limits obtaining complete equilibrium. However, unlike fixed drugs, such degradation has little if any effect on the conduct or dosage requirements of the anesthetic. On the other hand, biotransformation of inhalation anesthetics may well be a vector of viscerotoxicity of the halogenated anesthetics.

3. *Diffusion through skin into bowel and air spaces.* Diffusion of anesthetic through the skin into the atmosphere is a source of loss preventing complete equilibrium. Typical losses include nitrous oxide ($F_I = 70\%$) 2.5 ml/min/M^2 and halothane ($F_I = 0.9\%$) 0.006 ml/min/M^2. Anesthetics given at a high F_I such as nitrous oxide replace nitrogen in bowel and air spaces (e.g., middle ear, pneumothorax, brain ventricular air from pneumoencephalography). Since nitrous oxide is more soluble than nitrogen at the same partial pressure, when it passes from a dissolved state in blood to an air space, it expands to a larger volume than the nitrogen it replaces. Enlargement of brain ventricles filled with air from pneumoencephalography can cause herniation through the foramen magnum. Enlargement of a preexisting pneumothorax can occur via the same mechanism. In this manner nitrous oxide anesthesia produces variable increases in bowel volume.

Basically, the concentration effect stipulates that the higher the inspired concentration of an anesthetic, the faster the rate of rise to equilibrium. In theory, the equilibrium curves in Fig. 32-3 should be independent of the concentration or partial pressure of the anesthetic inspired. In practice, this is not so. High concentrations give a more rapid initial rise toward an equilibrium state than low (subanesthetic) concentrations. To understand this effect, imagine an inspired concentration of an anesthetic to be 100% ($F_I = 1.0$). If this 100% concentration fills the alveoli, regardless of uptake into blood, the remaining end-tidal alveolar concentration will be 100% ($F_E = 1.0$) even though total lung volume is reduced. Actually, the concentration effect is seen only with nitrous oxide given in relatively high concentrations ($F_I = 0.5$ to 0.7). Under these circumstances there is rapid uptake of a significant portion of the anesthetic into the blood. In order to maintain lung volume there is literal sucking of anesthetic mixtures from the reservoir of the anesthesia machine into the lungs. The nitrous oxide from this source mixes with residual alveolar nitrous oxide to increase partial pressure of the anesthetic at end-tidal ventilation. Thus this mixing produces a higher F_E than would be expected, and the F_E/F_I ratio approaches 1.0 quickly.

Concentration effect

Uptake of large volumes of a first or primary gas given in high concentrations (the "concentration effect") accelerates the alveolar rate of rise for a second gas given simultaneously. Thus the second gas in low concentrations achieves equilibrium faster than if it were given in the absence of the primary, high-concentration gas. Clinically, nitrous oxide (the primary gas) is given in high concentrations ($F_I = 0.5$ to 0.7) with low concentrations of a potent anesthetic such as halothane or enflurane ($F_I = 0.005$ to 0.02). Because of the second gas effect, actually a spin-off of the concentration effect, the potent low-concentration anesthetic will reach equilibrium faster than if it had been administered in oxygen alone.

Second gas effect

Effects of ventilation

An increase in minute alveolar ventilation ($\dot{V}A$) obviously causes a more rapid rise in FE regardless of partition coefficients because more molecules of anesthetic are presented to the alveoli per unit time. However, uptake of anesthetics of high solubility is altered more than uptake of anesthetics of low solubility by increases in ventilation.

1. *High-solubility anesthetics ($\lambda > 1.0$).* Increasing $\dot{V}A$ causes a large increase in FE per unit time. The reason is that the blood has a large capacity for soluble anesthetics. When blood is exposed to more molecules of higher solubility anesthetics, more of these molecules can be taken up. This causes increases in the partial pressure of anesthetics in the blood manifested as an increase in FE partial pressure.

2. *Low-solubility drugs ($\lambda < 1.0$).* An increase in number of anesthetic molecules presented to pulmonary arterial blood per unit time with an agent of low solubility does not increase uptake (hence arterial blood partial pressure and FE) to a great extent. The insoluble anesthetic reaches equilibrium with blood rapidly with only a relatively small number of molecules. Being near saturation with the low capacity for these drugs, the blood can pick up only a few of the extra molecules presented to it with an increase in $\dot{V}A$.

The clinical corollary of uptake changes produced by increases in $\dot{V}A$ are obvious. Higher-solubility anesthetics are taken up rapidly with forced artificial ventilation. They may quickly reach dangerous concentration levels in tissues and blood. On the other hand, it is generally safe to hyperventilate patients with anesthetics of low solubility, since the effect is less with these insoluble anesthetics.

Effects of cardiac output

An increase in cardiac output ($\dot{Q}$) lowers FE, as there is more pulmonary arterial blood available for uptake of the anesthetic per unit time. Low-solubility anesthetics are altered to a lesser extent than are high-solubility anesthetics so that this latter group of anesthetics are more influenced by cardiac output changes. The clinical corollaries of this fact are (1) anesthetic depression of cardiac output can alter its own uptake as the alveolar end-tidal rate of rise (FE) is rapid with decreased cardiac output; and (2) highly soluble anesthetics rapidly reach equilibrium with depressed cardiac output. In shock states, use of soluble anesthetics can thus excessively depress an already compromised circulation if care is not taken.

To summarize the salient features of uptake and distribution of inhaled gases and vapors, the blood-gas partition coefficient is the most important physical constant establishing speed of induction of an anesthetic. The lower this coefficient, the faster pulmonary blood reaches equilibrium with a given anesthetic partial pressure and hence the faster the induction of anesthesia. Awakening from anesthesia is similar. The lower the solubility, the faster the awakening as the anesthetic rapidly dissipates from pulmonary venous blood into alveoli and is exhaled. The concentration and second gas effects hasten induction of an inhalation anesthetic. Changes in ventilation and cardiac output have opposite effects—increasing ventilation causes an increase in the rise to equilibrium (more prominent with soluble anesthetics) and increased cardiac output slows the rate of equilibrium. In clinical practice these and factors such as ventilation/perfusion inequalities, alterations of regional blood flow, volume status, degree of circulatory depression, and the pathophysiological status of the patient are taken into account during the conduct of general anesthesia.

Early pioneers in the field of anesthesia such as W.T.G. Morton, John Snow, and Arthur Guedel recognized that there is a progression of predictable physiological changes produced during anesthesia. The signs and stages of diethyl ether anesthesia with increasing depth were characterized by Guedel as follows:

STAGES AND SIGNS OF ANESTHESIA

Stage I Analgesia
Stage II Delirium
Stage III Surgical anesthesia
  Phase 1. Sleep and analgesia. Patient unresponsive to surgical stimulations. Pupils constricted and eyes moist. Intercostal ventilation (arterial blood concentration = 110 mg/100 ml).
  Phase 2. Pupils dilate and eyes dry. Beginning intercostal paralysis with increased diaphragmatic ventilation (arterial blood concentration = 120 mg/100 ml).
  Phase 3. Increasing skeletal muscle relaxation. Intercostal activity markedly decreased, diaphragmatic ventilation predominates. Tidal volume falls. Corneal reflexes absent with dilated pupils. (Arterial blood concentration = 130 mg/100 ml).
  Phase 4. Onset of complete intercostal paralysis; ends with diaphragmatic paralysis. Circulatory depression. Pupils maximally dilate. (Arterial blood concentration = 140 to 160 mg/100 ml).
Stage IV Medullary paralysis; failure of ventilation and circulation

Although evaluation of the patient anesthetized with diethyl ether is rather straightforward, newer more potent anesthetics with lower solubilities pass through these various phases faster. In addition, the overall pharmacological effects are somewhat different, although the end result is similar. Basically the new, more rapid anesthetics can be categorized into two stages: the stage of analgesia and delirium and the stage of surgical anesthesia. This latter stage is divided into light, moderate, and deep. With progressive deepening of surgical anesthesia there are parallel diminutions in ventilation and circulatory integrity. Death can occur from medullary paralysis and circulatory arrest in the absence of hypoxia with overdosage of potent anesthetics. As a general rule, deepening levels of the newer halogenated anesthetics produces the following effects in a dose-dependent fashion:

1. Decreased blood pressure caused by peripheral vasodilatation and/or direct cardiac contractility decrease
2. Decreased alveolar minute ventilation because of reduced tidal volumes (Ventilation becomes more diaphragmatic in nature as anesthesia deepens.)
3. Constriction and centering of the pupils in medium levels of surgical anesthesia that proceeds to pupillary dilatation with onset of deep anesthesia (Increased lacrimation is noted in light surgical levels of anesthesia, but the eyes are dry during deep levels.)

FIG. 32-4   *Schematic of, **A**, closed anesthesia system and **B**, pediatric valveless system. **A**, 1, Vaporizer for volatile liquid anesthetics; 2, compressed gas source; 3, inhalation unidirectional valve; 4, mask; 5, unidirectional exhalation valve; 6, rebreathing bag; and 7, carbon dioxide absorption chamber. **B**, 1, Vaporizer for volatile liquid anesthetics; 2, compressed gas source; 3, mask; 4, rebreathing bag; and 5, gas exhaust port.*

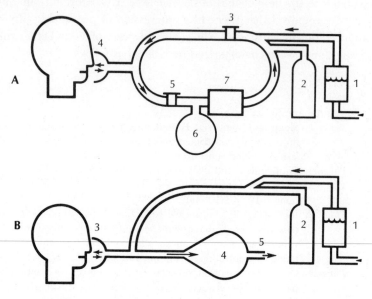

<table>
<tr><td>METHODS OF
ADMINISTRATION
OF GENERAL
ANESTHETICS</td></tr>
</table>

METHODS OF ADMINISTRATION OF GENERAL ANESTHETICS

The anesthetic gases and vapors are customarily administered to the lungs via an anesthesia machine. The basic components of an anesthesia machine include

1. Steel cylinders containing anesthetic gases and oxygen under pressure. Reduction valves lower the extremely high pressures of the cylinders to usable pressures conducive to flow gradients.
2. Flowmeters that accurately measure minute flow of gases.
3. Calibrated vaporizers. These are containers of a high heat capacity metal such as copper, filled with liquid anesthetic. A sintered bronze disk in the bottom of the vaporizer disperses in-flowing oxygen into small bubbles, which vaporize the liquid anesthetic in precision fashion. Volatile anesthetics such as halothane and enflurane are vaporized to permit the administration of precise amounts.
4. A carbon dioxide absorber.
5. A rebreathing bag.
6. Connecting tubing.
7. Unidirectional valves.

Although open drop and insufflation techniques were used in the past, they are only of historical interest now. The closed system and the semiclosed systems are used commonly for adult patients at present; the nonrebreathing, nonvalvular systems are used for pediatric patients. A description, including the advantages and disadvantages of these systems, follows:

1. *Closed system:* Economical; prevents excess anesthetics from polluting operating room; conserves heat and respiratory moisture; more difficult to calculate anesthetic dosage.
2. *Semiclosed system:* Easy to calculate anesthetic dose; not economical because gases are expelled into environment and system loses heat and moisture.
3. *Nonrebreathing, nonvalvular system:* Low resistance highly suitable for pediatric patients; loses heat and contributes to operating room pollution of trace anesthetic concentrations.

Fig. 32-4 illustrates the schematics of each of these systems. Administration of gases and vapors from the anesthesia machine is accomplished either by face mask or endotracheal tube.

The mechanism by which anesthetics work is not known. Inhaled anesthetics possess no unique molecular configuration that can be associated with a particular structure-activity relationship. Interaction with cellular components is by means of van der Waals forces only. The anesthetics are nonspecific and change the function of all cellular constituents.

THEORIES OF GENERAL ANESTHESIA

Effects of anesthetics have been attributed to blocks of ionic channels and alterations of neurotransmitter release, but these actions cannot be correlated well enough to evolve a unitary hypothesis of mechanism of action. Several theories of anesthesia have been postulated, but all have been found to be deficient in certain respects.

1. *Biochemical hypothesis.* Quastel theorized that anesthetics depress cellular respiration. This theory was postulated on the finding that certain anesthetics decrease adenosine triphosphate (ATP) production and cellular oxygen utilization in vitro. However, brain ATP concentration is not reduced by anesthetics in vivo.
2. *Hydrate theory.* Pauling and Miller postulated that anesthetic molecules form gas hydrates or structured water, which inhibit brain function at crucial sites. However, recent studies have demonstrated that correlation of hydrate formation and potency of inhalation anesthetics is very poor.
3. *Ionic pore theory.* Another theorized mechanism of anesthesia attributes the state to block of ionic channels by interaction of anesthetic molecules with membranes. In many cases, high pressures can reverse anesthetics, perhaps by changing membrane structure so that the anesthetics can no longer interact at these sites. However, this theory has poor correlation with the lipid solubility of anesthetics.

The Meyer-Overton correlation with fat solubility has stood the test of time. In general, the more lipid soluble an anesthetic, the more potent it is. However, this is a correlation only rather than a mechanism of the anesthesia state. It is difficult to imagine that anesthetics act on lipids only, and many organic solvents are quite fat soluble without appreciable anesthetic effects.

| INTRAVENOUS ANESTHETICS | Certain types of fixed drugs are classified as anesthetics, although it should be remembered that they are incomplete and do not have the controllability of the inhaled drugs. |

| Barbiturates | Barbiturates used intravenously to produce or supplement hypnosis during anesthesia are highly lipid-soluble molecules. They follow many of the distribution characteristics of the inhaled anesthetics. It must be remembered that barbiturates are hypnotics only and do not possess analgesic or muscle relaxant activity except with gross overdosage. Two barbiturates, thiopental and methohexital, are commonly employed. |

Thiopental sodium (Pentothal) is a potent ultrashort-acting thiobarbiturate, which is the sulfur analog of pentobarbital (Nembutal). The thio-group gives the drug greater lipid solubility, hence fosters penetration of the blood-brain barrier. Although barbiturates are organic acids, the pH has to be increased to 10 (as the sodium salt) to produce aqueous solubility.

Thiopental sodium

Thiopental is depressive to both circulation and ventilation. The drug is commonly used to produce a smooth, pleasant induction of anesthesia. It has no viscerotoxic effects, and overdosage is marked by an extension of pharmacological effects (i.e., marked circulatory and ventilatory depression with upper airway obstruction).

Termination of action of this, and other intravenously administered barbiturates, is due to both redistribution and metabolism. Plasma levels fall rapidly as the drug is taken up by richly perfused organs. It is then distributed to muscle and eventually to fatty tissues. Awakening occurs with normal therapeutic dosages within 15 minutes, about the time skeletal muscle is reaching saturation. Metabolism of the barbiturate is extensive, with less than 5% being excreted unchanged by the kidney. Metabolism begins as soon as the barbiturate is administered but is not as important in terminating activity as redistribution. **Thiamylal** (Surital) is a thiobarbiturate similar to thiopental.

Methohexital (Brevital) is an ultrashort-acting oxybarbiturate. It was designed to have a slightly shorter duration of hypnosis than thiopental, but clinically this difference is not always apparent.

Contraindications to the use of intravenous barbiturates include shock states and asthma. Barbiturates exacerbate the metabolic disease acute intermittent porphyria and should not be used in such patients. Inadvertent intraarterial injections of barbiturates can induce severe arterial spasm and thrombosis followed by gangrene of the extremities. Barbiturates are given intravenously in 1.0% to 2.5% solutions.

Innovar is a trade name for the combination of a narcotic analgesic, fentanyl, and *Innovar* a butyrophenone tranquilizer, droperidol. Each milliliter contains 0.05 mg fentanyl and 2.5 mg droperidol. The drug combination is used as a supplement to nitrous oxide anesthesia. Fentanyl has a relatively short duration of action and is used by itself as a narcotic-analgesic during anesthesia. Fentanyl is now use extensively as a major narcotic-analgesic for many open-heart procedures. The lack of cardiovascular effects of the narcotic underlies the reasons for such employment. Dosages employed for these techniques are large, approximately 50 µg/kg or higher, administered intravenously. Conventional doses of fentanyl for routine surgery vary from 3.0 to 5.0 µg/kg, administered intravenously.

The combination is a useful adjuvant to balanced anesthesia. Fentanyl, like all narcotics, severely depresses ventilation. A peculiar increase in chest wall muscle tone, termed *wooden rigidity*, is occasionally observed if the narcotic is injected rapidly intravenously. Rarely droperidol produces a parkinsonian-type extrapyramidal reaction in certain individuals. The anesthetic-like state produced by Innovar has been termed *neurolept-anesthesia*. Innovar, given by the intramuscular route, is also used for preoperative medication in certain patients.

Ketamine hydrochloride is a phencyclidine derivative capable of producing a *Ketamine* trance-like state with freedom from pain, termed *dissociative anesthesia*. The drug is given either intravenously or intramuscularly. Ketamine produces little to no muscular relaxation. Patients will respond to visceral pain but not to superficial pain under the influence of ketamine. It frequently produces psychic problems when used in adults. These have been described as terrifying dreams and severe distortions of reality. For that reason use of ketamine is usually limited to that of an anesthetic for superficial procedures in infants and children. Ketamine stimulates the sympathetic nervous system so that there may be an increase in blood pressure. It frequently increases salivation. Ketamine raises intracranial pressure and is thus relatively contraindicated in the presence of CNS tumors or space-occupying lesions. Ketamine is available in solutions of 10 mg/ml for intravenous use and 50 mg/ml for intramuscular administration.

Ketamine

Etomidate (Amidate) is an intravenous anesthetic induction drug recently intro- *Etomidate* duced into clinical practice in the United States. It is an imidazole congener and quite distinct from other drugs in this class. Etomidate is hypnotic only and possesses no analgesic properties. Intravenous dose is 0.3 to 0.4 mg/kg.

Hallmarks of the drug include rapid biotransformation by liver and kidney, which contributes to a very brief duration of action. Clinically there are essentially no cardiovascular or ventilatory depressive actions. Animal studies have demonstrated that the drug has a wider margin of safety than thiopental or methohexital. Thus etomidate may have desirable characteristics as an induction drug for certain poor risk pocedures. Disadvantages include involuntary skeletal muscle cotractions and painful injection, which can lead to thrombophlebitis. These adverse reactions limit use of etomidate for routine anesthetic induction. The venous irritant action is believed caused by the vehicle propylene glycol, which must be employed for solubility. Adrenal steroid depletion has recently been reported following administration and may limit the usefulness of this drug.

PREANESTHETIC MEDICATION

Several classes of drugs are frequently given before the induction of anesthesia. The primary objectives are to produce an anxiety-free, sedated patient. Additional reasons to give such medications include depression of vagal tone and as supplements to the anesthetic drugs. Individual drugs used for preanesthtic medication are describe in the following categories:

1. *Anticholinergics:* Atropine, scopolamine, and glycopyrrolate are frequently given intramuscularly before anesthesia to decrease vagal cardiac tone and to block bronchial secretions. The value of such muscarinic blockers is less now than when secretion-producing irritant anesthetics such as cyclopropane and diethyl ether were used.

2. *Narcotics:* Analgesics such as meperidine (Demerol), morphine, and fentanyl (Sublimaze) are given to decrease anxiety and as a narcotic supplement to anesthesia. These drugs all produce certain degrees of respiratory depression by themselves, which is increased when combined with anesthetics.

3. *Sedatives:* Barbiturates, primarily the short-acting drugs secobarbital (Seconal) and pentobarbital (Nembutal), are given to allay anxiety and produce a drowsy patient.

4. *Benzodiazepines:* Diazepam (Valium) given orally or intravenously produces sedation and some amnesia without significant detriments to circulation or to ventilation. For this reason, drugs of this class are now quite frequently employed as preanesthetic medications.

All the preanesthetic drugs possess certain disadvantages such as respiratory depression, and so on. Thus use is dependent on intimate pharmacological and pathological knowledge and clinical judgement. As important as the premedicant drugs are in allaying the patient's anxieties, of equal importance is the psychological rapport made by the anesthesiologist.

PHARMACOLOGICAL EFFECTS OF ANESTHETICS

Because of the ubiquitous nature of anesthetic distribution and the nonspecific effect on all cellular functions, discussion of the specific organ effects from these drugs is frequently incomplete. Although anesthetics in general are depressants to function, there are many quantitative differences in these actions. To add complexity, each of the anesthetics differs qualitatively in this regard.

Anesthetics depress all portions of the CNS. There is no single site or locus of effect; however, there are considerable regional differences. It is believed that the higher cortical centers and the ascending reticular activating system are the most susceptible portions of the brain to anesthetics. This is a dose-dependent phenomenon. As anesthetic concentration in the brain increases, lower centers are depressed. This eventually leads to respiratory and circulatory arrest, the mechanism of death with overdosage of general anesthetics. The neurons of the reticular activating system are depressed in a differential manner. For example, in very light planes of anesthesia, one commonly encounters clonus, hyperreflexia, and other neurological signs, which indicate that the depressor neurons of the reticular activating system are inhibited at lower dosages than the excitatory neurons.

Nervous system
CENTRAL NERVOUS
SYSTEM

Recent studies have indicated that profound effects on the spinal cord are produced by the general anesthetics. The gating area for pain impulses, the substantia gelantinosa of Rolando, is depressed in function, such that pain impulses ascending via pathways including the lateral, spinal, and thalamic tracts are depressed. Thus fewer pain impulses reach the brain during anesthesia. Many of the general anesthetics also produce skeletal muscle relaxation by an effect on the internuncial pool of the spinal cord. Although there are discernible effects of general anesthetics in the region of the myoneural junction, it is believed that the spinal cord effects are the ones responsible for most of the skeletal muscle relaxation seen with the administration of these drugs.

PERIPHERAL
NERVOUS SYSTEM

Here, there is a wide difference in action spectrum produced by the general anesthetics, differences made more complex by the profound dose relationships involved. Some of the inhalation anesthetics, particularly the older ones, such as diethyl ether and cyclopropane, appear to be sympathetic nervous system stimulants. Actually, rather than a stimulating effect, this may be due to quantitative differences in action on excitatory and inhibitory neurons controlling sympathetic nervous activity. Levels of plasma norepinephrine may increase threefold to tenfold during anesthesia with an anesthetic such as cyclopropane. This is one of the primary reasons that, until a decade or so ago, cyclopropane was considered to be the anesthetic of choice in shock states. Due to the release of norepinephrine, blood pressure was maintained with this anesthetic, although flow to organs was consequently diminished because of arteriolar constriction. Other sympathomimetic effects are revealed in the increased glycogenolysis seen with the anesthetic diethyl ether. Blood sugars may reach levels as high as 200 to 250 mg/100 ml with this anesthetic. Nitrous oxide, alone of presently employed anesthetics, possesses some sympathetic excitatory actions. By contrast, modern halogenated anesthetics such as halothane cause total inhibition of the sympathetic nervous system and a reduced plasma catecholamine content.

AUTONOMIC
NERVOUS SYSTEM

These agents also do not produce glycogenolysis. Effects of general inhalation anesthetics on parasympathetic activity are quite variable. Some of the anesthetics, such as cyclopropane and halothane, have been adjudged to be vagal stimulants, particuarly in lighter planes of anesthesia. The evidence for this is scanty, but both anesthetics seem to produce a mild degree of bradycardia, which can be overcome by the muscarinic-blocking drug atropine. Further evidence for enhanced vagal activity comes from the clinical reports implicating cyclopropane in possibly triggering bronchial constriction in asthmatics. On the other hand, halothane and the other halogenated hydrocarbon anesthetics do not have this effect on bronchial smooth muscle and are therefore considered to be drugs of choice for the patient with constrictive bronchiolar disease.

Respiration   With deep levels of anesthesia, respiratory depression is common with all general anesthetics. Diethyl ether produces a clear-cut depression of tidal volume due to intercostal muscle paralysis and finally diaphragmatic paralysis. With other anesthetics, such as halothane, this differential effect on muscle activity to depress respiration is less clear. Certainly, at all planes of anesthesia there is a graded depression of medullary activity. Classically, ventilation during anesthesia shows lowered tidal volume and increased frequency of respiration with a net reduction in alveolar minute ventilation. Response to arterial and alveolar carbon dioxide tensions is decreased, so that there is a classic rightward shift and decreased slope of the carbon dioxide response curve. This is a dose-dependent phenomenon. In lighter planes of surgical anesthesia, some anesthetics, such as diethyl ether, have less effects on respiration, such that normal or near normal carbon dioxide tension is maintained. However, with most of the halogenated anesthetics, the drop in alveolar ventilation and alveolar minute ventilation ($\dot{V}A$) will produce an increased $PaCO_2$. For this reason, the administration of a general anesthetic is frequently performed with assisted or controlled ventilation. This may be done either by manual inflation of the rebreathing bag of the anesthesia machine or by the insertion of a mechanical ventilator into the circuit. Some of the older anesthetics, such as diethyl ether, cause increased bronchial secretions. These can be blocked with atropine, scopolamine, or glycopyrrolate and are one of the reasons why anticholinergics were frequently given as preoperative medications. The present-day anesthetics do not normally cause an increase in pulmonary secretions, so use of the anticholinergics for this reason is waning.

Circulation   Anesthetics affect both the heart and the peripheral circulation. All the drugs in this category affect the heart by producing a dose-related, negative inotropic effect. In isolated animal preparations, this can be seen as a depression of twitch height in isolated papillary muscles and in intact humans by a fall in cardiac output. The anesthetics differ from a quantitative point of view in this action. Halothane, for example, depresses the myocardium to a greater extent in equally anesthetic dosages than does diethyl ether. There are subtle autonomic differences, which change the situation in intact humans also. For example, with those anesthetics that stimulate norepinephrine release from adrenergic nerves, there is less negative inotropic effect because increases in sympathetic transmitter indirectly stimulate the myocardium.

The anesthetics, particularly the halogenated ones, depress peripheral sympathetic nerves by affecting the ganglia. For this reason, peripheral vasodilatation usually occurs during anesthesia. The overall effect of the negative inotropic effects and the depression of peripheral circulation is a drop in blood pressure in a dose-dependent fashion. Systolic blood pressure seems to be affected to a greater degree than does diastolic blood pressure, so that during clinical anesthesia there is a tendency for the pulse pressure to narrow.

Changes in cardiac rhythm and conduction are not uncommon during anesthesia. The most common arrhythmia seen is a downward displacement of the pacemaker, progressing from wandering pacemaker to nodal rhythm. This arrhythmia is usually benign. The second most common form of arrhythmias is premature ventricular contractions. Many anesthetics are capable of interacting with plasma epinephrine or norepinephrine concentration elevation to produce the so-called hydrocarbon anesthetic arrhythmias. Probably as a result of changes in automaticity, the threshold to premature ventricular contractions is lowered by many anesthetics. In light planes of anesthesia, if there is sympathetic stimulation or if exogenous sympathomimetic amines are administered, troublesome ventricular arrhythmias can be produced. For example, the cyclopropane-epinephrine sequence is used in pharmacology in testing cardiac antifibrillatory drugs. Since hypercapnia can lead to increased release of catecholamines, these may interact with the myocardium "sensitized" to a lower arrhythmia threshold by hydrocarbon anesthetics to produce ventricular arrhythmias. These arrhythmias are frequently clues to the clinician that ventilation is not adequate. Injection of catecholamines during anesthesia with certain of these anesthetics should be done with caution, if at all. There have been minimal dose schedules of drugs such as epinephrine, which can be safely injected during the course of halothane anesthesia. The agents most likely to produce these catecholamine anesthetic arrhythmias are the straight chain hydrocarbons, namely cyclopropane and halothane. The ether series of anesthetics, halogenated or not, seems to present far fewer problems in this regard.

Uterus

The halogenated anesthetics inhibit the contractile response of the gravid uterus when oxytocic drugs are administered. Thus they may produce or allow certain degrees of uterine relaxation, which may be advantageous for version extractions or other intrauterine manipulations. This is a two-edged sword, however, as these anesthetics will also permit sufficient degrees of uterine relaxation to increase postpartum bleeding. The gaseous and vapor anesthetics pass the placenta into the fetus with a great deal of ease. These effects must be taken into consideration during obstetrical anesthesia.

Hepatic and metabolic actions

Anesthetics have several effects on the liver. Experimental evidence indicates that anesthetics depress mitochondrial function such that total body oxygen consumption is reduced. Actually, this has a certain advantage since, if there is reduction in flow due to altered peripheral circulation and cardiac effects, in the anesthetized state less oxygen will be required, the delivery of which may be somewhat impaired. Splanchnic blood flow is diminished by most of the anesthetics, such that total hepatic blood flow is decreased. In addition, the anesthetics seem to have an "antiinsulin effect," which decreases the ability of the liver to take up glucose and incorporate it into glucose-6-phosphate. For example, if an exogenous glucose load is administered during the course of general anesthesia, a diabetic type of prolonged tolerance curve will result because of this effect. The hepatic microsomal enzymes responsible for the biotransformation of various drugs are diminished in activity during clinical anesthesia. Combined with the drop in hepatic blood flow limiting access of drugs to the liver, there will be prolonged half-lives of drugs seen during clinical anesthesia. Recent evidence indicates that during the high dose levels of clinical anesthesia there is impairment of certain synthetic pathways, such as the urea cycle, and of bilirubin conjunction. These effects quickly dissipate as the anesthetic is terminated. Because of the transient action, they cannot be considered as toxic.

Biotransformation and toxicity

Until 1965 it was thought that the general inhalation anesthetics were inert and were not extensively biotransformed in the body. This concept has proved to be fallacious. The anesthetics are metabolized to various degrees, depending on the molecular structure and partition coefficients. Low partition coefficients limit the time that the anesthetic is in contact with the enzymes of biotransformation. Thus an anesthetic of rather low partition coefficient would not be expected to undergo as much biotransformation as one that persists in the body for a long period of time. The extremes are seen in the case of isoflurane, which is only 1% to 2% metabolized in the body, as compared to methoxyflurane. Methoxyflurane has a rather high degree of metabolism; over 50% of the drug absorbed by the body is biotransformed. The biotransformation of certain anesthetics may be responsible for cases of viscerotoxicity reported following anesthesia. For example, methoxyflurane is converted to free fluoride ion. High fluoride concentrations greater than 80 μm/L may give rise to renal damage and the so-called high output renal failure syndrome. Biotransformation of chloroform, an older anesthetic no longer clinically employed, has definitely been implicated in hepatic toxicity. The mechanism of this effect is that biotransformation produces free radicals or reactive intermediates, which combine with liver macromolecules to form covalent bonds. The altered proteins and lipoproteins are no longer capable of function and may actually undergo necrosis. Halothane, ordinarily a very safe anesthetic, has been implicated in unpredictable hepatic toxicity. This is a rare, sporadic event, which probably occurs no more often than 1:20,000 administrations. Although there is a possibility that this may represent an allergy, evidence is accumulating that the biotransformation of halothane to reactive intermediates may be the proximate vector of liver damage in these rare individuals. Abnormal biotransformation may be via a reductive rather than the customary oxidative pathway, controlled by genetic and/or environmental (drug induction) factors. This results in

TABLE 32-3   Clinical characteristics of general anesthetics

Anesthetic	Analgesia	Hypnosis	Skeletal muscle relaxation	Depression of reflexes	Flammability	Compatibility with epinephrine
Nitrous oxide	+	+	0	+	No	Yes
Cyclopropane	+ +	+ + + +	+	+ +	Yes	No
Diethyl ether	+ + + +	+ + + +	+ + + +	+ + + +	Yes	Yes
Methoxyflurane	+ + + +	+ + + +	+ + + +	+ + + +	No	Yes
Halothane	+ +	+ + + +	+ +	+ + + +	No	No
Enflurane	+ + +	+ + + +	+ + +	+ + + +	No	Yes
Isoflurane	+ + +	+ + + +	+ + +	+ + + +	No	Yes

+ + + +, Maximum effect; +, minimum effect.

minor hepatic damage. In some individuals antibodies to these metabolite-protein complexes may form to produce severe hepatic necrosis. Closely repeated halothane anesthetics seem more likely to produce this event, particularly in obese, middle-aged women.

Reduction in renal function is commonly seen during the course of anesthesia. This occurs primarily by a reduction in renal blood flow and leads to decreases in glomerular infiltration rate. Nausea and vomiting may follow the administration of general anesthetics. Although this effect may have a CNS etiology, it must be kept in mind that surgical pain and stimulation probably play a role in this side effect. Certain of the older anesthetics, such as cyclopropane and diethyl ether, seem to cause postoperative nausea and vomiting to a greater degree than some of the newer anesthetics such as halothane. Because of hypothalamic depression, generally patients' temperatures decrease slightly during anesthesia. Certain anesthetics, such as halothane, seem to trigger a catastrophic disease known as malignant hyperpyrexia in genetically susceptible individuals. This sudden and highly lethal event causes rises in temperatures to 42° C or higher with severe tissue acidosis.

Miscellaneous effects

The inhalation anesthetics are divided into two broad categories: gaseous anesthetics and volatile liquid anesthetics (Table 32-3). The gaseous anesthetics are defined as those with boiling points below room temperature and critical pressures greater than 760 torr. They are usually marketed as compressed gases, are in the liquid or gaseous state, and are under high pressures in steel cylinders. The cylinders are colored differently for each gas, such as blue for nitrous oxide and orange for cyclopropane. The volatile liquid anesthetics are liquids at room temperature, are usually more potent than the gases, and are ethers or halogenated hydrocarbons. Gaseous anesthetics generally possess blood-air and oil-gas partition coefficients lower

CLINICAL PHARMACOLOGY OF INDIVIDUAL ANESTHETICS

than the volatile anesthetics, are consequently faster for induction and recovery, and are less potent. Selection of a particular anesthetic for a particular surgical patient is predicated on the pathophysiology and the type of surgical procedure involved. Selection of the appropriate anesthetic(s) is one of the critical factors involved in the presurgical rounds of the anesthesiologist.

Gaseous *anesthetics* NITROUS OXIDE	Nitrous oxide (N_2O) is a colorless, odorless, tasteless gas, which is not metabolized. It is carried in the body in physical solution only. Nitrous oxide is an impotent anesthetic. It must be supplemented and used in the so-called balanced anesthetic technique, which consists of additional hypnosis (usually by barbiturates or tranquilizers), analgesia, (accomplished by intravenous narcotics), and supplementary muscle relaxants produced by the curariform drugs. Nitrous oxide is not flammable and is compatible with all other drugs, including catecholamines. Analgesia occurs with inspired concentrations of greater than 20% and hypnosis at concentrations of about 40% at sea level. However, because of its lack of potency, it is impossible to achieve complete surgical anesthesia with nitrous oxide without depriving the patient of oxygen.

Nitrous oxide has no significant effects on the respiratory, hepatic, renal, or autonomic nervous systems, except for a very slight myocardial depressant action and sympathomimetic effect. Nitrous oxide has been called an "ideal anesthetic" because of supposed lack of depressive effects. Recent investigations indicate it may not be as benign as once thought. Nitrous oxide inhalation for only 2 hours can drastically lower levels of methionine synthetase used in vitamin B_{12} synthesis. Although surgical patients given an anesthetic with nitrous oxide do not manifest pernicious anemia, individuals abusing the drug over chronic periods have demonstrated the neurological picture of vitamin B_{12} deficiency.

In addition to use in the so called balanced technique, nitrous oxide is commonly administered simultaneously with the more powerful anesthetics such as halothane and diethyl ether. This is done to speed the equilibrium attainment of the more powerful agent and to add the analgesic potency of nitrous oxide to that of the more powerful agents without harmful systemic effects. For example, halothane is quite depressive to myocardial contractility. The MAC for halothane with oxygen only is 0.8%. If the halothane is administered in 70% nitrous oxide with 30% oxygen atmosphere, the MAC of halothane is reduced to 0.35%.

CYCLOPROPANE	Cyclopropane (C_3H_6) represents a potent gas, which can produce complete anesthesia without supplementation by intravenous anesthetics. The usual anesthetic dose at equilibrium is 10% to 20% inspired. Cyclopropane is no longer a popular anesthetic because of its flammability and explodability. It does stimulate the sympathoadrenal system and blood pressure is well maintained with this drug. However, this blood pressure maintenance is performed at the expense of critical alterations in peripheral flow. Cyclopropane is the classic drug that is incompatible with catecholamines. It is rarely used at present.

Diethyl ether ($[C_2H_5]_2O$) is a pungent, volatile liquid, which is irritating to respiratory mucosa and may reflexively stimulate ventilation. Diethyl ether was the first general anesthetic to be employed clinically. It is rarely used now, primarily because of its flammability when mixed with air or oxygen. The hallmark of diethyl ether is that it is more benign to the cardiovascular system than any other complete anesthetic. Although it does cause a certain degree of negative inotropic effect, this is countered in humans by the reflex release of catecholamines. The net effect is only a slight fall in cardiac output. Ether does not lower the threshold of the ventricular myocardium to catecholamines. Diethyl ether produces good skeletal muscle and uterine relaxation. Because of its high partition coefficients and because there are good clinical signs of depth of ether anesthesia, following the planes of anesthesia with this drug is easier than with many of anesthetics of lower solubility. For this reason, ether has often been termed the safest anesthetic.

The major disadvantages of diethyl ether, in addition to its flammability, are the high incidence of nausea and vomiting during recovery and its slow induction and emergence. Similarly to cyclopropane, diethyl ether is rarely used because of its flammability.

Volatile liquid anesthetics
DIETHYL ETHER

Halothane (C_2F_3HBrCl) was the first of the truly modern, nonflammable halogenated inhalation anesthetics. It is rapid, pleasant for patients, and an exceptional anesthetic. The unresolved problem of hepatotoxicity has caused a decline in its use presently; however, it has been proven in all other categories to be a very safe anesthetic.

Halothane produces marked depression of alveolar minute ventilation with the classical decrease in tidal volume but increase in inspiratory rate. Therefore assisted or controlled ventilation is commonly employed when halothane is administered. It is nonirritating to the respiratory tract and does not cause increased pulmonary secretions.

Halothane is an example of an anesthetic with depressant effects on the heart with no increase in sympathetic nervous activity to secondarily augment contractility. Cardiac output, contractile force, and blood pressure all fall during the administration of halothane. Part of the blood pressure fall results from a decrease in the sympathetic nervous system activity with a decline in peripheral resistance. Some degree of bradycardia is frequently seen during anesthesia with halothane. Halothane does lower the threshold of ventricular muscle to catecholamine-induced arrhythmias. However, this effect is not as great as with cyclopropane but still warrants extreme caution when epinephrine or other sympathomimetic amines are to be administered to a patient during the course of halothane anesthesia. Uterine relaxation is good with halothane anesthesia.

Because of its low-solubility characteristics, it is considered a rapid anesthetic. It is commonly given together with nitrous oxide, although it may be given alone in oxygen. At the present time, it is regarded as the premier drug for pediatric anesthesia due to its ease of induction and rapid awakening characteristics. Although there is

HALOTHANE

the spectre of hepatic damage, which is occasionally reported following its use, this viscerotoxic effect does not seem to occur in infants and children.

METHOXYFLURANE

Methoxyflurane ($CCl_2HCF_2OCH_3$; Penthrane) is a potent, nonflammable anesthetic, which was one of the first of a series of halogenated ethers. Its hallmark is that it produces excellent skeletal muscle relaxation. A difficulty with it, however, is the rather high solubility characteristics, which make for slow induction and awakening. Unlike halothane, methoxyflurane does not sensitize the myocardium to catecholamines to a very high degree. Again, this may be a function of the ether link of the anesthetic. It is a rather pleasant smelling liquid of low volatility, which is only slightly irritating to the respiratory tracts. Although it does depress ventilation, depression of cardiac contractility is probably less than that of halothane at equally effective dosages.

The great drawback to methoxyflurane, which has decreased its clinical use over the last few years, is its biotransformation to free fluoride ions that contribute to high output renal failure. It has fairly extensive biotransformation due to its molecular configuration and its highly lipophilic nature. To reduce the amount of free fluoride form from biotransformation, it has been suggested that methoxyflurane anesthesia be limited in humans to 2 MAC hours.

ENFLURANE

Enflurane (CF_2HOCF_2CFClH; Ethrane) is one of the most popular potent anesthetics in clinical use at this time. It is a halogenated ether, which combines many of the virtues of both halothane and methoxyflurane without some of their disadvantages. It is a potent, volatile liquid, which is usually administered with nitrous oxide or solely in oxygen. It produces depression of myocardial contractility to a degree about equal to halothane. However, because of its ether link, it does not sensitize the myocardium to endogenous and exogenous catecholamines to the degree that halothane does. This link also gives enflurane its excellent skeletal muscle relaxant properties.

Because of lower solubility parameters, the anesthetic is not extensively biotransformed in the body. Perhaps 1% to 2%, and no more than 2% to 3%, of an absorbed dose is metabolized. Even though a metabolic product is free fluoride ion, this halogen does not achieve blood levels sufficient to produce renal disease. Its degree of sporadic hepatic damage seems to be far less than that of halothane so that repeat doses are not contraindicated. Clinically, the drug may be a little more difficult to use than halothane, but it seems to be replacing that anesthetic in adult anesthesia.

A major problem associated with enflurane is that the combination of high concentrations of the anesthetic and hypocapnia foster grand mal seizures. Under such circumstances, the EEG reveals classical spike and dome traces. This effect does not seem to be a deleterious one and can be avoided by maintaining normocapnia and employing just those concentrations necessary at the time for the surgery.

Isoflurane ($CF_3CHClOCHF_2$; Forane) is an isomer of enflurane. It is the newest in the long line of halogenated ether compounds, so clinical experience with it is not as extensive as with halothane and enflurane. The drug is even more resistant to biotransformation than is enflurane; less than 1% of the total absorbed is metabolized. Therefore it may have the virtue of less viscerotoxicity than any other commonly employed anesthetic. Many of its features are quite similar to that of enflurane. However, there is evidence to support the fact that its respiratory depressant effect may be slightly greater than that of enflurane but its cardiovascular depressant effect less than that of enflurane. It also does not tend to foster convulsive activity. The drug is nonflammable and is compatible, to a certain degree, with catecholamines similar to enflurane. Skeletal muscle and uterine relaxation properties appear to be good. Because of a somewhat pungent odor, inhalation inductions are often not as smooth as with halothane. Although it does not cause a significant negative inotropic action, the anesthetic does produce rather profound peripheral vasodilatation with concomitant drops in blood pressure. A resulting tachycardia can occur, which may be bothersome in patients with coronary artery disease.

ISOFLURANE

REFERENCES

1. Banker, J.P., Forrest, W.H., Jr., Mostellar, F., and Vandam, L.D.: The National Halothane Study, Bethesda, Maryland, NIH, NIGMS, 1969.
2. Brown, B.R., Jr., and Crout, J.R., Jr.: A comparative study of the effects of five general anesthetics on myocardial contractility. I. Isometric conditions, Anestesiology **34**:236, 1971.
3. DeJong, R.H., Robles, R., Corbin, R.W., and Nace, R.A.: Effect of inhalational anesthetics on monosynaptic and polysynaptic transmission in the spinal cord, J. Pharmacol. Exp. Ther. **162**:326, 1960.
4. Eger, E.I. II: Anesthetic uptake and action, Baltimore, 1974, The Williams & Williams Co.
5. Eger, E.I. II, and Lanson, C.P., Jr.: Anesthetic solubility in blood and tissues: values and significance, Br. J. Anaesth. **36**:140, 1964.
6. Katz, R.L., and Epstein, R.A.: the interaction of anesthetic agents and adrenergic drugs to produce cardiac arrhythmias, Anesthesiology **29**:763, 1968.
7. McLain, G.E., Sipes, I.G., and Brown, B.R., Jr.: An animal model of halothane hepatotoxicity: role of enzyme induction and hypoxia, Anesthesiology **51**:321, 1979.
8. Price, H.L., Kornat, P.J., Safer, J.N., Conner, E.H., and Price, M.L.: The uptake of thiopental by body tissues and its relation to the duration of narcosis, Clin. Pharmacol. Ther. **1**:16, 1960.
9. Saidman, L.J., Eger, E.I. II, Munson, E.S., Babad, A.A., and Mualleni, M.: Minimum alveolar concentration of methoxyflurane, halothane, ether, and cycloproprane in man: correlation with theories of anesthesia, Anesthesiology **28**:994, 1967.
10. Smith, N.T., Miller, R.D., Corbascio, A.N., editors: Drug Interactions in Anesthesia, Philadelphia, 1981, Lea & Febiger.
11. Van Dyke, R.A., Chenoweth, M.B., and Van Poznak, A.: Metabolism of volatile anesthetics. I. Conversion in vivo of several anesthetics to $14Co_2$ and chloride, Biochem. Pharmacol. **13**:1239, 1964.

Chapter 33

Pharmacology of local anesthesia

GENERAL CONCEPT   Local anesthetics are drugs employed to produce a transient and reversible loss of sensation in a circumscribed area of the body. They achieve this effect by interfering with nerve conduction.

In 1884 Köller, who had studied *cocaine* with Sigmund Freud, introduced the drug into medicine as a topical anesthetic in ophthalmology. This was the beginning of the first era in the history of local anesthesia.

The second era began in 1904 with the introduction of *procaine* by Einhorn. This was the first safe local anesthesia suitable for injection. Procaine remained the most widely used local anesthetic until the introduction of *lidocaine* (Xylocaine), which is considered the agent of choice for infiltration at present. Other local anesthetics of importance are *tetracaine, mepivacaine, prilocaine,* and *bupivacaine*. All these drugs are either esters or amides, and they differ from each other in their toxicity, metabolism, onset, and duration of action. Lidocaine, in addition to being an important local anesthetic, has important uses as an antiarrhythmic agent (p. 445).

Electrophysiological studies indicate that the local anesthetics interfere with the rate of rise of the depolarization phase of the action potential. As a consequence the cell does not depolarize sufficiently after excitation to fire. Thus the propagated action potential is blocked by these drugs.

CLASSIFICATION   Local anesthetics may be classified according to their chemistry or on the basis of their clinical usage.

According to chemistry   Local anesthetics are either esters or amides. They consist of an aromatic portion, an intermediate chain, and an amine portion. The aromatic portion confers lipophilic properties to the molecule, whereas the amine portion is hydrophilic. The ester or amide components of the molecule determine the characteristics of metabolic degradation. The esters are mostly hydrolyzed in plasma by pseudocholinesterase, whereas the amides are destroyed largely in the liver.

Esters of benzoic acid
    Cocaine
    Tetracaine (Pontocaine)
    Piperocaine (Metycaine)
    Hexylcaine (Cyclaine)
    Ethyl aminobenzoate (Benzocaine)
    Butacaine (Butyn)
Esters of meta-aminobenzoic acid
    Cyclomethycaine (Surfacaine)
    Metabutoxycaine (Primacaine)

Esters of p-aminobenzoic acid
    Procaine (Novocain)
    Butethamine (Monocaine)
    Chloroprocaine (Nesacaine)
    Proparacaine (Ophthaine)
Amides
    Lidocaine (Xylocaine)
    Dibucaine (Nupercaine)
    Mepivacaine (Carbocaine)
    Prilocaine (Citanest)
    Bupivacaine (Marcaine)

Local anesthetics have several types of clinical applications, and their suitability for these varies with their pharmacological properties. Some of these applications are (1) infiltration and block anesthesia, (2) surface anesthesia, (3) spinal anesthesia (4) epidural and caudal anesthesia, and (5) intravenous anesthesia. In the following list the drugs of greatest interest are italicized. *According to clinical usage*

Infiltration and block anesthesia: *procaine, chloroprocaine, hexylcaine, lidocaine,* mepivacaine, *bupivacaine,* piperocaine, prilocaine, propoxycaine, and tetracaine; also, in dentistry: butethamine, metabutethamine, isobucaine, meprylcaine, and pyrrocaine

Surface anesthesia: *benzocaine, benoxinate, butacaine, butyl aminobenzoate, cocaine,* cyclomethycaine, dibucaine, dimethisoquin, diperodon, dyclonine, hexylcaine, lidocaine, phenacaine, piperocaine, pramoxine, proparacaine, and tetracaine; also, benzyl alcohol, phenol, and ethyl chloride

Spinal anesthesia (subarachnoid or intrathecal): *tetracaine,* procaine, dibucaine, lidocaine, mepivacaine, and piperocaine

Epidural and caudal anesthesia: *lidocaine, prilocaine,* and *mepivacaine;* also, procaine, chloroprocaine, piperocaine, and tetracaine

Intravenous anesthesia: *lidocaine* and *procaine* (seldom used for anesthesia but for other indications)

Electrophysiological studies indicate that the local anesthetics do not alter the resting membrane potential or threshold potential of nerves. They act on the rate of rise of the depolarization phase of the action potential. Since depolarization does not reach the point at which firing occurs, propagated action potential fails to occur. *MODE OF ACTION*

The effects of local anesthetics on ionic fluxes are of great interest, and recent studies emphasize the relationships between these drugs and the calcium ion with secondary effects on sodium fluxes. Although no detailed discussion will be attempted, local anesthetic agents appear to compete with calcium for a site in the nerve membrane that controls the passage of sodium across the memrane. It is believed at present that calcium is bound to phospholipids in the cell membrane. A fair correlation could be found between local anesthetic potency and their ability to prevent the binding of calcium by phosphatidylserine in artificial membranes.

Experimental studies indicate also that an increase in calcium concentration is able to overcome the nerve block produced by local anesthetics.

Active form

PROBLEM 33-1. *When the hydrochloride of a local anesthetic is injected, which is the active form, the uncharged base or the charged cation? When dealing with an intact isolated nerve, the local anesthetics such as lidocaine are more potent in an alkaline solution, suggesting the uncharged base as the active form. On the other hand, when a desheathed nerve is used, the less alkaline preparations are more efficacious. It is believed at present that the uncharged base penetrates better across the nerve sheath, but it is the charged cation that exerts its pharmacological effect. The problem is complicated by the fact that the results are not applicable to all members of the series of local anesthetics.*

Action on various nerve fibers

According to diameter, myelination, and conduction velocities, nerve fibers can be classified into three types—A, B, and C fibers. The A fibers have a diameter of 1 to 20 μm, are myelinated, and have conduction velocities up to 100 m/sec. Somatic motor and some sensory fibers fall into this classification. Blockade of these fibers results in skeletal muscle relaxation, loss of thermal and tactile sensation, proprioceptive loss, and loss of the sensation of sharp pain. B fibers vary in diameter from 1 to 3 μm, are myelinated, and conduct at intermediate velocities. Preganglionic fibers fall into this group, and their blockade obviously results in autonomic paralysis. C fibers are usually under 1 μm in diameter and are not myelinated, and conduction velocity is approximately 1 m/sec. Postganglionic fibers as well as more somatic sensory fibers fall into this classification. Blockade results in autonomic paralysis; loss of the sensation of itch, tickle, and dull pain and loss of much of the thermal sensation.

Clinically the general order of loss of function is as follows: (1) pain, (2) temperature, (3) touch, (4) proprioception, and (5) skeletal muscle tone. If pressure is exerted on a mixed nerve, the fibers are depressed in somewhat the reverse order.

In summary, local anesthetic drugs depress the small, unmyelinated fibers first and the larger, myelinated fibers last. The time for the onset of action is shorter for the smaller fibers, and the concentration of drug required is less.

ABSORPTION, FATE, AND EXCRETION

Absorption of the various local anesthetics depends on the site of injection, the degree of vasodilatation caused by the agent itself, the dose, and the presence of a vasoconstrictor in the solution. Epinephrine added to a procaine hydrochloride solution greatly increases its duration of action as an infiltration agent.

The onset and duration of action of various local anesthetics as determined by a standardized ulnar block technique are shown in Table 33-1.

Local anesthetics of the ester type are hydrolyzed by plasma pseudocholinesterase. Those having the amide linkage are largely destroyed in the liver (Table 33-2).

In human beings, procaine is broken down to *p*-aminobenzoic acid, 80% of which is excreted in the urine, and diethylaminoethanol, 30% of which is excreted in the urine. Only 2% is excreted unchanged in the urine. Only 10% to 20% of lidocaine appears unchanged, the rest being metabolized, presumably mainly in the liver.

Procaine is hydrolyzed in spinal fluid 150 times more slowly than in plasma, there being very little esterase present. The hydrolysis results from the alkalinity of the spinal fluid and is approximately the same as with a buffer having the same pH.

TABLE 33-1 Onset and duration of action of various local anesthetics determined by a standardized ulnar block technique

Drug	Concentration	Relative potency	Onset in minutes	Duration of action in minutes
Procaine	1	1	7	19
Lidocaine	1	4	5	40
Mepivacaine	1	4	4	99
Prilocaine	1	4	3	98
Tetracaine*	0.25	16	7	135
Bupivacaine*	0.25	16	8	415

Modified from Covino, B.G.: N. Engl. J. Med. **286**:975, 1035, 1972; based on data from Albert, J., and Löfström, B.: Acta Anesth. Scand. **5**;99, 1961.
*Solutions contain epinephrine 1:200,000.

TABLE 33-2 Relative hydrolysis rates of local anesthetics by plasma esterase

Local anesthetic	Rate of hydrolysis
Piperocaine	6.5
Chloroprocaine	5.0
Procaine	1.0
Tetracaine	0.2
Dibucaine	0

Lidocaine is metabolized in the liver by removal of one or both ethyl groups from the molecule. The resulting metabolites, monoethylglycinexylidide (MEGX) and glycinexilidine (GX), still have pharmacological activity and may contribute to CNS toxicity.

METHODS OF ADMINISTRATION

Local anesthetics may be administered by topical application, by infiltration of tissues to bathe fine nerve elements, by injection adjacent to nerves and their branches, and by injection into the epidural or subarachnoid spaces. Occasionally, intravenous injections are utilized to control certain pain situations. The details of subarachnoid and epidural anesthesia are outside the intended scope of this discussion.

SYSTEMIC ACTIONS

Local anesthetics exert their effect largely on a circumscribed area. Nevertheless, they are absorbed from the site of injection and may exert systemic effects, particularly on the cardiovascular system and the CNS and particularly when an excessive dose is utilized.

Cardiovascular effects	Since lidocaine is widely used as an antiarrhythmic drug, much has been learned about its effect on the heart, and this information is generally also applicable to the other local anesthetics. At nontoxic concentrations lidocaine alters or abolishes the rate of slow diastolic depolarization in Purkinje's fibers and may shorten the effective refractory period as well as the duration of the action potential. In toxic doses lidocaine decreases the maximal depolarization of Purkinje's fibers and reduces conduction velocity. Such doses may also have a direct negative inotropic effect.

The local anesthetics tend to relax the vascular smooth muscle, but cocaine can cause vasoconstriction by blocking the reuptake of norepinephrine.

CNS effects	Although the usual local anesthesia produces no CNS effects, increased doses may cause excitatory effects resulting in convulsions and eventually respiratory depression. It is believed on the basis of animal experiments that the local anesthetics may block inhibitory cortical synapses. This leads to excitation. Larger doses depress both inhibitory and facilitory neurons, leading to depression.

Miscellaneous effects	Compared with their actions on the cardiovascular system and the CNS, the local anesthetics have few additional effects. They may depress ganglionic transmission and neuromuscular transmission. These actions are unimportant unless some other potent agent is used concomitantly. For example, lidocaine may enhance the action of neuromuscular blocking agents.

Vasoconstrictors and local anesthetics	Vasoconstrictors, particularly epinephrine, are commonly added to local anesthetic solutions that are to be used for infiltration or nerve block. The purpose is to prevent absorption of the drug and thereby prolong its action locally and reduce systemic reactions. Concentrations of epinephrine used for this purpose in local anesthesia vary from 2 to 10 μg/ml, or 1:500,000 to 1:100,000.

Although the addition of epinephrine to such drugs as procaine is sound, other drugs such as lidocaine, prilocaine, mepivacaine, and bupivacaine may be used without the addition of vasoconstrictors.

Epinephrine may contribute to the systemic effects of local anesthetics and may be responsible for symptoms such as anxiety, tachycardia, and hypertension.

TOXICITY	The ester-type local anesthetics, such as procaine and tetracaine, may produce true allergic reactions manifested as skin rashes or bronchospasm. Allergic reactions to the amides, such as lidocaine, are very rare.

The majority of toxic reactions are a result of overdosage. The figures given in Table 33-3 refer to maximum safe dosages, determined in milligrams per kilogram of body weight, administered to healthy adults without inadvertent intravascular or subarachnoid injection.

In general the true pharmacological signs of toxicity from local anesthetics are CNS stimulation followed by depression and peripheral cardiovascular depression. Salivation and tremor, convulsion, and coma, associated with hypertension and tachy-

TABLE 33-3	Maximum safe dosages of local anesthetics administered to healthy adults without inadvertent intravascular or subarachnoid injection	
Anesthetic	mg/kg of body weight
4% cocaine	1 (topical)
1% procaine	10 (injection)
0.15% tetracaine	1 (injection)
1% lidocaine	1 (injection)
0.5% bupivacaine	2.5 (injection)

cardia and followed by hypotension, all occurring in a few minutes, represent the full-blown picture.

The treatment is symptomatic and essentially involves restoration of normal ventilation and circulation. Barbiturates in doses greater than hypnotic are effective in the *prevention* of CNS stimulation caused by local anesthetics. Diazepam (Valium) is being used increasingly for the same purpose.

CLINICAL CHARACTERISTICS

Cocaine

Cocaine is too toxic to be injected into the tissues and is therefore used only topically. It produces excellent topical anesthesia and vasoconstriction, which results in shrinkage of mucous membranes. Absorption from the urinary mucous membranes is rapid, and cocaine should not be used in this area. Some clinicians believe that vasoconstriction with 10% cocaine is better than with a 4% solution and that toxicity will be less with the stronger preparation because the cocaine will be more slowly absorbed. This may be dangerous, however. The vasoconstrictor effect of cocaine and potentiation by this local anesthetic of the actions of catecholamines are most likely consequences of inhibition of the uptake of catecholamines by adrenergic nerve terminals. Cocaine abuse is discussed on p. 350. Acute cocaine poisoning is probably best treated with chlorpromazine.

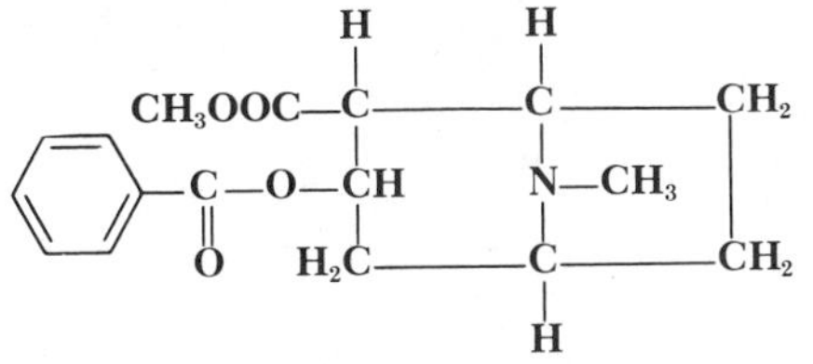

Cocaine

Ethyl aminobenzoate

Ethyl aminobenzoate (Benzocaine) is so poorly soluble that it is not absorbed from mucous membranes. Ointments containing 5% to 10% concentrations of ethyl aminobenzoate provide potent, safe topical anesthesia.

$$H_2N—\langle\ \rangle—\overset{\displaystyle C}{\underset{\displaystyle O}{\|}}—O—CH_2CH_3$$

Ethyl aminobenzoate

Procaine

Procaine (Novocain) was the standard against which all local anesthetics were compared. However, it has the disadvantage of producing poor topical anesthesia. Its duration of action is approximately 1 hour but can be significantly prolonged by the addition of epinephrine. Onset of anesthesia occurs rapidly. Afterward the patient often notes only the soreness produced by the needle used for injection. Procaine will block small to large nerve fibers in concentrations of 0.5% to 2%.

Chloroprocaine (Nesacaine) is a derivative of procaine that has a much shorter duration of action because of its more rapid hydrolysis.

$$H_2N\langle\ \rangle—\overset{\displaystyle C}{\underset{\displaystyle O}{\|}}—O—CH_2CH_2N\begin{smallmatrix}C_2H_5\\[4pt]\\[4pt]C_2H_5\end{smallmatrix}\ \cdot HCl$$

Procaine hydrochloride

Lidocaine

Lidocaine (Xylocaine) has supplanted procaine as the standard of comparison for local anesthetics. It is more potent and more versatile, being suitable not only for infiltration and nerve block but for surface anesthesia as well. This results in a rapid, potent anesthetic effect. It is used in concentrations of 0.5% to 2% and is more potent than equivalent solutions of procaine. Lidocaine has one other characteristic that distinguishes it from procaine and other local anesthetics—it very often produces sedation along with the local anesthesia. Lidocaine differs from most drugs in this group in being an amide rather than an ester. Lidocaine is metabolized in the liver by *N*-dealkylation. Two of the metabolites still have pharmacological activity and may contribute to toxic reactions in patients with altered metabolism.

$$\begin{array}{c} CH_3 \\ \\ \overset{\displaystyle H}{N}—\overset{\displaystyle C}{\underset{\displaystyle O}{\|}}—CH_2—N\begin{smallmatrix}C_2H_5\\[4pt]\\[4pt]C_2H_5\end{smallmatrix} \\ \\ CH_3 \end{array}$$

Lidocaine

Tetracaine

The chief differences between tetracaine (Pontocaine) and procaine and lidocaine are tetracaine's longer time required for full onset of action (10 minutes or more), longer duration of action (approximately 50%), and greater potency. For injection anesthesia, tetracaine is available in 0.15% solution. For topical anesthesia it is used in 1% and 2% concentrations. Tetracaine should not be sprayed into the airway in concentrations greater than 2%. The total dose should be carefully calculated and probably should not, in this situation, exceed 0.5 mg/kg of body weight. It is rapidly absorbed topically and has resulted in several fatalities from topical misuse. The chief disadvantage of tetracaine is slowness in onset of action.

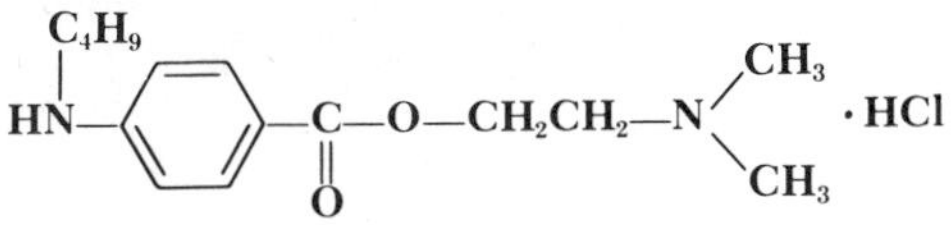

Tetracaine hydrochloride

Mepivacaine

Mepivacaine (Carbocaine) has essentially the same clinical effects as lidocaine except for two particular points. It does not spread in the tissues quite as well, and its duration of action is longer.

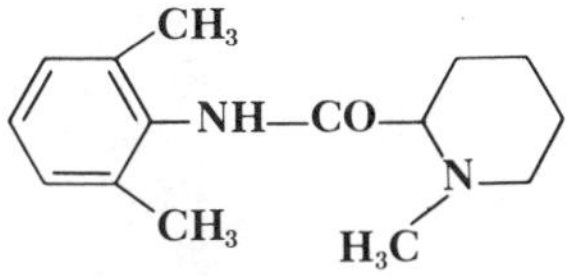

Mepivacaine

Bupivacaine

Bupivacaine (Marcaine) is an amide chemically related to mepivacaine. It has a long duration of action and its potency is four times greater than that of mepivacaine. Bupivacaine is used for infiltration, nerve block, and peridural anesthesia. Adverse effects of bupivacaine are similar to those produced by other local anesthetics. Bupivacaine is available in solutions containing 0.25%, 0.5%, and 0.75% of the drug.

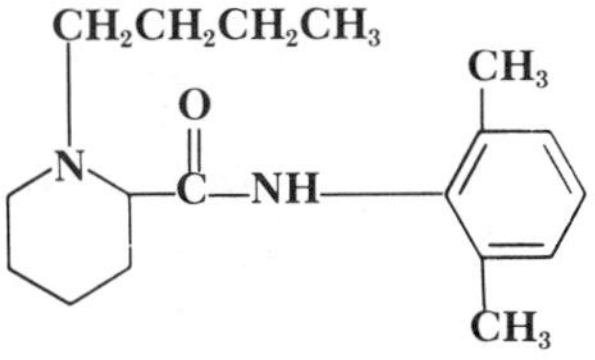

Bupivacaine

Dibucaine

Dibucaine (Nupercaine) is a very potent local anesthetic having a long duration of action. It is from 10 to 20 times as active and toxic as procaine. As a consequence, it is employed in a more dilute solution for injection than procaine (0.05% to 0.1%). It is suitable for topical use and also for spinal anesthesia.

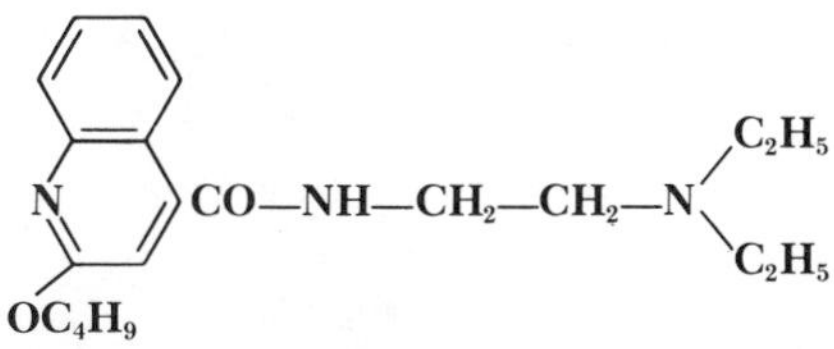

Dibucaine

CHOICE OF LOCAL ANESTHETICS

The needs of most physicians can be met by a few of the available local anesthetics. For infiltration lidocaine and bupivacaine are preferred. For spinal anesthesia, tetracaine appears to be the best. It has a duration of action of 2 hours or more and is hydrolyzed by plasma cholinesterase. For epidural anesthesia lidocaine (short duration) or bupivacaine (long duration) are often employed. Cocaine still has some uses for topical anesthesia.

REFERENCES

1. Aceves, J., and Machne, X.: The action of calcium and local anesthetics on nerve cells and their interaction during excitation, J. Pharmacol. Exp. Ther. **140**:136, 1963.
2. Adriani, J., and Zeperwick, R.: Clinical effectiveness of drugs used for topical anesthesia, JAMA **188**:711, 1964.
3. Alper, M.H.: Toxicity of local anesthetics, N. Engl. J. Med. **295**:1432, 1976.
4. Covino, B.G.: Local anesthesia, N. Engl. J. Med. **286:975, 1972.**
5. de Jong, R.H., and Wagman, I.H.: Physiological mechanisms of peripheral nerve block by local anesthetics, Anesthesiology **24**:484, 1963.
6. Dykes, M.H.M.: Evaluation of a local anesthetic agent: bupivacaine hydrochloride (Marcaine), JAMA **224**:1035, 1973.
7. Foldes, F.F., Davidson, G.M., Duncalf, D., and Shigeo, K.: The intravenous toxicity of local anesthetic agents in man, Clin. Pharmacol. Ther. **6**:328, 1965.
8. Ritchie, J.M., and Greengard, P.: On the active structure of local anesthetics, J. Pharmacol. Exp. Ther. **133**:241, 1961.
9. Strong, J.M., Parker, M., and Atkinson, A.J.: Identification of glycinexylidide in patients treated with intravenous lidocaine, Clin. Pharmacol. Ther. **146**:67, 1973.

section six

Drugs used in cardiovascular disease

Although many drugs exert an effect on the heart, five groups of agents will be discussed in this section either because they act selectively on the heart or because they are particularly useful in the treatment of cardiac disease: digitalis glycosides, antiarrhythmic drugs, coronary vasodilator drugs, anticoagulant drugs, and diuretic drugs. In addition, the hypocholesterolemic agents are briefly discussed. Antihypertensive drugs are considered in Chapter 18.

Chapter 34

Digitalis

WILLIAM WITHERING, 1785 *It has the power over the motion of the heart to a degree yet unobserved in any other medicine, and this power may be converted to salutary ends.*

Certain steroids and their glycosides have characteristic effects on the contractility and electrophysiology of the heart. Most of these glycosides are obtained from the leaves of the foxglove, *Digitalis purpurea* or *Digitalis lanata*, or from the seeds of *Strophanthus gratus*. These cardioactive steroids are widely used in the treatment of heart failure and in the management of certain arrhythmias. They are collectively referred to as digitalis.

Although catecholamines, methylxanthines, and glucagon also increase the contractility of the myocardium, digitalis must accomplish its effect by a unique mechanism and is an important drug in the treatment of heart failure.

At the molecular level digitalis is a powerful inhibitor of sodium–potassium–adenosine triphosphatase (Na^+-K^+-ATPase). It is possible, although not proved, that the cardiac effects of the glycosides are a consequence of ATPase inhibition with changes in ion distribution.

Digitalis exerts striking effects on the *electrophysiology* of the heart. These effects are not the same in all portions of the organ. Most significant are more rapid repolarization of the ventricles (shortened electric systole) and, in higher concentrations, increased automaticity or increased rate of diastolic depolarization with appearance of ectopic activity. The atrioventricular (AV) node is markedly affected by the glycosides. Digitalis slows conduction and prolongs the refractory period of this node.

Digitalis poisoning is surprisingly common in clinical practice.[3] However, with the development of radioimmunoassays to monitor serum levels, and as special problems with the drug in specific disease states have been noted, management has improved and the occurrence of digitalis intoxication has decreased.[17,30] The therapeutic index of the drug is small, and it is dangerous in certain circumstances. For example, either hypokalemia or hypercalcemia greatly increases the possibility of fatal arrhythmias during digitalis administration.

GENERAL CONCEPT

HISTORY   The history of digitalis is a remarkable example of the discovery of an important drug in a folk remedy. William Withering,[38] having heard of a mixture of herbs that an old woman of Shropshire used successfully in the treatment of dropsy (congestive heart failure), suspected that its beneficial properties must have been caused by the foxglove. In testing it in patients with congestive failure, Withering was greatly impressed with the diuretic effect of the foxglove and believed that the drug probably acted on the kidney. On the other hand, he also stated that the drug had a remarkable "power over the heart."

Over the years digitalis has become the most important drug in the treatment of congestive failure, atrial flutter, and fibrillation. Its position is being challenged by the more intensive use of diuretics, by reduction of afterload and preload, and by newer inotropic agents. Nevertheless, digitalis remains one of the most important drugs in medicine.

EFFECTS ON HEART   Digitalis increases the contractility of the heart muscle and influences its electrophysiological properties such as conductivity, refractory period, and automaticity. It is increasingly recognized that the effectiveness of digitalis in the treatment of congestive failure is a consequence of its positive inotropic effect. On the other hand, some of its electrophysiological influences make the drug highly useful in the treatment of a variety of arrhythmias.

Contractility is influenced by digitalis in both the normal and the failing heart. In a now classic study (Fig. 34-1), Braunwald demonstrated this effect in humans by attaching a Walton-Brodie strain gauge arch to the right ventricular myocardium of patients undergoing cardiac surgery. The effect of digitalis on contractility has also been shown in the isolated heart (Fig. 34-2).

Digitalis increases both the force and the velocity of myocardial contraction, and it shortens the duration of systole. It promotes more complete emptying of the ventricles and decreases the size of the heart in failure. This reduction in heart size results in a decrease in cardiac wall tension, thereby lowering the energy requirements and the rate of oxygen consumption by the cardiac muscle. The final result is therefore an overall beneficial increase in the supply/demand ratio for the myocardium.

PROBLEM 34-1. Although digitalis increases the contractility of the normal as well as the failing heart, its effect on cardiac output is much greater in congestive failure. In fact, its ability to increase cardiac output in normal individuals has been questioned for many years.

The explanation of this paradox is related to hemodynamic adjustments. In the normal individual, digitalis not only increases cardiac contractility but it also causes constriction of peripheral vessels. It may also decrease venous pressure and may slow the sinus rate. Under these circumstances no increase in cardiac output can be demonstrated despite the positive inotropic effect.

The situation is different in the failing heart. In patients with congestive failure, the peripheral resistance is already high because the falling cardiac output leads to increased sympathetic tone. Under these circumstances the positive inotropic effect of digitalis increases cardiac output because the tone of peripheral vessels is lowered as a result of decreased sympathetic tone.

FIG. 34-1

Contractile force and arterial pressure recordings immediately and 20 minutes after injection of 1.4 mg acetylstrophanthidin in a 28-year-old woman with an atrial septal defect. The lower tracings show contractile force recordings before injection and at intervals after acetylstrophanthidin. Note that the drug augments the contractile force of the nonfailing human heart and constricts the systemic vascular bed as manifested by an increase in arterial pressure.

From Braunwald, E., Bloodwell, R.D., Goldberg, L.I., and Morrow, A.G.: J. Clin. Invest. *40*:52, 1961.

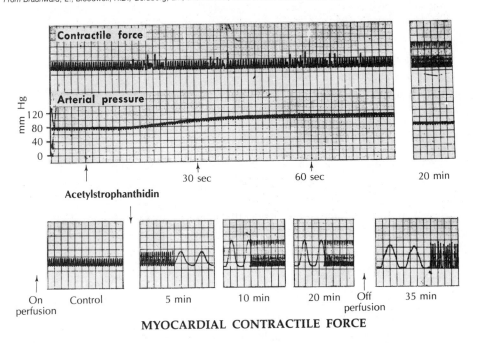

MYOCARDIAL CONTRACTILE FORCE

FIG. 34-2

Effect of digitalis on left ventricular function curves. Left ventricular stroke work is a measure of ventricular performance. Note that digitalis shifts the ventricular function curve upward and to the left; that is, myocardial contractility is increased. (CHF, Congestive heart failure.)

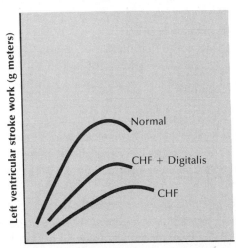

PROBLEM 34-2. *Does digitalis increase the efficiency of the failing heart? It has been observed that digitalis will increase cardiac output in the failing heart without a corresponding increase in oxygen consumption. At first glance this could be interpreted as an increase in efficiency, since more work is performed by the heart per unit of oxygen consumed.*[26]

The problem is much more complicated, however. The ventricular radius of the failing heart is reduced by digitalis. Oxygen consumption should be reduced as the ventricular radius becomes smaller. It is becoming clear that if heart size remained constant, digitalis would increase oxygen consumption as it increased contractility. On the other hand, the reduction of ventricular radius leads to a decrease in oxygen utilization, and the two effects cancel each other out.

Electrophysiological effects	The electrophysiological effects of digitalis provide the basis of its actions on *conductivity, refractory period,* and *automaticity*. These effects must be examined separately on the conducting tissue and the ventricular and atrial muscle cells. The problem is made complex by the existence of both *autonomic* and *direct* actions of the glycosides and by differences in the sensitivity of normal and diseased heart to the electrophysiological effects of digitalis.

Conducting tissue	At low doses, digitalis slows atrioventricular conduction. Since this action is reversed by atropine, it is commonly referred to as a "vagal effect." The direct effect of the drug that is not reversible by atropine becomes evident with higher doses.

AV node conduction is prolonged by digitalis. Prolongation of the P-R interval and varying degrees of block are electrocardiographic evidences of this action when the supraventricular rate is slow.

AV refractory period is also prolonged by digitalis. This action becomes important when the supraventricular rate is rapid, such as in atrial flutter and fibrillation when the purpose in using digitalis is to decrease the number of impulses reaching the ventricles.

Purkinje's fibers and to a lesser extent ventricular muscle respond to digitalis with a shortening of the action potential, decreased refractory period, and the appearance of pacemaker activity as a result of increased rate of diastolic depolarization (Fig. 34-3). Recent evidence suggests that increased automaticity is more likely if the fibers are stretched or potassium is low.[32]

Although it is generally accepted that digitalis increases ventricular automaticity in normal hearts, there are some observations that indicate an antiarrhythmic action of the drug in patients with ventricular premature beats.[25] Further studies are needed on this point.

Ventricular and atrial muscle	In the ventricle, digitalis shortens the refractory period and the duration of the action potential. Thus the Q-T interval shortens. Isolated tissue studies show that low concentrations of digitalis increase contractility prior to a sigificant change in transmembrane action potential.

In the atrium, the actions of digitalis are complicated by vagal effects. Digitalis may increase the release of acetylcholine and may also increase the sensitivity of the fibers to the released mediator.[33] In a normally innervated atrium without atropine,

FIG. 34-3

Diagram of the effect of digitalis on isolated Purkinje fibers. Note that digitalis decreases the duration of the action potential as it shortens the plateau. Refractory period is shortened. Increased rate of diastolic depolarization can result in the development of ectopic pacemaker activity.

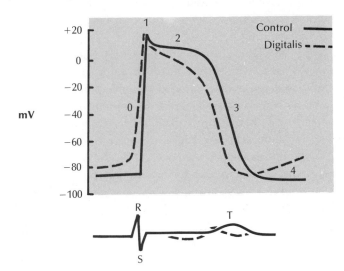

digitalis shortens the refractory period. On the other hand, in the denervated or atropine-treated atrium, digitalis may cause an increase in the refractory period.

EFFECT ON HEART RATE

In normal individuals, digitalis has little effect on heart rate. In congestive failure, digitalis slows the rapid sinus rhythm primarily by an indirect mechanism. The tachycardia in this case is a consequence of increased sympathetic activity brought about by decreased cardiac output. As digitalis increases cardiac output, the sympathetic drive to the sinoatrial node is reduced. Digitalis is not useful in the treatment of sinus tachycardia caused by fever and other conditions, since it has essentially no effect on the S-A node.

Other factors that may play a role in the cardiac slowing caused by digitalis are (1) prolongation of the refractory period of the AV node when atrial rate is rapid, (2) slowing of AV conduction (a partial block may be converted to complete block), and (3) reflex vagal stimulation elicited by digitalis. These mechanisms are discussed further in connection with the antiarrhythmic drugs.

Electrocardiographic effects

The effects of digitalis reflect the more rapid repolarization of the ventricle, changes in AV nodal conduction and refractory period, and increased ectopic activity. They are characterized by S-T segment depression, inversion of the T wave, shortened Q-T interval, prolongation of the P-R interval, AV dissociation, and ventricular arrhythmias such as premature ventricular contractions, bigeminal rhythm, and ventricular fibrillation.

FUNDAMENTAL
CELLULAR
EFFECTS

Digitalis has two striking effects that are probably related to its inotropic, electrophysiological, and toxic actions. One is related to Na^+-K^+-ATPase inhibition, the other to calcium metabolism.

Inhibition of the Na^+-K^+-ATPase should increase intracellular sodium. This sodium in turn may exchange with extracellular calcium.[1] It is possible, however, that the enzyme inhibition decreases the outward pumping of both sodium and calcium, thus increasing the calcium pool available for excitation-contraction coupling.

There are many reasons to believe that some connection exists between the digitalis effect and calcium. The two drugs are synergistic,[29] and calcium administration can be dangerous in digitalized patients. On the other hand, hypocalcemia has been shown to result in insensitivity to digoxin.[8] Furthermore, digitalis may increase the availability of intracellular calcium for the process of excitation-contraction coupling.

EXTRACARDIAC
EFFECTS

When used in therapeutic doses, the effects of digitalis are exerted largely on the heart. Some of the extracardiac effects may be important, however, as an aid to recognizing impending digitalis-induced cardiac toxicity.

The *gastrointestinal effects* manifest themselves commonly in the form of nausea and anorexia. These effects are central or reflex in origin when the purified glycosides are used. With powdered digitalis or digitalis tincture, a local effect contributes to nausea and anorexia. The intravenously administered glycosides exert their emetic effect by acting on the chemoreceptor trigger zone.

The *neurological effects* consist of blurred vision, paresthesias, and toxic psychosis. These symptoms are often misdiagnosed in elderly patients.

Endocrinological changes such as gynecomastia occur rarely. Allergic reactions are extremely uncommon.

The "diuretic effect" is primarily a consequence of increased cardiac output and renal blood flow, although in large doses the various glycosides cause some inhibition of sodium reabsorption directly in the renal tubules.[28]

Some experiments suggest that an action of digitalis on the central nervous system (CNS) contributes to arrhythmia and ventricular fibrillation.[14,15,36] For example, the intravenous administration of large doses of digitalis glycoside induces ventricular fibrillation in the dog. Ventricular fibrillation did not occur, however, after bilateral cardiac sympathectomy and ligation of the adrenal glands.[27] In some definitive experiments,[14] electric activity was monitored in sympathetic, parasympathetic, and phrenic nerves before and after ouabain administration in cats. Ouabain increased traffic in these nerves. Spinal transection prevented these effects and increased the dose of ouabain needed for producing ventricular arrhythmias. It appears then that neural activation, probably at the level of the brain stem, plays a role in the development of ouabain-induced arrhythmias.

The cardioactive steroids and their glycosides are widely distributed in nature. **SOURCES AND** Since their effects on the heart are qualitatively the same, it is sufficient to utilize **CHEMISTRY** only a few of these in therapeutics. Some believe that most physicians would do well to utilize only one such as digoxin, an intermediate-acting glycoside, which can be given orally or intravenously. Nevertheless, there are several digitalis glycosides in current use, and their sources and chemistry will be briefly summarized.

The glycosides most commonly used are obtained from the foxglove or *Digitalis purpurea*, *Digitalis lanata*, or the seeds of the African tree, *Strophanthus gratus*. The most important glycosides obtained from these plants are as follows:

Digitalis purpurea	*Digitalis lanata*	*Strophanthus gratus*
Digitoxin	Digoxin	Ouabain
Digoxin	Lanatoside C	
Digitalis leaf	Deslanoside	

The structure of digitoxin is characterized by a steroid nucleus with an unsaturated lactone attached in the C-17 position. The three sugars attached to the C-3 position are unusual deoxyhexoses. The molecule without the sugars is called an *aglycone* or *genin*. The steroidal structure and the unsaturated lactone are essential for the characteristic cardioactive effect. The removal of the sugars results in generally weaker and more evanescent activity.

Digitoxose-digitoxose-digitoxose

Digitoxin

(Digoxin differs only in having an OH at C-12)

Ouabain

Digoxin differs from digitoxin only in the presence of an OH at the C-12 position. Lanatoside C (Cedilanid) is the parent compound of digoxin and differs only from the latter by having an additional glucose molecule and an acetyl group on the oligosaccharide side chain. Removal of the acetyl group by alkaline hydrolysis yields the deslanoside, and the further removal of glucose by enzymatic hydrolysis gives digoxin.

Ouabain, obtained from the seeds of *Strophanthus gratus*, differs somewhat in its steroidal portion from the previously discussed compounds. Its aglycone is known as G-strophanthidin, and the sugar to which it is attached in the glycoside is rhamnose.

The various clinically useful glycosides and genins differ mainly in their pharmacokinetic characteristics, which are reflections of their water or lipid solubility, gastrointestinal absorption, metabolism, and excretion. Digitoxin is highly lipid sol-

TABLE 34-1 Properties of digitalis preparations

Preparation	Gastro-intestinal absorption	Onset of action*	Half-life†	Peak effect	Excretion or metabolism	Digitalizing dose (mg) Oral	Digitalizing dose (mg) Intravenous	Oral maintenance dose (mg)
Digoxin	75%	15-30 min	36 hr	1½-5 hr	Renal; some GI	1.25-1.5	0.75-1.0	0.25-0.5
Digitoxin	95%	25-120 min	5 days	4-6 days	Hepatic‡	0.7-1.2	1.0	0.1
Ouabain	Unreliable	5-10 min	21 hr	½-2 hr	Renal; some GI	—	0.3-0.5	—
Deslanoside	Unreliable	10-30 min	33 hr	1-2 hr	Renal	—	0.8	—

Modified from Smith, T.W.: N. Engl. J. Med. **288:**721, 1973.
*Intravenous administration.
†For normal subjects.
‡Enterohepatic circulation exists.

uble, digoxin is less so, and ouabain is water soluble. As expected from their solubilities, digitoxin is completely absorbed from the gastrointestinal tract and persists in the body for a long time, having a half-life of 7 days. Digoxin is not as well absorbed and has a biological half-life of 1.5 days. Ouabain, a highly polar compound, is not well absorbed from the gastrointestinal tract and has a short duration of action (Table 34-1).

Digitoxin is highly bound to plasma proteins and is metabolized in the liver. It also undergoes enterohepatic circulation, being excreted in the bile and subsequently reabsorbed. Experimentally, hepatectomy increases the half-life of digitoxin, whereas renal failure increases the half-life of digoxin.

The essential feature of the pharmacokinetics of various digitalis compounds depends on the observation[19] that the total glycoside losses from the body are proportional to the total amount present; that is, the disappearance is a first-order reaction. The more glycoside there is in the body, the more is lost each day.

In the case of digoxin in a patient having normal renal function, the half-life of the drug is 1.6 days. This means that when such a patient is given a *loading dose* of digoxin, 65% of it will still be in the body 1 day later and 35% will be lost. Since the purpose of subsequent *maintenance doses* is to replace losses, the daily maintenance dose will be 35% of the loading dose. The loading dose is usually 0.75 to 1.5 mg of digoxin given in three divided doses approximately 5 hours apart.[19] The loading dose sets the total glycoside in the body to a desired level. Since the glycoside disappears logarithmically, after five glycoside half-lives only one thirty-second of the loading dose remains in the body. The purpose of the maintenance doses then is to keep the total amount of glycoside at the desired level. In the case of digoxin, urinary losses represent 86% of the total loss, and changes in renal function will greatly influence its dosages.

Accumulation of a digitalis glycoside on a fixed daily dose compared with its disappear-   *FIG. 34-4*
ance after dosage is stopped. Time is expressed in units of half-times.

From Jeliffe, R.W.: Ann. Intern. Med. **69**:703, 1968.

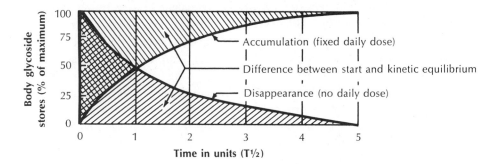

If no loading dose is given and the patient is placed on a fixed daily maintenance dose, the body stores of the glycoside will accumulate until the amount lost daily equals the maintenance dose. The curve of accumulation is a mirror image of the disappearance curve, and kinetic equilibrium will be reached in approximately 5 half-lives. Ninety percent of maximum will be reached in 3.3 half-lives (Fig. 34-4).

PREPARATIONS

Digoxin may be looked on as the prototype of digitalis glycosides. There are experts who believe that most physicians could limit themselves to this drug whenever a digitalis preparation is needed. Nevertheless, there are several glycosides in current use that differ largely in speed of onset, duration of action, gastrointestinal absorption, and suitability for intravenous administration.

It is essential to remember that all digitalis glycosides exert the same qualitative effects on the myocardium and that the therapeutic to toxic ratios are the same. Some are clearly more dangerous than others by virtue of differences in their durations of action. The patient poisoned with acetylstrophanthidin is not in jeopardy for as long a period as is one with digitoxin.

The modern trend is to use pure glycosides rather than the older digitalis powdered leaf or other impure compounds, which must be standardized by bioassay. In the bioassay techniques, the unknown preparation is compared with a USP reference standard with regard to lethal potency on cats, frogs, or pigeons or using the emetic effect on pigeons. The pure glycosides are measured spectrophotometrically.

Digoxin is becoming the most widely used digitalis glycoside.

Pharmacokinetics. Digoxin has an intermediate duration of action with a biological half-life of 36 hours. The drug may be administered orally or intravenously. When administered orally about 75% of it is absorbed.

It has previously been reported that there are marked differences in the bioavailability of various oral digoxin preparations depending on the manufacturer.[18] However, since 1974 the FDA has required manufacturers to meet minimum specifications for tablet dissolution rate and content. As a result, all forms of digoxin marketed in the United States are probably bioequivalent.

Gastrointestinal absorption of digoxin is influenced by several conditions. Patients with malabsorption syndromes may absorb the drug poorly. Cholestyramine and other resins interfere with digoxin absorption. Also, various antacids, kaolin, and pectin reduce the oral absorption of the glycoside.[7]

Digoxin is excreted by glomerular filtration and is not significantly reabsorbed by the tubules. Only 20% of the drug is bound by plasma proteins. The loss of digoxin from the body takes place in an exponential fashion. In other words, the loss of the glycoside is proportional to the amount present in the body. The half-life of tritiated digoxin is 1.6 days, which increases to 4.4 days in anuric patients.[12]

Oral preparations of digoxin (Lanoxin) include tablets of 0.125, 0.25, and 0.5 mg and an elixir of 0.05 mg/ml. It is also available in solution for injection, 0.1 and 0.25 mg/ml.

Like digoxin, deslanoside (Cedilanid-D) is derived from *D. lanata*. It is similar in action to digoxin, and its usual digitalizing intravenous dose is 1.4 mg. Deslanoside is a derivative of lanatoside C (Cedilanid), which is poorly absorbed from the gastrointestinal tract and is rarely used.

Digitoxin is the main active glycoside in digitalis leaf *(D. purpurea)*. On a weight basis it is a thousand times as active as the powdered leaf, so that 1 mg of digitoxin is equivalent to 1 g of the leaf.

Digitoxin is the least polar of the useful cardiac glycosides, and it is highly bound to plasma proteins (97%). In contrast with digoxin, digitoxin is largely metabolized by the liver, with renal excretion being a minor factor in its disposition. Digitoxin undergoes enterohepatic circulation and cholestyramine interferes with its reabsorption.

The physiological half-life of digitoxin is approximately 5 to 7 days. Anuria prolongs the half-time to 8 days. This prolongation is obviously relatively less than in the case of digoxin, which depends much more on renal excretion for its elimination.

A patient receiving digitoxin therapy loses about 10% of the amount in the body in a day. The drug accumulates until the peak stores represent 10 times the daily maintenance dose. A loading dose is generally given at the beginning of treatment, since on a daily maintenance dose a long time would be required for full digitalization. Because of its slow metabolic degradation, its toxic effects continue for a long time after the drug is discontinued. This is one of the reasons for the increasing popularity of digoxin in preference to digitoxin, although there is no unanimity on this question. The metabolic degradation of digitoxin is accelerated by drugs that stimulate the activity of hepatic microsomal enzymes, such as phenobarbital.

Transition from digoxin to digitoxin in a patient may lead to difficulties because of their different pharmacokinetics.[19] Transition from digoxin maintenance to digitoxin maintenance would lead to underdigitalization, whereas changing from digitoxin to digoxin without careful adjustment of dosages may lead to digitalis poisoning.

Oral preparations of digitoxin (Crystodigin; Digitalin Nativelle; Purodigin) include oral tablets containing 0.05, 0.1, 0.15, and 0.2 mg; elixir, 0.5 mg/ml; and injectable solution, 0.2 mg/ml.

Ouabain, a crystalline glycoside, is obtained from *S. gratus*. It is a highly polar glycoside, suitable for intravenous injection only, because it is poorly absorbed from the gastrointestinal tract. It is commonly used in experimental work. Its plasma half-life is 21 hours.

Gitalin is a mixture of glycosides obtained from *D. purpurea*. It has no advantages, although a more favorable therapeutic index has been claimed for it.

Digitalis is the principal drug of choice in the treatment of congestive failure and in certain arrhythmias. Some of the latter indications are absolute and others are controversial. *THERAPEUTIC INDICATIONS*

Congestive failure caused by a variety of underlying mechanisms responds well to digitalis treatment. By increasing contractility, the drug increases cardiac output and relieves the elevated ventricular pressures, pulmonary congestion, and venous pressure. Diuresis is brought about with relief of edema. *Congestive failure*

Controversy exists in relation to the use of digitalis in myocardial infarction with failure. The drug may aggravate the arrhythmias that commonly accompany the infarction. Some experts believe that this danger has been overemphasized. Other areas of controversy relate to the prophylactic use of digitalis, which is avoided by most clinicians.

Arrhythmias of certain types represent important indications for the use of digitalis. Among these the most prominent are atrial fibrillation, atrial flutter, and paroxysmal atrial tachycardia. *Arrhythmias*

The main purpose of using digitalis in atrial fibrillation in the absence of congestive failure is to slow the ventricular rate. This is achieved by the prolongation of the refractory period of the AV node, which allows fewer of the supraventricular impulses to get through. Digitalis does not generally stop the atrial fibrillation itself. *ATRIAL FIBRILLATION*

In atrial flutter, the rapid atrial rate is accompanied by a 2:1 or 3:1 AV block. Digitalis further increases the magnitude of the AV block, thus slowing the ventricular rate. As to the atrial flutter itself, digitalis tends to convert flutter to fibrillation. This effect is probably a consequence of decreasing the refractory period of the atria. Occasionally, after flutter is converted to fibrillation by digitalis and the drug is stopped, normal sinus rhythm may result. *ATRIAL FLUTTER*

Clinical factors modifying digitalis dosage

Clinical states that increase sensitivity to toxic effects

Acute myocardial infarction
Advanced ventricular failure
Latent disease of the AV node
Chronic pulmonary disease; hypoxemia
Decreased renal function
Hypokalemia
Hypothyroidism
Hypomagnesemia
Hypercalcemia
Advanced age

Clinical states that decrease sensitivity to toxic effects

Hyperthyroidism
Impaired gastrointestinal absorption
Enhanced digitoxin metabolism
Infancy
Hypocalcemia

From Lucchesi, B.R.: Inotropic agents and drugs used to support the failing heart. In Antonaccio, M., editor: Cardiovascular pharmacology, New York, 1977, Raven Press, p. 361.

PAROXYSMAL ATRIAL TACHYCARDIA
Paroxysmal atrial tachycardia often responds to increased vagal activity, which can be elicited by pressure on the carotid sinus. Digitalis may act by a similar mechanism, since it has a definite vagal effect.

Cor pulmonale
Digitalis treatment of persistent right-sided heart failure secondary to chronic obstructive lung disease is somewhat controversial. At best, digitalis should be considered as an adjunct to treatment of this disease. One major problem lies in the fact that these patients suffer from arterial hypoxemia, which contributes to digitalis sensitivity and therefore increased susceptibility to digitalis toxicity. Other factors predisposing to toxicity include electrolyte imbalance, respiratory acidosis, and concomitant treatment with sympathomimetic agents (see box, above). Thus digitalis appears to have a useful but limited role in the treatment of cor pulmonale.

DIGITALIS POISONING
Intoxication with digitalis is common and hazardous. In a survey carried out in a general hospital, digitalis intoxication was found to be the most common adverse drug reaction.[31]

The symptoms of digitalis poisoning include both extracardiac[24] and cardiac manifestations. In mild to moderate intoxication, the symptoms consist of anorexia, ventricular ectopic beats, and bradycardia. These may progress to nausea and vomiting, headache, malaise, and ventricular premature beats. In severe intoxication, the

Serum digoxin concentrations related in general to effects. *FIG. 34-5*

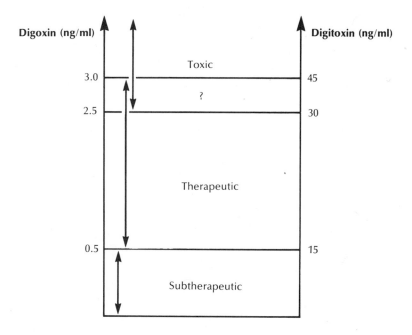

symptoms are characterized by blurring of vision, disorientation, diarrhea, ventricular tachycardia, and sinoatrial and AV block. This may progress to ventricular fibrillation.

There are several reasons for the frequency of digitalis intoxication. The therapeutic index of digitalis is low and highly variable in different patients. The common use of thiazide diruetics leads to hypokalemia, which aggravates digitalis toxicity.

The development of methods for determining serum concentrations of digoxin and digitoxin by radioimmunoassay may be important in the prevention of some cases of digitalis intoxication (Fig. 34-5). It should be stressed, however, that such determinations should not replace good clinical judgment, because numerous factors influence the significance of a given serum concentration. Some of these factors are the underlying heart disease, the serum concentration of potassium and magnesium, and endocrine factors. When digoxin plasma concentrations are determined, the blood sample should be obtained at least 5 hours after the oral dose to avoid sampling during the distribution phase.

The electrocardiographic changes observed in digitalis poisoning can be explained on the basis of the drug's electrophysiological effects. Ventricular arrhythmias are related to increased automaticity (increased rate of diastolic depolarization). AV dissociation is related to the actions of digitalis on conduction and refractory period at the AV node. The lowering of the S-T segment and inversion of the T wave commonly observed after digitalis may reflect rapid repolarization of the ventricle and perhaps a change in the initiation of the repolarization process.

TABLE 34-2   Drug interactions with digoxin

Drug	Effect*	Mechanism
Amphotericin B	↑	Induces hypokalemia
Cholestyramine; colestipol	↓	Binds digoxin in gastrointestinal tract; interferes with enterohepatic circulation
Quinidine	↑	Decreases renal clearance of digoxin
Reserpine	↑	See text
Spironolactone	↑	Inhibits tubular secretion of digoxin
Thiazides; furosemide; bumetanide	↑	Diuretic-induced hypokalemia potentiates digitalis effect
Verapamil; nifedipene	↑	Decreases renal clearance of digoxin

* ↑, Potentiates digitalis effect; ↓, impairs digitalis effect.

Drug interactions and digitalis intoxication

In addition to the potassium-losing diuretics that predispose to digitalis toxicity, there are other drug interactions of clinical significance (see Table 34-2). Calcium (parenteral) and catecholamines or sympathomimetic drugs may promote ectopic pacemaker activity in digitalized patients. Barbiturates such as phenobarbital may accelerate the metabolism of digitoxin. Cholestyramine resin binds digitoxin in the intestine and thus interferes with its enterohepatic circulation. Digitalis can be used in reserpinized patients, since the glycosides still exert their characteristic cardiotonic effect. On the other hand, the administration of parenteral reserpine to a digitalized patient may cause arrhythmias, probably as a consequence of sudden catecholamine release.[10]

Digoxin toxicity is enhanced by quinidine.[16] When therapeutic doses of quinidine are administered to patients maintained on digoxin, there is on the average a doubling of the serum digoxin concentration. The exact mechanism of this drug interaction remains controversial. However, most of these patients will have a decrease in the renal clearance of digoxin and many will have a decrease in the volume of distribution.[5,11] If it is judged clinically necessary to administer digoxin and quinidine concomitantly, then serum digoxin concentrations should be monitored closely so that appropriate adjustments can be made in the digoxin dosage.

Treatment of digitalis poisoning

The most important measure in the treatment of digitalis poisoning is the discontinuation of the drug administration. Potassium chloride by mouth or by slow intravenous infusion may be helpful in stopping the ventricular arrhythmias. It should be remembered, however, that elevated potassium concentrations may aggravate AV block, although potassium may improve it if serum potassium is low. It is believed by many investigators that the infusion of potassium in a digitalized patient may produce abnormally high serum concentrations because of the effect of the glycosides on the membrane ATPase in various tissues. Other drugs that are used occasionally in digitalis poisoning are the antiarrhythmic drugs such as phenytoin, lidocaine, and procainamide. Purified Fab fragments of digoxin specific antibodies have been used successfully to treat digitalis intoxication in animals and in patients with advanced, life-threatening toxicity.[35] However, this form of therapy is not generally available. Adsorptive hemoperfusion, a technique that passes the patient's blood over an absorbing substance such as charcoal, has been used to accelerate digitalis elimination in patients poisoned with digoxin[34] and digitoxin.[13]

The principles behind the loading dose and the maintenance dose have already been discussed in relation to pharmacokinetics of digitalis (p. 426). For practical purposes, initial digitalization is accomplished by either a *rapid method* or a *cumulative (slow) method*.

DIGITALIZATION AND MAINTENANCE

In the rapid method, the estimated loading dose is administered in a single dose or in two or three divided doses given a few hours apart, depending on the response. In the cumulative method, smaller doses are employed at greater intervals until full digitalization takes place by cumulation. For example, digitoxin may be given for initial digitalization in a single dose of 1.2 or 0.4 mg every 8 hours for three doses. This initial digitalization is followed in subsequent days by the maintenance dose, which in the case of digitoxin is 0.1 to 0.2 mg daily.

For details on digitalizing and maintenance doses of the various glycosides see Table 34-1.

Dobutamine hydrochloride (Dobutrex) is a synthetic derivative of isoproterenol. It increases myocardial contractility but causes less tachycardia or peripheral arterial effects.[37] Administered by intravenous infusion, the drug may be useful in relatively acute heart failure without severe hypotension. In cardiogenic shock with severe hypotension, dobutamine is not sufficient to elevate blood pressure adequately, since it does not increase peripheral resistance. Since the electrophysiological effects of dobutamine are similar to those of isoproterenol, the drug may cause an increase in heart rate, and in the presence of coronary artery disease ischemia may be aggravated.

NEWER INOTROPIC AGENTS

Amrinone is a new ionotropic agent that differs in its mode of action from digitalis and the β-adrenergic agonists.[20] It is a bipyridine derivative that has been shown to exert strong positive inotropic effects in a variety of experimental preparations. Amrinone has undergone limited therapeutic trials. In patients with congestive heart failure that did not respond well to digitalization, amrinone caused further increases in resting cardiac output while decreasing left ventricular end diastolic, pulmonary capillary wedge, and right atrial pressure as well as systemic vascular resistance. The exact mechanism of action of amrinone remains unclear, although it is thought to influence excitation-contraction coupling in cardiac muscle. It does not appear to act on the sodium-potassium pump or to alter cyclic AMP levels. The ultimate position of amrinone in relation to digitalis cannot be predicted.

REFERENCES

1. Akera, T., and Brody, T.M.: The role of Na$^+$, K$^+$-ATPase in the inotropic action of digitalis, Pharmacol. Rev. **29**:187, 1977.

2. Aronson, J.K.: Clinical pharmacokinetics of digoxin 1980, Clin. Pharmacokinet. **5**:137, 1980.

3. Beller, G.A., Smith, T.W., Abelmann, W.H., Haver, E., and Hood, W.B.: Digitalis intoxication: a prospective clinical study with serum level correlations, N. Engl. J. Med. **284**:989, 1971.

4. Benotti, J.R., Grossman, W., Braunwald, E., Dovolos, D.D., and Alouis, A.A.: Hemodynamic assessment of amrinone, a new inotropic agent, N. Engl. J. Med. **199**:1373, 1978.

5. Bigger, J.T., and Leahey, E.B., Jr.: Quinidine and digoxin—an important interaction, Drugs **24**:229, 1982.

6. Bresnahan, J.F., and Vliestra, R.E.: Clinical pharmacology—digitalis glycosides, Mayo Clin. Proc. **54**:675, 1979.

7. Brown, D.D., and Juhl, R.P.: Decreased bioavailability of digoxin due to antacids and kaolin-pectin, N. Engl. J. Med. **295**:1034, 1976.

8. Chopra, O., Janson, P., and Sawin, P.: Insensitivity to digoxin associated with hypocalcemia, N. Engl. J. Med. **196**:917, 1977.

9. Cohn, J.: Physiologic basis of vasodilator therapy for heart failure, Am. J. Med. **71**:135, 1981.

10. Dick, H.L.H., McCawley, E.L., and Fisher, W.A.: Reserpine-digitalis toxicity, Arch. Intern. Med. **109**:503, 1962.

11. Doering, W.: Quinidine-digoxin interaction: pharmacokinetics, underlying mechanism and clinical implications, N. Engl. J. Med. **301**:400, 1979.

12. Doherty, J.E., deSoyza, N., Kane, J.J., Bissett, J.K., and Murphy, M.L.: Clinical pharmacokinetics of digitalis glycosides, Prog. Cardiovasc. Dis. **21**:141, 1978.

13. Gilfrich, H.J., Kasper, W., Meinertz, T., Okonek, S., and Bork, R.: Treatment of massive digitoxin overdose by charcoal hemoperfusion, Lancet **1**:505, 1978.

14. Gillis, R.A., et al.: Neuroexcitatory effects of digitalis and heir role in the development of cardiac arrhythmias, J. Pharmacol. Exp. Ther. **183**:154, 1972.

15. Gillis, R.A., Pearle, D.R., and Levitt, B.: Digitalis: a neuroexcitatory drug, Circulation **52**:739, 1975.

16. Hager, W.D., Fenster, P., Mayersohn, M., Perrier, D., Graves, P., Marcus, F.I., and Goldman, S.: Digoxin-quinidine interaction, N. Engl. J. Med. **300**:1238, 1979.

17. Henry, D.A., Lowe, J.M., Lawson, D.H., and Whiting, B.: The changing pattern of toxicity to digoxin, Postgrad. Med. J. **57**:358, 1981.

18. Huffman, D.H., and Azarnoff, D.L.: Absorption of orally given digoxin preparations. JAMA **222**:957, 1972

19. Jeliffe, R.W.: An improved method for replacing one digitalis glycoside with another, Med. Times **98**:105, 1970.

20. Katz, A.M.: A new inotropic drug: its promise and a caution, N. Engl. J. Med. **299**:1409, 1978.

21. Klein, H.O., Lang, R., Weiss, E., Segni, E.D., Libhaber, C., Guerrero, J., and Kaplinsky, E.: The influence of verapamil on serum digoxin concentration, Circulation **65**:998, 1982.

22. Lathers, C.M., and Roberts, J.: Minireview—digitalis cardiotoxicity revisited, Life Sci. **27**:1713, 1980.

23. Lee, D.C., Johnson, R.A., Bingham, J.B., Lehy, M., Dinsmore, R.E., Goroll, A.H., Newell, J.B., Strauss, W., and Haber, E.: Heart failure in outpatients-a randomized trial of digoxin versus placebo. N. Engl. J. Med. **306**:699, 1982.

24. Lely, A.H., and Van Eter, C.H.J.: Noncardiac symptoms of digitalis intoxication, Am. Heart J. **83**:149, 1972.

25. Lown, B., Graboys, T.B., Pidrid, P.J., Cohen, B.H., Stockman, M.B., and Gaughan, C.E.: Effect of digitalis drug on ventricular premature beats, N. Engl. J. Med. **296**:301, 1977.

26. Mason, D.T.: Digitalis pharmacology and therapeutics: recent advances, Ann. Intern. Med. **80**:520, 1974.

27. Mendez, C., Aceves, J., and Mendez, R.: The antiadrenergic action of digitalis on the refractory period of the A-V transmission system, J. Pharmacol. Exp. Ther. **131**:199, 1961.

28. Nechay, B.R., and Nelson, J.A.: Renal ouabain-sensitive ATP-ase activity and Na$^+$ reabsorption, J. Pharmacol. Exp. Ther. **175**:717, 1970.

29. Nola, G.T., Pope, S., and Harrison, D.L.: Assessment of the synergistic relationship between serum calcium and digitalis, Am. Heart J. **79**:499, 1970.

30. Ochs, H.R., Greenblatt, D.J., Bodem, G., and Dengler, H.J.: Disease-related alterations in cardiac glycoside disposition, Clin. Pharmacokinet. **7**:434, 1982.

31. Oglive, R.I., and Ruedy, J.: An educational program in digitalis therapy, JAMA **222**:50, 1972.

32. Rosen, M.R., Gelband, H., Merker, C., and Hoffman, B.F.: Mechanisms of digitalis toxicity: effects of ouabain on phase four of canine Purkinje fiber transmembrane potentials, Circulation **47**:681, 1973.

33. Rosen, M.R., Wit, A.L., and Hoffman, B.: Electrophysiology and pharmacology of cardiac arrhythmias. IV. Cardiac antiarrhythmic and toxic effects of digitalis, Am. Heart J. **89**:391, 1975.

34. Smiley, J.W., March, N.M., and Del-Guercio, E.T.: Hemoperfusion in the management of digoxin toxicity, JAMA **240**:2736, 1978.

35. Smith, T.W., Butler, V.P., Jr., Haber, E., Fozzard, H., Marcus, F.I., Bremner, W.F., Schulman, I.C., and Phillips, A.: Treatment of life-threatening digitalis intoxication with digoxin-specific Fab antibody fragments: experience in 26 cases, N. Engl. J. Med. **307**:1357, 1982.

36. Somberg, J.L., and Smith, T.W.: Localization of the neurally mediated arrhythmogenic properties of digitalis, Science **204**:321, 1979.

37. Sonneblick, E.H., Frishman, W.H., and LeJemtel, T.H.: Dobutamine: a new synthetic cardioactive sympathetic amine, N. Engl. J. Med. **300**:17, 1979.

38. Withering, W.: An account of the foxglove, and some of its medicinal uses: with practical remarks on dropsy, and other diseases. London, 1785, C.G.J.&J. Robinson. (Reprinted in Medical Classics **2**:305, 1937.)

Chapter 35

Antiarrhythmic drugs

GENERAL CONCEPT　　The antiarrhythmic drugs are useful in the prevention and treatment of disorders of cardiac rhythm. Cardiac arrhythmias, or more properly dysrhythmias, have high morbidity and mortality. Major advances have taken place in our understanding of cardiac electrophysiology and of the mode of action of drugs used in the treatment of arrhythmias. In general, cardiac arrhythmias can be considered to arise from abnormal conduction, abnormal impulse initiation, or both.[22]

Although the classification of antiarrhythmic agents is controversial, the available drugs can be placed into four groups on the basis of their electrophysiological effects (Table 35-1). *Class I* drugs act by depressing the fast inward sodium current in cardiac muscle, resulting in prolongation of the effective refractory period and depression of phase 4 depolarization. *Class II* drugs are β-adrenergic blocking agents. They reduce sympathetic excitation to the heart and inhibit phase 4 depolarization, especially that augmented by catecholamines. *Class III* agents, represented by bretylium, prolong the action potential and refractory period. Finally, *Class IV* drugs selectively block the slow calcium channel; verapamil is representative of this series.

CARDIAC ELECTRO-PHYSIOLOGY　　An understanding of the pharmacology of antiarrhythmic drugs requires some background knowledge of cardiac electrophysiology. Fig. 35-1 depicts a normal cardiac action potential from a Purkinje fiber. The resting cell has a membrane potential of approximately -90 mV, with the inside of the cell being electronegative relative to the outside of the cell. This negative potential results primarily from a transmembrane potassium ion gradient maintained in part by a sodium-potassium adenosine triphosphatase (ATPase) pump that selectively moves Na^+ out of the cell and K^+ into the cell. If the cell is adequately stimulated, there is a rapid influx of sodium through specific membrane channels. This rapid depolarization (phase 0) of ventricular myocardial tissue corresponds to the familiar QRS complex of the surface electrocardiogram. As the sodium ion influx decreases, the cell membrane starts to repolarize (i.e., becomes more negative), resulting in phase 1 of the action potential. In addition,

TABLE 35-1	Classification of antiarrhythmic drugs		
I	II	III	IV
Quinidine	Propranolol	Bretylium	Verapamil
Procainamide	Metoprolol	Amiodarone*	Diltiazem
Disopyramide	Nadolol		
Lidocaine	Timolol		
Tocainide†	Atenolol		
Mexiletine†			
Aprindine†			
Phenytoin			

*Tentative classification—possible additional mechanisms.
†Investigational drug.

Cardiac action potential as recorded from a Purkinje fiber and a ventricular fiber electrogram. Phases of the action potential are indicated by 0, 1, 2, 3, and 4. g, Transmembrane conductance of an ion. FIG. 35-1

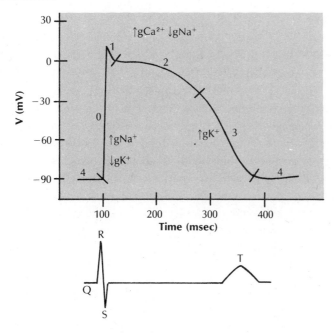

a second inward current, arising primarily from the movement of calcium, begins. This calcium influx maintains a depolarized state and is primarily responsible for phase 2 (plateau) of the action potential. Finally, both the inward sodium and the inward calcium currents decline, and rapid repolarization (phase 3) occurs as a result of potassium efflux. In essence, the action potential is a coordinated sequence of ion movements; initially sodium rapidly enters the cell, followed by a calcium influx, and finally a potassium efflux that returns the cell to its resting state. Several antiarrhythmic drugs exert their effects by altering these ion fluxes.

ELECTRO-PHYSIOLOGICAL BASIS OF ANTIARRHYTHMIC ACTION

Most tachyarrhythmias are consequences of two basic mechanisms[22,26]: (1) ectopic focal activity and/or (2) reentry. In ectopic focal activity a potential pacemaker fires independently because of an increase in the slope of diastolic depolarization, the threshold potential being more negative, or because of a decrease in the maximum diastolic potential.[25] Myocardial ischemia, excessive myocardial catecholamine release, stretching of the myocardium, and cardiac glycoside toxicity have been shown to produce some of these electrophysiological effects.

The conditions necessary for reentry to occur are as follows[26]: (1) the conduction pathway must be blocked, (2) there must be slow conduction over an alternate route to a point beyond the block, and (3) there must be delayed excitation beyond the block. With a sufficient delay in excitation beyond the block, the tissue proximal to the site of block may be excited from the opposite direction and the circuit is then established. These principles are illustrated in Fig. 35-2.

The various classes of antiarrhythmic drugs have characteristic electrophysiological effects on the myocardium, modified in some instances by extracardiac effects.

Class I drugs have local anesthetic properties. They reduce the maximum rate of depolarization, increase the threshold of excitability, depress conduction velocity, prolong the effective refractory period, and reduce the spontaneous diastolic depolarization in pacemaker cells. These effects are shown for quinidine in Fig. 35-3. The decrease in diastolic depolarization tends to suppress ectopic focal activity. Prolongation of refractory periods tends to abolish reentry. These drugs generally prolong the duration of the action potential with simultaneous prolongation of the effective refractory period. Lidocaine and phenytoin differ from other members of the class in shortening the action potential. The actions of quinidine, procainamide, and disopyramide are modified by their anticholinergic activity.

Class II antiarrhythmic drugs are β-adrenergic blocking agents such as propranolol. Their β-blocking effect is much more important than any local anesthetic activity they may have. Their mode of action is related to a depression of the slope of the spontaneous diastolic depolarization (phase 4).

Class III drugs, represented mainly by bretylium, appear to act by prolonging the action potential that is associated with a prolongation of the effective refractory period.

Class IV antiarrhythmic drugs are a group of agents best represented by verapamil. These agents selectively block the slow inward current (slow response) carried

Schematic representation of reentry in the Purkinje system. Purkinje fiber (P) in the distal **FIG. 35-2**
ventricular conducting system divides into two branches (a and b) before making contact
with ventricular muscle (VM) to form a loop. Panel A shows the sequence of activation
under normal conditions; the sinus impulse descends via the main Purkinje bundle leading
to the loop, conducts through both branches (a and b) into ventricular muscle, collides,
and terminates. Panel B shows the pattern of activation when an area of unidirectional
conduction block is present (shaded area in branch b). Conduction is blocked in the
antegrade direction in b but not in the retrograde direction (from VM to b). The impulse
in limb a conducts slowly around the loop and returns to the site of antegrade block in
limb b. Because of slowed conduction, this impulse arrives at the site of antegrade block
in b after the refractory period has passed and is able to conduct in a retrograde manner.
In panel C the impulse traveling retrogradely past the site of antegrade block into b
conducts into P, activating the ventricle giving rise to a reciprocal beat. It may also continue
the "circus" via limb a, producing repetitive reciprocal beats. The rate of this reciprocal
beating will be determined by the total conduction time around the loop.

From Vera, Z., and Mason, D.T.: Am. Heart J. 101:329, 1981.

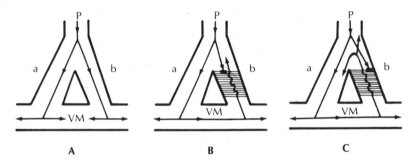

Diagrammatic representation of the effect of quinidine on the transmembrane electrical **FIG. 35-3**
potential of a spontaneously depolarizing conductive fiber in the ventricular myocar-
dium.

Modified from Mason, D.T., et al.: Clin. Pharmacol. Ther. 11:460, 1970.

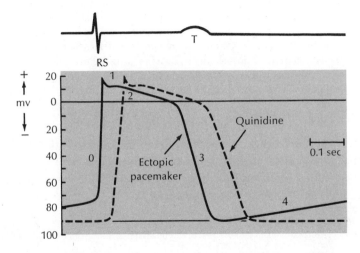

primarily by calcium and perhaps by sodium.[2,18] In cardiac muscle the fast inward current (fast response) is carried by sodium. The slow response, which mediates pacemaker potentials and may be an important factor in certain pathological conditions, such as ischemia or digitalis toxicity, is dependent primarily on the inward calcium current. The antiarrhythmic effect of verapamil appears to be largely caused by its blocking effect on this inward calcium current. Verapamil reduces the action potential amplitude in the upper- and mid-AV nodal regions and prolongs the time-dependent recovery of excitability and the effective refractory period of the AV nodal fibers. These effects block conduction of premature impulses in the AV node, thereby preventing the conduction delay that is necessary to allow AV nodal reentry and tachycardia. The ability of verapamil to prevent atrial arrhythmias may be a result of abolition of slow response activity in diseased atrial muscle and/or of suppression of propagation of the impulse through the AV node.

ANTIARRHYTHMIC DRUGS
Quinidine

Quinidine is the dextrorotatory isomer of quinine and has the following structure:

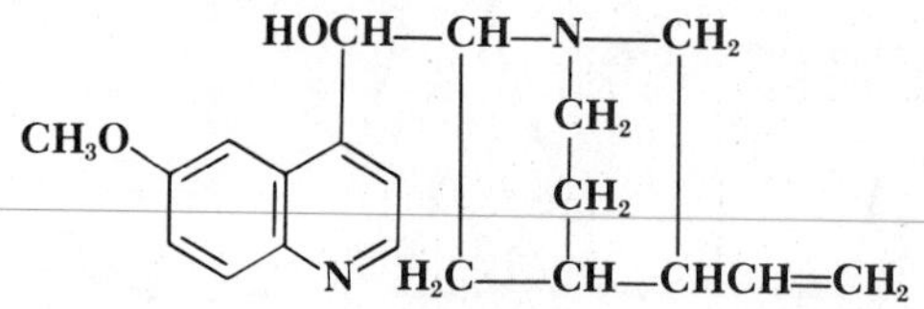

Quinidine

The introduction of quinidine into therapeutics is one of the classical stories of medical history. In 1914 the Viennese cardiologist Wenckebach[28] had a Dutch sea captain as a patient. The captain had a completely irregular pulse as a consequence of atrial fibrillation. Wenckebach described the situation in this way.

> He did not feel great discomfort during the attack, but, as he said, being a Dutch merchant, used to good order in his affairs, he would like to have good order in his heart business also, and asked why there were heart specialists if they could not abolish this very disagreeable phenomenon. On my telling him that I could promise him nothing, he told me that he knew himself how to get rid of his attacks, and as I did not believe him, he promised to come back the next morning with a regular pulse, and he did. It happens that quinine in many countries, especially in countries where there is a good deal of malaria, is a sort of drug for everything, just as one takes acetylsalicylic acid today if one does not feel well or is afraid of having taken a cold. Occasionally, taking the drug during an attack of fibrillation, the patient found that the attack was stopped within from twenty to twenty-five minutes, and later he found that a gram of quinine regularly abolished his irregularity.*

In 1918 Frey[6] tried drugs related to quinine in patients with atrial fibrillation and introduced quinidine, the dextro isomer of quinine, into cardiac therapy. During the succeeding years the antifibrillatory action of quinidine was confirmed, but its widespread use led to a number of sudden deaths.

---

*From Beckman, H.: Treatment in general practice, Philadelphia, 1934, W.B. Saunders Co.

Eventually it was recognized that there are definite contraindications to the use of the drug. In the presence of conduction defects it may produce cardiac standstill and should be avoided. Once the mode of action of the drug was understood and contraindications to its use were recognized, quinidine obtained its present position in cardiac therapy.

Quinidine is a Class I antiarrhythmic drug. Thus it reduces the maximum rate of depolarization, increases the threshold of excitability, depresses conduction velocity, prolongs the effective refractory period, and reduces the spontaneous diastolic depolarization in pacemaker cells (Fig. 35-3), thus depressing automaticity. The drug is useful in both supraventricular and ventricular tachyarrhythmias. Quinidine can convert atrial tachyarrhythmias to normal sinus rhythm, but cardioversion is replacing this use of the drug.

CARDIAC EFFECTS

A complicating factor in the action of quinidine is its "vagolytic" or anticholinergic effect. This anticholinergic action tends to predominate at lower plasma quinidine concentrations and may result in increased conduction velocity in the AV node. This

Effect of quinidine on electrocardiogram. Note changes in P wave, QRS complex, and T wave at varying dosage levels.   **FIG. 35-4**

From Burch, G.E., and Winsor, T.: *A primer of electrocardiography*, Philadelphia, 1960, Lea & Febiger.

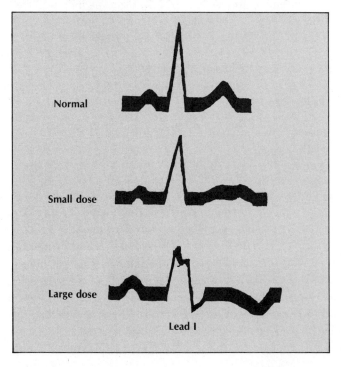

may counteract its direct effect and might explain the acceleration of heart rate that may be caused by the drug. The anticholinergic effect may also explain the paradoxical tachycardia seen in some cases during treatment of atrial flutter with block. At steady state therapeutic plasma concentrations the direct electrophysiological actions of quinidine predominate.

Electrocardiographic effects. Quinidine in higher doses prolongs the P-R, QRS, and Q-T intervals (Fig. 35-4). Widening of the QRS complex is related to slowing conduction in the His-Purkinje system and in the ventricular muscle. Changes in the Q-T interval and alteration in T waves are related to changes in repolarization. The direct effect of the drug on AV conduction and refractoriness of the AV system explains the prolongation of the P-R interval.

EXTRACARDIAC AND ADVERSE EFFECTS

Quinidine tends to depress all muscle tissue, including vascular smooth muscle and skeletal muscle. Particularly when injected intravenously, the drug can cause profound hypotension and shock. Its effect on skeletal muscle becomes particularly evident in patients with myasthenia gravis, in whom it causes profound weakness.

Cinchonism caused by quinidine is characterized by ringing of the ears and dizziness and is similar to what may be observed after the administration of quinine or salicylates.

Quinidine thrombocytopenia appears to occur on an immune basis. In a typical case a patient taking quinidine for several weeks notices the development of petechial hemorrhages in the buccal mucous membranes. The symptoms disappear when the drug is discontinued and reappear after reinstitution of therapy. This disorder is thought to be due to formation of a plasma protein–quinidine complex that evokes a circulating antibody ultimately resulting in platelet destruction.[9]

CARDIOTOXICITY AND ITS TREATMENT

Quinidine may cause ventricular arrhythmias and even ventricular fibrillation. The so-called quinidine syncope is probably a consequence of ventricular fibrillation.[27]

It may seem paradoxical that an antiarrhythmic drug can cause ventricular arrhythmias. Since quinidine depresses automaticity, the clinically observed ventricular arrhythmias after excessive doses of quinidine are probably caused by reentry mechanism rather than by increased automaticity.

Quinidine is particularly dangerous in patients having conduction defects. In such patients, when conduction is further impaired and automaticity of the Purkinje system is depressed, the ventricles may not take over when AV conduction fails, and cardiac standstill may ensue. The administration of the drug should be stopped when significant increases in P-R interval or QRS widenings supervene during treatment.

PHARMACOKINETICS

When given orally, quinidine produces its peak effect in 1.5 to 4 hours. Its half-life is about 4 to 6 hours. Quinidine sulfate is rapidly absorbed with peak levels in about 1.5 hours. By contrast, the gluconate is more slowly absorbed with peak levels about 4 hours after a dose.[8] The more prolonged absorption phase of the gluconate results in lower peak concentrations. Consequently, the gluconate can be administered less frequently than the sulfate.

About 10% to 50% of administered quinidine is excreted in unchanged form in the urine. The rest is transformed in the liver by hydroxylation. The amount excreted is influenced by the pH of the urine. Alkalinization with molar sodium lactate tends to decrease the excretion of quinidine, although it may improve some toxic effects of the drug.

Quinidine is bound to plasma proteins, a fact that may account for some lack of correlation between blood levels and therapeutic effect. Nevertheless, toxic manifestations correlate better with serum levels than with the dose of the drug.

Drug interactions occur with quinidine and will be discussed in Chapter 63.

Preparations of quinidine include: quinidine sulfate in tablets containing 200 and 300 mg and timed-release tablets of 300 mg (Quinidex Extentabs); and quinidine gluconate in tablets containing 324 mg (Quinaglute Dura-Tabs) or 330 mg (Duraquin). A 275 mg tablet of the polygalacturonate (Cardioquin) is also available.

The usual initial adult dosage of quinidine is 600 to 900 mg daily. The actual dose and dosage interval will vary depending on the formulation, the effects of disease, and individual variations in kinetics. Optimum therapy requires the monitoring of plasma levels. Moreover, interpretation of therapeutic concentrations depends on the analytical method employed. Older methods were less specific and measured active drug as well as active and inactive metabolites.[10,31] Using an assay that measured only active drug, Kessler et al.[11] determined the therapeutic range for quinidine to be 2.3 to 5 µg/ml, which is considerably lower than that obtained with older analytical methods.

Quinidine gluconate is available for intramuscular injection. Intravenous administration is dangerous and should not be undertaken without monitoring the electrocardiogram.

PREPARATIONS, ADMINISTRATION, AND DOSAGE

The commonly used local anesthetic procaine was shown by Mautz[17] in 1936 to elevate the threshold to electric stimulation when applied to the myocardium of animals. In subsequent years thoracic surgeons and anesthesiologists frequently used topical procaine in surgery to reduce premature ventricular and atrial contractions during surgery. Procaine was even administered intravenously for this purpose.

Procainamide DEVELOPMENT AS CARDIAC DRUG

Procaine hydrochloride

Procainamide hydrochloride

Encouraged by these studies, investigators studied the antifibrillatory activities of compounds related to procaine, including the effects of the two hydrolysis products of procaine, *p*-aminobenzoic acid and diethylaminoethanol. The most fruitful consequence of these studies was the finding that if the ester linkage in procaine was replaced by an amide linkage, the resulting compound had distinct advantages as an antiarrhythmic drug. The main advantages consist of greater stability in the body and fewer CNS effects. The greater stability results from the fact that the drug is an amide rather than an ester.

CARDIAC EFFECTS

Procainamide hydrochloride (Pronestyl) is so similar in its actions to quinidine that the two drugs could be used interchangeably. Quinidine is preferred by some physicians for prolonged oral use because procainamide can cause a drug-induced lupus erythematosus–like syndrome characterized by rheumatic symptoms, pleuropericardial involvement, and antinuclear antibodies.[4] On the other hand, procainamide is safer when used intravenously and is beneficial in the treatment of ventricular tachyarrhythmias that do not respond to lidocaine.

PHARMACOKINETICS

Procainamide is absorbed well from the gastrointestinal tract and is 15% protein bound. It is metabolized in the liver to its major metabolite *N*-acetylprocainamide, which has antiarrhythmic activity but does not appear to induce lupus erythematosus.[13] The rate of acetylation is genetically conditioned, and patients may be fast or slow acetylators. It has been demonstrated that genetically slow acetylators of procainamide have an earlier onset of, and a higher prevalence of, drug-induced lupus compared to rapid acetylators.[30] Renal disease prolongs the half-life of procainamide.

Procainamide hydrochloride (Pronestyl) is available in 250, 375, and 500 mg tablets and in injectable solutions containing 100 and 500 mg/ml. Sustained-release preparations of procainamide (Procan SR) are also available.

EXTRACARDIAC EFFECTS AND TOXICITY

Procainamide may cause a marked fall of blood pressure after the administration of large intravenous doses. This is probably a consequence of its action on vascular smooth muscle and on contractility of the myocardium, although ganglionic blocking effects have also been described. The drug has local anesthetic properties but is not useful for nerve block.

Nausea, anorexia, mental confusion, hallucinations, skin rashes, agranulocytosis, chills, and fever have been reported after the use of procainamide, in addition to the lupus erythematosus–like syndrome.

Disopyramide

Disopyramide phosphate (Norpace) is a Class I antiarrhythmic drug, which resembles quinidine and procainamide in its action. It is used for the prevention of ventricular premature beats and also atrial tachyarrhythmias. The drug has anticholinergic activity. Disopyramide is absorbed well from the gastrointestinal tract and has a plasma half-life of 4 to 5 hours. Renal impairment prolongs the half-life.

Disopyramide may cause or worsen congestive heart failure or produce severe hypotension as a consequence of its negative inotropic properties. This is most likely to occur in patients with marginally compensated underlying cardiac failure.[21] Rarely, disopyramide prolongs the QRS or Q-T interval. This is an indication to either reduce the dosage or consider stopping the medication. Its anticholinergic action can result in adverse effects. For this reason disopyramide should not be given to patients with glaucoma, myasthenia gravis, or urinary retention.

Disopyramide phosphate (Norpace) is available in 100 and 150 mg capsules, which are administered every 6 hours in patients with normal renal function.

Lidocaine hydrochloride (Xylocaine hydrochloride) is a Class I antiarrhythmic drug, which has become the most widely used agent for the treatment and prevention of ventricular ectopic activity associated with myocardial infarction. In many centers lidocaine is used for the prophylaxis of primary ventricular fibrillation occurring after myocardial infarction and even with suspected acute myocardial infarction.

Lidocaine differs in some important aspects from most other members of the Class I antiarrhythmic drugs. Although it depresses automaticity and diastolic depolarization, it does not slow conduction and has little effect on atrial function. It does not prolong the action potential and refractory period.

Lidocaine must be injected intravenously or intramuscularly because when given orally it shows the first-pass effect, with the liver inactivating it very rapidly. For the same reason, liver damage or impaired hepatic blood flow increases the half-life of lidocaine.

Lidocaine

The distribution half-life of lidocaine is 8.3 minutes. Its disposition half-life is 107 minutes. The volume of distribution is 530 ml/kg, and its clearance is 10 ml/kg/min. The clearance of lidocaine is reduced in patients with chronic liver disease or congestive heart failure (because of decreased hepatic blood flow).

Lidocaine is given as a loading dose (1 mg/kg) followed by a continuous infusion (1 to 4 mg/min). There is, however, significant variability among patients in the plasma concentration resulting from a given dose.[33] In many instances this variation can be accounted for by changes in αl-acid glycoprotein (AAG), an important plasma protein binding site for lidocaine.[23] For example, AAG concentrations rise after myocardial infarction, resulting in marked increases in total plasma lidocaine concentrations, while the free (nonprotein bound) fraction rises much less.[24] Rapid, clinically useful methods for measuring free (and presumably active) lidocaine concentrations are needed to monitor therapy most effectively.

Adverse effects of lidocaine include drowsiness, convulsions, and coma. Very large doses have adverse effects on the heart, manifested by depression of AV conduction and a negative inotropic effect.

Lidocaine hydrochloride is available as Xylocaine Intravenous Injection in solution containing 20, 40, or 200 mg/ml. A loading dose of 50 to 100 mg is recommended,

PHARMACO-KINETICS

given over a period of 2 to 5 minutes. The dose may be repeated after 5 minutes, not to exceed 300 mg/hour.

| Mexiletine | Mexiletine (Mexitil) is very similar to lidocaine in its electrophysiological effects, chemical structure, and clinical spectrum of antiarrhythmic actions.[19,20] It differs from lidocaine mainly in its suitability for oral administration, its pharmacokinetics, and its side effects. Unlike lidocaine, mexiletine has high systemic availability following oral ingestion. Peak plasma levels are obtained 2 to 4 hours after giving the dose. The elimination half-life in healthy volunteers is about 11.5 hours. Mexiletine is extensively metabolized, and the renal clearance of the drug is increased by urinary acidosis. Therapeutic blood concentrations range from 0.5 to 2 μg/ml with side effects being more frequent at higher levels. |

Mexiletine has minimum hemodynamic effects and only a mild negative inotropic action. However, its myocardial depressant action can be more pronounced in patients with poorly compensated congestive heart failure. The major therapeutic indication for mexiletine is in the long-term prophylaxis of recurrent ventricular arrhythmias, particularly those associated with previous myocardial infarction.

The major adverse effects of mexiletine are neurological and include tremors, nystagmus, diplopia, ataxia, and confusion. Nausea and vomiting may also be seen. Nevertheless, mexiletine is well tolerated by many patients. The usual dose of mexiletine (Mexitil) is 600 to 1000 mg every 8 to 12 hours.

| Tocainide | Tocainide (Tonocard) is also a lidocaine congener that is similar to mexiletine in its electrophysiological properties and antiarrhythmic action.[19] Tocainide is active following oral ingestion with peak serum concentrations occurring within 60 to 90 minutes. Its elimination half-life is about 14 hours in patients. Effective plasma concentrations between 3.5 and 7 μg/ml can usually be achieved with a total daily dose of between 400 and 1100 mg of tocainide hydrochloride given in two or three divided doses. The major clinical indication for tocainide is in the prophylaxis of ventricular tachyarrhythmias.[29] Tocainide can produce the same neurological and gastrointestinal side effects as mexiletine. |

| Aprindine | Aprindine (Fibocil) is a powerful Class I antiarrhythmic drug, which may be effective in both supraventricular and ventricular arrhythmias. It is orally active and has a very long half-life but may cause neurological side effects in a small percentage of patients.[19] |

| Phenytoin | The antiepileptic drug phenytoin (Dilantin) was found to decrease ventricular arrhythmias in dogs after coronary ligation in 1950. More recently it has become widely used as an antiarrhythmic drug, especially in digitalis-induced tachyarrhythmias, which may be its only real indication. |

Phenytoin depresses automaticity in ventricular and atrial tissues and may actually improve AV conduction. Generally it is not a useful antiarrhythmic drug, and even in digitalis toxicity lidocaine is usually preferred.

The effective level of phenytoin for antiarrhythmic activity is about 6 to 18 µg/ml, which is about the same as for its anticonvulsant effectiveness.

Phenytoin is absorbed slowly when given by mouth, and peak levels are not obtained for several hours. The drug should not be given intramuscularly, since its absorption is erratic.[27] The drug is metabolized by liver microsomal enzymes, being parahydroxylated. The disappearance of phenytoin does not follow first-order kinetics because of saturation of the microsomal enzymes at therapeutic serum levels. With this reservation, it is useful to know that within the usual therapeutically effective concentration, serum levels fall to one half in 18 to 24 hours.

PHARMACOKINETICS

For oral administration to obtain a prompt effect, phenytoin may be administered in a dose of 1000 mg the first day, 500 to 600 mg the second and third days, and 400 to 500 mg thereafter.[27]

Intravenous phenytoin should be given by infusion only to severely ill patients. Infusion rate should be 25 to 50 mg/min. A total dose of 500 mg to 1 g should not be exceeded.

DOSAGE

Phenytoin (Dilantin) is available in capsules containing 100 mg. It is also available as a powder to make a solution for injection, 50 mg/ml.

PREPARATIONS

Propranolol (Inderal) exerts its antiarrhythmic activity by acting on β-adrenergic receptors. Its membrane-stabilizing effect is not as important because plasma concentrations are not high enough to achieve such an effect.

Propranolol depresses automaticity, prolongs AV conduction, reduces heart rate, and also decreases contractility. The drug is particularly effective in the treatment of tachyarrhythmias caused by increased sympathetic activity. It prevents the reflex tachycardia caused by vasodilator antihypertensive drugs. Along with digitalis it slows ventricular rate in atrial flutter and fibrillation. It has been used in digitalis toxicity, but lidocaine or phenytoin are preferred.

Adverse effects of propranolol include bronchospasm, congestive heart failure, and cardiac arrest. Bradycardia is common but is not a contraindication to the continued use of propranolol. Sudden withdrawal of propranolol may lead to a recurrence of angina and even sudden death. It is tempting to speculate about the possibility of β-receptor up regulation caused by prolonged exposure to the blocking agent.

Propranolol

Propranolol (Inderal) may be given orally or intravenously. The oral dose is 10 to 40 mg two or three times a day. Intravenously, 0.1 to 0.15 mg/kg should be administered in divided doses of 0.5 to 0.75 mg every 1 or 2 minutes with appropriate monitoring. The patient should be observed for myocardial depression and brady-

DOSAGE

cardia. Atropine or isoproterenol will reverse excessive bradycardia. It may require relatively large doses of isoproterenol by intravenous infusion to counteract the bradycardia, since propranolol blocks the β receptors.

Bretylium tosylate

Bretylium tosylate (Bretylol) is an adrenergic neuronal blocking drug, which was originally developed as an antihypertensive agent. Troublesome side effects made it essentially useless as an antihypertensive drug, but its antiarrhythmic properties brought it back into clinical use.

Bretylium exerts its effect as an antiarrhythmic by prolonging the action potential with simultaneous prolongation of the effective refractory period. The drug is used to treat severe ventricular tachyarrhythmias that are unresponsive to other drugs. Even after intravenous injection, the effect of the drug may be delayed for several minutes or hours. Initially, the drug causes norepinephrine release and an increase in blood pressure. This is followed by a fall in blood pressure.

In addition to changes in blood pressure, adverse effects of bretylium include nausea, bradycardia, angina, diarrhea, skin rash, and others. The drug should be administered slowly.

Bretylium tosylate is a quaternary ammonium compound, and it is eliminated unchanged by the kidney.

Bretylium tosylate (Bretylol) is available in solution containing 50 mg/ml. The drug is administered intravenously or intramuscularly.

Verapamil

Verapamil (Isoptin, Calan) is a *papaverine* derivative, which appears to be of value in certain atrial tachyarrhythmias and also in the management of angina pectoris. The drug has a unique mechanism of action and may represent the first of a series of new antiarrhythmic drugs. Verapamil inhibits transmembrane fluxes of calcium[25] and acts on the slow channel. Since the slow channel is involved in the action potential in pacemaker cells, verapamil acts on the SA node, prolongs AV refractoriness, depresses potential or latent pacemaker cells, and produces vasodilatation.

Intravenous verapamil is effective in converting reentrant paroxysmal supraventricular tachycardia (PSVT) to normal sinus rhythm.[18] Long-term oral therapy with verapamil may decrease the frequency and duration of PSVT and severity of symptoms.[16] Verapamil, because of its ability to slow AV conduction and hence ventricular responses, is also useful for patients with atrial fibrillation. The slower heart rate is maintained with exercise, and many patients experience subjective improvement as manifested by increased effort tolerance and decreased palpitations during exertion.[12]

Verapamil (Isoptin, Calan) is available as an intravenous preparation, 2.5 mg/ml, and in tablets, 80 and 120 mg.

SELECTION OF DRUGS

There are several principles that should be remembered before selecting a drug for the treatment of a cardiac arrhythmia. (1) Many arrhythmias do not require drug treatment. (2) Most antiarrhythmic drugs can be dangerous. (3) Cardioversion (DC countershock) has changed many of the indications for the use of antiarrhythmic medications.

With these limitations, the use of antiarrhythmic drugs in various arrhythmias will be briefly summarized.

Paroxysmal atrial tachycardia may occur in otherwise normal individuals. It may terminate spontaneously but may recur. It may also occur as a manifestation of digitalis toxicity.

Vagal maneuvers, such as carotid massage, may terminate the attack. Anticholinesterase drugs such as edrophonium and neostigmine may be used. Vasoconstrictors, such as methoxamine or phenylephrine, may terminate an attack by causing reflex vagal activity as a consequence of elevation of the blood pressure. Digitalis may be effective and is commonly used in atrial tachycardias in children.

Verapamil is being used more extensively for supraventricular tachyarrhythmias, and, finally, propranolol may also be of use in the treatment of such rhythm disturbances.

Supraventricular arrhythmias
PAROXYSMAL ATRIAL TACHYCARDIA

Digitalis is the most important drug in the treatment of atrial flutter. It acts primarily by increasing the degree of AV block, thereby decreasing the ventricular rate. As for the flutter itself, digitalis tends to convert it to fibrillation. The explanation resides in the ability of digitalis to shorten the refractory period in the atrial muscle. Occasionally quinidine is used for the conversion of flutter to normal sinus rhythm. In this case digitalis should be employed first to prevent excessive tachycardia, a consequence of the vagolytic action of quinidine. Cardioversion finds increasing usefulness in the treatment of atrial flutter.

If digitalis is not effective, the addition of propranolol may be useful.

Intravenous verapamil converts atrial flutter to a normal sinus rhythm in about 30% of cases.;[18] As with digitalis, verapamil often converts atrial flutter to atrial fibrillation which, in turn, may convert to sinus rhythm.

ATRIAL FLUTTER

Digitalis is the most important drug in the treatment of atrial fibrillation. It does not convert atrial fibrillation to normal sinus rhythm, but it slows the ventricular rate by increasing AV block, and it corrects cardiac failure if it is present. Quinidine can convert atrial fibrillation to normal sinus rhythm, but the newer tendency is to use cardioversion for this purpose. Even when DC countershock is employed, quinidine may be helpful in preventing the recurrence of atrial fibrillation.

When quinidine is added to digoxin treatment, the plasma level of the glycoside may rise to dangerous levels.[3] Administration of quinidine is often started before cardioversion, and it may terminate the fibrillation by itself. Disopyramide may be used in the same manner.

Verapamil can also be used in atrial fibrillation because of its ability to slow the ventricular response by blocking AV conduction.

ATRIAL FIBRILLATION

Ventricular arrhythmias

Occasional premature ventricular contractions generally do not require drug treatment. On the other hand, ventricular tachycardia may be a serious condition that requires intensive treatment. Although DC countershock is now commonly used for stopping ventricular tachycardia, it should not be employed if the arrhythmia is caused by digitalis.[15]

For premature ventricular beats lidocaine is the drug of choice, but procainamide may also be tried. For chronic treatment quinidine, procainamide, propranolol, or disopyramide are suitable. Lidocaine, procainamide, and propranolol are also commonly used in attempts to terminate ventricular tachycardia. Bretylium is also employed occasionally.

Digitalis-induced arrhythmias may be treated with lidocaine, phenytoin, or propranolol. Antibody fractions to digitalis have been used on an investigational basis.

Digitalis is generally considered to be dangerous in the management of ventricular arrhythmias. This concept has been challenged by some investigations.[15]

REFERENCES

1. Akhtar, M.: Management of ventricular tachyarrhythmias, JAMA **247**:671, 1982.
2. Antman, E.M., Stone, P.H., Mueller, J.E., and Braunswald, E.: Calcium channel blocking agents in the treatment of cardiovascular disorders. I. Basic and clinical electrophysiologic effects, Ann. Intern. Med. **93**:875, 1980.
3. Bigger, J.T., and Leahey, E.B., Jr.: Quinidine and digoxin—an important interaction, Drugs **24**:229, 1982.
4. Blomgren, S.E., Condemi, J.J., and Vaughan, J.H.: Procainamide-induced lupus erythematosus: clinical and laboratory observations, Am. J. Med. **52**:338, 1972.
5. Danilo, P., Jr.: Tocainide, Am. Heart J. **97**:259, 1979.
6. Frey, W.: Weitere Erfahrungen mit Chinidin bei absoluter Herz unregelmassigkeit, Klin. Wochenschr. **55**:849, 1918.
7. Gettes, L.S.: Physiology and pharmacology of antiarrhythmic drugs, Hosp. Pract. Oct. 1981, p. 89.
8. Greenblatt, D.J., Pfeifer, H.J., and Ochs, H.R., et al.: Pharmacokinetics of quinidine in humans after intravenous, intramuscular and oral administration, J. Pharmacol. Exp. Ther. **202**:365, 1977.

9. Hackett, T., Kelton, J.G., and Powers, P.: Drug-induced platelet destruction, Semin. Thromb. Hemostas. **8**:116, 1982.
10. Hartel, G., and Harganne, A.: Comparison of two methods for quinidine determination and chromatographic analysis of the difference, Clin. Chim. Acta **23**:289, 1969.
11. Kessler, K.M., Lowenthal, D.T., Warner, H., et a.: Quinidine elimination in patients with congestive heart failure or poor renal function, N. Engl. J. Med. **290**:706, 1974.
12. Klein, H.O., Paugner, H., DiSegni, E., David, O., and Kaplinsky, E.: The beneficial effects of verapamil on chronic atrial fibrillation, Arch. Intern. Med. **139**:747, 1979.
13. Kluger, J., Drayer, D.E., Reidenberg, M.M., and Lahita, R.: Acetylprocainamide therapy in patients with previous procainamide-induced lupus syndrome, Ann. Int. Med. **95**:18, 1981.
14. Koch-Weser, J.: Bretylium, N. Engl. J. Med. **300**:473, 1979.
15. Lown, B., Grabays, R.B., Podrid, P.J., Cohen, B.H., Stockman, M.B., and Gaughan, C.E.: Effect of digitalis drug on ventricular premature beats, N. Engl. J. Med. **296**:301, 1977.

16. Mauretson, D.R., Winneford, M.O., Walker, W.S., Rude, R.E., Cory, J.R., and Hills, L.D.: Oral verapamil for paroxysmal supraventricular tachycardia: a long-term, double blind randomized trial, Ann. Intern. Med. **96**:409, 1982.

17. Mautz, F.R.: The reduction of cardiac irritability by the epicardial and systemic administration of drugs as a protection in cardiac surgery, J. Thorac. Surg. **5**:612, 1936.

18. McGoon, M.D., Vlietstra, R.E., Holmes, D.R., Jr., and Osborn, J.E.: The clinical use of verapamil, Mayo Clin. Proc. **57**:485, 1982.

19. Nademanee, K., and Singh, B.N.: Advances in antiarrhythmic therapy: the role of newer antiarrhythmic drugs, JAMA **247**:217, 1982.

20. Podrid, P.J., and Lown, B.: Mexiletine for ventricular arrhythmias, Am. J. Cardiol. **47**:895, 1981.

21. Podrid, P.J., Schoeneberger, A., and Lown, B.: Congestive heart failure caused by oral disopyramide, N. Engl. J. Med. **302**:614, 1980.

22. Reder, R.F., and Rosen, M.R.: Mechanisms of cardiac arrhythmias, Cardiovasc. Rev. Rep. **2**:1007, 1981.

23. Routledge, P.A., Stargel, W.W., Barchowsky, A., Wagner, G.S., and Shand, D.G.: Control of lidocaine therapy: new perspectives, Ther. Drug Monit. **4**:265, 1982.

24. Routledge, P.A., Stargel, W.W., Wagner, G.S., and Shand, D.G.: Increased alpha-1-acid glycoprotein and lidocaine disposition in myocardial infarction, Ann. Intern. Med. **93**:701, 1980.

25. Singh, B.N., Collett, J.T., and Chew, C.Y.C.: New perspectives in the pharmacologic therapy of cardiac arrhythmias, Prog. Cardiovasc. Dis. **22**:243, 1980.

26. Vera, Z., and Mason, D.T.: Reentry versus automaticity: role in tachyarrhythmia genesis and antiarrhythmic therapy, Am. Heart J. **101**:329, 1981.

27. Wasserman, A.J., and Proctor, J.D.: Pharmacology of antiarrhythmics: quinidine, beta-blockers, diphenylhydantoin, bretylium, Med. Coll. Va. Q. **9**:53, 1978.

28. Wenckebach, K.F.: Die unregelmassige Harztatigkeit und ihre Klinische Bedeutung, Leipzig, 1914, W. Englemann.

29. Winkle, R.A., Mason, J.W., and Harrison, D.C.: Tocainide for drug-resistant ventricular arrhythmias: efficacy, side effects, and lidocaine responsiveness for predicting tocainide success, Am. Heart. J. **100**:1031, 1980.

30. Woosley, R.L., Drayer, D.E., Reidenberg, M.M., Nies, A.S., Carr, K., and Oates, J.A.: Effect of acetylator phenotype on the rate at which procainamide induces antinuclear antibodies and the lupus syndrome, N. Engl. J. Med. **198**:1157, 1978.

31. Woosley, R.L., and Shand, D.G.: Pharmacokinetics of antiarrhythmic drugs, Am. J. Cardiol. **41**:986, 1978.

32. Zipes, D.P.: New approaches to antiarrhythmic therapy, N. Engl. J. Med. **304**:475, 1981.

33. Zito, R.A., Reid, P.R., and Longstieth, J.S.: Variability of early lidocaine levels in patients, Am. Heart J. **94**:292, 1977.

Chapter 36

Antianginal drugs

GENERAL CONCEPT   It is an old empirical observation that amyl nitrite (1867) and nitroglycerin (1879) relieve the pain of angina pectoris. Since nitrates and nitrites dilate blood vessels, including the coronary arteries, the role of coronary vasodilatation in the relief of angina has been generally assumed.

The problem is much more complex, however. Angina results from an imbalance between oxygen demand and supply in ischemic areas of the myocardium. Drugs may improve angina theoretically by reducing the demand or by increasing the supply of oxygen. There is increasing evidence for a reduction of demand by an action on the peripheral circulation as a primary mechanism for the antianginal effect of the nitrates and nitrites. On the other hand, drugs that increase myocardial oxygen demand, such as the catecholamines, have adverse effects in patients with coronary disease. In addition to its use in angina pectoris, nitrate therapy is becoming routine in the vasodilator management of congestive heart failure. The use of nitrates has also expanded because of the availability of intravenous formulations and longer acting oral and topical preparations.

The β-adrenergic blocking agents, such as propranolol, are used extensively in the treatment of angina. Drugs of this class emphasize the importance of reduction of cardiac work in the relief of angina.

Calcium channel blocking drugs, such as verapamil, nifedipine, and diltiazem, are also effective antianginal agents. They dilate coronary arteries and are particularly useful in patients with Prinzmetal's angina resulting from coronary artery spasm. The calcium channel blockers can also be effective in chronic, exercise-induced angina, probably as a consequence of their systemic vasodilating action, which reduces myocardial oxygen requirements.

The clinically useful nitrites and nitrates exert qualitatively similar effects. The most interesting compounds in the group and their formulas are as follows:

Nitrates

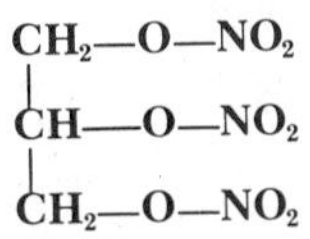

$$CH_2—O—NO_2$$
$$|$$
$$CH—O—NO_2$$
$$|$$
$$CH_2—O—NO_2$$

Glyceryl trinitrate

$$CH_2—O—NO_2$$
$$|$$
$$O_2N—O—CH_2—C—CH_2—O—NO_2$$
$$|$$
$$CH_2—O—NO_2$$

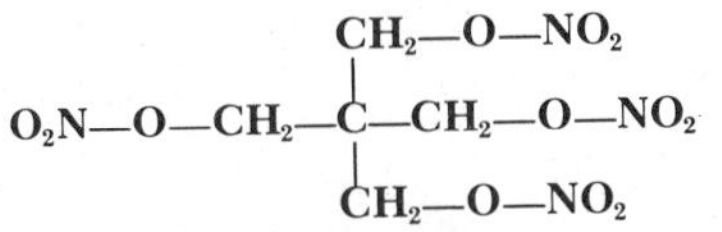

Pentaerythritol tetranitrate

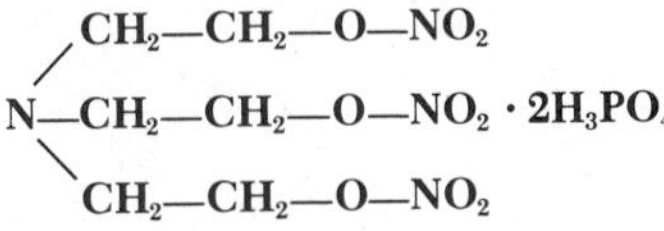

$$CH_2—CH_2—O—NO_2$$
$$/$$
$$N—CH_2—CH_2—O—NO_2 \cdot 2H_3PO_4$$
$$\backslash$$
$$CH_2—CH_2—O—NO_2$$

Triethanolamine trinitrate biphosphate

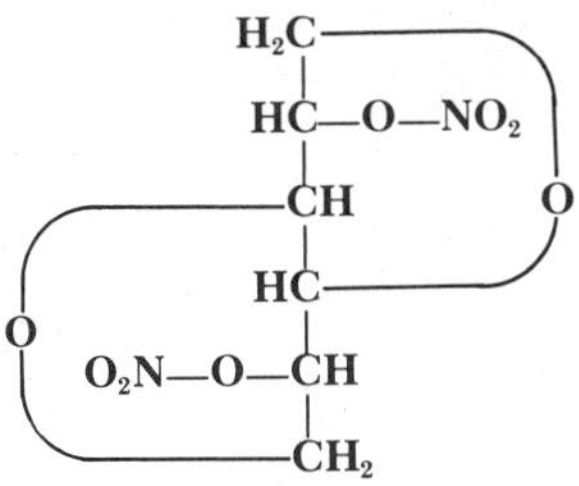

$$H_2C—$$
$$|$$
$$HC—O—NO_2$$
$$|$$
$$CH \quad O$$
$$|$$
$$HC—$$
$$|$$
$$O_2N—O—CH$$
$$|$$
$$—CH_2$$

Isosorbide dinitrate

$$CH_2—O—NO_2$$
$$|$$
$$CH—O—NO_2$$
$$|$$
$$CH—O—NO_2$$
$$|$$
$$CH_2—O—NO_2$$

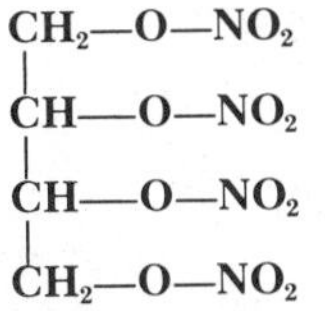

Erythrityl tetranitrate

Nitrites

$$H_3C$$
$$\backslash$$
$$CHCH_2CH_2NO_2$$
$$/$$
$$H_3C$$

$$NaNO_2$$

Sodium nitrite

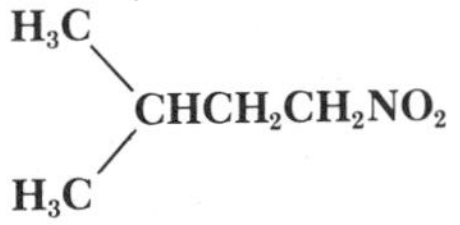

Amyl nitrite

The effects of nitrites, calcium blockers, and β-blockers on myocardial oxygen requirements and oxygen supply are shown in Table 36-1.

If a patient suffering from an attack of angina pectoris places a small 0.3 mg tablet of nitroglycerin under the tongue, the attack frequently subsides in a matter of minutes. Furthermore, the drug is often effective if taken prophylactically before the performance of some task that ordinarily produces angina.

This is not a placebo effect. Although a large proportion of patients suffering from angina pectoris claim benefit from placebo tablets, a significantly greater number derive benefit from nitroglycerin. Furthermore, if a patient between anginal attacks is asked to perform a standard exercise tolerance test such as the Master two-step test, precordial pain and T-wave inversion on the electrocardiogram may be developed, generally interpreted as consequences of myocardial ischemia. If the same patient has received prophylactic nitroglycerin, he or she is often protected against both the pain and the eletrocardiographic alterations during exercise.

The simplest interpretation of this remarkable effect of nitroglycerin would be that the drug improves blood flow to ischemic areas in the myocardium by dilating coronary vessels. This interpretation, however, appears to be untenable.

TABLE 36-1 Effects of nitrites, calcium blockers, and β-blockers on myocardial oxygen requirements and supply

| | Nitrates | Calcium blockers | | | β-blockers |
		NF	DZ	VP	
Determinants of myocardial oxygen requirements					
Heart rate	↑	↑	↓ —	—	↓ *
Left ventricular pressure	↓	↓	↓ —	↓	↓ *
Left ventricular volume/radius	↓ *	↓	↓	↑ —	↑
Velocity of contraction	↑	↑	—	↓	↓
Systolic ejection period	↓	↓	↑ —	—	↑
Determinants of myocardial oxygen supply					
Coronary vasodilatation	↑ *	↑ *	↑ *	↑ *	↓
Aortic diastolic pressure	↓	↓	↓	↓	↓
Diastolic perfusion time	↓	↓	↑		↑

*Most significant effects.
—, No changes; NF, nifedipine; DZ, diltiazem; VP, veparamil.

TABLE 36-2 Long-acting nitrates: recommended dosage and duration of action

Drug	Dosage	Duration of action (hr)
Oral nitroglycerin	6.5-19.5 mg every 4-6 hr*	4-6
2% nitroglycerin ointment	½-2 in (1.3-5 cm; 7.5-30 mg) every 4-6 hr	3-6
Isosorbide dinitrate		
Sublingual	2.5-10 mg every 2-4 hr	1.5-3†
Oral	10-60 mg every 4-6 hr*	4-6
Chewable	5-10 mg every 2-4 hr	2-3
Oral pentaerythritol tetranitrate	40-80 mg every 4-6 hr*	3-5

From Abrams, J.: N. Engl. J. Med. **302**:1234, 1980. Reprinted by permission of the New England Journal of Medicine.
*Large doses, often greater than manufacturers recommend, may be necessary to produce a therapeutic effect.
†Most studies indicate a duration of action for sublingual isosorbide dinitrate of 90 to 120 minutes; some indicate activity for 4 hours.

PROBLEM 36-1. *Would nitroglycerin administered directly into a coronary artery relieve angina? This has been tested by two clinical investigators.[7] In 25 patients undergoing cardiac catheterization as possible candidates for revascularization surgery, 0.075 mg of nitroglycerin was injected into the left coronary artery through the angiographic catheter at a time when angina was induced by pacing. The intracoronary injection was ineffective despite a significant increase in coronary sinus blood flow in many of the patients. Intravenous injection of 0.2 mg of nitroglycerin relieved the angina that was unaffected by the preceding intracoronary injection. This study indicates that it is the action of nitroglycerin on the systemic circulation that is responsible for its antianginal effect.*

The antianginal effect of nitroglycerin is believed to result from reduction of venous tone, diminished venous return, some peripheral arterial dilatation, and to a questionable extent from dilatation of those coronary arteries that are capable of responding to the drug. Nitroglycerin is a potent vasodilator. It exerts its greatest effect on the venous system (capacitance vessels) and a lesser effect on the arterial circulation (resistance vessels). All nitrate esters produce the same physiological effects as nitroglycerin.

In addition to the coronary vessels, certain other vascular areas are quite susceptible to the action of nitrites. The skin vessels of the face and neck, the so-called blush areas, may be markedly dilated. Meningeal vessels are dilated also, and this is the probable cause of the headache that may be produced by the nitrites.

Effects of nitroglycerin and nitrites on other smooth muscles

Probaby all smooth muscles can be made to relax by the nitrites, and some minor therapeutic applications of this effect have been made. The biliary tract can be relaxed with sublingual nitroglycerin, as evidenced by a measured decrease in biliary pressure. The nitrites also can relax the ureter. Although they have been shown to relax the bronchial smooth muscle, much more effective medications are available for this purpose.

Comparison of nitroglycerin with other nitrites and nitrates

Amyl nitrite is a volatile liquid that is available in small glass pearls containing 0.2 ml. These are crushed in a handkerchief by the patient and inhaled. Amyl nitrite has a short onset of action (less than 1 minute), but its duration of action is also short (not exceeding 10 minutes). It is particularly prone to cause cutaneous vasodilatation, marked lowering of systemic pressure, and even syncope and tachycardia. In addition, its odor is objectionable, particularly when used by ambulatory patients. For these reasons nitroglycerin is preferred.

Sodium nitrite has more toxicological than therapeutic importance. Although its smooth muscle effects are similar to those of other nitrites, its irritant effects on the gastric mucosa and its tendency to produce methemoglobin make it unsuitable as a coronary vasodilator.

Preparations

Nitroglycerin is available in oral, sublingual, topical, and intravenous formulations. In an attempt to achieve a longer duration of action, a variety of oral sustained-release preparations, nitroglycerin ointment, and a number of synthetic nitrate esters have been marketed (Table 36-2). The oral preparations often have to be given in large doses to overcome extensive first-pass hepatic metabolism.

In addition to the topical nitroglycerin ointment, a variety of transdermal nitroglycerin preparations are available (Table 36-3). These ready-to-wear adhesive bandages contain nitroglycerin on lactose in a viscous silicone fluid (Transderm) or nitroglycerin microsealed in a solid silicone polymer (Nitrodisc). These drug delivery systems are intended to release nitroglycerin continuously over about a 24-hour period. Some pharmacokinetic studies suggest that in certain patients once-a-day dosage is sufficient.

Tolerance to vascular actions of nitrites	Tolerance develops to headache produced by nitrates. Thus munitions workers when first exposed to nitrates complain of headaches, but they become tolerant in a few days. They may also develop nitrate dependence, since some workers, when they terminate their exposure to the chemical, may develop anginal attacks. Despite these observations, tolerance to the antianginal effects of the nitrates and nitrites apparently does not occur, and nitrate dependence is not a problem in patients who take these drugs by the oral route for long periods of time.
Toxic effects of nitrites and nitrates	The toxic effects of nitrites and nitrates are generally predictable from known pharmacological actions of these compounds. Severe fall of blood pressure with syncope, headaches, glaucoma, and elevated intracranial pressure can result from excessive dosage or unusual susceptibility of the patient. In addition, the nitrites can produce methemoglobinemia by oxidizing the iron of the hemoglobin molecule from the ferrous to the ferric state. This ability is used to advantage in the treatment of cyanide poisoning.

Nitrite poisoning may be acute or chronic. It may result from the therapeutic or accidental intake of nitrites or from the ingestion of some nitrate that may be converted to nitrites by intestinal bacteria, as has occurred following the ingestion of bismuth subnitrate. Increasing attention is paid to the fact that well water in some rural areas may contain enough nitrate to cause chronic intoxication with methemoglobinemia. Chronic poisoning from nitrates and nitrites is an industrial hazard, particularly in the explosives industry.

There is increasing concern also about the addition of nitrites and nitrates to meat products. The nitrites may be converted in the stomach to nitrosamines, which are carcinogenic.

Metabolism of organic nitrates	Organic nitrates are changed in the body to nitrites. Blood levels of nitrites, however, do not correlate well with antianginal activity. It has been suggested that coronary dilator activity depends on the intact molecule of the organic nitrate and not on reduction to nitrite.

The degradation of nitroglycerin occurs primarily in the liver by means of a glutathione-dependent organic nitrate reductase. The activity of the liver is largely responsible for the ineffectiveness of orally administered nitrates compared with the sublingually given tablets.

	TABLE 36-3	Transdermal nitroglycerin preparations	
Product name	Product surface area (cm²)	NTG content (mg)	NTG delivered over 24 hours (mg)
Transderm-Nitro 5	10	25	5.0
Transderm-Nitro 10	20	50	10.0
Nitro-Dur 5	5	26	2.5
Nitro-Dur 10	10	51	5.0
Nitro-Dur 15	15	77	10.0
Nitro-Dur 20	20	104	10.0
Nitrodisc 16	8	16	11 2
Nitrodisc 32	16	32	22.4

From Dasta, J.F., and Geraets, D.R. Copyright 1982 by the American Pharmaceutical Association. Originally published in the Journal of the American Pharmaceutical Association 22:29, 1982. Reprinted with permission of the American Pharmaceutical Association.

Therapeutic aims in use of nitrites and nitrates

The most important indication for the use of these compounds is the management of angina pectoris. If necessary, the nitrates can be used in combination with either β-adrenergc blocking agents or calcium channel blockers for this purpose.

The nitrates are also widely used in the management of congestive heart failure. Their benefit in failure is derived primarily from venodilatation (which decreases preload) and to a lesser extent from arteriolar dilatation (which decreases afterload).

Continuous intravenous nitroglycerin infusions have been used for unstable angina, congestive heart failure complicating acute myocardial infarction, perioperative control of blood pressure in patients undergoing coronary artery bypass surgery, and for controlled hypotension during noncardiac surgery. Because nitroglycerin can be absorbed into various plastics, care must be taken to use approved infusion sets when administering intravenous nitroglycerin. The infusion rate is generally begun at 5 μg/min and the dose titrated to the clinically desired endpoint (i.e., the desired blood pressure, cessation of chest pain, or the appropriate reduction in the pulmonary capillary wedge pressure).

β-ADRENERGIC BLOCKING AGENTS

The β-adrenergic antagonists are widely used in the management of angina pectoris. The general pharmacology of this class of drugs is discussed in Chapter 16. They are effective in angina because they reduce myocardial oxygen demand as a result of their negative chronotropic and inotropic effects and their ability to block catecholamine-induced increments in heart rate and blood pressure. Several β blockers, including propranolol, metoprolol, timolol, atenolol, and nadolol, are appropriate for use in angina pectoris. These agents must be used cautiously because of their ability to precipitate congestive heart failure or bronchospasm in susceptible patients.

TABLE 36-4   Side effects of antianginal drugs*

	Hypotension, flushing, headache	Left ventricular dysfunction	Decreased heart rate, atrioventricular block†	Gastrointestinal symptoms	Broncho-constriction‡
Beta blockers	0	+ +	+ + +	+	+ + +
Nitrates	+ + +	0	0	0	0
Diltiazem	+	+	+	0	0
Nifedipine	+ + +	0	0	0	0
Verapamil	+	+	+ +	+ +	0

From Braunwald, E.: N. Engl. J. Med. **307**:1618, 1982. Reprinted by permission of the New England Journal of Medicine.
*0, Absent; +, mild; + +, moderate; + + +, sometimes severe.
†In patients with sick-sinus-node syndrome or conduction-system disease.
‡In patients with obstructive lung disease.

DRUGS IN VARIANT ANGINA

Variant angina, or Prinzmetal's angina, is characterized by chest pain at rest rather than following exercise. Coronary artery spasm appears to be the cause of the chest pain and S-T segment elevation.

Attacks may be precipitated by the administration of epinephrine, norepinephrine, and sympathomimetic drugs in general. Propranolol may aggravate variant angina. Ergonovine maleate, a constrictor of vascular smooth muscle, is being used as a diagnostic agent for variant angina. However, the drug is not without danger, since it can cause prolonged spasm of the coronary arteries. Coronary artery spasm can be treated effectively with calcium channel blocking agents such as verapamil, nifedipine, and diltiazem. These drugs interfere with calcium entry into vascular smooth muscle resulting in coronary vasodilatation and relief of spasm. The vasodilatation also occurs in the peripheral vasculature resulting in decreased peripheral vascular resistance and hence decreased afterload. This is an additional mechanism that contributes to their antianginal effect and their efficacy in chronic effort-induced angina. Because of this latter action, the calcium blockers may prove effective in the treatment of hypertension as well.

The use of verapamil as an antiarrhythmic agent is discussed in Chapter 35. The side effects of the calcium blockers are summarized in Table 36-4. It should be noted that these agents, particularly verapamil, can induce left ventricular dysfunction. For this reason the calcium blockers should be used cautiously in patients with myocardial disease, especially if given in combination with β-blocking agents.

Preparations

Verapamil (Calan, Isoptin) is available in 80 and 120 mg tablets. The usual initial dose is 80 mg three times a day and may be increased to a total daily dose of 360 mg. Higher doses seem to offer no added benefit.

Nifedipine (Procardia) is available in 10 mg capsules. Therapy is usually initiated with 10 mg three times a day and may be increased to a maximum total daily dose of 120 mg.

Diltiazem (Cardizem) is available in 30 and 60 mg tablets. The usual initial dose is 30 mg three times a day. The maximum total daily dose is 240 mg.

REFERENCES

1. Abrams, M.: Nitroglycerin and long-acting nitrates, N. Engl. J. Med. **302**:1234, 1980.
2. Braunwald, E.: Mechanism of action of calcium-channel blocking agents, N. Engl. J. Med. **307**:1618, 1982.
3. Cohn, J.N., editor: Calcium-entry blockers in coronary artery disease, part 2, Circulation **65**:I1, 1982.
4. Flaim, S.F., and Zelis, R., editors: Calcium blockers: mechanisms of action and clinical applications, Baltimore, 1982, Urban & Schwarzenberg.
5. Frishman, W.H.: Beta-adrenoceptor antagonists: new drugs and new indicators, N. Engl. J. Med. **305**:500, 1981.
6. Frishman, W.H.: Beta-adrenergic blockade in clinical practice, Hosp. Prac. **17**:57, 1982.
7. Ganz, W., and Marcus, H.S.: Failure of intracoronary nitroglycerin to alleviate pacing-induced angina, Circulation **46**:880, 1972.
8. Hill, N.S., Antman, E.M., Green, L.H., and Alpert, J.S.: Intravenous nitroglycerin: a review of pharmacology, indications, therapeutic effects and complications, Chest **79**:69, 1981.
9. Schwartz, A., editor; Symposium on cardiovascular disease and calcium antagonists, Am. J. Cardiol. **49**:497, 1982.

Chapter 37

Anticoagulant, thrombolytic, and antiplatelet drugs

GENERAL
CONCEPT   Several hemostatic mechanisms have evolved to prevent excessive bleeding after injury. Blood clots are a multi-staged sequence that involves the endothelial cell, the blood platelet, the coagulation cascade, and the fibrinolytic system. This normal hemostatic defense is sometimes exaggerated so that unwanted clotting occurs. Such inappropriate clotting is thought to be involved in the pathogenesis of a variety of cardiovascular disorders including deep venous thrombosis and pulmonary embolism. Inappropriate activation of platelets has been postulated to contribute to the pathogenesis of stroke, myocardial infarction, and atherosclerosis. Hence anticoagulant, thrombolytic, and antiplatelet drugs are used extensively in clinical practice.

Heparin acts by binding to the plasma protein antithrombin III, thereby enhancing the ability of antithrombin to neutralize certain activated clotting factors.

The orally administered anticoagulants, derivatives of 4-hydroxycoumarin and indanedione, produce a delayed decrease in the activity of vitamin K–dependent coagulation factors such as factors VII, IX, X, and II. These drugs are thought to inhibit the conversion of glutamic acid to γ-carboxyglutamic acid on the end terminals of these proteins, thereby blocking their activation.

Nonsteroidal antiinflammatory drugs, such as aspirin and indomethacin, interfere with platelet function by inhibiting the cyclooxygenase enzyme, thereby blocking conversion of arachidonic acid to various prostaglandins and thromboxane A_2.

Streptokinase and urokinase activate plasminogen and may dissolve some intravascular thrombi.

Heparin is antagonized by protamine sulfate and coumarin anticoagulants by vitamin K. Heparin therapy may be monitored by whole blood clotting time or the partial thromboplastin time (PTT), whereas the coumarin and indanedione anticoagulants require determination of the prothrombin time (PT).

The fundamental component of a clot is fibrin. Fibrin is an insoluble protein generated from a soluble plasma precursor (fibrinogen) by the action of thrombin. Thrombin can be produced by two convergent series of reactions designated as the *intrinsic* and *extrinsic* pathways of thrombin formation (Fig. 37-1). In vitro the intrinsic system is triggered when plasma comes in contact with certain substances that have a negative surface charge (glass, kaolin, diatomaceous earth). This sets off a series of reactions, which is depicted in Fig. 37-1. It is not certain what activates factor XII (Hageman factor) in vivo, but damaged endothelial cells and some forms of collagen might serve as a local stimulus at sites of vascular injury. The extrinsic pathway bypasses several of the steps involved in the intrinsic pathway and is initiated

CLOTTING PROCESS AND DRUG ACTION

Scheme of blood coagulation. Reactions enclosed by solid lines are of the "intrinsic system," whereas those within the shaded box are of the "extrinsic system." PL, Phospholipid; Ca, calcium.

FIG. 37-1

From Williams, W.J.: Res. Staff Phys. *15:*39, 1969.

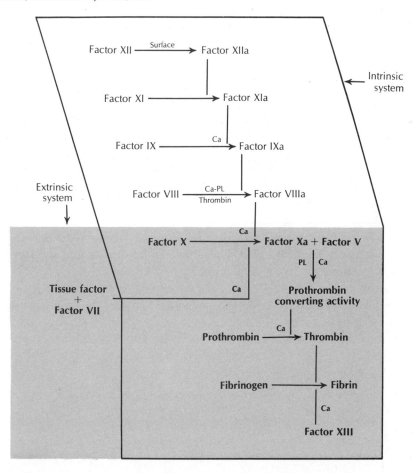

Blood coagulation factors

Factor I   Fibrinogen
Factor II   Prothrombin
Factor III   Tissue factor, tissue thromboplastin, thrombokinase
Factor IV   Calcium
Factor V   Proaccelerin, labile factor, plasma Ac-globulin
Factor VI
Factor VII   Proconvertin, stable factor, serum prothrombin conversion accelerator (SPCA)
Factor VIII Antihemophilic globulin (AHG), antihemophilic factor (AHF)
Factor IX   Plasma thromboplastin component (PTC), Christmas factor
Factor X   Stuart-Prower factor
Factor XI   Plasma thromboplastin antecedent (PTA), antihemophilic factor C
Factor XII   Hageman factor
Factor XIII Fibrin-stabilizing factor, fibrinase

Modified from Williams, W.J.: Res. Staff Phys. 15:39, 1969.

---

when plasma comes in contact with tissue thromboplastin. The nomenclature of the various coagulation factors has been a source of confusion. These are summarized in the box above.

Coagulation is vulnerable to drug action at several points. In vitro, inactivation of calcium by oxalate, citrate, or ethylenediaminetetraacetic acid (EDTA) will prevent clotting. This approach is not effective in vivo because ionized calcium levels sufficiently low to accomplish an anticoagulant effect are incompatible with life. Heparin and similar highly charged molecules can block clotting both in vitro and in vivo. Finally, compounds that block the production of some of the proteins that are essential in the scheme will prevent clotting in vivo but not in the test tube. This is the mode of action of the coumarins.

ANTICOAGULANTS
Heparin

Heparin is a sulfated mucopolysaccharide containing fractions varying in molecular weight between 6000 and 25,000. Commercial heparin is obtained from beef lung or hog intestinal mucosa.

From a chemical standpoint, heparin is a sulfated mucopolysaccharide composed of repeating units of sulfated glucosamine and glucuronic acid. It is a strong acid and is available in the form of its sodium salt.

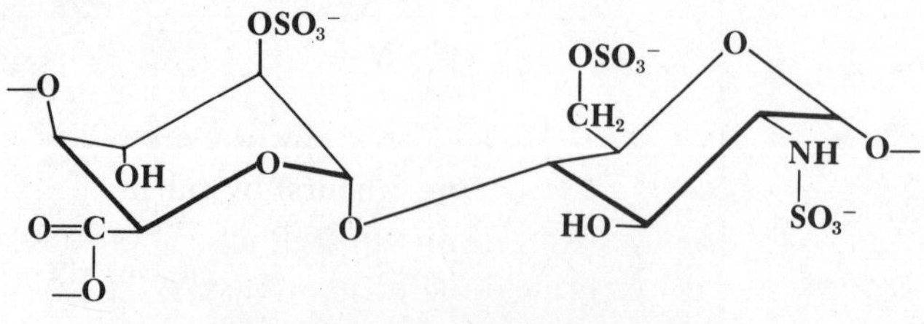

Configuration of disaccharides in heparin

Heparin inhibits clotting both in vitro and in vivo. It has been known for several years that heparin requires a plasma cofactor to exhibit its anticoagulant activity. This cofactor is now known to be antithrombin III (AT-III), an α_2 globulin capable of inactivating thrombin. AT-III binds heparin and undergoes a conformational change that in turn increases the rate of its inactivating effect on thrombin. **ANTICOAGULANT EFFECT**

The anticoagulant half-life of heparin injected intravenously varies from 1 to 2 hours. In extensive intravascular thrombosis an antiheparin, platelet factor 4, is released, which leads to increased heparin requirements.

In addition to its direct anticoagulant effect, heparin may be taken up by endothelial cells, altering the properties of the blood vessels.

Monitoring of anticoagulant activity following heparin administration has been done traditionally by the Lee-White clotting time. This is being abandoned because of poor reproducibility. Instead, the partial thromboplastin time and the thrombin time are being used.

Injected heparin has the remarkable ability of decreasing the turbidity of plasma following alimentary hyperlipemia. Interest in this phenomenon has been growing steadily. **LIPEMIA-CLEARING EFFECT**

When heparin is added in vitro to lipemic plasma, it causes no clearing. On the other hand, when lipemic plasma is added to clear plasma from an animal that has received heparin, clearing takes place.

The actual clearing factor appears to be a lipase that catalyzes the hydrolysis of triglycerides. The triglycerides of plasma are associated with proteins in the chylomicrons. Neutral fats that are split off by the enzyme from the chylomicrons are gradually dissolved in the plasma. Probably through the same mechanism, the β lipoproteins, which are of high molecular weight and low density, are transformed into α lipoproteins of lower molecular weight and high density.

The clearing factor is present in various tissues and appears to be released from its binding sites by heparin. Heparin is most probably an integral part of the lipase and may provide a link between enzyme and substrate.

The lipemia-clearing effect of heparin requires much smaller doses than those necessary for significant anticoagulant action. Lipemia is cleared by doses of less than 1 μg/kg in the rat and as little as 2 mg in humans. Larger doses of heparin, however, will release greater enzyme activity.

Heparin is not absorbed from the gastrointestinal tract. To obtain an anticoagulant effect the sodium or calcium salt of heparin is injected intravenously or subcutaneously. **ADMINISTRATION AND DOSAGE**

The dosage of heparin depends on the indication for its use. Heparin can be employed in low dosage (5,000 units every 12 hours) by subcutaneous injection for the prophylaxis of venous thrombosis. For the treatment of overt thromboembolism heparin should be given intravenously; the daily required dose is usually about 30,000 units. This total dose can be administered in divided intravenous boluses every 4 hours or as a continuous intravenous infusion. Some investigators believe that the incidence of hemorrhagic complications is less when heparin is administered by continuous infusion. Nevertheless, the physician should not rely on predetermined dosage schedules but should individualize the dose based on frequent determinations of the partial thromboplastin time.

Commercial preparations of heparin are bioassayed on the basis of anticoagulant action in comparison with a standard preparation. One hundred USP units corresponds to about 1 mg of heparin.

| PREPARATIONS | Heparin sodium USP is available as a suspension for injection, 1000, 5000, 10,000, 20,000, and 40,000 units/ml, and as a gel for repository injection, 20,000 units/ml. Heparin calcium (Calciparine) is also available in unit doses of 5000 units/0.2 ml, 12,500 units/0.5 ml, and 20,000 units/0.8 ml. |

| TOXICITY | Except for its anticoagulant effect, heparin is quite inert pharmacologically. An intravenous injection of 5 mg/kg is used routinely in experimental animals, and this large quantity has no significant effects on blood pressure, heart rate, or respiration. In its clinical use heparin may promote bleeding from open wounds and mucous membranes, especially when dosage is excessive. Some believe that cerebral hemorrhage may be precipitated in susceptible patients. Elderly women are especially susceptible to heparin. Hematomas can occur at subcutaneous injection sites. Some investigators feel that the incidence of this complication is less with calcium heparin than with sodium heparin.

In humans, long-term heparin treatment may result in osteoporosis. Also, symptoms suggesting hypersensitivity and inhibition of aldosterone secretion have been reported. |

| HEPARIN ANTAGONISTS | The effects of heparin overdosage will last only a relatively short time because the drug is metabolized in a few hours. If hemorrhage threatens during even a short waiting period, chemical antidotes are available.

Protamine sulfate will combine with heparin milligram for milligram to block its anticoagulant effect both in the test tube and in the patient. |

| METABOLISM AND EXCRETION | After intravenous injection, blood levels of heparin decline exponentially with a half-life of about 1 hour. Although most of the heparin is metabolized in the body, as much as 50% of a large intravenous dose may be excreted in the urine. |

| *Coumarin and indanedione anticoagulants* DEVELOPMENT | The story of the introduction of the coumarin compounds into therapeutics is unusually interesting. It has been known for many years that cattle can develop a hemorrhagic disease when they eat spoiled sweet clover. It has also been known that the hemorrhages are caused by lowered prothrombin levels in the animals. In |

1941 Link and associates at the University of Wisconsin showed that a coumarin compound was responsible for this hemorrhagic disease of cattle. They synthesized dicumarol, which has been used quite extensively in clinical practice and was the forerunner of a number of coumarin and indanedione derivatives.

The various coumarin anticoagulants act by the same basic mechanism. They inhibit the formation of prothrombin, factor VII (proconvertin), factor IX (Christmas), and factor X (Stuart-Prower factor).

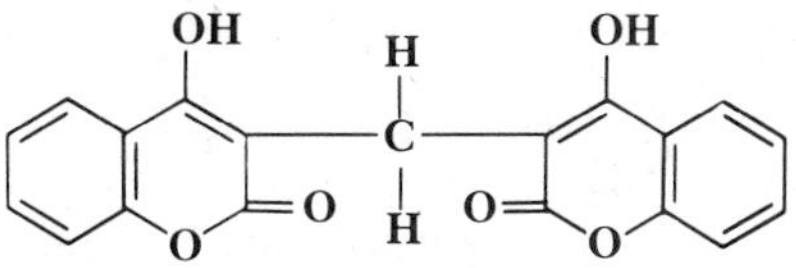

Dicumarol

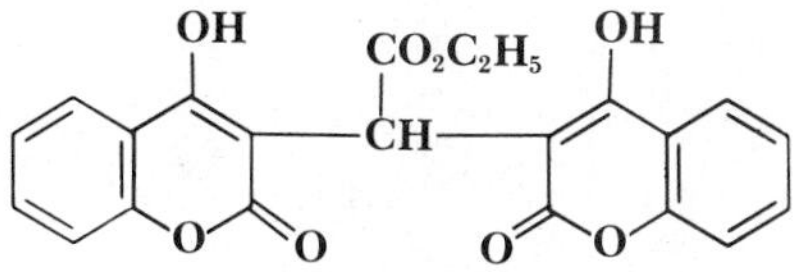

Ethyl biscoumacetate

The coumarin anticoagulants include, in addition to dicumarol, warfarin sodium (Coumadin sodium), warfarin potassium (Athrombin-K), acenocoumarol (Sintrom), and phenprocoumon (Liquamar). The available indanedione derivatives include phenindione (Hedulin) and anisindione (Miradon).

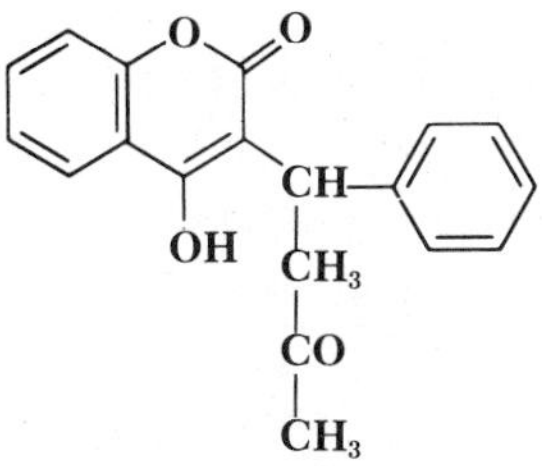

Warfarin

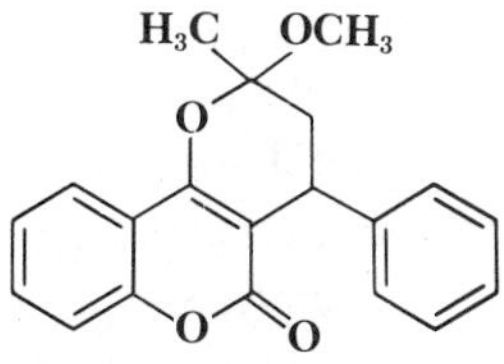

Cyclocumarol

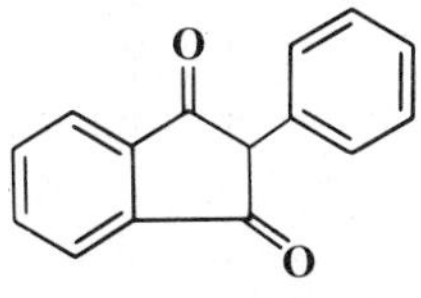

Phenindione

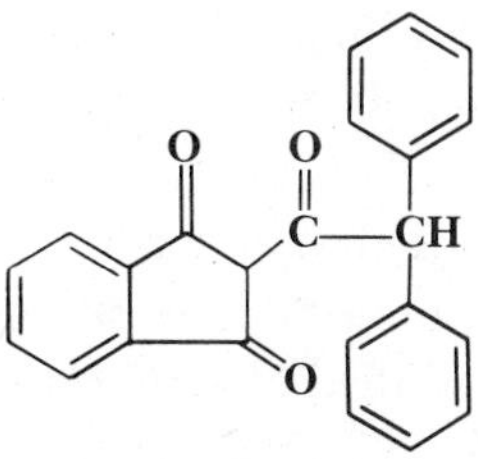

Diphenadione

FIG. 37-2   *Mechanism of coumarin action. Coumarin-type drugs interfere with the vitamin K cycle by blocking the enzyme that reduces vitamin K epoxide to vitamin K. Carboxylation of the glutamic acid residues of factors II, VII, IX, and X (left) is prevented, thereby inhibiting the activation of these factors.*

Modified from Walsh, P.N.: Hosp. Prac. 18(1):101, 1983.

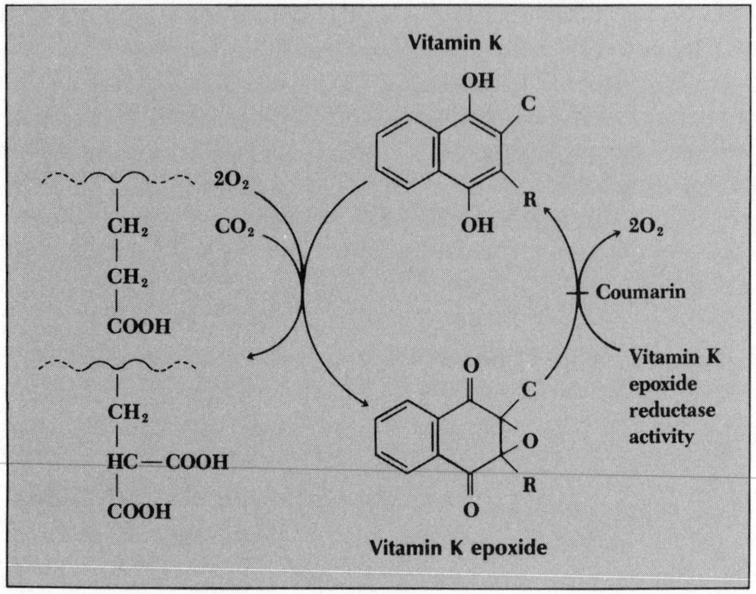

MODE OF ACTION

As illustrated in Fig. 37-2, the coumarin anticoagulants exert their effect by blocking carboxylation of various clotting factors, thereby inhibiting their activation. There is a characteristic delay in the action of these compounds. This is understandable because the normal prothrombin content of the plasma must decline before evidence of impaired synthesis can manifest itself. The coumarin compounds vary in speed of onset and duration of action, probably because of their varying speeds of absorption and metabolic degradation.

VARIATIONS IN SUSCEPTIBILITY

There is great individual variation in susceptibility to the coumarin anticoagulants. The variation is a consequence of many factors. Absorption from the intestine, metabolic transformation, diet, and genetically conditioned resistance may all contribute.

Prothrombin concentration during coumarin therapy is measured by comparing the prothrombin time of the patient's plasma with that of normal plasma. In the usual one-stage prothrombin test, thromboplastin is added to citrated plasma at 37° C. Calcium chloride is then added in excess, and the time for clotting is recorded. It is known now that the test measures not only prothrombin but also other components such as factor VII.

During therapy with the coumarin drugs it is desirable to maintain prothrombin concentration at 20% of normal, and dosage is adjusted to achieve this aim. Without such laboratory control, use of the coumarins would be dangerous. Severe depression of prothrombin concentration may be associated with bleeding, which can manifest itself as microscopic hematuria or even such severe bleeding as cerebral hemorrhage.

Two methods are available for counteracting the action of the coumarin drug and their congeners: fresh whole blood transfusion and use of vitamin K preparations.

Among the most effective antidotes for coumarin poisoning is phytonadione (vitamin K_1, AquaMEPHYTON), which is water soluble and may be administered intravenously. Anaphylactic reactions, including fatalities, have occurred following intravenous injection of phytonadione. Therefore this route of administration should be restricted to those situations where other routes are not feasible. To correct an excessively prolonged prothrombin time caused by oral anticoagulant therapy, 2.5 to 10 mg is recommended. It should be injected slowly, not exceeding 1 mg/min. In rare instances higher doses may be required. When used in large doses as antidotes, the vitamin K preparations have a prolonged action and have prevented reinstitution of coumarin or indanedione therapy for as long as 2 weeks. Vitamin K preparations have no affect on the anticoagulant action of heparin.

VITAMIN K AS ANTIDOTE TO PROTHROMBIN-DEPRESSANT DRUGS

Subcutaneous heparin and coumarin-type anticoagulants are used for the prevention of deep venous thrombosis (DVT) and pulmonary emboli (PE) in high-risk patients. Because of its rapid onset of action, intravenous heparin (followed by coumarin therapy) is used in the initial treatment of acute DVT and PE. The intravenous heparin is usually given for 7 to 10 days while adequate anticoagulation with coumarin is achieved. Most physicians continue the oral anticoagulant for 3 to 6 months in patients with documented DVT or PE.

Heparin is also used to maintain the fluidity of the blood in extracorporeal circulations such as heart-lung machines and artificial kidney machines. Often, so-called regional heparinization is employed in these settings. This is a technique whereby heparin is infused into the patient's blood just before it enters the extracorporeal device, and protamine is infused into the blood to neutralize the heparin just before the blood is returned to the patient. As a result, the blood is anticoagulated only while it is in the machine and the patient avoids the risks of systemic anticoagulation. In certain instances, heparin is also employed in the management of disseminated intravascular coagulation (DIC).

The use of anticoagulants in acute myocardial infarction remains controversial. Although long-term anticoagulation after myocardial infarction seems to offer little benefit, some physicians will prescribe subcutaneous heparin while patients are in a coronary care unit. The role of anticoagulation in cerebrovascular disease represents another area of controversy.

CLINICAL PHARMACOLOGY AND DRUG INTERACTIONS

TABLE 37-1   Average doses of various coumarin and indanedione
anticoagulants

Preparation	Average initial dose (mg)	Average maintenance dose (mg)
Dicumarol	300	25-120
Warfarin sodium (Coumadin sodium)	10-15	6
Acenocoumarin (Sintrom)	15-25	2-10
Phenprocoumon (Liquamar)	20-30	1-5
Phenindione (Hedulin)	100-200	25-50

Oral anticoagulants are used to prevent systemic embolization in patients with mitral stenosis, particularly if they have supraventricular tachyarrhythmias such as atrial fibrillation.

Several of the oral anticoagulants and their dosages are listed in Table 37-1. The earlier practice of initiating therapy with a large loading dose is no longer recommended. The use of a loading dose does not bring about more rapid anticoagulation and can expose the patient to a transient but significant risk of hemorrhage.

Phenindione has caused serious toxic effects such as agranulocytosis and liver damage. Most clinical investigators in the United States prefer the coumarins and find that warfarin is one of the best from the standpoint of ease of regulation. It is a good rule for physicians to use the anticoagulant with which they are thoroughly familiar and only if they have facilities for one-stage prothrombin time determinations.

Drug interactions in the clinical use of coumarin anticoagulants are of great importance (see also Chapter 63). Some drugs stimulate the metabolic degradation of the coumarins and thus decrease their effectiveness. Other drugs increase the effectiveness of the anticoagulants by blocking their metabolism or by interfering with their binding to plasma proteins.

Drug effects on the response to coumarin anticoagulants are as follows:

Drugs that increase the effect of coumarin anticoagulants
   Antibiotics affecting the intestinal flora
   Phenylbutazone and some other acidic drugs
   Salicylates (large doses)
   Chloral hydrate
   Clofibrate
   Disulfiram
   Adrogenic anabolic steroids
   Methylphenidate
   Propylthiouracil
   d-Thyroxine

Drugs that decrease the effect of coumarin anticoagulants
   Barbiturates
   Ethchlorvynol
   Glutethimide
   Cimetidine
Coumarin potentiation of other drugs
   Tolbutamide
   Phenytoin

Blood has the inherent capacity of dissolving clots by means of the fibrinolytic system. There are reasons to believe that this system functions under normal circumstances to remove minor fibrin depositions that occur in small vessels. Clotted blood may be injected repeatedly into rabbits without being demonstrable at autopsy. It is presumably dissolved through fibrinolysis.

FIBRINOLYSIN

Fibrinolysin, also called *plasmin* by some investigators, is a proteolytic enzyme that attacks a variety of proteins but has a great affinity for fibrinogen or fibrin. A schematic representation of the human fibrinolytic system is shown below.

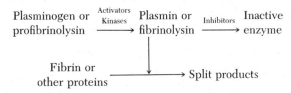

Plasminogen, or profibrinolysin, occurs in plasma as the inactive precursor of fibrinolysin. Plasmin has the ability to lyse fresh fibrin clots with the generation of fibrin split products. Streptokinase and urokinase are plasminogen activators.

Streptokinase (Streptase) is an enzyme produced by certain strains of streptococci. It is a foreign protein and therefore antigenic. Since most patients have antibodies directed against streptococci, an antigen-antibody complex is formed when streptokinase is infused. Consequently, when streptokinase therapy is initiated, a sufficient loading dose must be given to neutralize or inhibit circulating antibodies. Because of this problem of antigenicity, streptokinase should generally not be readministered for 6 to 12 months after a course of therapy.

Streptokinase and urokinase

Urokinase (Abbokinase, Breokinase) is a plasminogen activator that was initially isolated from human urine. It can now also be produced from tissue cultures of human embryonic kidney cells. It lacks the antigenicity problems of streptokinase but is considerably more expensive.

The Food and Drug Administration has approved streptokinase for treatment of acute pulmonary embolism and deep-vein thrombosis (within 7 days of onset of symptoms), acute myocardial infarction, acute arterial thrombosis, and occlusion of access shunts and intravascular catheters. As expected, fresh clots are more susceptible to the action of both streptokinase and urokinase.

INDICATIONS

Streptokinase and urokinase therapy should be initiated with a loading dose. The usual loading dose of streptokinase is 250,000 units, given over 20 to 30 minutes by means of a constant infusion pump through a peripheral vein. The usual loading dose of urokinase is 4400 IU/kg of body weight, administered over 10 minutes. The following maintenance doses have been recommended: streptokinase, 100,000 units/ hour for 24 hours in pulmonary embolism and for 48 to 72 hours in deep-vein

Dosages

thrombosis; urokinase, 4400 IU/kg/hour for 12 to 24 hours in pulmonary embolism.[4] Intraarterial infusions have been employed to lyse arterial clots, but more commonly these agents are used intravenously. After thrombolytic therapy is completed, systemic heparin should be continued for 5 to 10 days followed by oral anticoagulation.

Monitoring fibrinolytic therapy	The whole-blood euglobulin lysis time or the thrombin time should be monitored to determine whether some degree of systemic fibrinolysis has been established. If these tests are not available, then fibrin degradation products or the partial thromboplastin time and prothrombin time can be measured. These tests should be performed during a control period and after 3 to 4 hours of lytic treatment. It can be inferred that systemic lysis has been established as long as the test values during thrombolytic infusion are greater than the control values (except for the euglobulin lysis time, which is shortened). It is particularly important to document a systemic effect with these tests during streptokinase therapy because high levels of antistreptococcal antibodies can render the streptokinase ineffective.
Complications of thrombolytic therapy	Bleeding, fever, and allergic reactions have been reported as complications of streptokinase and urokinase therapy. Active internal bleeding, a cerebrovascular process, or a neurosurgical procedure within 2 months are absolute contraindications to thrombolytic therapy.

Streptokinase-streptodornase (Varidase) is a mixture of enzymes used topically for dissolving blood clots (streptokinase) and the viscous nucleoproteins of pus (streptodornase). It is useful in evacuating the contents of hemothorax and empyema and as an aid in surgical debridement.

Adverse effects to the enzyme mixture include fever and local irritation. Active hemorrhage is a contraindication to its use. The usefulness of streptokinase-streptodornase in the form of buccal tablets or the intramuscular route for a systemic antiinflammatory effect is not certain.

Streptokinase-streptodornase (Varidase) is available as a powder for topical use containing 100,000 units of streptokinase and 25,000 units of streptodornase per vial. Streptokinase-streptodornase should not be injected intravenously because of hazardous impurities present in the preparation.

ε-Aminocaproic acid (Amicar) inhibits plasminogen activators and to a lesser extent plasmin. The drug has been used to decrease hemorrhage associated with certain surgical procedures.

ANTIPLATELET DRUGS Platelets and hemostasis	When a blood vessel is injured, there is an initial vasoconstriction that results in diminution of flow from the severed vessels and a reduction in the area that must be occluded by the hemostatic plug. Blood platelets adhere to the exposed subendothelial constituents (collagen, basement membrane), resulting in formation of an initial layer of platelets. During this process, platelets can release a number of substances (thromboxane A_2, ADP, serotonin) that can enhance the reflex vasoconstriction and cause additional platelets to aggregate. The growing mass of platelets

can eventually occlude the vessel. The injured tissue releases tissue thromboplastin, which activates the clotting mechanism, resulting in the eventual production of thrombin. This increases platelet aggregation further and results in production of a network of fibrin that interconnects the platelet plug. The platelet may be involved in vascular disorders through these mechanisms. In addition, platelets can release a growth factor that stimulates proliferation of intimal smooth muscle cells. Smooth muscle proliferation is thought to be one of the earliest steps in the atherosclerotic process. Thus the platelet has been postulated to have a pivotal role in the pathogenesis of several vascular disorders, including myocardial infarction, stroke, and atherosclerosis.

Aspirin and nonsteroidal antiinflammatory agents

Several drugs exert antiplatelet effects. Nonsteroidal antiinflammatory agents, such as aspirin and indomethacin, inhibit platelet function by blocking the cyclooxygenase enzyme, which converts arachidonic acid to the endoperoxide PGG_2. PGG_2 can be converted in the platelet to thromboxane A_2, a potent vasoconstrictor that also promotes platelet aggregation. Aspirin irreversibly acetylates the platelet cyclooxygenase, and since the platelet is unable to synthesize new enzyme, the effect persists for the life span of the platelet. Other nonsteroidal antiinflammatory agents are reversible cyclooxygenase inhibitors.

Dipyridamole

Platelet aggregation is associated with a decrease in platelet cyclic AMP. Conversely, agents that increase cyclic AMP levels inhibit platelet adhesion, aggregation, and the release reaction. Prostacyclin, produced by vascular endothelium, stimulates adenylate cyclase when it binds to platelet membranes. This is thought to account for its ability to inhibit platelet aggregation. Dipyridamole inhibits platelet phosphodiesterase, the enzyme that breaks down cyclic AMP. By inhibiting this enzyme, dipyridamole potentiates the increase in cyclic AMP and platelet inhibition caused by aspirin or prostacyclin. Hence aspirin has been used in combination with dipyridamole in a variety of clinical studies. Dipyridamole also inhibits adhesion of platelets to damaged endothelium and to artificial surfaces. For this reason it has been used to prevent embolic phenomena in patients with artificial heart valves.

Sulfinpyrazone

Sulfinpyrazone is also a reversible cyclooxygenase inhibitor. Unlike aspirin, however, it neither prolongs the bleeding time nor affects platelet aggregation in normal individuals. Nevertheless, sulfinpyrazone normalizes platelet survival, whereas aspirin does not. The mechanism of this action is unknown.

Several drugs possessing so-called membrane-stabilizing or local anesthetic properties inhibit platelet aggregation. β-Adrenergic blockers (such as propranolol), some tranquilizers, local anesthetics, and the antimalarial drug mepacrine are examples of such agents. The mechanism of these platelet effects is unknown but might relate to an inhibition of calcium action in the platelet. Some studies have shown that propranolol normalizes hyperaggregable platelet responses in patients with angina.

Clinical trials   Although use of antiplatelet drugs in cardiovascular disease has aroused considerable interest, clinical trials produced equivocal results. Aspirin, aspirin and dipyridamole in combination, and sulfinpyrazone have been evaluated in several large-scale clinical trials to determine if these agents are of benefit in preventing reinfarction and sudden death in patients with heart disease or in the prevention of stroke or transient ischemic attacks (TIAs) in patients with cerebrovascular disease. Although favorable trends were suggested in several of these studies, at this time antiplatelet therapy has been officially approved only in respect to the use of aspirin in preventing TIAs and stroke in males following an initial cerebrovascular event. Despite six clinical trials with aspirin following acute myocardial infarction, there is no definitive proof that mortality is reduced with this form of therapy. Perhaps with development of more specific agents (thromboxane synthetase inhibitors) or with development of better methods to identify subgroups of patients likely to respond, antiplatelet therapy will become a more effective treatment modality in cardiovascular disease.

REFERENCES

1. Deykin, D.: Current status of anticoagulant therapy, Am. J. Med. **72:**659, 1982.
2. Frishman, W.H.: Antiplatelet therapy in coronary heart disease, Hosp. Pract. **17**(5):73, 1982.
3. Link, K.P.: The anticoagulant from spoiled sweet clover hay, Harvey Lect. **39:**162, 1944.
4. Sharma, G.V.R.K., Cella, G., Parisi, A.F., and Sashara, A.A.: Thrombolytic therapy, N. Engl. J. Med. **306:**1268, 1982.
5. Thomas, D.P.: Heparin, Clin. Haematol. **10:**443, 1981.
6. Walsh, P.N.: Oral anticoagulant therapy, Hosp. Pract. **18**(1):101, 1982.

Chapter 38

Diuretic drugs

Diuretic agents increase the renal excretion of solute and water. Most of them do this by decreasing renal tubular reabsorption of sodium, chloride, and water. Excretion of potassium and bicarbonate, and to a much lesser extent divalent cations such as calcium and magnesium, may also be increased. Diuretics do not affect directly either glomerular filtration or the action of the antidiuretic hormone (ADH) on the distal portion of the nephron.

Reduction in water reabsorption by diuretic drugs is dependent on their ability to increase solute excretion. This reduction in water reabsorption can be accomplished by the glomerular ultrafiltration of a substance that the tubules may have limited or no ability to reabsorb (an osmotic diuretic) or by a drug that decreases reabsorption of sodium and preferably chloride (a saluretic agent). The electrolyte carries with it an osmotic equivalent of water more or less, depending on how and where the drug acts. The types of diuretics that will be considered in some detail include (1) osmotic diuretics; (2) organomercurial diuretics; (3) carbonic anhydrase inhibitors that act predominantly in the distal cortical portion of the renal tubules; (4) carbonic anhydrase inhibitors that act predominantly in the proximal segment; (5) diuretics that act on the loop of Henle; and (6) antikaliuretic diuretics, which decrease the exchange of sodium (reabsorption) for potassium (secretion) in the distal cortical segment of the nephron.

If one is to use a diuretic drug effectively, the status of both renal and extrarenal factors involved in diuresis needs to be understood. For instance, the more restricted glomerular filtration becomes, by disease or reduction in systemic blood pressure, the less diuresis such an agent is likely to have. On the other hand, a diuretic agent may induce only limited diuresis by even normal kidneys if the return of edema fluid for glomerular filtration is restricted by low plasma proteins (hypoproteinemia, usually hypoalbuminemia) or by heart failure.

FIG. 38-1   *The concentration of electrolytes essential to water balance is essentially the same in extracellular fluid, plasma, and glomerular ultrafiltrate.*

Reprinted by permission from Figure 2, page 73 in Discovery, development and delivery of new drugs by Karl H. Beyer, Jr. Copyright 1978, Spectrum Publications, Inc., Jamaica, New York.

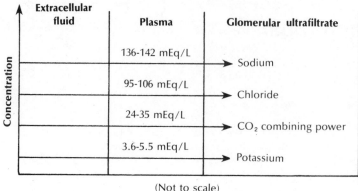

(Not to scale)

<table>
<tr><td></td><td></td><td></td></tr>
</table>

EXTRARENAL ASPECTS

The use of diuretic drugs for the relief of edema (extravascular accumulation of fluid in tissues) requires an understanding of the factors influencing movement of plasma water from the vascular system to the extravascular space (for exchange with tissue fluids) and its return to the vascular system for perfusion of nephron. Salient features of these factors follow.

1. Extracellular-extravascular fluid, plasma and glomerular ultrafiltrate have essentially the same electrolyte composition (Fig. 38-1). Thus although the site of action of the diuretic agent on the renal tubules may seem remote, as it inhibits the reabsorption of salt and water the drug reduces commensurately the composition and volume of extracellular fluid and ultimately reduces total body water.

2. Even seemingly slight changes in the hemodynamic forces relating cardiac output to vascular peripheral resistance can profoundly alter the quantitative action of diuretics. For instance, simply putting an edematous patient at bed rest and restricting salt intake may be sufficient under some circumstances to bring about an impressive loss of edema fluid, as reflected in body weight, illustrated by the example in Fig. 38-2.

3. Either an increase in cardiac function of a failing heart induced by a cardiotonic agent such as digitalis or a decrease in electrolyte and water reabsorption by a diuretic may increase urine volume and reduce edema. Employed together properly, the therapeutic efficacy of these two mechanisms is enhanced to an extent neither can cause alone (Fig. 38-3).

4. Even though the foregoing three factors are accounted for, diuresis may be unsatisfactory unless the concentration, hence osmotic force, of plasma protein is adequate to return extravascular fluid to the vascular system to sustain plasma volume

Effect of bed rest and low sodium diet on loss of weight (edema) and sodium in a cirrhotic   *FIG. 38-2*
patient.

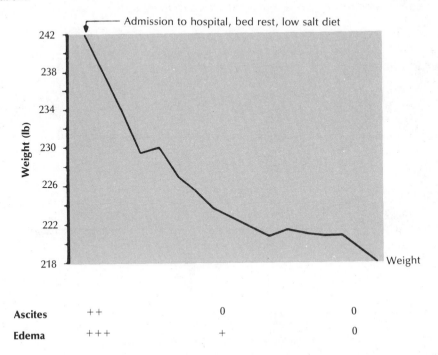

Ascites	+ +	0	0
Edema	+ + +	+	0

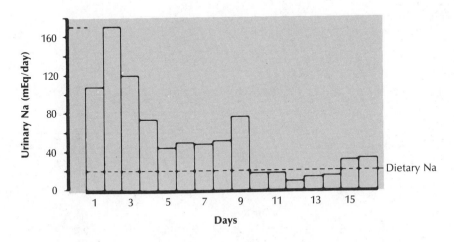

FIG. 38-3   *Decrease in circulation time and weight reduction in patients with congestive heart failure when **A**, a cardiotonic agent is administered alone, **B**, a cardiotonic and a diuretic agent are coadministered, and **C**, the diuretic agent is administered alone.*

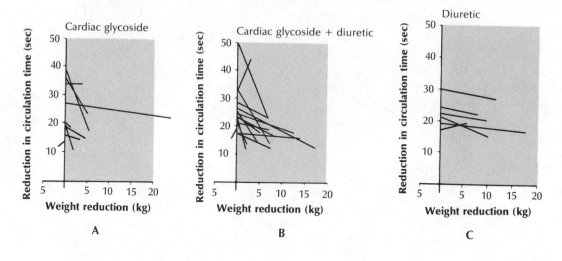

A

B

C

FIG. 38-4   *Effect of intermittent transfusions of whole blood and/or albumin on (increased) diuretic response to the daily oral administration of ethacrynic acid.*

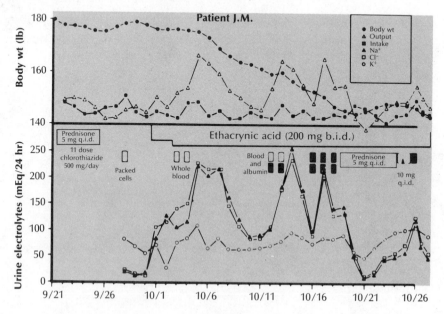

and to influence the perfusion of renal tubules favorably. As illustrated in Fig. 38-4, frequent transfusions of whole blood or albumin to a hypoproteinemic patient markedly increase response to a diuretic agent.

It is beyond the scope of this chapter to present in detail the physiological basis for the actions of diuretic agents. Fig. 38-6 may be helpful, together with Table 38-1, which lists normal values of the principal solutes with which we will be concerned in glomerular ultrafiltrate (plasma water) and urine.

The rate of glomerular ultrafiltration can be increased by plasma volume expansion and/or increased systemic blood pressure. It can be reduced by (1) decreased systemic arterial pressure; (2) renal afferent arteriolar constriction caused by adrenergic stimulation and/or by increased renin production; (3) obstruction of the afferent arteriole,

INTRARENAL ASPECTS

Effect of coadministration of an adrenocorticoid and a diuretic agent on reduction of urinary protein, BUN, and weight and increase in sodium and chloride excretion by a patient with nephrotic syndrome.

FIG. 38-5

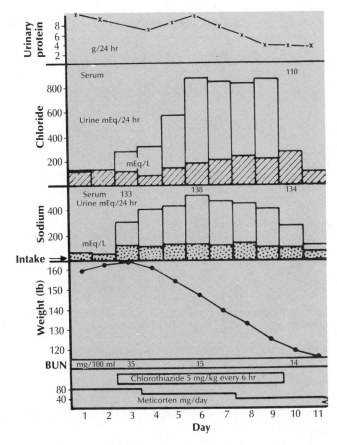

TABLE 38-1	Important constituents of glomerular ultrafiltrate (plasma water), that relate to urine formation	
	Approximate amount/24 hr	
	Glomerular ultrafiltrate	Urine
Urea	40 g	20 g
Sodium	600 g	6 g
Potassium	7 g	3 g
Chloride	640 g	9 g
Bicarbonate	0.7 g	± g
Water	180 L	1.5 L

FIG. 38-6 *Diagram of a nephron to illustrate electrolyte and water transport across the cells and the site(s) of action of some diuretic drugs.*

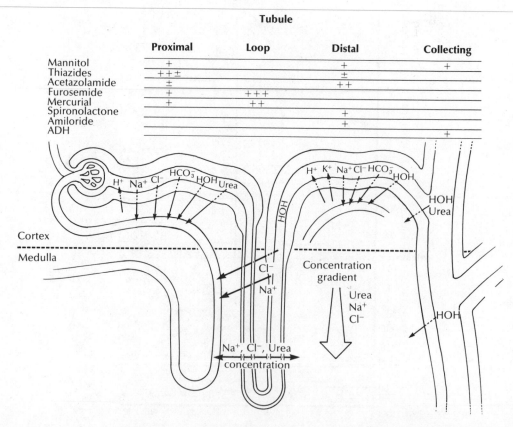

as by embolization; or (4) reduction of filtration due to glomerulitis or more general glomerulonephritis, in which case both kidneys are usually involved (as in examples 1 and 2) but not necessarily to the same extent. If the integrity of ultrafiltration by the glomerular membrane is altered by disease, plasma proteins may be filtered and lost more rapidly than they can be replaced. Diuretic agents do not affect glomerular filtration directly, although their use together with a glucocorticoid such as prednisolone may be beneficial for repair of glomerular membranes and management of glomerulonephritis (Fig. 38-5).

The proximal portion of the renal tubules is responsible for reabsorption of 70% or more of filtered monovalent electrolytes and water. This was first demonstrated convincingly by micropuncture of renal tubules in the frog kidney by Richards and his associates[13] during the 1920s and early 1930s and has since been amply confirmed in several mammalian species.

The proximal tubules actively reabsorb sodium ions in exchange for hydrogen ions (Fig. 38-6). The hydrogen ion is made available by dissociation of $H_2CO_3 \leftrightharpoons H^+ \pm HCO_3^-$ and the influence of an enzyme, carbonic anhydrase, located on the lumenal side of the cell membrane ($H^+ \pm HCO_3^- \xrightarrow{A} H^+ + OH^- + CO_2$). This exchange can be blocked by suitable carbonic anhydrase inhibitors with a characteristic NH_2SO_2 — R structure. H^+ may also be made available for exchange with NA^+ by the action of the cell's sulfhydryl-catalyzed dehydrogenases. These dehydrogenases can be inhibited by organomercurial diuretics and by ethacrynic acid, both of which are capable of forming sulfhydryl adducts. Potassium ions are thought to be exchanged for H^+ in the manner of Na^+ in the proximal portion of the nephron. The monovalent anions Cl^- and HCO_3^- undergo back-diffusion equivalent to reabsorption of cation. However, Cl^- diffuses more slowly than HCO_3^-, and as the fluid becomes more acidic in its passage through the proximal section, CO_2 is released, which can diffuse still more rapidly ($H^+ + HCO_3^- \rightarrow H^+ + OH^- + CO_2$). Na^+ and K^+ balance within the cells is sustained by the action of Na^+/K^+-dependent ATPase located at the interstitial border of the cell. Water is not actively reabsorbed but undergoes back-diffusion with the electrolyte so as to maintain an isoosmotic relationship. Urea is also substantially reabsorbed proximally, but its transport is even less well understood.

The loop of Henle is important to the conservation of salt and water. Its permeability and physical characteristics combine with those of the vasa recta to sustain an increasing concentration gradient of Na^+, Cl^-, and urea (but not K^+) from cortex to the papilla of the medulla (Fig. 38-6). The contributions to this phenomenon of close proximity of descending and ascending limbs of the loop and vasa recta are variously explained in terms of the counter-current multiplier and countercurrent exchange theories of function, respectively. Most critical to this concentration gradient of Na^+ and Cl^- is the fact that they are reabsorbed to the extent of 15% or so of glomerular filtrate, predominantly by the thick segment of the ascending limb of the loop, which is impermeable to water. Because it is impermeable to water, it is called the diluting segment. Thus the luminal fluid enters the distal portion of the nephron in a hypotonic state, that is, reduced osmotic pressure.

Reabsorption of electrolyte by the thick segment is unique in that Na^+ is thought to attend the reabsorption of Cl^-. It is Cl^- reabsorption that is the determinant, the opposite of the cortical relationship of Na^+ and Cl^- reabsorption. The loop appears to be permeable to the diffusion of urea into the interstitium in such a manner that the countercurrent mechanism can sustain its increasing gradient from cortex to inner medulla.

In the distal cortical portion of the tubule Na^+ can undergo active reabsorption by exchange with H^+ made available by the action of carbonic anhydrase. In addition, active reabsorption of Na^+ is facilitated by the action of aldosterone, the hormone of the adrenal cortex that influences Na^+ exchange with K^+, which is secreted at this site. Ordinarily, the reabsorption of Na^+ is almost complete at this site, removing with it by diffusion an osmotic equivalent of water. The H^+ contributes to urine acidification under which condition little or no HCO_3^- escapes reabsorption and Cl^- remains as the principal anion in this process.

In the collecting tubules antidiuretic hormone (ADH) facilitates back-diffusion of urea and of water to the net extent of some 99% of the amount filtered. This back-diffusion of water is dependent on the high osmotic gradient of Na^+ and Cl^- in the medulla, to which urea also contributes. If secretion of ADH by the hypothalamus is depressed by alcohol or by water diuresis (a high consumption of water), urine flow increases.

OSMOTIC DIURETICS   **Mannitol** is the prototype today of an osmotic diuretic. Its chemical structure resembles that of glucose. Like glucose it is completely filtered at the glomeruli and is tolerated by intravenous injection in larger amounts, but there the resemblance ends. Mannitol is not absorbed to any useful extent when given orally, its distribution in the body is limited to extracellular fluid, and when filtered, it is not reabsorbed by the renal tubules. Consequently, since it is not reabsorbed, an osmotic equivalent of water passes with mannitol along the renal tubules to increase the volume of urine excreted. Since mannitol is neither secreted nor reabsorbed by the renal tubules, it may be used to measure glomerular filtration rate.

$$
\begin{array}{c}
CH_2OH \\
| \\
H - C - OH \\
| \\
H - C - OH \\
| \\
HO - C - H \\
| \\
HO - C - H \\
| \\
CH_2OH
\end{array}
$$

Mannitol

Mannitol is not ordinarily employed for reduction of edema associated with heart failure, for example. **Mannitol** is administered in hypertonic concentrations, greater than 5% and up to 25% in from 50 to 1000 ml distilled water intravenously, to rid the body of excess fluid administered at the time of general or intracranial surgery. If mannitol diuresis is sufficient to increase urine flow by perhaps threefold or more, it may increase the excretion of sodium, chloride, and urea somewhat as a result of reduced transit time for their reabsorption, but its diuretic effect is not contingent thereon. Its duration of action is short (2 or 3 hours), depending on concentration, volume administered, and the duration of infusion, if glomerular filtration rate is normal. If cardiovascular-renal function is sufficiently impaired so that edema is obviously present, a diuretic that acts directly on the tubules to increase salt and water excretion may be more effective.

Other agents, such as urea and ammonium chloride, have been employed as osmotic diuretics in the past, but urea is not as effective, mole for mole, since it is reabsorbed to a considerable extent (perhaps half the amount filtered by humans). Ammonium chloride is irritating regardless of how administered and may induce hyperchloremic acidosis if employed to excess.

ORGANOMERCURIAL DIURETICS

Until the 1950s, the organomercurials were the only diuretics that could be relied on when they were most needed. (Also available, although clinically less useful because much less active, were the xanthines [e.g., caffeine and theophylline], which were orally active, safe, and had the right spectrum of electrolyte and water excretion.)

The organomercurials, with their many faults, were the mainstay of diuretic therapy for 30 years from 1920. In 1920 Saxl and Heilig[14] reported that when syphilitic patients were injected with the antisyphilitic drug merbaphen (Novasurol), they tended to excrete more urine.

Mercaptomerin sodium (Thiomerin) is still available and may be administered in solution intramuscularly or subcutaneously. Each ml of **mercaptomerin sodium** (Thiomerin) for injection contains 125 mg, equivalent to approximately 40 mg mercury in water for injection, and 0.1 mg disodium edetate.

Mercaptomerin sodium

The disuse of organomercurials today may be illustrated by the omission of all such drugs from the 1983 *Physician's Desk Reference*. Nevertheless, a general discussion of organomercurials is included to provide a perspective for more modern diuretic therapy.

In general, organomercurials are administered intramuscularly, although they have been given orally (usually irritating and not well absorbed), intravenously (contraindicated because of rare but acute cardiac fibrillation), or subcutaneously (no better absorbed, occasional slough). The onset of action is delayed, requiring perhaps 2 hours for maximum effect, and the duration is prolonged (a day or two, depending on dose, edema state, and renal function). Ordinarily, they are administered intermittently, every few days or more frequently if needed to control edema.

Typically, organomercurials increase the excretion (inhibit reabsorption) of sodium and chloride. Their effect on potassium is variable. Water excretion is in excess of electrolyte, thereby producing increased free water clearance. They exist in the body and urine as cysteine adducts and are secreted by the proximal portion of the tubules by the same active transport system as for *p*-aminohippuric and certain other organic acids.

Whereas they have been thought to act by inhibiting the availability of sulfhydryl-catalyzed hydrogen from dehydrogenases for exchange with sodium in the proximal tubules, more recent evidence supports their preponderant action on the thick segment of the loop of Henle, in the manner of loop diuretics (see discussion of loop diuretics). Their effectiveness is enhanced by acidifying agents such as ammonium chloride and depressed by sodium bicarbonate alkalinization of urine.

Apart from the inherent irritation induced in varying degree by these compounds, their propensity to cause renal tubular toxicity to the point of necrosis, if administered in too high dosage too frequently, limits their utility. In other words, when they are most needed, their use at effective dosage is attended by gravest risk to the patient. Fortunately, there are safer potent diuretics today that are more convenient to use.

CARBONIC ANHYDRASE INHIBITORS

Shortly after sulfanilamide introduced the modern era of chemotherapy, it was noted to cause alkaline urine and a metabolic acidosis in patients.[17] Mann and Keilin[10] showed that sulfanilamide inhibited the ubiquitous enzyme carbonic anhydrase, which had been found to be present in the cortex but not the medulla of the kidney. In 1945 Pitts and Alexander[12] made use of sulfanilamide-induced carbonic anhydrase inhibition in dogs to set forth the present theory of urine acidification. From this background, Schwartz[15] reported in 1949 the clinical use of sulfanilamide for relief of edema in cardiac decompensated patients, although the increased excretion of bicarbonate limited its utility. The stage was set for modern diuretic therapy by this report and by a publication of Krebs[9] on chemical structure-activity relationships to the effect that (1) irreversible substitution of the sulfamoyl-nitrogen of sulfanilamide destroyed activity (previously noted by Mann and Keilin[10]), (2) heterocyclic sulfonamides were the more active, and (3) acetylation of the *p*-amino group enhanced activity of sufanilamide.

$$H_2N - C_6H_4 - \overset{\displaystyle O}{\underset{\displaystyle O}{S}} - NH_2$$

Sulfanilamide

From this background the development of diuretics based on carbonic anhydrase inhibition took two directions: (1) the search for more potent carbonic anhydrase inhibitors per se and (2) the search for carbonic anhydrase inhibitors that would increase chloride excretion as the predominant anion with sodium—a saluretic compound.

The search for more potent carbonic anhydrase inhibitors culminated in **acetazolamide** (Diamox), a heterocyclic acetylaminosulfonamide. Its in vitro activity is about 1000 times greater than sulfanilamide; their pharmacodynamic effects are otherwise similar. Its clinical utility as a diuretic was reported in 1953.

Predominantly distal carbonic anhydrase diuretics

Acetazolamide

Acetazolamide is the first potent diuretic to be well absorbed and well tolerated when administered orally. It is filtered at the glomeruli and actively secreted by the proximal renal tubules. It is reabsorbed by the renal tubules; reabsorption is pH-sensitive, being least at alkaline pH.

Typically, it increases excretion of Na^+, K^+, and HCO_3^-, and water and urinary pH. Under its influence little or no Cl^- appears in urine. Whereas its site of action was thought to be the proximal tubules, subsequent comparisons of the relationship of structure and physical characteristics to pattern of electrolyte excretion for other sulfonamides, including the thiazides, have been interpreted to place its predominant site of action in the distal cortical portion of the nephron, though some proximal effect cannot be excluded. Since the compound inhibits exchange of Na^+ for H^+ but does not decrease Na^+ for K^+ exchange in the distal segment, the increase in potassium excretion seems a compensatory effort by the nephron to conserve (reabsorb) sodium.

Acetazolamide (Diamox) tablets are available containing 125 and 250 mg and as a 500 mg sustained-release formulation. It is also available for parenteral use as 500 mg vials of the cryodesiccated sodium powder.

When acetazolamide or the closely related **ethoxzolamide** (Cardrase) is administered as a diuretic, it should be given intermittently to permit recovery of plasma HCO_3^- levels between doses. Otherwise, continuous effective therapy soon induces a metabolic (hyperchloremic) acidosis, under which conditions such compounds are ineffective.

Ethoxzolamide   Dichlorphenamide

Ethoxzolamide (Cardrase) is available as 125 mg tablets.

In present practice, reduction of intraocular tension in glaucoma is the main indication for these carbonic anhydrase inhibitors. Their volume of distribution permits their access to carbonic anhydrase in other tissues, as in the eye.

Dichlorphenamide (Daranide), like acetazolamide, is a potent carbonic anhydrase inhibitor. Its more lipophilic physical characteristic places the balance of its action and site of action in the renal cortex intermediate between chlorothiazide and acetazolamide. It is as natriuretic as, but less kaliuretic than, acetazolamide. It increases excretion of both chloride and bicarbonate with the diuresis. It is believed to act both proximally and on the distal cortical segment of the nephron, predominantly the latter.

Dichlorphenamide is employed more in management of respiratory acidosis and glaucoma than as a diuretic.

Dichlorphenamide (Daranide) is available as 50 mg tablets.

Because of the ubiquitous distribution of carbonic anhydrase in the nervous system, as well as in erythrocytes, the renal cortex, and elsewhere, side effects of drugs of this type may include parasthesia, which is reversible on withdrawing the agent.

Predominantly proximal carbonic anhydrase diuretics

The search for a saluretic carbonic anhydrase culminated in **chlorothiazide** (Diuril) and still more potent compounds. At the time that search was begun, it was evident that chloride output should closely approximate sodium excretion (Fig. 38-1). It was unclear how this could be accomplished with a carbonic anhydrase inhibitor. Fortunately, it was found early among sulfanilamide analogs that its *p*-carboxy congener was weakly chloruretic. This long-term search anticipated discovery of the thiazides by a few years. Described in 1957, chlorothiazide increases the excretion of predominantly Na^+, Cl^-, and water. Chlorothiazide is some 10 times more active as a carbonic anhydrase inhibitor than sulfanilamide.

Chlorothiazide (Diuril) is available as 250 and 500 mg tablets and as a suspension of 250 mg/5 ml. It is supplied for intravenous use as the sodium salt in white dry powder form equivalent to 0.5 g chlorothiazide.

Hydrochlorothiazide (HydroDiuril) is slightly more than equiactive as a carbonic anhydrase inhibitor compared with sulfanilamide. HCO_3^- excretion may be enhanced

TABLE 38-2   Relationship of ether/water partition coefficient to the order of activity and inversely to the in vitro carbonic anhydrase inhibition of several thiazides

Compound	Natriuretic activity	Partition coefficient	CO_2-ase inhibition (M) $\times 10^{-5}$
Chlorothiazide	1	0.08	.17
Hydrochlorothiazide	10	0.37	2.3
Trichlormethiazide	100	1.53	5.5
Cyclopenthiazide	1000	10.2	1.3

From Beyer, K.H., and Baer, J.E.: Med. Clin. North Am. **59**:735, 1975.

sufficiently to increase urine pH slightly. K^+ is increased in a compensatory manner, since Na^+ exchange with H^+ is inhibited, not Na^+/K^+ exchange. **Hydrochlorothiazide** (HydroDiuril) is supplied as 25, 50, and 100 mg tablets.

Chlorothiazide   Hydrochlorothiazide

FIG. 38-7 *Single-dose response curve for trichlormethiazide, hydrochlorothiazide, and chlorothiazide.*

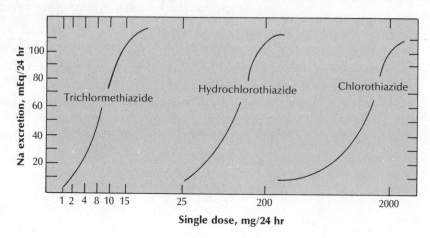

The thiazides and related compounds are secreted by the proximal portion of renal tubules, and to the extent that they are not bound to plasma albumin, they are filtered at the glomeruli, also. Dosage of individual compounds relates to their accumulation in the course of their secretion by the tubules and is inversely related to lipid solubility (Table 38-2) as is their efflux from the proximal tubule. Consequently, except for chlorothiazide (which is the least lipid soluble), they do not reach the distal convuluted tubules in sufficient concentration (considering their relatively weak inherent activity) to inhibit carbonic anhydrase at that distal site. They do not increase pH or bicarbonate excretion.

In general, the thiazides induce the same maximum natriuretic response regardless of dosage (Fig. 38-7), and their effect on salt and water excretion is not pH sensitive; activity is not increased or decreased by conditions sufficient to make urine more acid or alkaline.

The thiazides and **chlorthalidone** (Hygroton), which is a long-acting analog, are well tolerated and effective when administered orally or parenterally to edematous patients with normal or moderate impairment of renal function. They are also useful alone or as adjuncts to other antihypertensive therapy. **Chlorthalidone** (Hygroton) is supplied as 25 and 50 mg tablets.

Hypokalemia secondary to increased potassium excretion is a common occurrence. Complaint of weakness or fatigue from exertion may be sufficient to suggest potassium chloride supplementation. Patients on digitalis-like therapy are likely to manifest greater sensitivity to digitalis toxicity and/or electrocardiographic signs of conduction defect during hypokalemia. Ordinarily, patients with good renal function on a normal diet should manage their electrolyte balance spontaneously, although this may be compromised by hyperaldosteronism attending high-renin hypertension or cirrhosis (where diet may be compromised, also).

Hyperuricemia and increased BUN may relate more to pharmacodynamic effects of the drugs than to impaired renal function. Increased glucose tolerance tests may not be indicative of diabetes in the presence of thiazide therapy.

On balance, efficacy and tolerance make thiazides drugs of choice when they are adequate to manage edema and hypertension.

Presently, loop diuretics derive from two types of chemistry (other than the organomercurials mentioned previously in this text): (1) sulfonamides, in the instance of **furosemide** (Lasix) and **bumetanide** (Bumex) and (2) a sulfhydryl-reactive agent, **ethacrynic acid** (Edecrin). Both types of compound have much greater inherent activity or potency at optimum dosage than the thiazides. All three loop diuretics are well absorbed and active when administered by mouth or intravenously. The several loop diuretics are practically equipotent at optimum dosage. *LOOP DIURETICS*

Ethacrynic acid

Furosemide

Bumetanide

Their spectrum of electrolyte effect is essentially the same as for thiazides, but urine volume is likely to be greater and specific gravity less following administration of the loop diuretics. Thus these drugs extend therapy to edematous patients that may not be adequately controlled by thiazides, but in doing so they may require greater physician attention to patient care.

These compounds are secreted by the proximal segment of the renal tubules. This is their principal route of excretion by the kidney, since more than 90% of their plasma concentration is bound to albumin. Hence, their glomerular filtration is negligible. These compounds are considered to act on Na^+/H^+ exchange in the proximal segment of the nephron, but their principal site of action is the thick segment of the loop of Henle, hence their designation as *loop diuretics*. They must reach this thick segment of the loop from the luminal side of the tubule to be effective; thus their secretion by the proximal convoluted segment is essential to their effectiveness.

Ethacrynic acid and furosemide reduce or abolish the osmotic gradient of the medulla (depending on dosage) by inhibiting chloride and sodium reabsorption at the thick segment of the ascending limb. Whereas the thiazides act predominantly in the proximal cortical segments and do not affect the medullary concentration gradient, any amount of furosemide that increases salt excretion decreases Na^+, Cl^-, and urea gradients in the medulla. This distinction accounts for the essential difference in effect of thiazides and loop diuretics on the excretion of water.

The loop diuretics reduce the osmotic concentration gradient of the medulla. In so doing, these drugs decrease the osmotic force responsible for water reabsorption from the collecting duct to an extent that cannot be overcome by the facilitatory effect of ADH. Consequently, these compounds increase free water clearance. Since the thiazides do not affect the medullary concentration gradient, they do not depress its effect on water reabsorption as do the loop diuretics; thus the effects of the two categories of diuretics on clearance of "free water" are different for this reason.

Because of their impressive potency, these drugs can be lifesaving, as in acute pulmonary edema, or threatening if abused or neglected. Abused, they can induce hypochloremic alkalosis, hypokalemia, and hyponatremia, which, except for hypokalemia, are quite uncommon for the thiazides. Like the thiazides, they cause hyperuricemia. Furosemide can alter glucose tolerance, but this seems less well established for ethacrynic acid.

The fact that the duration of action of the loop diuretics is short (2 to 4 hours) contributes to their safe use ordinarily. However, when they are employed at high dosage and frequently as a lifesaving measure, as in an attempt to prevent acute renal failure, they may cause sufficient disturbance of endolymph to induce temporary or permanent reduction (loss) of hearing. Decreased hepatic function reduces the rate of metabolism of furosemide, and reduced renal function prolongs the duration of action of these drugs. They should not be used after renal failure is manifest.

Except for an equivalent dosage of bumetanide, being only one-fortieth that of furosemide, the two drugs seem essentially the same with respect to effect on electrolyte and water excretion, oral efficacy, duration of action, and side effects.

Furosemide (Lasix) is supplied as 20, 40, and 80 mg tablets. It is also supplied for parenteral use as a sterile solution containing 10 mg furosemide. The solution is supplied in 2, 4, and 10 ml amber ampules.

Ethacrynic acid (Edecrin) is supplied as 25 and 50 mg tablets. Intravenous sodium ethacrynic acid is a dry white material supplied in vials equivalent to 50 mg ethacrynic acid.

Bumetanide (Bumex) is supplied as 0.5 and 1.0 mg tablets. It is also available in sterile solution for intravenous or intramuscular administration as a 2 ml ampule containing 0.25 mg bumetanide/ml.

ANTIKALIURETIC
(POTASSIUM-
SPARING) AGENTS

The saluretic diuretic agents discussed to this point cause a compensatory increase in potassium excretion. Ordinarily, this may not be alarming, but in cirrhosis when aldosterone metabolism is reduced or when its production is increased markedly, the saluretic agents may actually cause a greater increase in potassium excretion than sodium.

The efforts to discover diuretics that would increase sodium excretion by inhibiting its exchange in the distal convoluted tubule with potassium have resulted in two subclasses of antikaliuretic agents: (1) aldosterone antagonists and (2) agents that act directly to inhibit Na^+/K^+ exchange.

Spironolactone (Aldactone) is the only available antagonist of the effect of aldosterone on Na^+/K^+ transport. It may be administered orally. A parenteral dosage form is not yet marketed in this country.

Aldosterone antagonists

Aldosterone   Spironolactone

As an aldosterone antagonist, it is most effective under conditions where enhancement of Na^+ reabsorption and increased K^+ excretion induced by aldosterone are greatest, cirrhosis of the liver and high renin hypertension being most frequent. (It is not active in adrenalectomized animals.) The action of aldosterone is comparatively slow to develop, and the inherent effect of Na^+/K^+ exchange is much less than for Na^+/H^+ exchange. Hence, the effect of spironolactone is slow to develop and is sustained but is not as great, acutely, as for the other categories of saluretic agents. The prolonged duration of action makes the net natriuretic effect useful.

The spectrum of saluretic effect is one of increased Na^+ and Cl^- and reduced K^+ excretion. Under edematous conditions there is no increase in HCO_3^- excretion. Water excretion is more or less equivalent to electrolyte output.

Side effects relate to both mode of action and the chemistry of progestational hormones from which spironolactone was developed. Perhaps the most common undesirable effect is hyperkalemia from excessive K^+ retention by the kidneys. The initial symptomatology may be similar to that of hypokalemia, weakness, and fatiguability, which may be sufficient to suggest the need for plasma potassium determination.

Spironolactone was developed from the chemistry of progesterone, which had been noted to have aldosterone antagonist activity. Although spironolactone is at most only very weakly progestational, it can cause gynecomastia (more frequently in men than women), which may or may not be reversible. It has been reported to be tumorigenic in chronic toxicity studies in rats.

Spironolactone (Aldactone) is supplied as 25 and 100 mg tablets.

Presently, two direct-acting antikaliuretic agents are available: **Triamterene** (Dyrenium) and **Amiloride** (Midamor). They are administered orally.

Triamterene   **Amiloride**

Unlike the aldosterone antagonist, these basic compounds promptly inhibit sodium reabsorption and potassium excretion (Na^+/K^+ exchange in the distal cortical segment of the nephron). Consequently, they are uniformly effective regardless of the status of aldosterone blood levels and are active in adrenalectomized animals. This tends to make them more reliable, though the spectrum of electrolyte and water excretion ($Na^+ \uparrow$, $Cl^- \uparrow$, $K^+ \downarrow$) identifies them as potassium-sparing saluretic agents. They are most useful by themselves under conditions of excessive aldosterone effect with loss of potassium.

They are filtered at the glomeruli and are secreted by the proximal convoluted tubules. This is essential to their activity, for they are effective only when presented to their distal site of action from the luminal side of the tubule.

Amiloride is the more potent compound in this category of potassium-sparing agents. Although amiloride is inherently less potent than the thiazides because of the lesser magnitude of Na^+/K^+ exchange than Na^+/H^+, its duration of action is sufficient that on a day-to-day basis it is about as effective as thiazide therapy.

These compounds are well tolerated except for their propensity to retain potassium, which can result in hyperkalemia.

Their saluretic, antikaliuretic characteristics make them natural adjuncts to thiazide therapy. The different modes of action of the two types of compounds make their combined saluretic effects additive or even synergistic, whereas the qualitatively different actions of the two classes of compounds on potassium excretion summate to offset the risk of potassium changes. This has resulted in the availability of a number of hydrochlorothiazide and amiloride or triamterene combined formulations. Although the basic rationale for combining a loop diuretic with one of these agents is the same as for thiazides, the greater difference in potency and duration of action between the loop and antikaliuretic drugs seems to preclude such a formulation (from a practical standpoint).

Triamterene (Dyrenium) is supplied as 50 mg capsules.

Amiloride (Midamor) is supplied as the hydrochloride in 5 mg tablets.

1. Baer, J.E., Jones, C.B., Spitzer, S.A., and Russo, H.F.: The potassium-sparing and natriuretic activity of *N*-amidino-3,5-diamino-6-chloro-pyrazine-carboxamide hydrochloride dihydrate (amiloride hydrochloride), J. Pharmacol. Exp. Ther. **157**:472, 1967.

2. Baer, J.E., Russo, H.F., and Beyer, K.H.: Saluretic activity of hydrochlorothiazide (6-chloro-7-sulfamyl-3,4-dihydro-1,2,4-benzothiadiazine-1,1-dioxide) in the dog, Proc. Soc. Exp. Biol. Med. **100**:442, 1959.

3. Beyer, K.H.: Chlorothiazide, Br. J. Clin. Pharmacol. **13**:15, 1982.

4. Beyer, K.H., and Baer, J.E.: The site and mode of action of some sulfonamide-derived diuretics, Med. Clin. North Am. **59**:735, 1975.

5. Beyer, K.H., Baer, J.E., Michelson, J.K., and Russo, H.F.: Renotropic characteristics of ethacrynic acid: a phenoxyacetic saluretic-diuretic agent, J. Pharmacol. Exp. Ther. **147**:1, 1965.

6. Beyer, K.H., and Peuler, J.D.: Hypertension: perspectives, Pharmacol. Rev. **34**:287, 1982.

7. Burg, M., and Green, N.: Effect of ethacrynic acid on the thick ascending limb of Henle's loop, Kidney Int. **4**:301, 1973.

8. Handley, C.A., and Lavik, P.S.: Inhibition of kidney succinic dehydrogenase system by mercurial diuretics, J. Pharmacol. Exp. Ther. **100**:115, 1950.

9. Krebs, H.A.: Inhibition of carbonic anhydrase by sulfonamides, Biochem. J. **43**:525, 1948.

10. Mann, T., and Keilin, D.: Sulfanilamide as a specific inhibitor of carbonic anhydrase, Nature, Lond. **146**:164, 1940.

11. Maren, T.H.: Symposium on carbonic anhydrase inhibition as a physiological tool: pharmacological and renal effects of Diamox (6063)—a new carbonic anhydrase inhibitor, Trans. N.Y. Acad. Sci. **15**:53, 1952.

12. Pitts, R.F., and Alexander, R.S.: The nature of the renal tubular mechanism for acidifying the urine, Am. J. Physiol. **144**:239, 1945.

13. Richards, A.N.: Urine formation in the amphibian kidney, Harvey Lectures, **30**:93, 1934-1935.

14. Saxyl, P., and Heilig, R.: Über die diuretische Wirkung von Novasurol und anderen Quecksilberinjectionen, Wien. Klin. Wochenschr. **33**:943, 1920.

15. Schwartz, W.B.: The effect of sulfanilamide on salt and water excretion in congestive heart failure, N. Engl. J. Med. **240**:173, 1949.

16. Sleisenger, M., Richard, J., Knowlessar, O.D., Clarkson, B., Thompson, D., and Peterson, R.E.: Effects of spirolactones on excretion of water and electrolytes and on aldosterone metabolism in cirrhosis, J. Clin. Invest. **38**:1043, 1959.

17. Southworth, H.: Acidosis associated with the administration of para-amino-benzene-sulfonamide (Prontylin), Proc. Soc. Exp. Biol. Med. **36**:58, 1937.

18. Suki, W.S., Rector, F.C., and Seldin, D.W.: The site of action of furosemide and other sulfonamide diuretics in the dog, J. Clin. Invest. **44**:1458, 1965.

19. Timmer, R.J., Springman, F.R., and Thoms, R.K.: Evaluation of furosemide, a new diuretic agent, Curr. Ther. Res. **6**:88, 1964.

20. Tuzel, I.H., editor: Perspectives on bumetanide (symposium), J. Clin. Pharmacol. **21**:531, 1981.

21. Wiebelhaus, V.D., Weinstock, J., Brennan, F.T., Sosnowski, G., and Larsen, T.J.: A potent non-steroid orally active antagonist of aldosterone, Fed. Proc. **20**:409, 1961.

REFERENCES

Chapter 39

Pharmacological approaches to atherosclerosis

GENERAL CONCEPTS   Research on atherosclerosis is dominated by concepts that envision some connection between hyperlipoproteinemias and the arterial disease. A major new concept invokes a receptor-mediated control of cholesterol metabolism.[3] According to this concept, mammalian cells have a low-density lipoprotein (LDL) receptor on their surface, which mediates the internalization of the cholesterol-rich lipoprotein. Cholesterol is then removed and utilized within the cell. In familial hypercholesterolemia the receptor is deficient, and atherosclerosis is common.[2] In other approaches the high-density lipoproteins (HDL) are viewed as protective and useful cholesterol carriers.

Although there is no conclusive evidence for a beneficial effect of correction of hyperlipoproteinemia, several drugs have been introduced for the purpose of lowering abnormally elevated serum lipid concentrations.

Clofibrate may inhibit the release of lipoproteins from the liver and does inhibit cholesterol biosynthesis. *Cholestyramine* and *colestipol* are resins that bind bile acids and prevent their absorption. *Dextrothyroxine* increases the catabolism of apoprotein B. *Nicotinic acid* depresses the synthesis of LDL and apoprotein B. *Probucol* reduces LDL cholesterol as well as HDL cholesterol and apolipoprotein A-1. Because lowering HDL could be theoretically detrimental, the ultimate role of probucol in the treatment of hypercholesterolemia is uncertain. *Estrogens* are no longer used in the treatment of hyperlipidemias, but *norethindrone acetate,* a progestational agent, and some anabolic steroids are used in some patients investigationally. *Sitosterols* from plants compete with cholesterol for absorption. In addition, neomycin sulfate precipitates cholesterol in the intestine and prevents its absorption.

CLOFIBRATE

Clofibrate (Atromid-S), the ethyl ester of chlorophenoxyisobutyric acid, is hydrolyzed in association with its gastrointestinal absorption. The resulting anion is transported in plasma bound largely to albumin. Clofibrate was first used in combination with or as a vehicle for androsterone, which is known to decrease cholesterol synthesis in the liver. Further studies revealed that clofibrate alone, when administered orally in doses of 500 mg four times daily, lowers the concentration of trigylcerides, lipoproteins, and cholesterol in plasma in a few weeks.

Clofibrate

Although several mechanisms of action have been suggested, clofibrate's chief effect on very low density lipoprotein (VLDL) is probably to increase the clearance of triglyceride-rich lipoproteins by increasing the activity of lipoprotein lipase.[3] Body cholesterol pools are reduced in association with increased biliary and fecal excretion of cholesterol. In some patients clofibrate may inhibit cholesterol biosynthesis. Clofibrate therapy may increase HDL cholesterol levels in patients with hypertriglyceridemia but not in most patients with normal triglyceride levels. The drug can be useful in hyperlipidemia types III, IV, and V and is less effective in type II. Except for the treatment of primary dysbetalipoproteinemia (type III), other antilipidemic drugs may prove more effective in individual patients. Its gastrointestinal effects and other side effects and its many drug interactions limit its usefulness. The drug should be given only to patients who are not adequately controlled with dietary therapy. Clofibrate is available in 500 mg capsules. The usual dose is one capsule four times a day.

BILE ACID–BINDING RESINS

Cholestyramine (Questran; Cuemid) and colestipol (Colestid) are anion-exchange resins that bind bile acids in the intestinal lumen, exchanging them for chloride. Since the resin is not absorbed, it promotes the fecal excretion of bile acids. To replace the lost bile acids, the liver increases its rate of bile acid synthesis. Since cholesterol is the precursor for the bile acids, the net result is an increased utilization of cholesterol and usually a lowering of the serum level. The effectiveness of bile acid–binding resins in lowering LDL cholesterol levels in plasma appears to depend on the ability of the liver to increase the population of LDL receptors to supply cholesterol in support of increased bile acid synthesis.[4]

Cholestyramine is used primarily for relief of pruritus associated with biliary tract obstruction. The bile acid–binding resins are also useful in the treatment of hyperlipidemias characterized by high levels of LDL cholesterol. They may be used in combination with nicotinic acid.

Cholestyramine and colestipol are granular preparations that should be mixed with juice or other liquid, allowed to hydrate for a few minutes, and then taken with meals. They are available in bulk or in individual packets containing 4 g (Cholestyramine) or 5 g (Colestipol). The usual starting dose is 20 g/day, and this may be increased to 30 or 32 g/day for maximum effect. The major side effects of these preparations are constipation and bloating. They interfere with the absorption of fat-soluble vitamins and numerous drugs including digitalis, thiazide diuretics, warfarin, thyroxine, phenobarbital, tetracycline, iron salts, and phenylbutazone.

DEXTRO-THYROXINE

It is generally known that a reciprocal relationship exists between thyroid function and serum cholesterol. Among the thyroxine analogs that have been synthesized, dextrothyroxine (Chloxin) has received the most attention in the treatment of hyperlipoproteinemias. It is estimated that levothyroxine is 10 to 20 times as calorigenic as dextrothyroxine, but the latter has about 20% of the hypocholesterolemic action of levothyroxine.

Dextrothyroxine may promote the catabolism of apoprotein B, thus reducing LDL. The drug is probably useful in type II hyperlipoproteinemia.

Side effects of dextrothyroxine are a consequence of its metabolic stimulating action. They include angina and arrhythmias. In the large Coronary Drug Research Project,[4] dextrothyroxine at 6 mg/day produced sufficient adverse effects and suspicion of excess mortality that the drug was eliminated from the study.

NICOTINIC ACID

Nicotinic acid has been used in the treatment of several hyperlipidemic disorders. Its primary mechanism of action is to inhibit the secretion of VLDL.[4] This in turn results in a decreased production of LDL. Another pharmacological effect of nicotinic acid that may be of therapeutic benefit is a decrease in the fractional catabolic rate for HDL, which results in higher levels of HDL cholesterol and apolipoprotein A-1. Nicotinic acid is the only agent of those studied in the Coronary Drug Project that produced a significant decrease in coronary events.[4]

The usefulness of nicotinic acid can be limited by troublesome side effects. Flushing occurs in practically all patients initially and may persist in some. This side effect appears to be prostaglandin mediated and can be blocked by pretreatment with aspirin. Activation of peptic ulcer and hepatic dysfunction are other toxic effects of large doses. Nicotinic acid is available in tablets of 100 and 500 mg. Occasionally it is used in combination with bile acid–binding resins.[3]

Probucol (Lorelco) is a cholesterol-lowering agent that is unrelated chemically to other lipid-lowering drugs. Its mechanism of action is still uncertain. It reduces serum cholesterol levels in laboratory animals by inhibiting cholesterol synthesis.[1] It has also been shown to increase the fecal excretion of bile acids in some human studies. Patients treated with probucol demonstrate reductions in both LDL and HDL cholesterol. Since HDL is thought to exert a protective effect in terms of atherosclerotic disease, a reduced level could be theoretically detrimental. Consequently, the ultimate role of probucol in the treatment of hypercholesterolemia remains controversial.

PROBUCOL

Absorption of cholesterol from the gastrointestinal tract is interfered with by certain plant sterols, known as sitosterols (Cytellin). These sterols are not significantly absorbed but have many disadvantages. They must be administered frequently, and they are unpalatable. As a consequence, they have not become widely used.

SITOSTEROLS

Although estrogens may lower serum cholesterol, they elevate serum triglycerides. Studies of women taking oral contraceptives often reveal an elevation of serum trigylcerides.

Some reports claimed that conjugated estrogenic substances (Premarin) increased the chances of survival of men having coronary disease. Other studies in which ethinyl estradiol was used failed to show any benefit in patients who had a previous myocardial infarction.

FEMALE SEX HORMONES

Norethindrone acetate (Norlutate), a progestational agent, may be useful in some women with type V hyperlipoproteinemia. The drug apparently decreases the concentrations of LDL and apoprotein A.

Oxandrolone (Anavar) may be useful in some men for the reduction of triglyceride concentrations. This drug, which is an anabolic steroid, is a derivative of testosterone.

NORETHINDRONE ACETATE AND OXANDROLONE

This aminoglycoside given orally is not well absorbed from the gastrointestinal tract. It precipitates cholesterol and prevents its absorption; thus it acts in a manner similar to cholestyramine. The drug may be useful in some forms of type II hyperlipoproteinemia.

NEOMYCIN SULFATE

Atherosclerosis is common and severe in some types of hyperlipoproteinemia, and the aim of management is to lower the concentration of lipids. The use of lipid-lowering agents depends on the type of hyperlipoproteinemia. Current recommendations are summarized in Table 39-1.

MANAGEMENT OF HYPERLIPO- PROTEINEMIAS

TABLE 39-1   Nondietary treatment of primary hyperlipidemias

Disorder	Drugs
Monogenic or oligogenic	
Familial hypercholesterolemia	
Heterozygous	Resin + nicotinic acid*
	Resin + neomycin
Homozygous	Resin + nicotinic acid
Familial multiple-type hyperlipoproteinemia	
Elevated LDL	Resin, nicotinic acid, or combination
Elevated VLDL	Nicotinic acid or clofibrate
Elevated VLDL + LDL	Resin, nicotinic acid, or combination
Familial hypertrigylceridemia	
Mild	Clofibrate or nicotinic acid
Severe (with chylomicronemia)	Nicotinic acid*
Familial dysbetalipoproteinemia	Clofibrate (small doses)*
	Nicotinic acid
Familial lipoprotein lipase of apolipoprotein C-II deficiency	None
Other	
Polygenic or unclassified hypercholesterolemia	Resin*
	Nicotinic acid or clofibrate
Exogenous hypercholesterolemia	β-Sitosterol
Sporadic or unclassified hypertriglyceridemia	Clofibrate or nicotinic acid

Reproduced with permission, from the Annual Review of Medicine, Volume 33. © 1982 by Annual Reviews, Inc.
*Drug of choice.

REFERENCES

1. Glueck, C.J.: Colestipol and probucol: treatment of primary and familial hypercholesterolemia and amelioration of atherosclerosis, Ann. Int. Med. **96:**475, 1982.
2. Goldstein, J.L., and Brown, M.S.: The LDL receptor defect in familial hypercholesterolemia, Med. Clin. North Am. **66:**335, 1982.
3. Havel, R.J., and Kane, J.P.: Therapy of hyperlipidemic states, Ann. Rev. Med. **33:**417, 1982.
4. Kane, J.P., and Malloy, M.J.: Treatment of hypercholesterolemia, Med. Clin. North Am. **66:**537, 1982.

section seven

Drug effects on the respiratory and gastrointestinal tracts

Chapter 40

Drug effects on the respiratory tract

Numerous drugs, along with other measures, contribute to the effective management of pulmonary disorders, particularly in chronic obstructive lung disease. The *bronchodilators* are helpful in opening blocked airways; the *mucolytic drugs* aid in altering the characteristics of respiratory tract fluid; the *antibiotics* are useful in dealing with infections; the *corticosteroids* reduce the inflammatory process. In addition to these useful drug effects, the hazardous nature of sedative drugs and oxygen at high concentration is increasingly recognized. It is also becoming clear that the lung is a metabolic organ that contributes to the elaboration and destruction of a variety of endogenous compounds of great pharmacological activity. Drug-induced pulmonary diseases are also receiving increased attention.

The groups of drugs that will be discussed at this point are the bronchodilators, expectorants, and mucolytic agents. In addition, current concepts on the metabolic functions of the lung of pharmacological interest and drug-induced pulmonary diseases will also be considered.

Numerous drugs are capable of causing contraction or relaxation of the bronchial smooth muscle. The more important ones are enumerated in Table 40-1.

The bronchial constrictors listed in Table 40-1 are of experimental interest only and have no therapeutic importance. Histamine and methacholine are said to have a greater constrictor effect in asthmatic than in normal individuals, and these compounds are sometimes used by clinical investigators for testing the potency of bronchodilator drugs.

The bronchodilators listed in Table 40-1 vary greatly in their usefulness. Atropine and other anticholinergics traditionally have been avoided because they decrease bronchial secretions, leading to inspissated mucus. However, recent studies indicate that atropine or its *N*-isopropyl derivative, ipratropium, may be quite effective when given by inhalation. At the present time the useful bronchodilators are limited to the β-adrenergic agonists and the methylxanthines.

PHARMACOLOGY OF BRONCHIAL SMOOTH MUSCLE

TABLE 40-1   Drugs acting on bronchial smooth muscle

Causing contraction	Causing relaxation or opposing contraction
Acetylcholine and related drugs	Atropine and other anticholinergic drugs
Histamine	Antihistaminics
β-Adrenergic blockers	β-Adrenergic agonists
α-Adrenergic agonists	Dimethylxanthine (theophylline)
Slow-reacting substance of anaphylaxis	Inhibitors of the immunological release of mediators of anaphylaxis
Bradykinin	Prostaglandins E
Prostaglandin $F_{2\alpha}$	Antagonists of slow-reacting substances of anaphylaxis and prostaglandins F

BRONCHO-DILATORS
β-Adrenergic agonists and methylxanthines

The effectiveness of epinephrine, sympathomimetic drugs, and theophylline derivatives such as aminophylline in bronchial asthma has been known for many years. Increased knowledge of the mode of action of these compounds is of more recent origin, and schemes of their influence on the bronchi are shown in Fig. 40-1.

With the postulation of α and β receptors it became clear that β receptor agonists and the methylxanthines or phosphodiesterase inhibitors are especially potent in dilating the bronchial smooth muscle. It is most likely that the effectiveness of both groups of drugs is based on their common property of increasing the levels of adenosine 3':5'-cyclic phosphate (cyclic AMP) in the smooth muscle of the bronchioles (Fig. 40-1).

The pure, direct-acting β-adrenergic agonist isoproterenol has become one of the most widely used bronchodilators. Its administration by a specially constructed inhaler has contributed to its popularity. It has some disadvantages, however. As expected from its pharmacology, isoproterenol causes considerable cardiac stimulation and its action is short. Furthermore, it has been suggested that the use of isoproterenol may have contributed to the annual increase in mortality of asthmatic individuals in England and Wales. The deaths have been attributed to various causes, such as alterations in the viscosity of bronchial secretions, decreased arterial oxygen tensions, and increased ventricular irritability with arrhythmias.

With the postulation by Lands[8] of two types of β-adrenergic receptors, efforts have been directed at synthesizing drugs that would have a more specific effect on the bronchial smooth muscle and would also have a more prolonged action, thus avoiding the disadvantages of isoproterenol.

Lands termed β_1 those receptors responsible for cardiac stimulation and lipolysis, whereas those responsible for bronchodilation and vasodepression were referred to as β_2. If two types of β receptors indeed exist, it should be possible to synthesize β agonists that have marked bronchodilator activity without much cardiac stimulation. Salbutamol and terbutaline appear to have such characteristics.

Bronchodilatation and bronchoconstriction as influenced by cyclic 3'5' AMP tissue con-   *FIG. 40-1*
centrations. (Schematic representation of a working hypothesis. For details see Problem
40-2.)

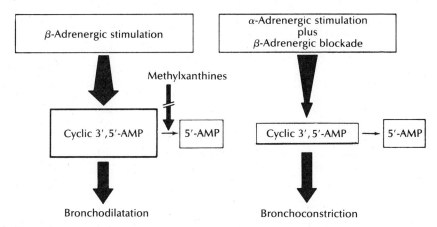

*PROBLEM 40-1. Is it possible to increase bronchodilator activity without a corresponding increase
in cardiac stimulant effect in β-adrenergic agonists? Salbutamol and isoproterenol were compared
on asthmatic subjects and in normal individuals in a double-blind trial to compare bronchodilator and
cardiovascular activity.[12]*

*Aerosols containing salbutamol (100 γg/inhalation) or isoproterenol (500 γg/inhalation) were pro-
vided for a double-blind trial in identical containers. Forced expiratory spirograms were analyzed for
forced expiratory volume in 1 second (FEV₁) and forced vital capacity (FVC) as well as by other
criteria. Heart rate was measured from a continuous electrocardiogram.*

*In asthmatic subjects the FEV₁ showed a similar increase with both drugs initially, but 3 and 4
hours later the values were significantly higher for salbutamol. Heart rate did not increase with salbutamol but showed a rise with isoproterenol. In normal subjects, salbutamol produced a small
increase in heart rate, whereas isoproterenol increased heart rate on the average by 33 beats a
minute and caused palpitation.*

It may be concluded from this clinical study that for comparable bronchodilator
activity salbutamol produces much less cardiac stimulation. It appears, then, that
the β receptors in bronchial smooth muscle and the heart are somewhat different.
Animal experiments point to the same conclusion.

Since β-adrenergic receptors mediate bronchodilatation, the question remains:
are there α-adrenergic receptors in the bronchial smooth muscle and do they have
any function in drug effects?

*PROBLEM 40-2. Do α-adrenergic receptors play a role in drug-induced bronchoconstriction? In
a recent experimental study, isolated strips of human bronchi were tested for their response to a
variety of drugs. The bronchodilating effect of epinephrine was abolished by propranolol. After β-
receptor blockade, epinephrine produced bronchoconstriction. However, the dose of epinephrine
required for the constrictor effect was 10 times greater than the dose that caused bronchial dilatation
before β-receptor blockade. The constriction caused by epinephrine could be abolished by phentolamine, an α-adrenergic blocking drug. It may be concluded from this study and from other evidence*

that α-adrenergic agonists may cause bronchoconstriction in high doses. Such bronchoconstriction becomes evident after the β receptors are blocked. Whether the α receptor—mediated bronchoconstriction has any clinical significance remains to be demonstrated. It is not known, for example, if it is related to tachyphylaxis to epinephrine, the so-called epinephrine fastness *in asthmatic individuals.*

Although the adrenergic drugs are most effective, the methylxanthines such as theophylline and its double salt aminophylline are useful. This is especially true in patients in whom some contraindication exists to the adrenergic drugs or in those who are tolerant to them. Intravenously administered aminophylline may be effective in terminating an asthmatic attack.

In addition to the adrenergic drugs and the methylxanthines, the adrenal corticosteroids are used in severe asthma. It is believed that the corticosteroids prevent the release of arachidonic acid by inhibiting phospholipases. In this connection, it is of great interest that the leukotrienes, which are produced from arachidonic acid by the enzyme lipoxygenase, are potent bronchial constrictors in humans.

Adverse effects

Epinephrine and isoproterenol have all the cardiovascular side effects predictable from their pharmacology, and patients may manifest tachycardia, palpitations, and arrhythmias. Ephedrine, which acts by releasing endogenous catecholamines, crosses the blood-brain barrier and causes nervousness and wakefulness in addition to the peripheral sympathomimetic effects.

Orally administered theophylline or aminophylline causes gastric irritation, and these drugs are irregularly absorbed from the gastrointestinal tract. It is claimed that theophylline in 20% alcohol is less likely to cause gastric irritation and is better absorbed. Aminophylline suppositories are irregularly absorbed and may lead to rectal irritation. Intravenously administered aminophylline may lead to CNS stimulation and convulsions.

Individual bronchodilators

Epinephrine is highly effective in the treatment of acute asthma. It may be injected subcutaneously for a short duration of action, intramuscularly, or as a suspension in oil. It may be administered as an inhalant. When issued frequently, it may produce tachyphylaxis, the mechanism of which is not understood. Perhaps it is a rebound phenomenon.

Ephedrine is highly useful in the prevention and treatment of asthma. It is effective when given orally, and it has a duration of action that last several hours. It acts by releasing endogenous catecholamines, and tachyphylaxis may develop to its continued use. CNS stimulation is a common side effect caused by ephedrine. For this reason there are combinations of ephedrine and phenobarbital available. The latter is usually present in doses too small to counteract the wakefulness caused by ephedrine. The usual dosage of ephedrine for adults is 15 to 50 mg, which may be given as often as every hour if needed. **Pseudoephedrine hydrochloride** (Sudafed) is an active stereoisomer of ephedrine used in a manner similar to the latter.

Isoproterenol as the hydrochloride or sulfate is administered preferably by inhalation. The drug may also be given intravenously. Sublingual tablets of the drug are available, but absorption of these is irregular. Cardiovascular side effects are common after the administration of isoproterenol. Sudden death has occurred under these circumstances.

Albuterol (salbutamol, Ventolin) is a relatively selective β_2-adrenergic bronchodilator. Albuterol is one-half to one-fourth as potent as isoproterenol in producing increases in heart rate. It is available in inhalers. Each inhalation delivers 90 μg of the drug. It is also supplied in the form of tablets as the sulfate containing 4 mg/tablet. The usual dose is 2 to 4 mg three or four times a day.

Metaproterenol sulfate, also known as orciprenaline, is a β receptor agonist with a moderately long duration of action. It differs from isoproterenol only in its two hydroxyl groups attached in meta position on the benzene ring.

It is claimed that the oral administration of a single dose of 20 mg exerts a bronchodilator effect that may last up to 4 hours. Its main contraindications are in patients with cardiac arrhythmias associated with tachycardia.

Metaproterenol sulfate (Alupen) is available in tablets, 20 mg, and in metered dose inhalers. Each metered dose delivers at the mouthpiece approximately 0.65 mg of metaproterenol sulfate.

Terbutaline sulfate (Brethine) is closely related to metaproterenol and may have a greater preference for β_2 receptors. It is available in 5 mg tablets.

Aminophylline (theophylline ethylenediamine) may be administered by slow intravenous injection, orally, or rectally. Its absorption from the gastrointestinal tract is variable. Irritation of the rectum may result from suppositories. Excessive blood levels such as may occur from intravenous injections may lead to convulsions, shock, and death. About 85% of aminophylline is theophylline. For blood levels of theophylline after its intravenous injection, see Mitenko and Ogilvie.[10]

Oxtriphylline (Choledyl) is the choline salt of theophylline containing 64% theophylline. It is more soluble than theophylline and may be better absorbed after oral administration.

Dyphylline (Dilor, Lufyllin, Neothylline) is 7(2,3-dihydroxypropyl) theophylline, a neutral derivative. It corresponds to 70% anhydrous theophylline. It is more soluble than the parent compound and is less irritating. It may even be injected intramuscularly.

Theophylline is also available in timed-release tablets (Theo-Dur) and timed-release capsules (Slo-Phyllin).

Pharmacokinetics of theophylline. Ideal serum concentrations of theophylline vary from 5 to 20 μg/ml. The drug is adequately absorbed from the gastrointestinal tract, and dosage is determined by the clearance rate. Half-life of the drug varies from 3 to 13 hours and is more rapid in children than in adults.

Although widely used, the expectorants and mucolytic drugs hardly constitute one of the brilliant chapters of pharmacology. These drugs presumably alter the viscosity of the sputum, change the volume of respiratory tract fluid, and facilitate expectoration. The mode of action of some of these drugs is understood. In many

EXPECTORANTS AND MUCOLYTIC DRUGS

cases, however, there is much doubt about their mechanism of action and their effectiveness.

Acetylcysteine (Mucomyst) reduces the viscosity of sputum, presumably by depolymerizing mucopolysaccharides. It is used by nebulization or by instillation of the upper respiratory tract and the mouth. The drug reacts with rubber and metals.

Terpin hydrate is volatile oil believed to act on bronchial secretory cells. It is commonly used as a vehicle for cough mixtures in the form of the elixir.

A number of expectorants are believed to stimulate respiratory tract secretion by a reflex through irritation of the stomach. These include **potassium iodide, syrup of ipecac, glyceryl guaiacolate,** and **ammonium chloride.** Proof for the effectiveness of these drugs is hard to find.

Pancreatic dornase is pancreatic deoxyribonuclease that hydrolyzes the deoxyribonucleoprotein of purulent sputum and thereby reduces its viscosity.

It is the belief of competent authorities that the inhalation of nebulized water, sodium chloride solutions, and hygroscopic agents may be more valuable than the use of other inhalants in the treatment of diseases of the respiratory tract complicated by difficulties in expectoration.

ELABORATION AND DESTRUCTION OF PHARMACO- LOGICAL AGENTS BY THE LUNGS

It is increasingly recognized that the lungs are involved in the elaboration and destruction of a variety of pharmacological agents. Histamine has long been known to be present in high concentration in the mast cells of the lungs, and its release by anaphylaxis has been studied by many workers.

In addition to histamine, other pharmacological agents are released during anaphylaxis. According to a study on the perfused guinea pig lung, in addition to histamine, the lipid slow-reacting substance, prostaglandins, serotonin, and certain polypeptides such as bradykinin may also be released or elaborated.

The prostaglandins are receiving much attention for a number of reasons. The lungs are a major site of prostaglandin synthesis. In addition, mechanical stimulation of the lungs or simply hyperinflation may lead to increased synthesis or release of prostaglandins. The significance of this is still not clear. In addition to the prostaglandins, a number of peptides such as bradykinin and others may be elaborated by the lungs.

The potential of the lung for synthesizing hormonal agents is best seen in cases of bronchogenic carcinoma, which may lead to endocrine syndromes with elaboration of many different polypeptide hormones.

The lungs are highly efficient in inactivating a number of pharmacologically active compounds. PGE and PGF are rapidly removed and inactivated during one circulation through the lungs. Bradykinin is almost completely removed in one circulation through the lungs. This is achieved by kininases, which act on the nonapeptide by splitting off a C-terminal dipeptide.

Drugs may influence pulmonary function directly or indirectly. An example of a direct adverse effect is oxygen toxicity. Drugs alter pulmonary function indirectly by various mechanisms. Sedative drugs are an important cause of acute ventilatory failure. Pulmonary edema may be caused by salt and water overload or by depression of cardiac output. Intravenous medications causing thrombophlebitis contribute to pulmonary embolism. Finally, drug allergies may cause bronchospasm.

The directly acting drugs that may induce pulmonary disease encompass a variety of classes, such as inhalants, cancer chemotherapeutic agents, analgesics, antimicrobial drugs, and a miscellaneous category.

DRUG-INDUCED PULMONARY DISEASES

Several inhalants may lead to altered pulmonary function. They include oxygen, acetylcysteine, and isoproterenol. In addition, aspiration of mineral oil and iodinated oils used for bronchography can lead to adverse effects.

It may seem surprising that *oxygen* is toxic in high concentrations, but the tendency of premature infants to develop retrolental fibroplasia and blindness after the prolonged administration of the gas at greater than 40% concentration is well documented. In addition, adults who inhale oxygen at greater than 60% concentrations may develop pulmonary irritation, congestion, atelectasis, and decreased vital capacity. CNS changes manifested by paresthesias also occur. The pulmonary toxic effect of oxygen in humans under hyperbaric conditions has been studied in great detail. Breathing oxygen at 2 atmospheres, symptoms began within 3 to 8 hours and consisted of mild tracheal irritation and decreased vital capacity. After 8 to 10 hours, symptoms were characterized by uncontrollable coughing, dyspnea at rest, and a tracheobronchial burning sensation. Recovery of vital capacity occurred generally in 1 to 3 days.

Mineral oil, when aspirated, causes acute or chronic pneumonitis. *Iodinated* oils employed in bronchography may have adverse effects on a pulmonary reserve that is already impaired.

The bronchoconstrictor effect of acetylcysteine has already been mentioned (p. 504). *Isoproterenol* has been implicated by association in cases of sudden death in asthmatic persons. It has been suggested that in some individuals the drug is converted to 3-methoxyisoproterenol, which is a weak antagonist of the β-adrenergic receptor. *Disodium cromoglycate* may also cause some bronchospasm when given by nebulization.

Inhalants

Cancer chemotherapeutic agents may in some cases cause pulmonary diseases. Diffuse pulmonary disease has been associated with the use of *busulfan* and *cyclophosphamide*. *Methotrexate* has also been implicated in some cases of pulmonary disease.

Cancer chemotherapeutic agents

The narcotic analgesics *heroin* and *methadone* may produce pulmonary edema by mechanisms that are obscure (p. 338). *Propoxyphene* poisoning has also been associated with pulmonary edema.

Analgesics

Aspirin may cause bronchoconstriction in some individuals. Although this is often referred to as aspirin allergy, its immunological basis is unlikely. Often aspirin-sensitive persons fail to show similar reactions to sodium salicylate, whereas they may react to chemically unrelated antiinflammatory drugs such as indomethacin. The mechanism of this aspirin hypersensitivity remains a mystery.

Antimicrobial drugs

A variety of antimicrobial drugs may cause pulmonary diseases. *Nitrofurantoin* administration may lead to a pleuropneumonic reaction. *Sulfonamides* may cause vasculitis, which may include the pulmonary vessels. Sulfonamides, para-aminosalicylate, and penicillin may produce pulmonary infiltration with eosinophilia, usually referred to as Löffler's syndrome. The *aminoglycosides* may cause muscle weakness, which with involvement of respiratory muscles may lead to respiratory paralysis. *Polymyxin B* given by aerosol can cause bronchospasm. This antibiotic is a well-known histamine releaser.

Miscellaneous drugs causing pulmonary disease

Methysergide can produce chronic pleural effusion. *Corticosteroids* may lead to the development of opportunistic pulmonary infections, particularly *Pneumocystis carinii* pneumonia.

REFERENCES

1. Barton, A.D., and Lourenco, R.V.: Bronchial secretions and mucociliary clearance, Arch. Intern. Med. **131**:140, 1973.
2. Dolovich, J., and Hargreave, F.E.: Strategies in the control of asthma, Med. Clin. North Am. **65**:1033, 1981.
3. Gillis, C.N., and Roth, J.A.: Pulmonary disposition of circulating vasoactive hormones, Biochem. Pharmacol. **25**:2547, 1976.
4. Greenberger, P.A.: Theophylline, Ration. Drug Ther. **14**:1, 1980.
5. Henderson, W.R., Shelhamer, J.H., Reingold, D.B., Smith, L.J., Evans, R., and Kaliner, M.: Alpha-adrenergic hyper-responsiveness in asthma, N. Engl. J. Med. **300**:642, 1979.
6. Holroyde, M.C., Altounian, R.E.C., Cole, M., Dixon, M., and Elliot, E.V.: Bronchoconstriction produced in man by leukotrienes C and D, Lancet **2**:17, 1981.
7. Irwin, R.S., Rosen, M.J., and Braman, S.S.: Cough—a comprehensive review, Arch. Intern. Med. **137**:1186, 1977.
8. Lands, A.M., et al.: Differentiation of receptor systems activated by sympathomimetic amines, Nature **214**:597, 1967.
9. Miller, W.F.: Aerosol therapy in acute and chronic respiratory disease, Arch. Intern. Med. **131**:148, 1973.
10. Mitenko, P.A., and Ogilvie, R.I.: Rational intravenous doses of theophylline, N. Engl. J. Med. **289**:600, 1973.
11. Piafsky, K.M., and Ogilvie, R.I.: Dosage of theophylline in bronchial asthma, N. Engl. J. Med. **292**:1218, 1975.
12. Tattersfield, A.E., and McNicol, M.W.: Salbutamol and isoproterenol; a double-blind trial to compare bronchodilator and cardiovascular activity, N. Engl. J. Med. **281**:1323, 1969.
13. Tinkelman, D.G., and Avner, S.E.: Ephedrine therapy in asthmatic children, JAMA **237**:553, 1977.
14. Weinberger, M.: Theophylline for treatment of asthma, J. Pediatr. **92**:1, 1978.
15. Weinberger, M., and Riegelman, S.: Rational use of theophylline for broncho-

dilatation, N. Engl. J. Med. **291**:151, 1974.

16. Wilson, A.F.: Drug treatment of acute asthma, JAMA **237**:1141, 1977.

17. Wolfe, J.D., Tashkin, D.P., Calverese, B., and Simmons, M.: Bronchodilator effects of terbutaline and aminophylline alone and in combination in asthmatic patients, N. Engl. J. Med. **298**:363, 1978.

18. Zaske, D.E., Miller, K.W., Strem, E.L., Austrian, S., and Johnson, P.B.: Oral aminophylline therapy: increased dosage requirements in children, JAMA **237**:1453, 1977.

Chapter 41

Drug effects on the gastrointestinal tract

Drugs that exert a useful effect on the gastrointestinal tract may be best grouped according to their therapeutic indications. Since the most common medical problems in relation to the gastrointestinal tract are the management of peptic ulcer, constipation, diarrhea, and deficiencies of digestive factors, the various drugs used in gastroenterology are discussed under the following headings: anticholinergics, gastric antacids, and cathartics, laxatives, and antidiarrheal agents. The histamine H_2-receptor antagonists are discussed on p. 223.

ANTI-CHOLINERGICS

An effective dose of an anticholinergic drug decreases nocturnal acid secretion by about 50%.[6] It also decreases gastric acid secretion stimulated by histamine or pentagastrin or a meal by about 30% to 50%. The duration of action of an anticholinergic drug is longer if it is administered 1 hour after a meal, but effectiveness can be demonstrated even when it is given 30 minutes before a meal. Dosage should be carefully titrated in each patient by increasing the dose until side effects such as dryness of the mouth are noted. Contraindications to the use of anticholinergic drugs include glaucoma, prostatic hyperplasia, and gastric retention.

Some of the most commonly used antispasmodics are propantheline (Pro-Banthine), diphemanil (Prantal), oxphenonium (Antrenyl), penthienate (Monodral), tricyclamol (Co-Elorine), methscopolamine bromide (Pamine), dicyclomine (Bentyl), and glycopyrrolate (Robinul). Although none of these drugs is perfect, their administration to the point of tolerance along with antacids provides dramatic relief of pain in ulcer patients.

GASTRIC ANTACIDS

Many experimental and clinical observations suggest that antacids are among the most important drugs in the treatment of peptic ulcer. Although used for many years, important aspects of their pharmacology have only been worked out recently.[6]

When administered during the fasting state, the duration of action of the antacids is only 30 minutes. However, when administered after meals, their action may last

TABLE 41-1   Characteristics of various antacids

Antacid	Composition	Buffering capacity (mEq of hydrochloride per ml)	Sodium content (mg/5 ml)
Aludrox	Magnesium and aluminum hydroxides, simethicone	2.81	4.5
Amphojel	Aluminum hydroxide gel	1.93	8.1
Gelusil	Aluminum hydroxide gel, magnesium trisilicate	1.33	6.5
Gelusil M	Aluminum hydroxide gel, magnesium hydroxide, and trisilicate	2.23	5.7
Maalox	Aluminum hydroxide gel, magnesium hydroxide	2.58	2.5
Magaldrate (Riopan)	Magnesium and aluminum hydroxides	2.23	0.7
Mylanta	Magnesium and aluminum hydroxides, simethicone	2.38	3.9
WinGel	Aluminum hydroxide gel, magnesium hydroxide, stabilized with hexitol	2.25	1.25

Modified from Fordtran, J.S., Morawski, S.G., and Richardson, C.T.: N. Engl. J. Med. **288**:923, 1973.

3 to 4 hours. The buffering action of the various antacids varies greatly depending on the preparation and the patient.

As shown in Table 41-1, the potency of the antacids varies considerably as does their sodium content. Effective doses require 75 to 150 mEq buffer. In addition, the hypersecretors, such as patients with duodenal ulcer, require larger quantities of antacid than patients who are not hypersecretors, such as persons with a gastric ulcer.

Gastric antacids are generally classified as *systemic* and *nonsystemic*, depending on the amount of systemic absorption of the cation responsible for the neutralization of gastric hydrochloric acid. Sodium bicarbonate (baking soda) is the only systemic antacid that has been used medically. It is now entirely abandoned except for its use by the lay public. Sodium bicarbonate is a very effective and rapid-acting neutralizer of gastric acid. Its disadvantage is that systemic absorption of the sodium ion causes alkalosis, which is characterized by elevated carbon dioxide content and pH of the plasma, loss of appetite, weakness, mental confusion, and, rarely, tetany. Renal insufficiency and calcinosis have been described in patients who have been taking systemic antacids for long periods of time.

The gastric antacids preferred at present are the drugs whose cationic portion is not absorbed from the intestine and that raise the pH of the gastric contents only to about 4. These drugs are often referred to as *nonsystemic buffer antacids*. Various aluminum and magnesium salts have this property. The antacids containing calcium carbonate are very potent, but they cause an increase in gastric secretion after their action is terminated. For this reason, the antacids that do not contain calcium are preferable.

Inhibition of gastric secretion by H_2-receptor antagonists is of great interest. Burimamide, metiamide, cimetidine, and ranitidine are discussed on pp. 223-225.

NONSYSTEMIC GASTRIC ANTACIDS

Among the poorly absorbed gastric antacids, calcium carbonate is the most effective but has many disadvantages, such as hypercalcemia, constipation, and acid rebound. Magnesium compounds are potent and useful in counteracting the constipating effects of calcium carbonate and aluminum hydroxide. Aluminum hydroxide is not absorbed and is constipating. It is useful in removing phosphate when such a measure is indicated.

Aluminum hydroxide gel and dihydroxyaluminum aminoacetate. Aluminum hydroxide gel (Amphojel) is a colloidal suspension that is available in a liquid preparation or in tablets. In the acid stomach, aluminum chloride is formed, but in the alkaline intestine, aluminum hydroxide is again formed and the chloride reabsorbed. As a consequence, no alteration in systemic acid-base balance occurs. This drug has been widely used in liquid and tablet form and also by continuous drip through a gastric tube in treating peptic ulcer.

$$Al(OH)_3$$

Aluminum hydroxide

$$(HO)_2Al-O-\overset{\overset{\displaystyle O}{\|}}{C}CH_2NH_2$$

Dihydroxyaluminum aminoacetate

Aluminum hydroxide gel will raise the pH of the stomach contents to only about 4. Its only disadvantages are a constipating effect and the possibility of causing some loss of phosphate in the feces. The former difficulty may be prevented by the addition of certain magnesium salts. The phosphate loss is not likely to be serious with moderate doses in patients receiving an adequate diet. However, aluminum phosphate gel may be used, which will obviate this difficulty, although it has a lesser capacity to neutralize acid. The binding of phosphate by aluminum salts may be beneficial in the management of patients with renal phosphatic calculi.

Dihydroxyaluminum aminoacetate is comparable to aluminum hydroxide gel on the basis of available clinical experience. In the test tube the buffering action of this antacid in a solid form is comparable to that of liquid preparations of aluminum hydroxide gel. There is not enough clinical evidence to allow a clear-cut decision on the possible superiority of one of these drugs over the others.

Magnesium trisilicate. In the stomach this drug is changed to magnesium chloride and silicon dioxide. In the alkaline intestine, magnesium remains as the carbonate, whereas chloride is reabsorbed.

In contrast to the aluminum salts, magnesium trisilicate not only does not cause constipation but in large doses may even produce some diarrhea. In many very popular preparations, aluminum hydroxide gel and magnesium trisilicate are combined in a single tablet. One of the most popular contains 0.5 g of magnesium trisilicate and 0.25 g of aluminum hydroxide. Apparently some silica may be absorbed, since in rare cases kidney stones containing silicon compounds have been reported.

Other nonabsorbed antacids. Magnesium oxide, magnesium hydroxide, and calcium carbonate are gastric antacids that differ from the previous group in that they can elevate the pH of the gastric contents to 7 or above. An 8% aqueous suspension of magnesium hydroxide, widely known as milk of magnesia, is probably the most potent antacid in common practice. The addition of aluminum hydroxide to magnesium hydroxide tends to decrease the neutralizing power of the magnesium salt.[10]

The absorption of magnesium may be of significance. As much as 15% to 30% of the magnesium chloride formed is available for absorption. The absorbed magnesium is rapidly cleared through the kidney and represents no danger to a normal person. However, magnesium salts should not be given to patients with poor renal function since dangerous toxicity may occur.

Magaldrate (Riopan) is a hydrated magnesium aluminate, a buffer-antacid that is not absorbed. Among advantages claimed for it is its low sodium content. Some of the commonly used antacids have a surprising amount of sodium, a disadvantage in some patients.

Sucrasulfate (Carafate) is a complex of sulfated sucrose and aluminum hydroxide. It is highly effective in the treatment of peptic ulcer. Its mode of action is a protective one on the ulcer site, where it forms a protective barrier to further injury by acid and pepsin. Sucrasulfate (Carafate) is supplied in 1 g tablets, which are administered four times a day on an empty stomach.

Metoclopramide hydrochloride (Reglan) is a dopamine antagonist that stimulates the motility of the upper gastrointestinal tract. Its action is abolished by anticholinergic drugs. The drug is widely used as an antiemetic. It increases the resting tone of the esophagus.

Adverse reactions of metoclopramide include drowsiness, fatigue, insomnia, dizziness, and bowel disturbances. The drug is contraindicated in pheochromocytoma because it may cause hypertensive reactions. It is also contraindicated in any clinical condition in which hypermotility of the gastrointestinal tract is undesirable.

Although the pharmacology of metoclopramide is extremely complex, it is widely used in the treatment of diabetic gastric stasis, in prophylaxis of vomiting in cancer chemotherapy, and to facilitate small bowel intubation and radiological examination where delayed gastric emptying interferes with the procedure. Metoclopramide hydrochloride (Reglan) is supplied in the form of tablets of 10 mg and in ampules of 2 ml containing 10 mg.

In contrast with older concepts, cathartic and laxative action is being attributed to an increase in fecal water excretion, resulting in most instances from alterations in the transport of fluid and electrolytes in the intestine.[1]

Constipation, when not due to organic causes, is generally attributed today to poor dietary habits, lack of bulk-producing foods, and inattention to the stimulus for defecation. Correction of these poor habits will often take care of the problem of chronic constipation without the necessity of prescribing laxatives.

Nevertheless, cathartics and laxatives have some valid uses in medicine. Soft

CATHARTICS, LAXATIVES, AND ANTIDIARRHEAL AGENTS

stools and lack of straining during defecation are desirable after hemorrhoidectomy and in persons with myocardial infarction. Cathartics are also prescribed for the purpose of speeding the elimination of various toxic materials such as some of the anthelmintics. By itself, however, chronic constipation should not be an indication for continual use of cathartics.

In diarrheal states the correction of fluid and electrolyte changes is today considered to be the primary therapeutic goal. Small doses of opiates in the form of paregoric (camphorated tincture of opium) or codeine may be employed to slow intestinal motility. Astringents and absorbents are also used but are not very effective. Determination of the cause of the diarrheal state—whether bacterial, parasitic, or toxic—is most important, and the specific cause should be corrected whenever possible.

Mechanism of cathartic action	The various cathartics may act by several different mechanisms:

1. Hydrophylic and osmotic properties may cause an increase in bulk of the intestinal contents and an increased rate of transit.
2. The contact cathartics may cause a direct effect on the intestinal mucosa through an action on cyclic AMP, causing increased secretions.
3. Lubricants and stool softeners act by mechanisms that are self-evident.

BULK CATHARTICS	Bulk cathartics promote intestinal evacuation because they are not significantly absorbed from the intestine. As a consequence, they retain a considerable amount of water, distend the colon, and promote the expulsion of liquid stools.

Magnesium sulfate is widely used in medicine. It is generally administered in doses of 15 g. Little of it is absorbed under normal circumstances, and the effects of the small amount absorbed are minimized by rapid renal excretion. If there is prolonged intestinal retention of the drug and renal function is simultaneously impaired, some systemic effects such as CNS depression may occur. It may be estimated that 15 g of magnesium sulfate requires 400 ml of water in order to make an isotonic solution. If the drug is given in a more concentrated form, it will abstract water from the tissues.

Magnesium hydroxide, usually administered as magnesia magma (milk of magnesia), is considerably more pleasant than the bitter sulfate. It is also considerably less effective.

The hydrophilic colloids are not absorbed from the gastrointestinal tract and retain considerable quantities of water. They are widely used, but simple dietary measures such as inclusion of prunes and bran-containing cereals can generally serve the purpose equally well.

LACTULOSE	This semisynthetic disaccharide is not hydrolyzed in the small intestine but is metabolized by bacteria in the large intestine to lactate and other organic compounds that are not well absorbed. The drug acts slowly as a laxative. In addition to its

laxative effect, lactulose has been found useful in portal systemic encephalopathy, where it causes up to 50% reduction of blood ammonia. This effect is related to bacterial action on lactulose and a reduction in the pH of the feces. Lactulose is supplied in the form of a syrup. Each 15 ml contains 10 g of the disaccharide with some other sugars. For a laxative, the drug is administered in a dose of 10 g. For encephalopathy, as much as 20 to 30 g must be administered.

The anthraquinone cathartics, or emodin compounds, phenolphthalein, castor oil, bisacodyl, cascara, aloe, senna, and rhubarb, are believed to act on the intestinal mucosa, causing changes in transport mechanisms. They are used more commonly in proprietary mixtures than in physician-prescribed formulations. *CONTACT CATHARTICS*

Phenolphthalein is also more commonly used in proprietary preparations than on a physician's prescription. The history of the discovery of the cathartic action of phenolphthalein is interesting. It was used for making adulterated wine in Hungary, and its cathartic properties were soon appreciated.

There is a delay of some 6 to 8 hours in the cathartic action of phenolphthalein, although the time may be less in children. The drug is believed to act on the large intestine, its exact mode of action being unknown. It is partially absorbed, and although its toxicity is low, it can cause very undesirable skin eruptions and persistent discoloration. The phenomenon of fixed eruption caused by phenolphthalein probably has a true allergic basis because the involved areas of skin flare up again when doses of phenolphthalein are taken that would exert no effect in a normal person.

Oxyphenisatin and its acetate salt are related to phenolphthalein. They can cause hepatic damage and should not be used.

Castor oil is obtained from the seeds of *Ricinus communis,* or castor bean. The oil itself is nonirritating, but when it is hydrolyzed in the intestine to ricinoleic acid, a cathartic effect is produced. This action is exerted especially on the small intestine. The usual dose of castor oil is 15 ml.

Bisacodyl (Dulcolax) in the form of oral tablets and suppositories appears to be useful for bowel evacuation. It stimulates the contraction of the large intestine and is apparently not absorbed from the intestine.

Bisacodyl has an effect on fluid and electrolyte absorption in the intestine[1]; its exact mechanism of action is not well understood.

Preparations of bisacodyl (Dulcolax) include enteric-coated tablets containing 5 mg that should be swallowed whole and suppositories containing 10 mg. The suppositories should not be used in patients in whom absorption may be facilitated by the presence of fissures or ulcerations.

Dioctyl sodium sulfosuccinate (Doxinate; Colace) was introduced as a fecal softener. The drug acts as a dispersing or wetting agent and appears to be inert from a pharmacological standpoint. It is used in daily doses of 10 to 20 mg in children and in larger doses in adults.[14] *Surface-active agents*

Antidiarrheal agents   The management of diarrhea is based on elimination of the cause when possible and administration of proper fluids and electrolytes. In addition, a variety of absorbents are employed on an empirical basis such as bismuth subcarbonate, kaolin, activated charcoal, and pectin.

It is recognized that increasing intestinal absorption and inhibiting the secretory process are the most effective bases of antidiarrheal action. The opiates, in addition to their action on motility, exert important influences on stimulating fluid absorption and interfering with secretion. Clonidine is highly effective in stimulating sodium and chloride absorption. Glucose solutions and the corticosteroids decrease inflammation and stimulate absorption.

The camphorated tincture of opium (paregoric) is a traditional antidiarrheal compound. The usual dose is 4 ml. Codeine sulfate is also highly effective when used in doses of 16 to 32 mg. The narcotics may obscure the diagnosis and should not be used if the cause of the disease can be eliminated, such as in amebic dysentery.

The opiate-like drug **diphenoxylate** (with atropine sulfate as Lomotil) has considerable efficacy as an antidiarrheal agent. A relatively low daily dosage (2.5 to 7.5 mg) usually gives good results. Diphenoxylate has been particularly recommended for chronic diarrhea when the more addictive opiates are undesirable. Each Lomotil tablet and each 5 ml of liquid contains 2.5 mg of diphenoxylate and 0.025 mg of atropine sulfate. Diphenoxylate has a low potential for producing physical dependence, but it may increase the effect of other CNS depressants. It should be used with caution in persons with liver disease as well as in those who have severe colitis.

Loperamide hydrochloride (Imodium) has recently been introduced as an antiperistaltic antidiarrheal agent. In contrast with Lomotil, the drug does not contain atropine but has some opiate-like properties, since it can cause morphine-like dependence in monkeys, and naloxone is recommended as a possible antidote. The drug is available in 2 mg capsules. Loperamide is a very effective drug, but it should not be used in persons with infectious diarrheas where the causative organism may invade the intestinal wall.

Cholestyramine may be an effective antidiarrheal agent whenever there is malabsorption of bile acids that contribute to the diarrhea. Such conditions include ileal resection or the irritable bowel syndrome. Cholestyramine therapy proved ineffective in tropical diarrhea in Vietnam.[8]

1. Binder, H.J.: Pharmacology of laxatives, Annu. Rev. Pharmacol. Toxicol. **17**:355, 1977.

2. Christensen, J.: The controls of gastrointestinal movements: some old and new views, N. Engl. J. Med. **285**:85, 1971.

3. Cohen, S., and Snape, W.J.: The pathophysiology and treatment of gastroesophageal reflux disease, Arch. Intern. Med. **138**:1398, 1978.

4. Fordtran, J.S., Morawski, S.G., and Richardson, C.T.: In vivo and in vitro evaluation of liquid antacids, N. Engl. J. Med. **288**:923, 1973.

5. Grady, G.F., and Keusch, G.T.: Pathogenesis of bacterial diarrheas, N. Engl. J. Med. **285**:831, 891, 1971.

6. Isenberg, J.I.: Therapy of peptic ulcer, JAMA **233**:540, 1975.

7. McCarthy, D.M.: Peptic ulcer: antacids or cimetidine? Hosp. Prac. Dec. 1979, p. 52.

8. McCloy, R.M., and Hofmann, A.F.: Tropical diarrhea in Vietnam—a controlled study of cholestyramine therapy, N. Engl. J. Med. **284**:139, 1971.

9. McHardy, G., and Balart, L.A.: Jaundice and oxyphenisatin, JAMA **211**:83, 1970.

10. Morrissey, J.F., and Barreras, R.F.: Antacid therapy, N. Engl. J. Med. **290**:550, 1974.

11. Nelson, D.C., McGrew, W.R.G., and Hoyumpa, A.M.: Hypernatremia and lactulose therapy, JAMA **249**:1295, 1983.

12. Netchvolodoff, C.V., and Hargrove, M.D.: Recent advances in the treatment of diarrhea, Arch. Intern. Med. **139**:813, 1979.

13. Schulze-Delrieu, K.: Metoclopropamide, Gastroenterology **77**:768, 1979.

14. Wilson, J.L., and Dickinson, D.G.: Use of dioctyl sodium sulfosuccinate (aerosol O.T.) for severe constipation, JAMA **158**:261, 1955.

REFERENCES

section eight

Drugs that influence metabolic and endocrine functions

Chapter 42

Insulin, glucagon, and oral hypoglycemic agents

Insulin, the hormone elaborated by the β cells of the pancreas, is a key regulator of metabolic processes. Although its action on carbohydrate metabolism has received the most attention, its absolute or relative deficiency results in many other serious metabolic consequences. *Glucagon*, the hormone produced by the α cells of the pancreatic islets, has some actions such as glycogenolysis and hyperglycemia that are opposed to those of insulin. The ratio of the two hormones may determine their overall effect on the liver. Glucagon has positive inotropic effects on the heart, probably as a consequence of stimulating cyclic AMP production. The *hypoglycemic sulfonylureas* promote the release of insulin from β cells. *Phenformin* is also used occasionally for lowering the blood sugar in diabetic persons, but the drug acts by some mechanism other than the promotion of insulin release.

Insulin is elaborated in the β cells as part of a larger peptide known as *proinsulin*. The release of insulin is stimulated not only by glucose but also by certain amino acids, gastrointestinal hormones, ketone bodies, and α-receptor blockers such as phentolamine. Inhibitors of insulin release include α-adrenergic agonists such as norepinephrine and epinephrine, unusual sugars (mannoheptulose), and diazoxide. The action of insulin is exerted on specific receptors in cell membranes.

In 1889 the surgical removal of the pancreas in the dog was shown to result in experimental diabetes, and in 1922 insulin was isolated from a dog's pancreas. The introduction of insulin revolutionized the treatment of diabetes and greatly prolonged the lives of juvenile diabetic patients. Subsequent work was directed at developing injectable forms of insulin that would delay the absorption of the hormone and would thereby prolong its action in the body.

Studies on insulin and diabetes were facilitated by the demonstration that alloxan could selectively destroy the β cells of the pancreas. This discovery provided a simple method for making experimental animals diabetic, compared with the previous and more laborious procedure of almost complete pancreatectomy.

Advances in insulin
research

β Cell function can be measured by determining the C-peptide in the circulation. The human insulin gene can be inserted into bacteria, and mass production of the hormone can be achieved by DNA technology. Insulin pumps with or without glucose sensors can be implanted in diabetics. The insulin receptor and postreceptor events provide explanations for previously unexplained observations such as insulin resistance in some diabetics and in obesity.

Glucagon is a physiological antagonist to insulin. It is a single-chain polypeptide of 3500 molecular weight that is secreted by the pancreas in the form of a prohormone. It antagonizes the actions of insulin and produces hyperglycemia, glycogenolysis, and ketogenesis. It acts through stimulation of cyclic AMP, and in high concentrations it has a positive inotropic effect.

The secretion of glucagon is stimulated by amino acids and is inhibited by glucose, free fatty acids, and ketones. Also, intestinal polypeptides and sympathetic stimulation promote its secretion. Somatostatin inhibits both glucagon and insulin release and is present in the pancreas.

Glucagon is available as the hydrochloride for the treatment of insulin reactions. It is administered subcutaneously or intramuscularly in doses of 0.5 to 2 mg. Its positive inotropic action differs from those of the catecholamines in that it is not accompanied by ventricular irritability or increased peripheral resistance.

Chemistry and
standardization

Insulin consists of two chains of polypeptides, the A and B chains joined by 2 disulfide bridges. In addition, the A chain contains another disulfide bridge. It circulates as free hormone with a half-life of 9 minutes. It is degraded by the liver and kidney.

Proinsulin, the biosynthetic precursor of insulin, is a single-chain polypeptide (Fig. 42-1). Its molecular weight is about 1.5 times that of insulin. Cleavage of proinsulin occurs within the β cells, resulting in insulin and the connecting fragment known as C-peptide.

Proinsulin is important in two clinical situations. Normally about 6% to 8% of plasma insulin consists of proinsulin. In some islet cell adenomas this concentration is much higher. The other clinical situation is related to the C-peptide. The C-peptide has no biological activity but can be measured. This is important in individuals who develop antibodies to insulin after taking it for a long time. In these individuals the antibodies interfere with the determination of plasma insulin. On the other hand, the C-peptide can be measured as an indicator of endogenous insulin release, since it is released along with insulin and no antibodies are formed to it in humans.

Insulin is *standardized* on the basis of its ability to lower the blood sugar in experimental animals, usually in the rabbit. An international unit of insulin should lower the blood sugar 45 mg/100 ml when injected into a fasting 2 kg rabbit. The international standard insulin contains 22 IU/mg.

Structure of bovine proinsulin showing A and B chains and C-peptide. Human proinsulin   FIG. 42-1
differs in three amino acids in the chains and several amino acids in the C-peptide.

From Steiner, D.F.: TRIANGLE, the Sandoz Journal of Medical Science, vol. II, no. 2, 1972, p. 52.

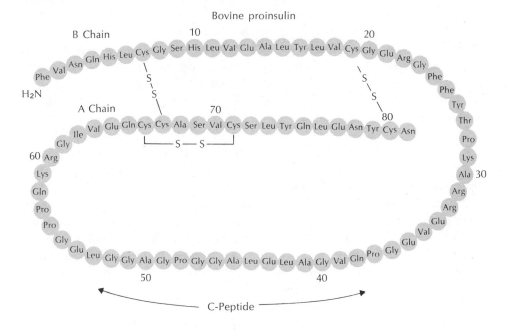

Bovine proinsulin

Electron microscopic studies indicate that insulin is present in β cells of the   *Release and*
pancreas in a particulate form. The most important stimulus for insulin release is   *metabolism*
glucose, but there are many other factors that can increase or decrease the release
of insulin.

Factors that *promote* the release of insulin are *glucose, leucine, arginine* or a
mixture of amino acids, *glucagon, ketone bodies, sulfonylureas, gastrin, secretin,*
pancreozymin, isoproterenol, and *α-receptor blockers,* such as phentolamine.

Factors that *inhibit* the release of insulin are *norepinephrine* and *epinephrine*
(α-adrenergic effects), unusual sugars such as *mannoheptulose,* and *diazoxide* (p.
196).

Once released, insulin reaches the liver first, where much of it is retained.

When insulin is injected into a normal or diabetic individual, the following changes   *Mode of action*
may be observed in the blood chemistry: (1) blood sugar decreases, (2) blood pyruvate
and lactate increase, (3) inorganic phosphate decreases, and (4) potassium decreases.

Lowering of the blood sugar may be explained on the basis of an increased uptake
of sugar by tissues such as muscle and fat. There is evidence indicating a decreased
hepatic output of glucose through the action of insulin. It has been shown by hepatic

vein catheterization in humans that the injection of insulin causes decreased hepatic output of glucose.

Increases in blood pyruvate and lactate are generally attributed to the increased rate of glucose utilization. As more glucose-6-phosphate is produced, more will pass through the various triose states to pyruvate and lactate.

Fall of inorganic phosphate levels may be assumed to reflect the increased rate of phosphorylation of glucose, which results in greater consumption of phosphate. Finally, for reasons that are not well understood, whenever glycogen is deposited in the liver, potassium is also deposited. This would explain the *lowering of the plasma potassium*.

In addition to these effects, insulin causes a fall in free amino acids in the plasma. It has also been shown that the incorporation of ^{35}S-labeled methionine into muscle was reduced in diabetic dogs but could be restored to normal with insulin. Thus insulin has an effect on protein metabolism, also.

When insulin is inadequate, as in most diabetic persons, counterregulatory events occur that seem to have a purpose of providing the fuels needed, such as glucose, free fatty acids, and ketone bodies. Thus low insulin plasma levels lead to an increase in epinephrine, glucagon, growth hormone, and cortisol. These hormones mobilize free fatty acids, which are converted into ketone bodies by the liver. They also accelerate gluconeogenesis in the liver.

Glucagon plasma concentrations are consistently elevated in diabetic individuals in relation to insulin, and diabetes is increasingly viewed as a bihormonal disease.

It appears likely from studies on the red cell that a non-lipid-soluble compound such as glucose is transported across the cell membrane through some carrier mechanism. Certain tissues such as muscle differ from erythrocytes in having a superimposed mechanism that opposes the penetration of glucose. This appears to be the site at which insulin acts. As a consequence, insulin promotes the entry of glucose into skeletal and heart muscle, fat, and leukocytes, whereas it is not required for sugar transport into the red cells, brain, or liver.

Preparations and clinical uses

Various insulin preparations differ mainly in their rate of absorption following subcutaneous injection. The rapidly absorbed regular insulin has been modified to form suspensions by two different procedures. The basic protamine has been added to raise the isoelectric point of the acidic insulin. In the newer procedure, the use of high concentrations of zinc and acetate buffer made it possible to prepare insulin suspensions having varying particle size. The most widely used insulins are regular insulin, which is rapid-acting, and isophane insulin suspension (NPH) or insulin zinc suspension (lente), which are intermediate-acting. The various properties of the available insulins are summarized in Table 42-1.

In addition to the USP insulins, which are not pure and may contain 6% proinsulin, there are single peak and single component insulins available, which are more than 99% pure and have 26 to 30 units of activity per milligram. The single component

TABLE 42-1   Insulin preparations

Action	Preparation	Hours after subcutaneous injection		Units/ml
		Peak action	Duration of action	
Rapid	Insulin injection (regular, crystalline zinc)	2-3	5-7	40, 80, 100, 500
	Prompt insulin zinc suspension (semilente)	4-6	12-16	40, 80
Intermediate	Isophane insulin suspension (NPH)	8-12	18-24	40, 80, 100
	Insulin zinc suspension (lente)	8-12	18-24	40, 80, 100
	Globulin zinc insulin injection (globin)	6-10	12-18	40, 80
Long	Protamine zinc insulin suspension	16-18	24-36	40, 80, 100
	Extended insulin zinc suspension (ultralente)	16-18	24-36	40, 80, 100

insulins are not as likely to induce the formation of antibodies, thus reducing the likelihood of insulin resistance.

Adverse effects

Adverse effects of insulin include hypoglycemia, local or systemic allergic reactions, lipoatrophy, and visual disturbances. Hypoglycemia is especially dangerous, since it can cause brain damage. Insulin resistance is caused by either a decrease in insulin receptors or postreceptor molecules involved in glucose transport. Interestingly, the obese person has hyperglycemia and hyperinsulinemia, suggesting insulin resistance; after weight loss this abnormality will disappear.

ORAL ANTIDIABETIC DRUGS
Hypoglycemic sulfonylurea compounds

The introduction of the hypoglycemic sulfonylurea compounds represents a notable development in the management of diabetes. Loubatières observed in 1942 in France that certain sulfonamides, when administered experimentally to patients suffering from typhoid fever, produced symptoms and signs of hypoglycemia. Extensive investigations done subsequently in many laboratories established that certain sulfonylureas can indeed produce hypoglycemia in normal animals but not in those made diabetic through the administration of alloxan. The most commonly used preparations in the United States are tolbutamide, chlorpropamide, acetohexamide, and tolazamide.

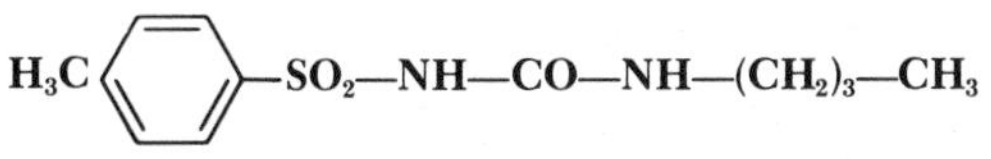

Tolbutamide

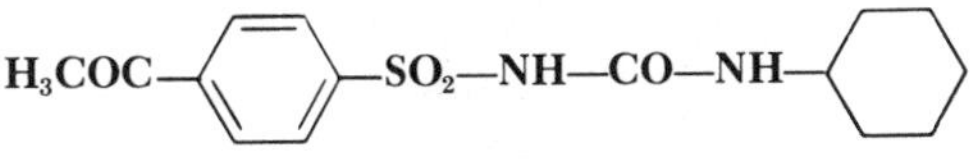

Acetohexamide

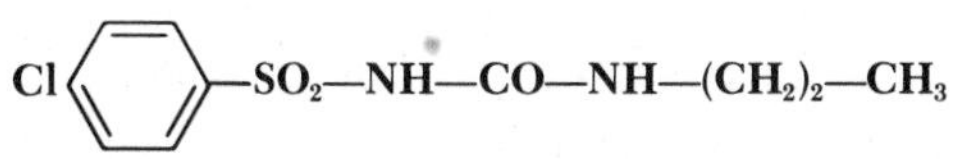

Chlorpropamide

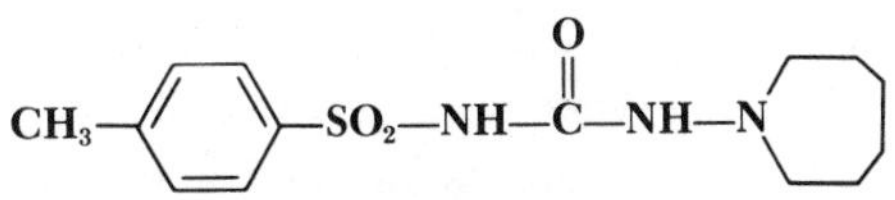

Tolazamide

MODE OF ACTION

Despite earlier arguments to the contrary, the pancreas is essential for the hypoglycemic action of the sulfonylureas. The degree of granulation of the islet cells is related to the insulin content of the pancreas, and the sulfonylureas cause a decrease in the granulation of the β cells.

Advantages of the hypoglycemic sulfonylureas over insulin in the management of diabetes are as follows:

1. *Ease of administration*. The sulfonylureas are taken in tablet form, whereas insulin must be injected.
2. *Endogenous release*. Release of insulin by the sulfonylureas resembles the physiological process in that the hormone first reaches the liver, where much of it is retained and exerts an effect on hepatic output of glucose. In contrast, injected insulin floods the peripheral tissues before it reaches the liver.
3. *Less allergic reaction*. Patients who are allergic to exogenous insulin obtained from animal sources or who have antibodies against such insulins may be managed more satisfactorily by promoting endogenous insulin release by means of the sulfonylureas.

TOLBUTAMIDE
CONTROVERSY

In a recent cooperative study at 12 university medical centers, a group of more than 800 diabetic persons was followed on one of four treatment schedules for 3 to 8 years.[10] During that time 89 patients died, 61 of them from heart attacks or other cardiovascular causes. Of the deaths, 30 occurred in the tolbutamide-treated group. The findings were interpreted as an indication that diet and tolbutamide therapy are no more effective than diet alone in prolonging life or even that diet and tolbutamide may be less effective than diet and insulin or diet alone insofar as cardiovascular mortality is concerned. Because of these findings, it has been recommended to physicians that sulfonylurea agents be used only in patients with adult-onset, non-ketotic diabetes that cannot be controlled by diet or weight loss and in whom the use of insulin is impractical.

Many competent diabetologists have criticized the study and the conclusions on the basis of deficiencies in design, and it is quite possible that a more extensive study would not support the same conclusions. Until such information is available, some caution in the use of the sulfonylureas is advisable.

PREPARATIONS AND
CLINICAL USES

The major characteristics of the oral hypoglycemic drugs are shown in Table 42-2. The differences in oral agent activity are determined by their fate in the body. Thus tolbutamide and tolazamide are rapidly metabolized. Acetohexamide is also rapidly metabolized, but its metabolite is more potent than the original drug. Chlorpropamide is long-acting because it is metabolized to a negligible extent.

ADVERSE EFFECTS

Hypoglycemia with sulfonylureas is generally not as great a danger as that after the use of insulin, but it may be serious and of long duration. An intolerance to alcohol similar to the disulfiram (Antabuse) reaction may occur, and gastrointestinal and allergic skin reactions have been reported.

Chemical type	Name	Half-life (hours)	Duration of action (hours)	Tablet size (mg)
TABLE 42-2 Characteristics of oral hypoglycemic drugs				
Sulfonylurea	Tolbutamide (Orinase)	4-6	6-12	500
	Acetohexamide (Dymelor)	6-18	12-24	250, 500
	Chloropropamide (Diabenese)	30-36	60	100, 250
	Tolazamide (Tolinase)	7	10-14	100, 250
Biguanide	Phenformin hydrochloride (DBI)	3	4-6	25
	Phenformin hydrochloride, timed-release (DBI-TD)	3	8-14	50 (capsules)

Phenformin

Phenformin (phenethylbiguanide; DBI) has been used in the management of some diabetic persons. It lowers blood sugar probably by increasing the number of insulin receptors and lowers blood sugar. Since the drug can cause serious or even fatal lactic acidosis, it is no longer used in the United States.

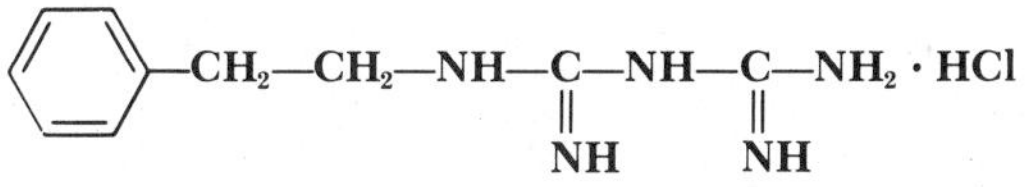

$$\text{C}_6\text{H}_5-\text{CH}_2-\text{CH}_2-\text{NH}-\underset{\underset{\text{NH}}{\|}}{\text{C}}-\text{NH}-\underset{\underset{\text{NH}}{\|}}{\text{C}}-\text{NH}_2 \cdot \text{HCl}$$

Phenformin hydrochloride

Clinical pharmacology

Extensive clinical experience indicates that the sulfonylureas just discussed are of about equal effectiveness in the treatment of adult-onset, ketosis-resistant diabetic persons. These drugs differ from each other mainly in duration of action and in recommended dosage.

The *oral hypoglycemic agents* should be used only in maturity-onset, nonketotic diabetic persons whose blood glucose cannot be controlled by diet alone and in whom insulin cannot be used.

Drug interactions complicate the clinical use of the sulfonylureas. Tolbutamide is strongly bound to plasma proteins, where it can displace dicumarol, thus leading to an increased anticoagulant effect. The interactions of tolbutamide and anticoagulants in patients may be quite complex. Although some reports indicate that administration of tolbutamide to patients on dicumarol therapy resulted in an increased anticoagulant effect, others find that diabetic patients on long-term tolbutamide treatment reacted normally to dicumarol and warfarin. Perhaps the order of administration is important. Thiazide diuretics oppose the action of the sulfonylureas.

REFERENCES

1. Cautrecasas, P.: Hormone-receptor interactions and the plasma membrane, Hosp. Pract. July, 1974.
2. Flier, J.S., Kahn, R., and Roth, J.: Receptors, antireceptor antibodies and mechanisms of insulin resistance, N. Engl. J. Med. **300**:413, 1979.
3. Goodner, C.J.: Somatostatin leads to glucagon's renaissance, N. Engl. J. Med. **292**:1022, 1975.
4. Loubatières, A.: The hypoglycemic sulfonamides: history and development of the problem from 1942 to 1955, Ann. N.Y. Acad. Sci. **71**:4, 1957.
5. McGarry, J.D., and Foster, D.W.: Hormonal control of ketogenesis, Arch. Intern. Med. **137**:495, 1977.
6. Poffenbarger, P.L., and Diess, W.P.: Insulin therapy for diabetic ketoacidosis, Tex. Med. **75**:42, 1979.
7. Salans, L.B.: Diabetes mellitus: a disease that is coming into focus, JAMA **247**: 590, 1982.
8. Shen, S.W., and Bressler, R.: Clinical pharmacology of oral antidiabetic agents, N. Engl. J. Med. **296**:787, 1977.
9. Unger, R.H., and Orci, L.: Glucagon and the A cell, N. Engl. J. Med. **304**:1518, 1575, 1981.
10. University Group Diabetes Program: A study of the effects of hypoglycemic agents on vascular complications in patients with adult-onset diabetes, Diabetes **19**(suppl. 2):747, 1970.

Chapter 43

Adrenal steroids

Since the observation by Hench in 1949 of a dramatic response to cortisone in a patient with rheumatoid arthritis, adrenal steroids and synthetic corticosteroids have become widely used and sometimes overused in medicine. *Cortisone* and related corticosteroids owe their popularity to their anti-inflammatory effect. More rarely, these drugs are useful for substitution therapy in adrenal insufficiency, which is often iatrogenic.

Aldosterone, the main mineralocorticoid of the adrenal gland, is largely of research interest. On the other hand, the *aldosterone antagonists* have important therapeutic applications.

During the decade following 1930 there was an intensive search for the active principles that could account for the essential role of the adrenal glands. In 1937 Reichstein and von Euw[13] prepared desoxycorticosterone synthetically and later demonstrated it in the adrenal glands. Although this steroid had powerful effects on salt and water metabolism and became useful in the management of Addison's disease, it was obvious that extracts of adrenal cortex also contained some other compounds that could influence not only salt metabolism but also the handling of carbohydrates and proteins as well.

World War II stimulated interest in the glucocorticoids, previously isolated by Kendall at the Mayo Clinic. It was suspected that such compounds might be valuable in the treatment of shock and exhaustion, although the scarcity of these compounds did not permit their evaluation in humans.

A milestone in the history of the adrenal steroids was the report of Hench and co-workers[10] on the effectiveness of cortisone and corticotropin in rheumatoid arthritis. Hench had been impressed for years with the potential reversibility of rheumatoid arthritis on the basis of the observation that patients tended to improve when jaundiced and also during pregnancy.

Results of the clinical trials in rheumatoid arthritis were dramatic, and soon cortisone and also corticotropin were found to cause symptomatic improvement in an amazing number of disease conditions. It was recognized at the same time that cortisone was not a cure for these many diseases. It seemed to "provide the susceptible tissues with a shieldlike buffer against the irritant."[9]

Although cortisol was largely responsible for the glucocorticoid activity of adrenal extracts, it was suspected that the amorphous fraction of such extracts still contained some material whose mineralocorticoid activity was much greater than that of desoxycorticosterone. The compound responsible for this was isolated in 1953 and was named *aldosterone*.

Subsequent research on the glucocorticoids led to the development of a variety of new steroids that have significantly greater antiinflammatory potency than cortisone, although their influence on carbohydrate metabolism generally parallels their antiinflammatory activity. A significant advantage of the newer steroids such as prednisone, methylprednisolone, triamcinolone, and dexamethasone is that these antiinflammatory steroids exert little effect on renal sodium reabsorption while possessing potent antiinflammatory activity.

PITUITARY-ADRENAL RELATIONSHIPS
Corticotropin

Corticotropin (adrenocorticotropic hormone; ACTH) from the anterior pituitary gland stimulates adrenal steroid synthesis from cholesterol and is necessary for normal cortical structure and function. Although corticotropin stimulates primarily the formation of glucocorticoids, it has a basic influence on the formation of all adrenal steroids.

Corticotropin release from the anterior pituitary gland is promoted by polypeptides isolated from the hypothalamus, sometimes referred to as corticotropin-releasing factor (CRF) (Fig. 43-1).

Regulation of corticotropin release is determined largely by the influence of cortisol levels on CRF production through a negative feedback. Stressful stimuli, including drugs such as epinephrine, can override the feedback inhibition and elevate cortisol blood levels. In addition to these important regulatory influences, there is a diurnal variation in corticotropin release that will be discussed subsequently.

The basic effect of corticotropin on the adrenal cortex is mediated by adenosine 3':5'-cyclic phosphate (cyclic AMP). Cyclic AMP acts similarly to corticotropin both in vitro and on the perfused dog adrenal gland, whereas phosphorylase activity of beef adrenal slices is increased by corticotropin. Corticotropin may stimulate steroid synthesis by the system involving adenyl cyclase.

The polypeptide corticotropin was isolated from the anterior pituitary and eventually synthesized. Human corticotropin consists of 39 amino acids, but not all amino acids are essential for biological activity, since the first 19 (counting from the N-terminal end) are sufficient for stimulating cortisol production. The first 13 amino acids in corticotropin are the same as those in melanocyte-stimulating hormone (α-MSH), so it is not surprising that corticotropin exerts an effect on melanocytes.

Preparations of corticotropin are available for intravenous and intramuscular ad-

Diagrammatic summary of the principal factors regulating ACTH secretion.   FIG. 43-1

From Ganong, W.F., Alpert, L.C., and Lee, T.C.: Review of medical physiology, ed. 6, Los Altos, Calif., 1973, Lange Medical Publications.

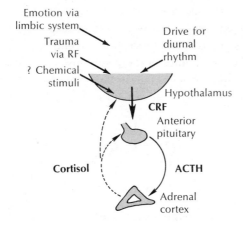

Pituitary-adrenal feedback system and its inhibition by metyrapone.   FIG. 43-2

Modified from Coppage, W.S., Jr., Island, D., Smith, M., and Liddle, G.W.: J. Clin. Invest. **38:**2101, 1959.

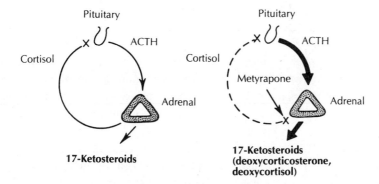

ministration. Oral administration is ineffective. When injected intravenously, corticotropin is rapidly destroyed in a matter of minutes. For this reason the hormone is administered either by intravenous infusion or by the intramuscular route as a repository corticotropin injection USP or sterile corticotropin zinc hydroxide suspension USP.

Corticotropin has some valid uses in the diagnosis of disturbed adrenocortical function. An intravenous infusion of the hormone will result in an increase in the excretion of cortisol metabolites if the adrenal glands are normal or hyperplastic.

Lowering of the 11-oxygenated (11-oxy) adrenal steroids in the body promotes corticotropin release by removal of the negative feedback. An interesting application of this knowledge is a test for anterior pituitary function by means of metyrapone (Fig. 43-2).

Metyrapone (Metopirone) inhibits the 11-β hydroxylation in the biosynthesis of cortisol, corticosterone, and aldosterone. The decrease in these 11-oxy steroids leads to intense corticotropin release from the anterior pituitary gland in normal individuals. Under these circumstances corticotropin stimulates the production of precursors of the 11-oxy steroids, 11-desoxyhydrocortisone (compound S) and 11-desoxycorticosterone (DOC). The metabolites of these steroids, 17-hydroxycorticosteroids and 17-ketogenic steroids, may be measured in the urine. In deficient anterior pituitary function, metyrapone administration will not increase these urinary metabolites.

Metyrapone

In adults, metyrapone is administered orally in doses of 750 mg every 4 hours for six doses. Urinary steroids are determined in the following 24 hours.

The metyrapone test is useless if adrenocortical function is defective. This is ascertained previously by determining the influence of corticotropin infusion on steroid output in the urine. Although the metyrapone test is still experimental, it is a remarkable example of the utilization of a new drug for probing body chemistry.

Androgens

In addition to the glucocorticoids and aldosterone, the adrenal cortex produces androgenic steroids such as dehydroepiandrosterone. The production of androgenic steroids is greatly increased in the adrenogenital syndrome, in which an enzymatic defect channels much of the steroid production toward androgens. Exogenous glucocorticoid administration tends to depress the androgen output through pituitary inhibition.

Adrenal suppressants

Certain toxic compounds such as amphenone B and the insecticide tetrachlorodiphenylethane (DDD) may damage the adrenal cortex. Amphenone B blocks several hydroxylations in addition to the one inhibited by metyrapone. Aminoglutethimide (Elipten) also blocks steroidogenesis by interfering with the conversion of cholesterol to pregnenolone.

GLUCOCORTI-COIDS
Cortisol and corticosterone

Cortisol (hydrocortisone) and corticosterone are the principal glucocorticoids of the adrenal cortex.

In the human adrenal cortex, cortisol predominates, whereas in some species such as the rat, corticosterone has greater quantitative importance. Human adrenal glands contain 2.3 to 5.5 μg of cortisol per gram of wet tissue. In the plasma of normal persons its concentration is about 8 μg/100 ml. The rate of secretion shows a characteristic rhythm or diurnal variation. Secretion begins in the early hours of the morning, before the individual awakens, and gradually declines toward late evening. The reasons for this anticipatory secretion before daily activities begin are not known. Normal daily output of cortisol in human beings is about 25 mg.

Cortisol   Corticosterone

The adrenal steroids are not stored in the adrenal cortex but are synthesized as needed. In the zona fasciculata and reticularis, cholesterol is changed to pregnenolone, which is metabolized to desoxycortisol and eventually cortisol. In the zona glomerulosa, the sequence of events is cholesterol → pregnenolone → desoxycorticosterone → aldosterone. Finally, in the zona fasciculata and reticularis, cholesterol is changed to pregnenolone and finally androstenedione.

BIOSYNTHESIS OF ADRENAL STEROIDS

Cortisol binds to a cytosolic receptor and is translocated to the nucleus where it stimulates transcription of messenger RNA and ultimately protein synthesis.

The three major effects of the steroid are on (1) carbohydrate, protein, and fat metabolism; (2) mineral metabolism; and (3) inflammation.

PHARMACOLOGICAL EFFECTS

Effect on carbohydrate and protein metabolism. The essential effects of cortisol on carbohydrate and protein metabolism are:

1. Increased gluconeogenesis from protein
2. Increased plasma glucose
3. Increased liver glycogen
4. Increased nitrogen excretion in the urine
5. Decreased peripheral glucose utilization

Little is known about the basic action of cortisol on fat metabolism. Unusual accumulations of fat (buffalo hump) occur in the patient treated with glucocorticoids. The adrenal glucocorticoids promote fat mobilization[10] and exert complex effects on ketone metabolism. Cortisol has a *permissive* effect on free fatty acid release from adipose tissue by catecholamines.

Effect on electrolyte and water metabolism. Although the glucocorticoids exert much less effect on renal handling of electrolytes than do desoxycorticosterone and aldosterone, administration of cortisol or cortisone still results in increased sodium retention, increased potassium excretion, and hypokalemic alkalosis in patients receiving prolonged treatment. On the other hand, patients with Addison's disease cannot be kept in electrolyte balance with glucocorticoids alone.

The adrenalectomized animal cannot excrete a large water load. Cortisone will restore this particular function (Table 43-1).

TABLE 43-1	Effects of bilateral adrenalectomy
Circulatory	Decreased blood pressure Decreased blood volume Hyponatremia, hypochloremia, hypoglycemia, and hyperkalemia Increased nonprotein nitrogen
Renal	Increased excretion of sodium and chloride Decreased excretion of potassium
Digestive	Loss of appetite, nausea, and vomiting
Muscular	Weakness Decreased sodium and increased potassium and water in muscle
Miscellaneous	Decreased resistance to all forms of stress Hypertrophy of lymphoid tissue and thymus Death unless treatment is instituted

In addition to an influence on renal handling of electrolytes, adrenal steroids may influence the distribution of electrolytes between cells and extracellular fluid.

Calcium metabolism is also affected by cortisol. It promotes the renal excretion of calcium, and it may reduce calcium absorption from the intestine.

Antiinflammatory action. Most of the clinical uses of the glucocorticoids and of ACTH may be attributed to the remarkable ability of the steroids to inhibit the inflammatory process.

The *mechanism of the antiinflammatory action* of the corticosteroids remains mysterious, although there is no lack of theories on this subject. The antiinflammatory action has been attributed to suppression of migration of polymorphonuclear leukocytes, suppression of reparative processes and functions of fibroblasts, reversal of enhanced capillary permeability, and lysosomal stabilization.

PROBLEM 43-1. Since there are both steroidal and nonsteroidal antiinflammatory drugs, do they act by the same mechanism? This is not likely for several reasons. Clinical experience indicates that the corticosteroids are much more effective in asthma, whereas the nonsteroidal drugs are efficacious in rheumatoid arthritis. Experimentally, the nonsteroidal antiinflammatory drugs such as aspirin or indomethacin inhibit prostaglandin synthesis, whereas cortisone has no such effect.

Although cortisol does not block the synthesis of prostaglandins from arachidonic acid, it prevents the release of arachidonic acid itself from phospholipids.[11] Thus its effect is most likely on phospholipase A_2 or on the production of a peptide, which then blocks the enzyme.[7]

Miscellaneous effects. The cortisone-like steroids exert a striking effect on the number of circulating eosinophils. These elements may completely disappear from the blood following the administration of the glucocorticoids or on the injection of corticotropin.

In addition to the eosinopenic effect, cortisone produces a marked decrease in circulating lymphocytes and an involution of lymphoid tissue.

There is little doubt that cortisone exerts effects on the CNS. Euphoria and other behavioral abnormalities may occur that cannot be explained by the clinical improvement of the primary disease. There is also evidence that glucocorticoid treatment may lower convulsive thresholds.

The glucocorticoids improve muscle strength in adrenalectomized animals. On the other hand, they can cause muscle weakness in prolonged treatment, which perhaps results from potassium loss and other metabolic actions on the muscle.

The effect of corticosteroid treatment on infections is quite complex. Animal experiments suggest that cortisone exerts an adverse effect on the course of a variety of experimental infections, particularly fungal diseases. It must be remembered, however, that very large doses of the steroids are used in such experiments. With reasonable doses, antibody production is not decreased, opsonins remain normal, and leukocytes ingest and destroy microorganisms, even in experimental infections. In humans, varicella and herpes of the eye may be more severe, and fungal diseases may develop after prolonged steroid therapy. On the other hand, there is every reason to believe that the danger of using corticosteroids in infections has been exaggerated. Infection must be viewed as an added factor, rather than as an absolute contraindication, when the risks of using corticosteroids are appraised.

Adverse effects. Excessive doses of glucocorticoids after prolonged administration produce the various manifestations of Cushing's disease, including moon face, hirsutism, acne, amenorrhea, osteoporosis, muscle wasting, variable hypernatremia and hypokalemia, hypertension, aggravation of diabetes mellitus, necrotizing arteritis in rheumatoid patients, aggravation of peptic ulcer, psychotic manifestations, and adrenal atrophy. The *most serious* systematic complications that may result from the clinical use of high doses of steroids are the diabetogenic and ulcerogenic effects; dissolution of supporting tissues such as bone, muscle, and skin; the hypertensive effect; and impairment of defense mechanisms against serious infections.

METABOLISM

Cortisone and other synthetic corticosteroids are absorbed rapidly and completely from the gastrointestinal tract. After oral administration, maximum plasma concentrations are reached in 1 to 2 hours. Hepatic degradation of the corticosteroids leads to a fairly rapid fall in plasma levels so that after 8 hours only 25% of the peak value can be demonstrated and the active drugs disappear completely in about 12 hours.

Drugs that promote the activity of microsomal enzymes in the liver tend to accelerate the metabolism of the corticosteroids. These drugs, which include phenobarbital, phenytoin, and others, may make it necessary to increase the dosage of the corticosteroids.

PREPARATIONS AND CLINICAL USES

Cortisol is available in oral tablets containing 10 or 20 mg. It is also available for intravenous injection and in various lotions and ointments for topical application.

Cortisone is used almost entirely in the tablet form or in suspension for intramuscular injection.

The large number of diseases in which cortisone and cortisol have been tried may be classified as follows on the basis of the degree of beneficial effect that may be expected from existing experience.

Favorable responses	*Transient beneficial effects*
Addison's disease	Acute leukemia
Hypopituitarism	Multiple myeloma
Adrenogenital syndrome	Lymphosarcoma
Severe bronchial asthma	Chronic lymphatic leukemia
Acute ocular inflammations	
Rheumatoid arthritis	
Acute bursitis	
Acute rheumatic fever	
Acute gouty arthritis	
Acquired hemolytic anemia	
Severe atopic dermatitis	
Acute lupus erythematosus	
Severe penicillin reactions	

Certain principles may be derived from the accumulated experience in the therapeutic use of the adrenal steroids.

1. These drugs do not cure any disease. They do not represent replacement therapy, as does insulin in diabetes, except in the rare case of Addison's disease of induced hypoadrenocorticism.

2. The antiinflammatory adrenal steroids are particularly useful in disease processes that occur in episodes and so require no extended therapy. They are also very useful in conditions in which topical application may suffice.

3. Every effort should be made to use other drugs or procedures before prolonged steroid treatment is undertaken. With continued use, hyperadrenocorticism resembling Cushing's syndrome may be inevitable. Cessation of treatment with these steroids may precipitate acute exacerbations of various diseases. Their suppression of the function of the adrenal glands may represent a serious danger if the patient meets with stressful situations.

4. Despite their many disadvantages, the adrenal glucocorticoids are of great therapeutic importance in self-limiting diseases and in chronic disabling processes that fail to respond to any other treatment. The systemic use of these drugs is always a calculated risk that is often worth taking in the presence of incapacitating and otherwise incurable disease.

Comparison of various glucocorticoids

Several glucocorticoids have been introduced into therapeutics on the basis of having antiinflammatory potency greater than cortisol without also having a corresponding increase in their tendency to retain sodium.

The chemical relationships among these newer glucocorticoids may be summarized in comparison with the structural formula of cortisone.

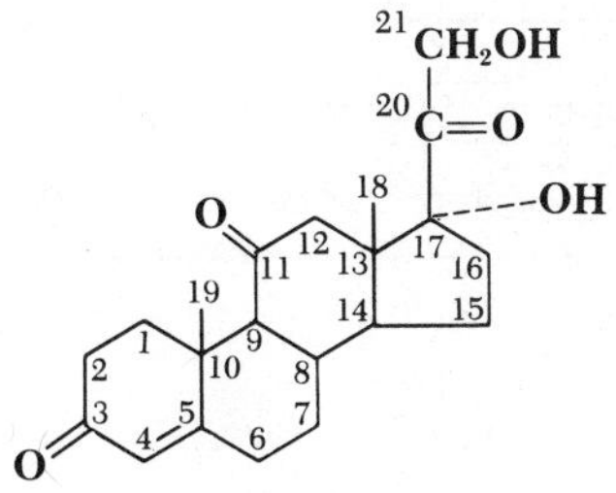

Cortisone

Cortisol has the same structural formulin as cortisone except that OH is in position 11.

Prednisone (Meticorten) is the same as cortisone except that there is a double bond between positions 1 and 2.

Prednisolone (Meticortelone) is the same as prednisone except that OH is in position 11.

Methylprednisolone (Medrol) is the same as prednisolone except that CH_3 is in position 6.

Triamcinolone (Aristocort) is the same as prednisolone except that F (α) is in position 9 and there is an additional α OH in position 16.

Dexamethasone (Decadron) is the same as triamcinolone except that α CH_3 instead of OH is in position 16.

Betamethasone (Celestone) is the same as dexamethasone except that CH_3 is in position 16 β instead of in α.

Fludrocortisone (9-α-fluorohydrocortisone) is the same as cortisol except that α F is in position 9.

Paramethasone (Haldrone) is the same as dexamethasone except that α F moves to position 6.

Halcinonide acetonide differs from triamcinolone acetonide by substitution of chlorine for the hydroxyl group in position 21 and reduction of a double bond at positions 1 and 2 in ring A. The new steroid has dermatological applications.

The introduction of prednisone and prednisolone into therapeutics was of great practical importance, since their high antiinflammatory action was not coupled with a correspondingly high sodium-retaining potency. This separation of effects allowed the physician to use these compounds without special salt-free diets and potassium supplementation (Table 43-2).

The synthetic analogs of cortisol are usually administered in the form of oral tablets. Suspensions of some of the drugs are available for intramuscular and intra-articular administration. Although they are of low solubility, water-soluble preparations of some of the steroids are available for intravenous use, such as the succinates or 21-phosphates.

The topical treatment of dermatological diseases has been revolutionized by the introduction of the antiinflammatory corticosteroids. These drugs applied to the skin

Dermatological applications

TABLE 43-2	Comparison of potencies of various steroids		
Steroid	Antiinflammatory potency	Daily dose (mg)	Sodium retention
Cortisone acetate (Cortone)	0.8	50-100	0.8
Cortisol (Cortef)	1	50-100	1
Prednisone (Meticorten)	2.5	10-20	0.8
Prednisolone (Meticortelone)	3	10-20	0.8
Methylprednisolone (Medrol)	4	10-20	0
Triamcinolone (Aristocort)	5	5-20	0
Dexamethasone (Decadron)	20	0.75-3	0
Paramethasone (Haldrone)	6	4-6	0
Betamethasone (Celestone)	20	0.6-3	0
Desoxycorticosterone (DOC)	0	1-3	10-25
Fludrocortisone (Florinef)	12	0.1	100
Aldosterone	0.2		250

cause vasoconstriction, and this effect has been useful in developing dermatological preparations.[12] The percutaneous absorption, particle size, and vehicle composition are important determinants of topical activity of corticosteroids.[12]

Beclomethasone   Beclomethasone dipropionate (Vanceril) was recently introduced for inhalation in asthmatic persons. The drug is related to prednisolone. Vanceril inhaler is a metered dose aerosol unit, which delivers 50 μg of the drug on each actuation. The usual dosage is two inhalations (100 μg) three or four times a day. The drug appears to be a satisfactory alternative to systemic glucocorticoids in patients with chronic bronchial asthma.[3]

MINERALO-CORTICOIDS
Aldosterone   Aldosterone is the main mineralocorticoid of the adrenal cortex. Extensive studies have been carried out on the role of this hormone in health and disease. A new disease entity, *primary aldosteronism,* has been described as a consequence of such studies. Despite the great interest of such investigations, aldosterone has no therapeutic importance since desoxycorticosterone is available for the correction of electrolyte abnormalities in adrenal insufficiency.

Aldosterone   **Desoxycorticosterone**

Aldosterone has an oxygen atom in position 11 and produces some effect on carbohydrate metabolism. However, its salt-retaining potency is so great and its concentration in the blood so small in relation to cortisol that its physiological function must have little to do with organic metabolism.

Release of aldosterone is promoted by a decrease in circulating blood volume. Stimulation of aldosterone release by angiotensin is of great interest and suggests a connection between aldosterone secretion and the kidney with its juxtaglomerular apparatus. This problem is discussed in Chapter 18. ACTH is necessary for aldosterone synthesis, but the final modulation of its production must be under the influence of other humoral factors, perhaps angiotensin.

Conditions in which aldosterone production is increased are as follows:

1. Primary aldosteronism, characterized by arterial hypertension, muscular weakness, tetany, hypokalemic alkalosis, negative potassium balance, hypomagnesemia, high serum sodium levels, and alkaline urine. This may be caused by adenoma or hyperplasia of the adrenal glands.

2. Secondary hyperaldosteronism, occurring in renal artery constriction with hypertension, malignant hypertension, pregnancy and toxemia of pregnancy, cirrhosis of the liver, nephrotic edema, and less certainly essential hypertension. In many patients with congestive heart failure, aldosterone output is within normal limits.

ALDOSTERONE ANTAGONISTS

Spironolactone (Aldactone) and triamterene antagonize aldosterone at the level of the renal tubules.

Spironolactone is a synthetic steroid that competes with aldosterone for the distal tubular receptor involved in sodium-potassium exchange. Triamterene, on the other hand, does not compete with aldosterone but has a direct effect on the renal tubules. Both drugs favor sodium excretion and potassium retention (pp. 489-490).

Desoxycorticosterone

Desoxycorticosterone acetate is available in solution in sesame oil for intramuscular injection. There are also microcrystalline suspensions of desoxycorticosterone trimethyl acetate for the same purpose. Pellets are available for subcutaneous implantation, which allows release of the steroid over a period of several months.

The main effect of desoxycorticosterone is exerted on the renal tubules. It promotes increased reabsorption of sodium and loss of potassium. Prolonged, intensive treatment with desoxycorticosterone in experimental animals can produce hypertension and necrotic changes in the heart and skeletal muscle. It is believed that these actions result from potassium loss and sodium retention.

REFERENCES

1. Abrass, I.B., Scarpace, P.J.: Glucocorticoid regulation of myocardial β-adrenergic receptors, Endocrinology **108**:977, 1981.

2. Ballin, J.C.: Evaluation of a new aerosolized steroid for asthma therapy: Beclomethasone dipropionate (Vanceril Inhaler), JAMA **236**:2891, 1976.

3. Bondarevsky, E., Shapiro, M.S., Schey, G., Shahor, J., and Bruderman, I.: Beclomethasone dipropionate use in chronic asthmatic patients, JAMA **236**:1969, 1976.

4. Cline, M.J.: Drugs and phagocytosis, N. Engl. J. Med. **291**:1187, 1974.

5. David, D.S., Grieco, M.H., and Cushman, P.: Adrenal glucocorticoids after twenty years, J. Chron. Dis. **22**:637, 1970.

6. Edelman, I.S.: Mechanism of action of aldosterone: energetic and permeability factors, J. Endocrinol. **81**:49, 1979.

7. Flower, R.J., and Blackwell, G.J.: Antiinflammatory steroids induce biosynthesis of a phospholipase A_2 inhibitor which prevents prostaglandin generation, Nature **278**:456, 1979.

8. Ganong, W.F., Alpert, L.C., and Lee, T.C.: ACTH and the regulation of adrenocortical secretion, N. Engl. J. Med. **290**:1006, 1974.

9. Hench, P.S.: Introduction: cortisone and ACTH in clinical medicine, Mayo Clin. Proc. **25**:474, 1950.

10. Hench, P.S., Slocumb, C.H., Barnes, A.R., Smith, H.L., Polley, H.L., and Kendall, E.C.: The effects of adrenal cortical hormone 17-hydroxy-11-dehydrocorticosterone (compound E) on the acute phase of rheumatic fever, Mayo Clin. Proc. **24**:277, 1949.

11. Hong, S.L., and Levine, L.: Inhibition of arachidonic acid release from cells as the biochemical action of antiinflammatory corticosteroids, Proc. Natl. Acad. Sci. U.S.A. **73**:1730, 1976.

12. Leibsohn, E., and Bagatell, F.K.: Halcinonide in the treatment of corticosteroid responsive dermatoses, Br. J. Dermatol. **90**:435, 1974.

13. Reichstein, T., and von Euw, J.: Constitutents of the adrenal cortex: isolation of substance Q (desoxycorticosterone) and R with other materials, Helv. Chim. Acta **21**:1181, 1938.

Chapter 44

Thyroid hormones and antithyroid drugs

GENERAL CONCEPT

The normal thyroid gland stores 15 times as much thyroxine (T_4) as triiodothyronine (T_3). It releases about 1% of the stored hormones daily, which are bound to a thyroid hormone–binding globulin and albumin. Only the free, unbound hormones are active and the ratio of free T_4 to T_3 is about 10:1. All of the circulating T_4 originates from the thyroid, whereas about 80% of T_3 is the product of deiodination of T_4 in the tissues.

The main effects of the thyroid hormones are exerted on metabolism and growth. They have calorigenic and protein anabolic effects.

Hypothyroidism is treated with replacement therapy, for which levothyroxine sodium (T_4) and desiccated thyroid (thyroid USP) are commonly employed. Occasionally liothyronine (T_3) is useful. *Hyperthyroidism* is treated with the thioamide drugs, propylthiouracil or methimazole, which inhibit the incorporation of iodine into thyroglobulin. Radioactive iodine ^{131}I and surgery have important indications also. Finally, propranolol is beneficial in the management of hyperthyroidism.

THYROID HORMONES
Nature and synthesis

In normal subjects the secretion of the thyroid hormones, thyroxine (T_4) and triiodothyronine (T_3), is regulated by the hypothalamus and the pituitary gland. The hypothalamus produces thyrotropin-releasing hormone (TRH), which stimulates the pituitary gland to synthesize and release the thyroid-stimulating hormone (TSH). The thyroid-stimulating hormone promotes the uptake of iodide by the thyroid, the synthesis of thyroglobulin and the release of T_4 and T_3. Increased concentrations of the thyroid hormones reduce TSH secretion by a negative feedback mechanism.

In hyperthyroidism the thyroid functions at an excessive rate and does so autonomously. Under these circumstances TSH levels become very low and the pituitary becomes unresponsive to TRH.

Circulation of thyroid hormones   The major circulating thyroid hormone is T_4, which is present in plasma at a concentration of 5 to 10 µg/100 ml. Serum triiodothyronine level is only about 0.1 µg/100 ml. Only about 0.03% of the T_4 is free. The rest is bound to thyroid-binding globulin and albumin. The free T_3 concentration is 0.3%.

The long half-lives of the thyroid hormones are a result of this binding. The half-life for T_4 is 6 to 7 days. The corresponding value for T_3 is about 2 days. Radioimmunoassay is used for the determintion of total T_4. Clinically, the T_3 resin uptake is employed. In many conditions the binding globulin concentrations are altered and may change the radioimmunoassay values even in the absence of thyroid disease. *Increased thyroid-binding globulin* is seen in pregnancy and oral contraceptive use. *Decreased thyroid-binding globulin* is produced by large doses of corticosteroids and by androgenic or anabolic steroids.

Certain drugs decrease the binding of the thyroid hormones to the binding globulin. These drugs include the salicylates and phenytoin.

Steps in synthesis of thyroxine   The structural formulas of the various organic iodine compounds of the thyroid gland are shown below.

The following steps may be distinguished in the elaboration of thyroxine: (1) concentration of inorganic iodide (iodide trapping), (2) oxidation of iodide to free iodine or hypoiodite, (3) formation of monoiodotyrosine and diiodotyrosine, and (4) coupling of two diiodotyrosines to form thyroxine, or tetraiodothyronine.

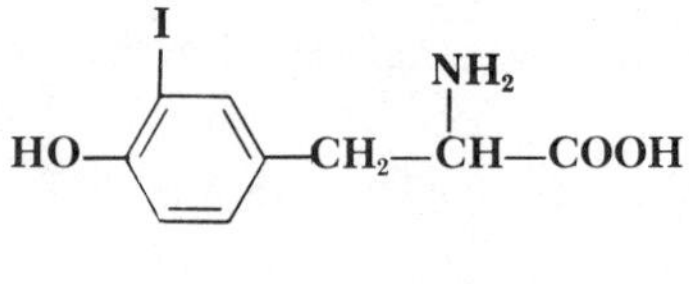

Monoiodotyrosine 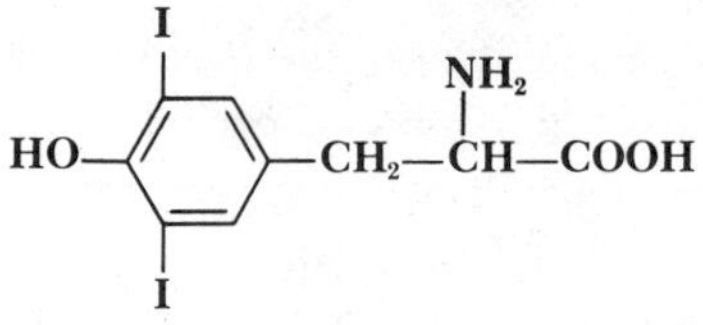   Diiodotyrosine

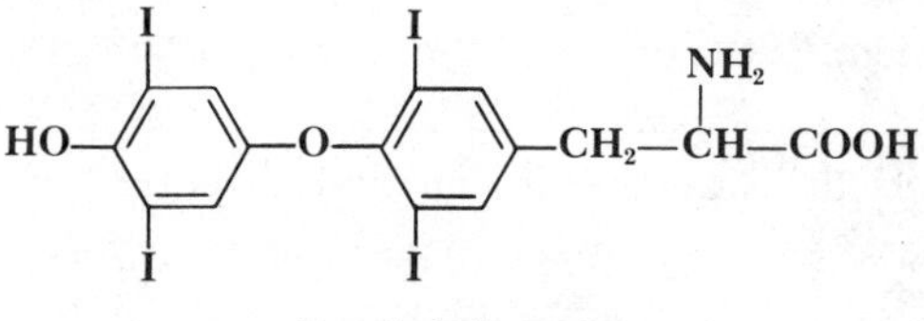

Tetraiodothyronine

The ability of the thyroid gland to concentrate iodide can be demonstrated if the rapid formation of organic iodine compounds is simultaneously blocked by such antithyroid drugs as propylthiouracil or methimazole. Under these conditions the concentration of iodide in the gland may be 30 to 200 times greater than that in plasma. This iodide-trapping mechanism can be blocked by thiocyanate or perchlorate.

It is believed that tyrosine is iodinated while it is attached in peptide linkage to thyroglobulin. The release of thyroxine from the storage protein probably involves the activity of a proteolytic enzyme.

Effects

A deficiency of thyroid hormones results in decreased metabolic rate, alterations in growth and development, disturbances in water and electrolyte metabolism, altered functions of the CNS, skeletal muscles, and circulation, and changes in cholesterol metabolism. Clinical conditions that may be attributed to thyroid deficiency are cretinism and myxedema of the adult and juvenile types.

The actions of the thyroid hormones may be exerted on the following functions:

1. Calorigenesis and thermoregulation
2. Metabolism of lipids, proteins, and carbohydrates
3. Reproduction
4. Growth and development
5. Cardiovascular system
6. Water and electrolyte handling
7. Nervous system

An excess of thyroid hormones produces many of the symptoms and signs of thyrotoxicosis such as nervousness and mental instability, tachycardia, elevated pulse pressure, sweating, and hypersusceptibility to epinephrine. The basal metabolic rate is elevated, the plasma PBI is above normal limits, and ^{131}I uptake by the thyroid is increased. By radioimmunoassay, serum T_3 and T_4 concentrations are shown to be elevated, the former more than the latter. The T_3 concentration falls more rapidly during the treatment of thyrotoxicosis.

The thermogenic effect of the thyroid hormones may be mediated at the level of RNA synthesis. A speculative postulate of the events is as follows[2]: binding of the thyroid hormone to a receptor, augmented synthesis of specific classes of RNA, induction of a protein that may be a part of the sodium pump or may activate the sodium pump in the membrane. The result is an increased ATP hydrolysis, increased formation of ADP and inorganic phosphate, and a higher mitochondrial oxidative phosphorylation.

Thyroxine and catecholamines

It is a common belief in medicine that the myocardium of the hyperthyroid patient is hypersensitive to catecholamines, and many symptoms of the disease resemble sympathetic hyperactivity. There is good evidence that an excess of thyroid hormone increases the number of β-adrenergic receptors in the myocardium. Because of these considerations, propranolol is very useful as an adjunct therapy in thyrotoxicosis, although it does not replace the treatment with the antithyroid drugs or surgery.

The β-adrenergic blocking drugs, such as propranolol, have become very important in the treatment of hyperthyroidism and are more effective than reserpine and guanethidine.[2]

Thyrotropic hormone

The activities of the thyroid gland are greatly influenced by the thyrotropic hormone of the anterior lobe of the pituitary body, which promotes the synthesis and release of thyroxine by the thyroid gland.

The rate of secretion of the thyrotropic hormone is normally inhibited by increased levels of thyroxine or triiodothyronine. When the synthesis of thyroxine is inhibited by the goitrogenic drugs, the thyroid gland becomes enlarged and its vascularity is increased; these changes are attributed to increased levels of circulating thyroid-stimulating hormone as a consequence of lower thyroxine levels.

Graves' disease is an autoimmune disease. The thyroid hyperactivity may be attributed to a thyroid-stimulating antibody and not to the thyrotrophic hormone. Measurement of the thyroid-stimulating antibody gives some indication for the likelihood of relapse when the disease is brought under control by treatment with the antithyroid drugs.

The thyroid suppression test is used in the diagnosis of Graves' disease. TSH secretion is normally suppressible by T_4 or T_3. In Graves' disease the TSH secretion and thyroid hyperactivity cannot be suppressed by the thyroid hormones, since the gland is driven by the thyroid-stimulating antibody. This test is useful in predicting if the patient will stay in remission after successful treatment.

Clinical uses and preparations

Indications for the use of thyroid preparations include hypothyroidism and conditions in which suppression of thyrotropin secretion is desirable. These include nontoxic goiter and chronic thyroiditis (Hashimoto's disease). Thyroid preparations may also have various diagnostic uses. Their employment in the treatment of obesity and dysmenorrhea is not based on good evidence.

Several preparations are available when treatment with thyroid hormones is indicated.

Thyroid USP is the cleaned, dried, and powdered thyroid gland of animals used for food by humans. It is standardized only by chemical and not by biological assay. It should contain 0.17% to 0.23% of iodine in organic combination. Variability in response may result from reliance on chemical assay alone.

Preparations include tablets containing 15, 30, 60, 120, 200, 250, and 300 mg and enteric-coated tablets of 30, 60, 120, and 200 mg.

Thyroid extract (Proloid) is a purified extract of the thyroid gland, assayed chemically and biologically. It is available in tablets containing 15, 30, 60, 100, 200, and 300 mg.

Levothyroxine sodium (Synthroid sodium) is the synthetic sodium salt of levothyroxine, with actions and uses similar to those of thyroid extract except that it may be injected intravenously in emergencies such as myxedema coma. The potency of 0.1 mg of levothyroxine is equal to that of 60 mg of thyroid USP from the standpoint of a clinical response.

Preparations include tablets containing 0.025, 0.05, 0.1, 0.15, 0.2, 0.3 mg and powder to make an injectable solution, 0.05 mg/ml.

Liothyronine sodium (Cytomel) is the synthetic sodium salt of levotriiodothyronine. It may be injected intravenously in myxedema coma, for which it is the drug of choice. Other uses are similar to those of thyroid extracts. The potency of 0.025 mg of liothyronine sodium is equivalent to that of 60 mg of thyroid USP.

Preparations include tablets containing 5, 25, and 50 μg and powder to make injectable solution, 114 μg/ml.

Liotrix (Euthyroid; Thyrolar) is a mixture of levothyroxine sodium and liothyronine sodium in the ratio of 4:1.

The tripeptide pyroglutamylhistidyl-prolinamide or TRH has been synthesized and is undergoing various clinical applications.[4] The drug causes release of thyrotropin and prolactin in normal persons. It may be useful as a diagnostic agent in evaluation of pituitary reserve and differentiation of hypothalamic hypothyroidism from that resulting from pituitary destruction and as a substitute for the thyroid suppression test and others. Hypothyroid patients respond to TRH with a marked elevation of serum thyrotropin. Patients with hyperthyroidism do not respond to TRH.

Thyrotropin-releasing hormone (TRH)

The development of the antithyroid drugs is the result of a series of interesting experimental observations. Perhaps the first indication of antithyroid action was the finding that rabbits on a cabbage diet developed goiter. Numerous studies followed in the antithyroid principles in plants of the *Brassica* genus. Interest in this field was further stimulated when it was found that rats on sulfaguanidine administration also developed hyperplastic thyroid glands. A systemic study of this problem led eventually to the clinical trial of thiourea and thiouracil in thyrotoxicosis.

ANTITHYROID DRUGS

Drugs that depress thyroid function can be placed in one of several categories on the basis of their mode of action.

Classification

Inhibitors of thyroxine synthesis
Thiourea (obsolete)
Thiouracil (obsolete)
Propylthiouracil
Methylthiouracil
Methimazole

Inhibitors of iodide trapping
Thiocyanates (obsolete)
Perchlorate (obsolete)
Drugs whose mode of action is uncertain
Iodides
Drugs that destroy thyroid tissue
Radioactive iodine (^{131}I)

The antithyroid drugs, also known as thioureylenes, block the thyroid peroxidase–catalyzed iodination of thyroglobulin. They compete with tyrosyl residues of thyroglobulin for active iodine. They also inactivate thyroid peroxidase.

Inhibitors of thyroxine synthesis

When these inhibitors of thyroxine formation are administered to humans or experimental animals, the preformed thyroxine continues to be secreted. However, thyroxine secretion diminishes as the stored organic iodine becomes exhausted because of a lack of resynthesis. This brings forth increased secretion of the thyroid-stimulating hormone, which produces a hyperplastic, highly vascularized thyroid gland that has a greatly increased capacity for iodide trapping. The individual becomes myxedematous.

Thiourea   Thiouracil   Propylthiouracil

Methimazole

Thiouracil was the first antithyroid drug used extensively. Its use led to numerous cases of drug allergy and agranulocytosis, and it was soon replaced by propylthiouracil. This drug is used in doses of 50 to 100 mg three or four times a day in tablet form. It causes allergic reactions and blood dyscrasias much less frequently than does thiouracil and is one of the most popular antithyroid drugs. Methylthiouracil has about the same potency as propylthiouracil but is less desirable in view of the more frequent allergic side effects observed following its use. Methimazole (Tapazole) is a highly potent antithyroid drug with a long duration of action. It is used in the form of 5 to 10 mg tablets, which are administered three times a day.

ACTIVITY   Considering thiouracil as 100, the activity of these drugs in humans is compared as follows:

Thiouracil	100
6-*N*-Propylthiouracil	75
6-Methylthiouracil	100
Methimazole	1000

METABOLISM   All these thioamide drugs are absorbed rapidly from the gastrointestinal tract. They are also excreted and metabolized fairly rapidly, necessitating frequent administration. The distribution of thiouracil in the body is unequal, with several organs, including the thyroid gland, containing more of the drug than the average of other tissues.

CLINICAL APPLICATIONS   Propylthiouracil and methimazole have the following indications: preparation of patients for surgery, chronic treatment of hyperthyroidism until spontaneous remission occurs, and management of thyrotoxic crisis (thyroid storm) along with propranolol and other drugs.

The thioamide drugs have a short half-life, about 1½ hours. As a consequence they must be administered several times a day. In long-term therapy it may be possible to reduce the frequency of administration, and the drugs may be given once a day.

The usual daily oral dosages for adults of the inhibitors of thyroxine synthesis are 200 and 300 mg of propylthiouracil, 15 to 30 mg of methimazole (Tapazole), and 200 mg of methylthiouracil.

Drugs such as thiocyanate, perchlorate, and nitrate can block the iodide-concentrating ability of the thyroid gland. Perchlorate has undergone clinical trial. It is quite effective, but agranulocytosis has been reported following its use.

Inhibitors of iodide trapping

Although a daily intake of about 150 μg of iodide is essential for normal thyroxine synthesis and although low intakes of iodide lead to goiter and cretinism, in large doses iodides can decrease the functional activity of the thyroid in Graves' disease.

Iodides

Recent evidence suggests that iodide administered to thyrotoxic patients causes an abrupt inhibition of the release of thyroxine, an effect that may be causally related to its beneficial therapeutic action.

Radioactive iodine (^{131}I) emits γ and β radiation and has a half-life of 8 days. Since it is handled by the body in the same manner as ordinary iodine, it has become extremely useful in the diagnosis of thyroid disease and in the treatment of hyperthyroidism and carcinoma of the thyroid.

Radioactive iodine

The destructive effect of ^{131}I on thyroid tissue is caused by the β radiation. The gamma rays are useful for estimating the quantity of the radioactive material in the gland by placing suitable counting equipment in front of the neck.

The isotope is available as sodium radioiodide. It is generally taken orally, but intravenous preparations are available. For diagnostic purposes the drug is given in doses of about 30 microcuries (μCi), whereas in the treatment of hyperthyroidism about a thousand times as much radioactivity is administered, in other words, 15 to 30 millicuries (mCi). The purpose of the treatment is the same as that of subtotal thyroidectomy.

^{131}I is contraindicated in pregnancy. It is customarily used in patients over 20 years of age. Thyroidectomy is preferred in younger hyperthyroid patients unless surgery represents an unusual hazard, for example, in the presence of heart disease. The most important complications following the use of radioiodine is hypothyroidism.

REFERENCES

1. Blum, A.S.: The medical management of hyperthyroidism, Ration. Drug. Ther. 8:1, 1974.
2. Edelman, I.S.: Thyroid thermogenesis, N. Engl. J. Med. 290:1303, 1974.
3. Haibich, H.: Hyperthyroidism in Graves disease, Arch. Intern. Med. 136:725, 1976.
4. Hershman, J.M.: Clinical application of thyrotropin-releasing hormone, N. Engl. J. Med. 290:886, 1974.
5. Oppenheimer, J.H.: Thyroid hormone action at the cellular level, Science 203:971, 1979.
6. Reynolds, L.R., and Kotchen, T.A.: Antithyroid drugs and radioactive iodine.

Fifteen years' experience with Graves' disease, Arch. Intern. Med. **139:**651, 1979.

7. Rosenberg, I.N.: Evaluation of thyroid function, N. Engl. J. Med. **286:**924, 1972.

8. Sterling, K.: Thyroid hormone action at the cell level, N. Engl. J. Med. **300:**117, 1979.

9. Taurog, A.: The mechanism of action of the thioureylene antithyroid drugs, Endocrinology **98:**1031, 1976.

10. Van Herle, A.J., Vassart, G., and Dumont, J.E.: Control of thyroglobulin synthesis and secretion, N. Engl. J. Med. **301:**307, 1979.

Chapter 45

Parathyroid extract and vitamin D

The concentration of ionized calcium in plasma is maintained by rapid exchange with bone calcium, excretion by the kidney, and absorption from the intestine. Parathyroid hormone, vitamin D, and calcitonin contribute in a major way to calcium homeostasis.

A fall in plasma calcium promotes a parathyroid secretion, whereas a rise in calcium inhibits it. The parathyroid hormone not only influences osteoclastic and osteocytic activity, but also stimulates the renal reabsorption of calcium and the formation of 1,25-dihydroxyvitamin D_3, a major regulator of intestinal absorption of calcium and phosphate.

Hypercalcemia is treated with furosemide and saline, phosphate, calcitonin, and glucocorticoids. Hypocalcemia is treated with calcium salts intravenously or orally, vitamin D, or its metabolite calcitriol (1,25-dihydroxyvitamin D_3). The diphosphonate, etidronate sodium has some uses in hypercalcemia also.

The parathyroid hormone is a polypeptide that is seldom used because it is antigenic. It mobilizes calcium from bone, promotes the renal reabsorption of calcium, decreases the renal reabsorption of phosphate, and stimulates the synthesis of 1,25-dihydroxyvitamin D_3.

The secretion of parathyroid is under negative feedback regulation by the serum ionized calcium concentrations.

As shown in Fig. 45-1, the injection of parathyroid extract in patients having idiopathic hypoparathyroidism results in phosphaturia, lowering of serum phosphorus, and gradual elevation of serum calcium. This sequence of events has been interpreted by Albright and Ellsworth[1] as indicative of a primary action of the parathyroid extract on phosphate excretion.

Although parathyroid extract does promote renal excretion of phosphate, there is much experimental evidence to indicate that the most important action of the parathyroid hormones is direct mobilization of calcium from bones. The action of

547

FIG. 45-1   *Effect of parathyroid extract (PTE) on serum inorganic phosphorus and calcium in patient with idiopathic hypoparathyroidism.*

From Munson, P.L.:Fed. Proc. 19:593, 1960

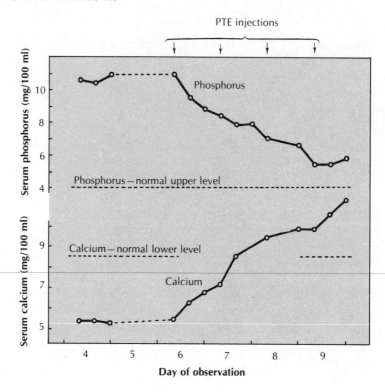

parathyroid extract on serum calcium has been demonstrated in nephrectomized animals. In addition, it has been shown that parathyroid transplants exert a local resorptive effect on bone. This effect has also been demonstrated in tissue cultures.

Calcium
homeostasis and
parathyroid extract

A variety of factors contribute to the maintenance of extracellular calcium within narrow limits. The daily diet contributes about 1 g of calcium, the absorption of which is influenced by vitamin D and to some extent by parathyroid hormone. Also, the phosphate, oxalate, and phytate content of the diet will decrease calcium absorption. Antacids containing $Al(OH)_3$ promote calcium absorption by binding phosphate to the intestine.

Extracellular calcium is in equilibrium with the exchangeable calcium of bone. When extracellular calcium falls, the exchangeable portion of bone calcium aids in returning it toward normal. In addition, renal reabsorption of calcium, renal excretion of phosphate, and resorption of nonexchangeable bone are important in opposing decreases in extracellular calcium levels. Bone resorption is promoted by the parathyroid hormone and by some steroids related to vitamin D. The release of parathyroid hormone is under the influence of the level of extracellular calcium.

The effects of the parathyroid hormone on bone reabsorption and phosphate excretion are mediated by the adenyl cyclase system and cyclic AMP.

Calcitonin, or thyrocalcitonin, is a second hormone involved in calcium homeostasis. Calcitonin is secreted by the parafollicular cells of the thyroid. These cells originate from the ultimobranchial body, a separate organ in some animals. Calcitonin produces hypocalcemia by inhibiting bone resorption. Calcitonin also promotes the urinary excretion of calcium and phosphate.

Calcitonin is normally present in the blood, and its concentration increases when calcium salts are administered. Its concentration is greatly increased in patients having medullary carcinoma of the thyroid. The function of calcitonin may be a protective one against hypercalcemia induced by increased calcium intake.

Calcitonin has been used clinically in Paget's disease, hypercalcemia, and osteoporosis. Its usefulness is limited by its short duration of action. In addition, resistance develops to its continued use, perhaps because of compensatory increase in the secretion of parathyroid hormone.

It was discovered more than 40 years ago that irradiation of plant sterols could yield antirachitic compounds. The active sterol produced by irradiation of ergosterol became known as vitamin D_2 or *ergocalciferol*. What was previously called vitamin D_1 was a mixture of active and inactive products. The vitamin that is produced in the skin by irradiation of 7-dehydrocholesterol was named vitamin D_3 or *cholecalciferol*. Although both vitamins D_2 and D_3 are active and undergo similar metabolic transformations, most of the circulating and stored vitamin D is ergocalciferol. This is a consequence of the high dietary intake of irradiated ergosterol. Vitamin D_3 differs from vitamin D_2 only in lacking a double bond between C-22 and C-23.

VITAMIN D

Current nomenclature

Vitamin D_2

Dihydrotachysterol

Both vitamins D_2 and D_3 must be hydroxylated in the C-25 position by the liver to become active. The resulting compounds are referred to as 25-hydroxyergocalciferol and 25-hydroxycholecalciferol, respectively. These compounds are carried in the circulation by a binding protein. Eventually, the microsomal enzymes of the liver convert them to inactive polar metabolites.

Metabolic activation

A further activating step occurs in the kidney for vitamin D_3. The 25-hydroxy-cholecalciferol is further hydroxylated to 1,25-hydroxycholecalciferol, which may be the final active form of vitamin D_3.

The first enzymatic hydroxylation of cholecalciferol in the liver is under feedback inhibition by the 25-hydroxylated compound. This feedback inhibition prevents over-production of this metabolite. The second hydroxylation, which takes place in the kidney, yields the product, 1,25-hydroxycholecalciferol, which is most potent in causing calcium reabsorption from the intestine and reabsorption from the bone. In severe renal disease it is possible to administer the dihydroxylated cholecalciferol, thus bypassing its lack of production by the failing kidney.

Dihydrotachysterol is also hydroxylated in the liver, but the 25-hydroxyl deriv-ative does not exert feedback inhibition on the reaction. The 25-hydroxyl derivative of dihydrotachysterol is the active form of the compound and does not require further activation in the kidney. For these reasons the drug is much more effective in promoting bone reabsorption than cholecalciferol and is commonly used in the treat-ment of hypoparathyroidism.

Drug interactions

Phenobarbital and phenytoin are known to increase microsomal hydroxylase ac-tivity in the liver. It is possible that the great frequency of rickets and osteomalacia in patients taking anticonvulsants is a consequence of increased enzymatic transfor-mation of vitamin D_2 and D_3 to inactive metabolites.[8]

The main function of vitamin D is to promote absorption of calcium and phos-phorus from the intestine. Deficiency of the vitamin in children leads to rickets, which may be prevented by the daily requirement of 800 units. Very rarely, osteo-malacia can occur in adults following vitamin D deficiency.

In the treatment of hypoparathyroidism, vitamin D_2 may be administered in large doses (400,000 IU) initially, and maintenance doses may vary from 100,000 to 200,000 IU/day. Dihydrotachysterol may be administered initially in doses of 3 to 8 mg (compared with 10 mg or more of vitamin D_2), and for maintenance a dose of about 1 mg/day is usually sufficient.

TOXIC EFFECTS OF PARATHYROID EXTRACT AND VITAMIN D

Toxic effects of parathyroid injection and of vitamin D are manifested as (1) hypercalcemia with numerous clinical consequences, (2) demineralization of bones, and (3) renal calculi and metastatic calcifications in soft tissues.

Hypercalcemia is associated with a number of clinical manifestations such as weakness, vomiting, diarrhea, and lack of muscle tone. The electrocardiographic changes that may occur at various levels of serum calcium are shown in Fig. 45-2. Serious toxic manifestations may be seen at calcium blood levels of 15 mg/100 ml. Signs of hypocalcemia are tetany, cataracts, and mental lethargy.

Effect of varying calcium levels on electrocardiogram.

FIG. 45-2

From Burch, G.E., and Winsor, T.: A primer of electrocardiography, Philadelphia, 1960, Lea & Febiger.

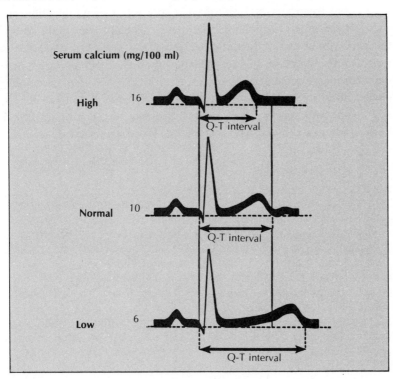

Phosphates, sodium sulfate, sodium citrate and **disodium edetate** (Endrate), when given by intravenous infusion, can lower calcium levels in the blood. Their administration should not be undertaken without considering their adverse effects.

Glucocorticoids antagonize the effects of vitamin D on calcium absorption from the intestine. They are useful in hypercalcemia caused by sarcoidosis or hypervitaminosis D. **Salmon calcitonin** (Calcimar) is a polypeptide, which is injected subcutaneously or intramuscularly for the occasional initial treatment of hyperparathyroidism, Paget's disease, and some malignancies. It loses its effectiveness in a few weeks.

Etidronate disodium (EHDP; Didronel) is a diphosphonate used in the treatment of Paget's disease. The drug seems to slow osteoblastic and osteoclastic activity. The drug lowers serum alkaline phosphatase and urinary hydroxyproline. The most serious adverse effect of etidronate is osteomalacia with fractures. Etidronate disodium (Didronel) is available in 200 mg tablets. The loop diuretics, such as **furosemide** (Lasix), tend to promote calcium excretion, whereas the **thiazides** cause hypercalcemia with chronic administration.

OTHER DRUGS INFLUENCING SERUM CALCIUM CONCENTRATIONS

Mithramycin, an antibiotic used in the treatment of testicular neoplasms, lowers calcium concentration, perhaps by a toxic effect on osteoclasts.

For the initial treatment of *hypocalcemia,* the intravenous injection of a 10% solution of **calcium gluconate** is highly effective. **Calcium gluceptate** may also be given intravenously or intramuscularly. Calcium salts used orally include calcium gluconate, calcium phosphate dibasic, calcium phosphate tribasic, calcium lactate, and calcium carbonate precipitated.

Calcitriol (Rocaltrol) is 1,25-dihydroxyvitamin D_3, a renal hormone. It promotes intestinal calcium absorption, and it may mobilize calcium from bone. It is used in hypocalcemic patients with chronic renal failure. Calcitriol (Rocaltrol) is available in 0.25 and 0.5 µg tablets.

REFERENCES

1. Albright, F., and Ellsworth, R.: Studies on the physiology of the parathyroid glands: calcium and phosphorus studies in a case of idiopathic hypoparathyroidism, J. Clin. Invest. 7:183, 1929.
2. Broadus, A.E., Horst, R.L., Lang, R., Littledike, E.T., and Rasmussen, H.: The importance of circulating 1,25-dihydroxyvitamin D in the pathogenesis of hypercalciuria and renal-stone formation in primary hyperparathyroidism, N. Engl. J. Med. 302:421, 1980.
3. DeLuca, H.F., and Suttie, J.W.: The fat-soluble vitamins, Madison, 1970, University of Wisconsin Press.
4. Haussler, M.R., and Cordy, P.E.: Metabolites and analogues of Vitamin D: which for what? JAMA 247:841, 1982.
5. Juan, D.: Hypocalcemia. Differential diagnosis and mechanisms. Arch. Intern. Med. 139:1166, 1979.
6. Lukert, B.P.: Vitamin D metabolism in man: effect of corticosteroids, Arch. Intern. Med. 136:1241, 1976.
7. Newmark, S.R.: Hypercalcemic and hypocalcemic crises, JAMA 230:1438, 1974.
8. Raisz, L.G.: A confusion of Vitamin D's, N. Engl. J. Med. 287:926, 1972.
9. Wills, M.R.: Intestinal absorption of calcium, Lancet 1:820, 1973.

Chapter 46

Posterior pituitary hormones—vasopressin and oxytocin

The posterior lobe of the pituitary body, the neurohypophysis, contains hormones having vasoactive, antidiuretic, and oxytocic properties. The original material was separated into two fractions. One contained most of the vasoactive and antidiuretic portion, whereas the other was predominantly oxytocic. Both active fractions, vasopressin and oxytocin, have been synthesized.

Both vasopressin and oxytocin are polypeptides containing eight amino acids. Vasopressin (in several species) contains the following amino acids: tyrosine, cystine, aspartic acid, glutamic acid, glycine, proline, arginine, and phenylalanine. In vasopressin obtained from hog pituitary, arginine is replaced by lysine.

Oxytocin resembles vasopressin in having six identical amino acids but contains leucine and isoleucine instead of arginine and phenylalanine.

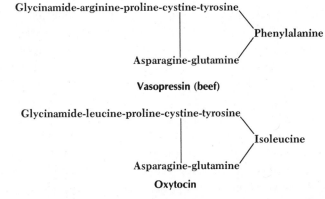

Preparations of these hormones are standardized by bioassay. Vasopressin preparations are standardized on the basis of the action of such preparations on the blood pressure of the dog. One USP unit is the activity present in 0.5 mg of standard powder of posterior pituitary. Oxytocic potency is determined by the depressor effect of oxytocin preparations on the blood pressure of the chicken.

VASOPRESSIN The most significant effect of vasopressin is exerted on the kidney. In addition, the hormone can constrict various blood vessels, including the coronary vessels. The only clearly established physiological function of vasopressin is its antidiuretic action.

The antidiuretic potency of vasopressin is very great. The infusion of less than 0.1 µg of vasopressin per hour produces maximum antidiuresis in humans. It is believed that the antidiuretic action of vasopressin is exerted on water reabsorption by the distal tubule and also by the collecting ducts. In physiological doses the hormone does not influence electrolyte absorption. Larger doses in some experiments have shown increased output of sodium and chloride, probably an indirect effect.

The antidiuretic hormone is elaborated by certain hypothalamic structures such as the supraoptic nuclei and is then transported to the neurohypophysis where it is stored. The release of the antidiuretic hormone is influenced by the osmolarity of the extracellular fluid and by many drugs. Endogenous neurohumoral agents also may play an important role in the release of antidiuretic hormones, since pain and emotions have important influences. It is generally accepted that some hypothalamic structures are sensitive to changes in the osmolarity of the extracellular fluid and act as osmoreceptors. Thus the ingestion of water and dilution of the extracellular fluid lead to inhibition of antidiuretic hormone secretion, whereas hypertonic solutions promote this process.

Diabetes insipidus, occurring spontaneously or produced experimentally by pituitary stalk section, is characterized by failure of distal tubular water reabsorption. As a consequence, persons with diabetes insipidus excrete large amounts of dilute urine and drink large quantities of water.

The mode of action of the antidiuretic hormone is now generally attributed to an increase in the size of pores or channels for the flow of water along osmotic gradients. There is evidence for this action on isolated systems such as the skin of toads and frogs.

The mechanism of action of vasopressin involves the activation of the adenyl cyclase system with the increase in the concentration of cyclic AMP.

Other drugs with antidiuretic effects in diabetes insipidus include clofibrate, chlorpropamide, and also the thiazides. Most of these are more likely to be useful in moderate forms of the disease, and the thiazides are useful especially in nephrogenic diabetes insipidus.

Effects on antidiuretic hormone release In addition to changes in osmolarity of the extracellular fluid, release of the antidiuretic hormone is influenced by a variety of drugs. The existence of a cholinergic mechanism for this process has been suggested on the basis of experiments showing that injections of *acetylcholine* or diisopropyl fluorophosphate into the supraoptic nuclei caused release of antidiuretic hormone. *Nicotine* has been shown to inhibit water diuresis in humans, probably through the release of antidiuretic hormone. *Alcohol* inhibits the release of antidiuretic hormone in response to dehydration and produces inappropriate water diuresis in a dehydrated individual. Alcohol does not block the action of nicotine on the release of the hormone.

Antidiuresis that occurs during general anesthesia and following the injection of histamine, morphine, and barbiturates (but not thiopental) has also been attributed to the release of antidiuretic hormone. Since muscular exercise, pain, and emotional excitement also cause inhibition of water diuresis, it is likely that some central control mechanism of antidiuretic hormone release is very susceptible to neural or neurohumoral influences. Of the large variety of drugs that can influence antidiuretic hormone release, many are known to alter neural activity or to act as stressful stimuli.

Certain hyponatremic syndromes are associated with "inappropriate" secretion of the antidiuretic hormone. They are characterized by primary water retention unassociated with sodium retention and edema. Some of the underlying diseases are bronchogenic carcinoma, head injury, and tuberculous meningitis.

Extrarenal effects

Although the main therapeutic advantage of vasopressin is its antidiuretic action, the hormone has stimulant effect on the smooth muscles of the blood vessels, intestine, and uterus. This action appears to be a direct musculotropic effect, not mediated by nerves or neurohumoral agents. When posterior pituitary preparations are used in the treatment of diabetes insipidus, the smooth muscle effects are undesirable side effects and usually indicate overdosage.

Preparations containing vasopressin constrict the coronary arteries and are therefore dangerous in persons who suffer from coronary disease. Although intravenous injection of posterior pituitary extract into animals causes marked peripheral vasoconstriction, blood pressure often increases only moderately. This is attributed to the fact that the coronary arteries are also constricted. Tachyphylaxis develops to the pressor action of vasopressin.

Antidiuretic preparations

Posterior pituitary USP is available as a powder for topical application, administered by inhalation or directly to the nasal mucosa. It may cause mucosal irritation. The duration of its antidiuretic effect is such that the drug must be used several times a day. Posterior pituitary is contraindicated in pregnancy and should be used with caution in patients with coronary artery disease. The dose is 40 to 60 mg topically three or four times daily.

Posterior pituitary injection is obsolete, being replaced by vasopressin injection.

Vasopressin injection (Pitressin) produces an antidiuretic effect lasting 2 to 8 hours when administered by subcutaneous or intramuscular injection. The solution may also be used topically. Vasopressin may cause fluid retention, hypertension, myocardial ischemia, gastrointestinal and uterine contractions, and allergic reactions. The available solution for injection contains 10 pressor units/ml.

Vasopressin tannate injection (Pitressin tannate) is a suspension in peanut oil of the insoluble tannate of the hormone, suitable for intramuscular administration. The duration of action is 2 to 3 days. Vasopressin tannate injection is available in oil, 5 pressor units/ml.

Desmopressin acetate (DDAVP) is a vasopressin analog, which has a prolonged action, and its antidiuretic effect in relation to its vasopressor effect is much greater than is the case for the other vasopressins. The drug is used topically by a nasal calibrated catheter. Its antidiuretic effect lasts 10 to 20 hours, and it may replace the other vasopressins in the management of severe diabetes insipidus. The drug is available in solutions containing 0.1 mg/ml of DDAVP.

Lypressin (Diapid) is a synthetic lysine vasopressin. It is administered by intranasal spray.

Clofibrate has an antidiuretic effect, probably by increasing the release of vasopressin from the neurohypophysis. **Chlorpropamide** apparently increases the sensitivity of the renal tubules to the action of vasopressin. The **thiazides** are generally ineffective in central diabetes insipidus but may be useful in the nephrogenic form of the disease.

Drugs acting on the uterus

The uterus receives sympathetic and parasympathetic innervation. The α-adrenergic receptors mediate stimulation, the β-receptors mediate inhibition. In addition, muscarinic receptors are also stimulatory. The uterus is susceptible to endocrine influences. Estrogens enhance responsiveness, whereas progesterone decreases the response.

The most commonly used drugs for enhancing the contractions of the uterus are *oxytocin*, the *prostaglandins*, and certain ergot preparations, particularly *ergonovine*.

Oxytocin

Oxytocin is a polypeptide amide that consists of eight amino acids and ammonia. Its molecular weight is 1007. Although the physiological functions of the hormone seem to be related to reproductive function in the female, its presence in the male suggests that it must have other functions also.

The separation of posterior pituitary extracts into the oxytocic and vasopressor-antidiuretic fractions was accomplished as early as 1928. More recently, oxytocin has been purified, chemically identified, and synthesized.

Oxytocin differs from vasopressin in the following respects:

1. It contains leucine and isoleucine instead of phenylalanine and arginine; the other six amino acids are identical in the two hormones.
2. It has no effect on water diuresis.
3. It is a potent stimulant of the gravid uterus at term and postpartum.
4. It does not produce vasoconstriction and may even lower blood pressure in certain species.
5. It may produce milk letdown during the postpartum period.
6. It has little effect on intestinal smooth muscle and coronary arteries.

BIOASSAY

Oxytocin preparations are bioassayed on the basis of the vasodepressor activity in chickens. The oxytocic activity associated with vasopressin preparations is assayed on the guinea pig uterus.

Oxytocin injection, synthetic (Pitocin; Syntocinon; Uteracon) is a synthetic preparation and used for induction of labor. It is also used to control postpartum uterine atony, but for the latter indication ergonovine is often preferred. The drug is available in solutions containing 5 units/0.5 ml or 10 units/ml. Dosage varies according to the indication. To control postpartum bleeding, oxytocin may be administered intramuscularly, 3 to 10 units. When given by intravenous injection for the same indication, its dosage should be reduced to 0.6 to 1.8 units. For intravenous infusion by the drip method, oxytocin, 2 units, is added to 500 ml of normal saline.

PREPARATIONS

Ergonovine maleate (Ergotrate Maleate) and **methylergonovine maleate** (Methergine) are used to decrease uterine bleeding by causing contraction of the uterine muscle after delivery of the placenta.

Prostaglandin preparations are used for producing abortions by the induction of uterine contractions. Carboprost tromethamine (Prostin/M15) is the 15-methyl derivative of prostaglandin F_2-Alpha. It is injected intramuscularly and is effective from the thirteenth to the twentieth week of pregnancy. Dinoprost tromethamine (Prostin F_2-Alpha) is usually administered intraamniotically. Dinoprostone (Prostin E_2) is available in the form of vaginal suppositories.

Other uterine stimulants

β-Adrenergic agonists, intravenous alcohol, and prostaglandin synthesis inhibitors, such as indomethacin, may be useful for the prevention of premature delivery.

Ritodrine hydrochloride (Yutopar), a β-adrenergic agonist, has been approved recently as an effective uterine relaxant for premature labor.

Uterine relaxants

1. Hays, R.M.: Antidiuretic hormone, N. Engl. J. Med. **295**:659, 1976.
2. Kosman, M.E.: Evaluation of a new antidiuretic agent, desmopressin acetate (DDAVP), JAMA **240**:1896, 1978.
3. Legros, J.J.: The neurohypophysial peptides: biosynthesis, biological role and prospects of use in neuropsychiatric therapy, Triangle **18**:17, 1979.
4. Taylor, A., Mamelak, M., Reaven, E., and Maffly, R.: Vasopressin: possible role of microtubules and microfilaments in its action, Science **181**:347, 1973.

REFERENCES

Chapter 47

Anterior pituitary gonadotropins and sex hormones

The anterior pituitary gland produces several polypeptide and glycoprotein hormones. The polypeptides are growth hormone (somatotropin), prolactin, corticotropin, and lipotropin. The glycoproteins are thyrotropin, luteinizing hormone (LH), and follicle-stimulating hormone (FSH). The cells of the anterior pituitary gland may secrete one or more of these hormones.

The secretion of these hormones is stimulated by hypothalamic-releasing factors (Fig. 47-1), also known as *hypophysiotropic hormones*, such as thyrotropin-releasing hormone (TRH), gonadotropin-releasing hormone (GnRH), prolactin-inhibiting factors (PIF), corticotropin-releasing factor (CRF), growth hormone–releasing factor (GHRF), and growth hormone release-inhibitory factor (somatostatin).

Several neuropharmacological agents alter anterior pituitary secretions by acting on the elaboration of hypothalamic releasing factors. It is believed that the neurons that secrete the releasing factors are located in the ventral hypothalamus, and various neurotransmitters regulate their functional activities. Among the possible transmitters, dopamine, norepinephrine, and serotonin have received the most consideration. Many drugs influence the elaboration of various releasing factors by interactions with their neurotransmitters. A brief summary based on a more extensive review will be attempted, classifying these drug effects according to the individual releasing factors.

Thyroid-stimulating hormone (TSH)–releasing factor. Protirelin (TRH) is a synthetic tripeptide (pyroglutamyl-histidyl-proline amide) available under the trade names Relefact or Thypinone in a solution containing 0.5 mg/ml of the hormone. Protirelin is used in the diagnosis of thyroid and pituitary disorders and in prolactinemic states, since it also stimulates prolactin secretion.

Corticotropin-releasing factor (CRF). Dextroamphetamine stimulates the release of CRF, which is blocked by an α-adrenergic blocking agent. Reserpine causes a transient increase in basal secretion. The phenothiazines such as chlorpromazine reduce the responses of CRF secretion to hypoglycemia, metyrapone, and pyrogens. These

Hypothalamic releasing factors. TRH, *TSH-releasing hormone;* CRF, *ACTH-releasing factor;* LRF, *LH-releasing factor;* FRF, *FSH-releasing factor;* MRF *and* MIF, *MSH-releasing and -inhibiting factors;* PIF *and* PRF, *prolactin-inhibiting and -releasing factors;* GRF *and* GIF, *GH-releasing and -inhibiting factors;* TSH, *thyroid-stimulating hormone;* ACTH, *adrenocorticotropic hormone;* LH, *luteinizing hormone;* FSH, *follicle-stimulating hormone;* MSH, *melanocyte-stimulating hormone;* PL, *prolactin;* GH, *growth hormone.*

FIG. 47-1

From Frohman, L.A.: N. Engl. J. Med. **286**:1391, 1972.

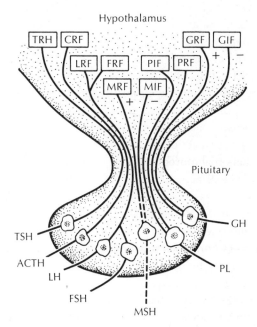

actions could be caused by an antiadrenergic, antidopaminergic, or antiserotoninergic effect of the phenothiazines.

Luteinizing hormone (LH)– and follicle-stimulating hormone (FSH)–releasing factors. Experimental studies indicate that dopamine is a stimulatory and serotonin is an inhibitory neurotransmitter involved in the release of LRF and FRF. The administration of L-dopa leads to a rise in plasma FSH and a more variable rise in plasma LH. The phenothiazines have been claimed to inhibit LRF secretion, whereas FRF was unaffected or even stimulated.

The semisynthetic ergot alkaloid **bromocriptine** (2-bromo-α-ergocryptine) is a drug that acts on dopamine receptors. It is being tried in the treatment of galactorrhea as well as in puerperal lactation, hyperprolactinemia, hypogonadism, acromegaly, and parkinsonism.[14]

Bromocriptine mesylate (Parlodel) is available in 2.5 mg tablets. As a dopaminergic drug, it lowers serum prolactin levels, and it is used in the management of reproductive disorders associated with hyperprolactinemia and suppression of postpartum lactation and in acromegaly. The drug is used also in the treatment of Parkinson's disease.

Prolactin-inhibiting factor (PIF). Galactorrhea is produced by a variety of psychotropic drugs, such as the phenothiazines, reserpine, methyldopa, and imipramine. It is believed that dopamine promotes the secretion of a PIF.

Growth hormone–releasing factor (GHRF). There is a strong suspicion of an adrenergic control of GHRF secretion. Dextroamphetamine stimulates GHRF, the effect being enhanced by propranolol. GHRF appears to be stimulated by α-adrenergic and inhibited by β-adrenergic mechanisms. Reserpine and chlorpromazine reduce the GHRF hypoglycemia. In an acromegalic patient, chlorpromazine caused a decrease in growth hormone levels.

Somatostatin, a tetradecapeptide, is found not only in the hypothalamus but also in the gastrointestinal tract and the pancreatic islets.[2] It inhibits the secretion of growth hormone, thyrotropin, glucagon, insulin, and some other hormones.

GROWTH HORMONE

Human growth hormone, also known as *somatotropin* (Asellacrin), although very scarce, is available for the treatment of hypopituitary drawfism. It is administered by intramuscular injection. Growth hormone produces gigantism or acromegaly, depending on the individual's age.

The growth hormone has antiinsulin effects and is diabetogenic. Some of its actions, however, are similar to those of insulin; for example, both promote the cellular uptake of amino acids.

Many of the actions of growth hormone require factors known as *somatomedins*, which are elaborated largely by the liver.

GONADOTROPINS AND SEX HORMONES

Gonadotropin secretion is regulated by hypothalamic centers that communicate with the anterior pituitary by means of releasing factors. Dopamine plays an important role in these central regulations. FSH promotes the growth of the follicle and the secretion of estrogens. LH, which is identical to the interstitial cell–stimulating hormone (ICSH), produces ovulation and promotes secretion of progesterone from the corpus luteum. Estrogens and progesterone exert a negative feedback on the secretion of gonadotropins.

Estrogens promote the growth of the reproductive organs in the female. They promote growth and cornification of the vaginal epithelium and stimulate cervical mucous secretion. Progesterone contributes to the differentiation in the female reproductive organs and is responsible for the secretions of the endometrium during the luteal phase of the menstrual cycle.

In the male, testosterone is secreted by the interstitial cells of Leydig. The anterior pituitary gland stimulates the activities of Leydig's cells by means of the hormone LH, also known as ICSH in the earlier literature.

Prolactin

Prolactin is unique among pituitary hormones, its secretion being controlled by a predominantly inhibitory influence from the hypothalamus. Dopamine is the primary inhibitory factor, whereas protirelin is a potent stimulus for secretion of prolactin. Estrogens also increase prolactin release. Patients with hyperprolactinemia have a syndrome of gonadal dysfunction, galactorrhea, hirsutism, and obesity. Drugs that lower prolactin concentration are the dopamine agonists such as bromocriptine mesylate, levodopa, apomorphine, and clonidine. Drugs that elevate prolactin concentrations are the dopamine antagonists or depletors such as reserpine, methyldopa, the phenothiazines, haloperidol, and metoclopramide.

The traditional schema of the hormonal control of menstruation is shown in Fig. 47-2, whereas the actual measurements of the serum concentrations of various hormones in normal women are depicted in Fig. 47-3.

OVULATORY CYCLE

The rise of serum FSH and LH concentrations in the early phase of the cycle is probably responsible for the initial growth and development of the follicles. FSH and LH act synergistically with regard to follicular maturation.

Ovulation is preceded by a surge of LH and also FSH. The LH surge is of primary importance in causing rupture of the follicle. Progesterone secretion follows the LH surge.

Hormonal control of menstruation.

FIG. 47-2

From Riley, G.M.: Gynecologic endocrinology, New York, 1959, Harper & Row, Publishers, Inc.

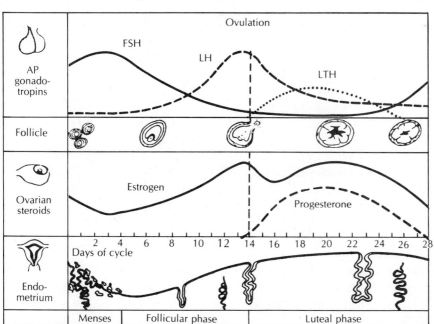

FIG. 47-3 *Serum concentrations of progesterone plotted against mean concentrations of FSH and LH determined in normal women. Centered according to day of LH peak (day 0).*

From Yen, S.S.C., Vela, P., Rankin, J., and Littell, A.S.: JAMA 211:1513, 1970.

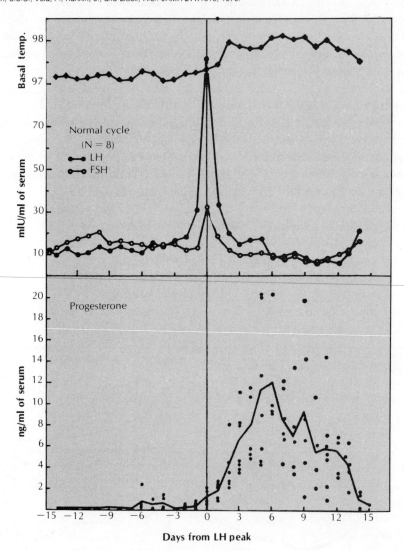

Estrogens, progesterone, and menstruation	The administration of estrogen to a woman without ovarian function can lead to withdrawal bleeding, breakthrough bleeding, or no bleeding, depending on dose and timing. Withdrawal bleeding occurs when the estrogen is employed in low doses for weeks and is suddenly stopped. Bleeding is like normal menstruation except that it is painless and more prolonged. Withdrawal bleeding can also be produced by administration of a single dose of estrogen.

Breakthrough bleeding occurs during the continued administration of a dose of estrogen that is *larger* than the amount necessary to induce withdrawal bleeding. Breakthrough bleeding is unpredictable in onset or amount. If the dose of estrogen is further increased, breakthrough bleeding will cease.

If progesterone is added to the continued administration of estrogen for a few days and then is stopped, menstruation that resembles normal menses will occur. Bleeding is predictable and painful and occurs 3 days after progesterone administration is stopped.

Human chorionic gonadotropin (HCG) is obtained from the urine of pregnant women. It has essentially the same activity as LH and is used for the treatment of cryptorchidism and for some diagnostic purposes. HCG may also be used in the treatment of infertility. Another drug used for the same purpose is **menotropins** (human menopausal gonadotropin [HMG]; Pergonal), which is extracted from the urine of postmenopausal women and contains both FSH and LH activity. Also, **clomiphene citrate** (Clomid), an antiestrogen may induce ovulation. **Danazol** (Danocrin), a derivative of ethisterone, is used for the treatment of endometriosis. It probably acts as an antigonadotropin.

CHORIONIC GONADOTROPIN

The gonadotropins are believed to promote the synthesis of enzymes, which in turn catalyze the various steps in steroidal biosynthesis. These steps in the formation of androstenedione are the same in testis, ovary, and adrenal cortex and may be summarized in the following manner:

Biosynthesis of steroids

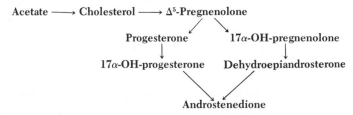

Androstenedione is converted by the ovary to testosterone and is then aromatized and demethylated to estrogens, the major product being estradiol. Estrone is also secreted by the ovary, with estriol being a metabolic product of the ovarian estrogens. Androstenedione may be converted to estrone in adipose tissue also, which may be a significant source of estrogens in premenopausal and particularly in postmenopausal women. In postmenopausal women, the source of androstenedione is principally the adrenal cortex. Estradiol and estrone are interconvertible in the body.

Testosterone may be found not only in the testis but also in the ovary and the adrenal cortex. Testosterone in women originates from these nontesticular sources. Plasma testosterone levels are about 10 times higher in males than in females.

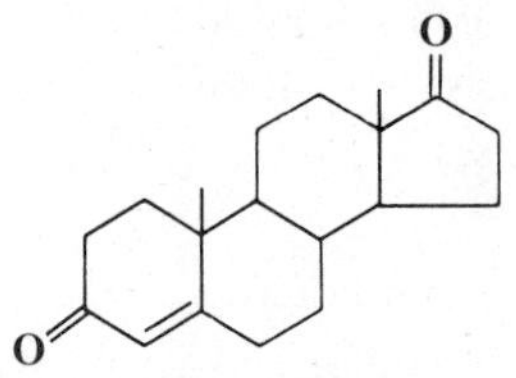

Androstenedione

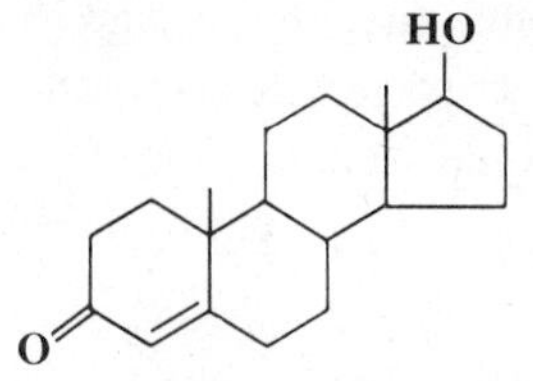

Testosterone

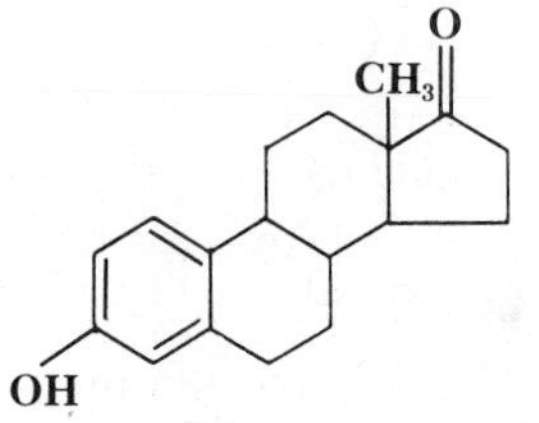

Estrone

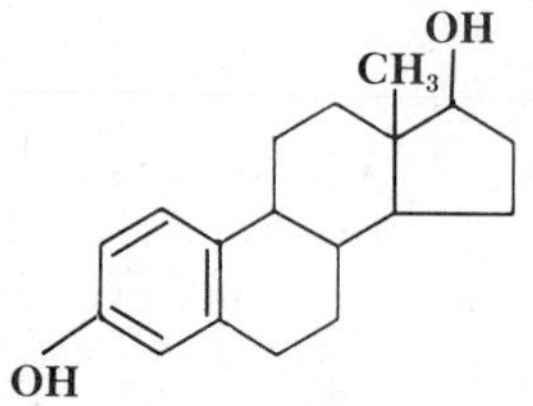

Estradiol

ESTROGENS

The estrogens have important effects on uterine development and cyclic endometrial changes associated with ovulation. They are also responsible for secondary sex characteristics in the female. Study of the estrogens has been greatly facilitated by the early development of a bioassay method based on changes the estrogens produce in the vaginal smear of the rat. The first estrogen isolated and synthesized was estrone, originally called *theelin*.

Estrogen receptor

Estrogens are bound and retained in their target organs by combining with a specific macromolecule—the estrogen receptor. High concentrations of estrogen-binding protein may be found in the uterus, vagina, and mammary gland, and the receptor is also present in many other tissues. It is believed that the receptor is in the cytosol fraction of cells.[4]

Since regulation of protein synthesis in the target tissue is the principal action of steroid hormones, the hormone-receptor complex must be transferred to the nucleus where it causes increased RNA synthesis followed by increased protein synthesis.

In metastatic breast cancer estrogen receptors are measured in the neoplasm to determine hormone sensitivity. Without estrogen receptors the tumor metastases will not respond to hormonal treatment. Response is more probable if receptors can be demonstrated in the tumor.

TYPES

The available estrogens are of two types: the natural and semisynthetic compounds and the synthetic estrogens. The members of the first group either occur naturally or represent slight chemical modifications of such natural compounds.

The synthetic drugs such as diethylstilbestrol appear to be quite different chemically.

Natural and semisynthetic estrogens. **Estradiol,** also known as α-estradol or 17β-estradiol, is the most potent estrogen produced by the ovary. It is used in doses of

0.1 to 0.5 mg three times a day in the form of tablets. It is also available in pellets of 0.4 mg for vaginal suppositories. Oily preparations can also be obtained for intramuscular injection.

Estradiol benzoate, estradiol cyclopentylpropionate, and estradiol dipropionate are available in solution in oil for intramuscular injection.

Estrone is used for intramuscular injection and vaginal suppositories.

Estrogenic substances, conjugated, contain a mixture of estrogens obtained from the urine of pregnant mares. The estrogens are in a conjugated form and are water soluble, whereas the previously mentioned preparations have low water solubility. This mixture is commonly used in the form of tablets, but solutions for parenteral administration are also available. These preparations contain sodium estrone sulfonate and equine estrogens. Their activity is expressed in terms of an equivalent amount of sodium estrone sulfonate. An example of this type of preparation is Premarin. Tablets of this preparation contain amounts varying from 0.3 to 2.5 mg. A synthetic conjugated estrogen is piperazine estrone sulfate.

Ethinyl estradiol is a semisynthetic estrogen of high potency. It is available in tablets and is administered in doses of 0.02 to 0.05 mg one to three times a day. The 3-methyl ether of ethinyl estradiol, known as *mestranol*, is commonly used in contraceptive progestin-estrogen combinations.

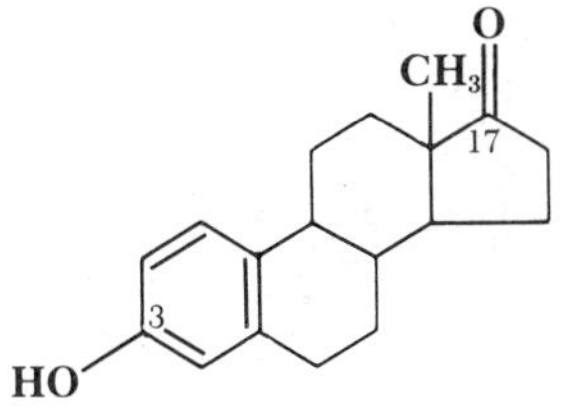

Estrone

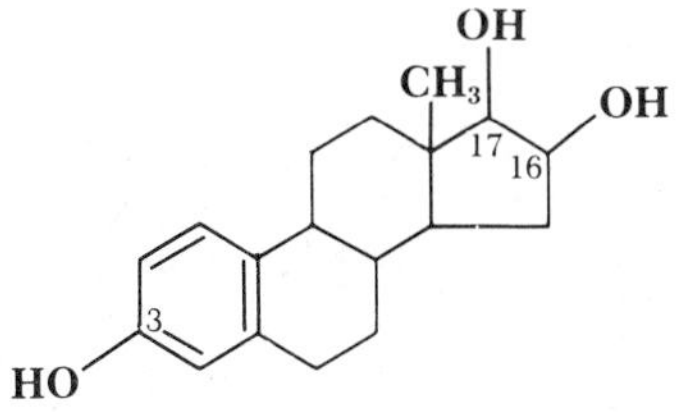

Estriol

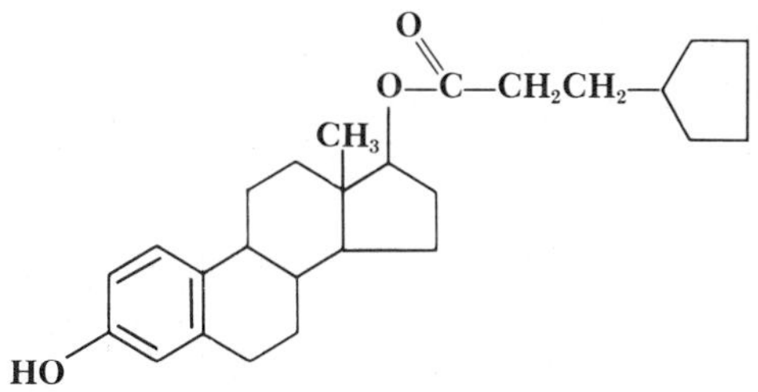

Estradiol cyclopentylpropionate

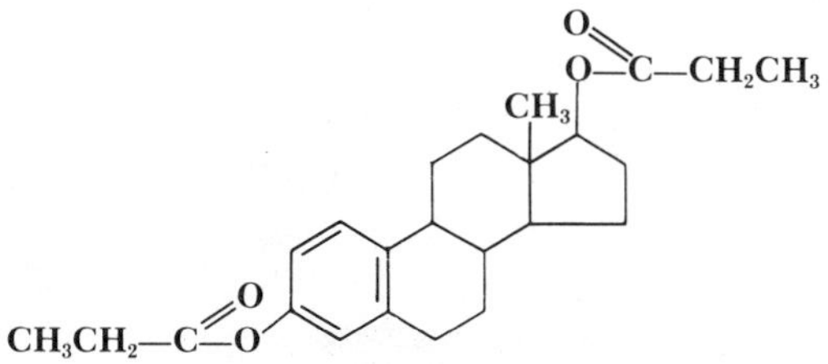

Estradiol dipropionate

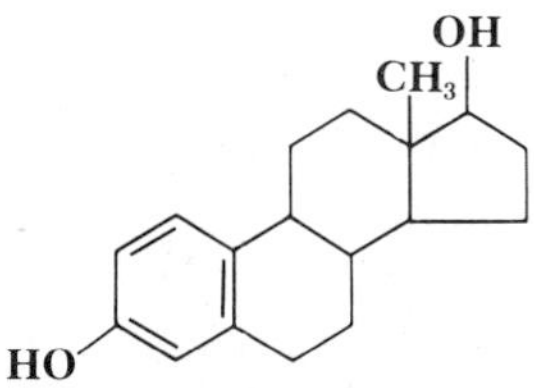

Estradiol

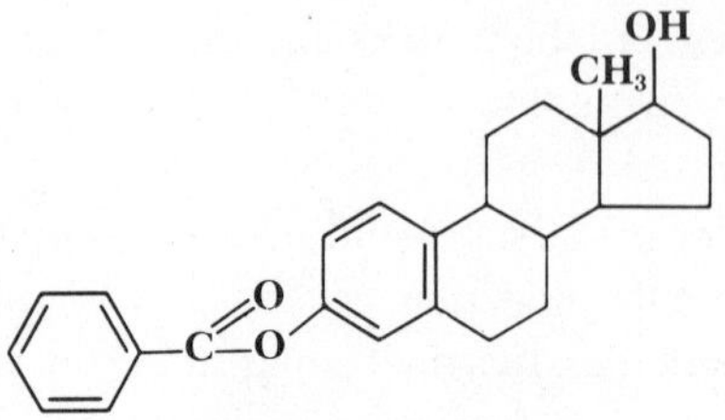

Estradiol benzoate

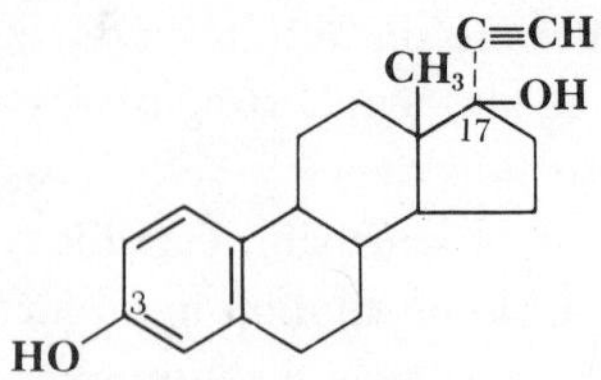

Ethinyl estradiol

Estriol may be a conversion product of estradiol. It is available in tablet form and is administered in doses of 0.06 to 0.12 mg one to four times a day.

Synthetic (nonsteroidal) estrogens. The synthesis of diethylstilbestrol led to recognition of the fact that simple derivatives of stilbene can produce all the effects of naturally occurring estrogens in the body. In addition, they are highly effective when administered by mouth. Many of the synthetic estrogens can be visualized as having basic structural similarities to estradiol. Others, termed *proestrogens*, must undergo metabolic alteration before they become active in the body. A prime example of a proestrogen is chlorotrianisene.

Diethylstilbestrol is used in tablet form, in ointments and suppositories, and in oily solutions for intramuscular injection. The usual dose is 0.5 to 1 mg/day.

Diethylstilbestrol administration during pregnancy is *strictly contraindicated*. A number of daughters of women who received diethylstilbestrol during pregnancy have developed vaginal adenosis or adenocarcinoma after puberty.

Other synthetic estrogens are dienestrol, hexestrol, benzestrol, and promethestrol dipropionate. The doses of these are of the same order of magnitude as those of diethylstilbestrol.

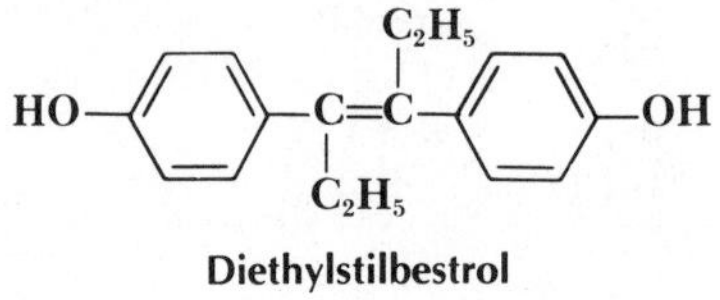

Diethylstilbestrol

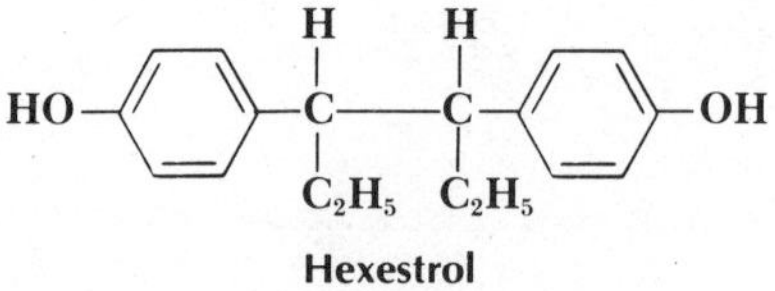

Hexestrol

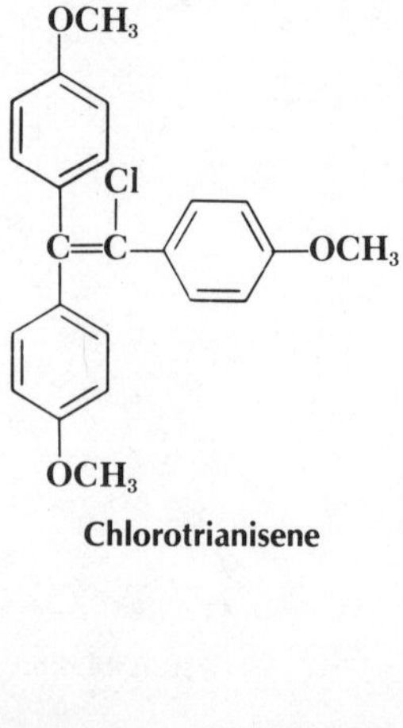

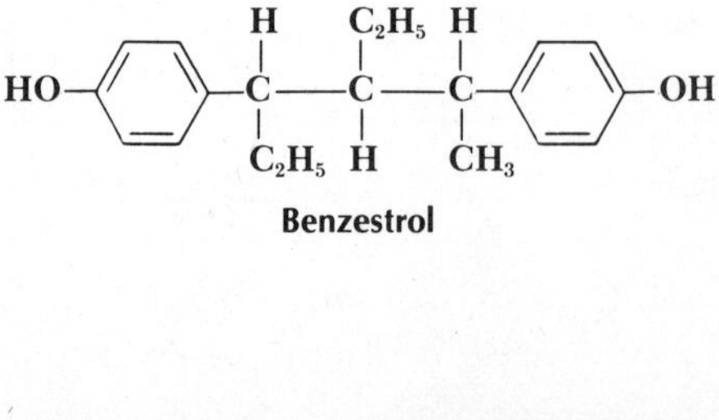

Benzestrol

Chlorotrianisene

Chlorotrianisene (Tace) has a very long duration of action, probably as a consequence of its storage in body fat. It is believed to be converted to an active compound in the body. It is available in capsules containing 12 mg in corn oil.

Clomiphene (Clomid), a drug structurally related to chlorotrianisene, appears to stimulate pituitary gonadotropin output in women, although it inhibits the pituitary gland in the rat. It is being tried with some success in treatment of some types of infertility. Clomiphene has been termed an *antiestrogen*. Its stimulant effect on gonadotropin output in women may be a consequence of removal of inhibition exerted by estrogens.

Clomiphene, available in 50 mg tablets, is used for promoting ovulation. Administered in courses of several days, the drug is highly effective. It can also have adverse effects, causing menopausal symptoms (hot flashes), enlargement of the ovaries, and multiple pregnancies that are more common than in normally ovulating women. This incidence has been estimated at 5% to 10%.

Other fertility drugs. It is of considerable investigational interest that extracts of the human pituitary gland or of menopausal urine (human menopausal gonadotropins) are highly effective in promoting ovulation. Given by injection, these investigational drugs cause considerable enlargement of the ovary and an abnormally high incidence of multiple pregnancies.

The preparation of **human menopausal gonadotropins (menotropins)** contains large amounts of FSH and LH. Its mode of action involves the ovary directly, whereas clomiphene acts indirectly as an antiestrogen on the production of the gonadotropins. Enlargement of the ovary occurs within 2 weeks after the administration of menotropins and may lead to ascites, bleeding, and rupture of ovarian cysts. Multiple births may occur in 20% of women who become pregnant after the use of menotropins.

The preparation is injected intramuscularly and is administered daily for 10 days. Menotropins (Pergonal) are available as a powder containing 75 IU of FSH and 75 IU of LH to make a solution for intramuscular injection.

The estrogens are responsible for the secondary sex characteristics in the female. They produce the proliferative endometrium. They have weak androgenic and anabolic actions. They exert a negative feedback on FSH secretion and when decreased, they cause the symptoms of menopause.

EFFECTS

Estrogens are used to replace the hormones in hypogonadal and hypopituitary states and in menopause. They may be useful in the treatment of osteoporosis. Other uses include the treatment of atrophic vaginitis, suppression of postpartum lactation, and prostatic carcinoma. They are also components of oral contraceptive agents.

CLINICAL USES

Persons with liver damage, as in cirrhosis, may excrete a much higher percentage of an estrogen than do normal persons. This hepatic inactivation is also the probable reason for the greater effectiveness of the natural estrogens when administered parenterally. Estrone, for example, may be 10 times as effective by the intramuscular

METABOLISM

route as by mouth. On the other hand, the synthetic estrogens are highly effective by mouth. This and other evidence indicate that synthetic estrogens are not degraded as rapidly or as completely as are the natural forms. Chlorotrianisene has a prolonged action because it is stored in body fat.

TOXICITY   The only adverse effects of the estrogens observed in a significant number of patients are anorexia, nausea, and vomiting. These symptoms are more likely to develop following the use of the synthetic compounds, diethylstilbestrol being the worst offender in this respect. It is likely, however, that some women become nauseated following the use of any of the estrogens.

PROGESTERONE   Progesterone is produced by the corpus luteum and has also been prepared synthetically.

Progesterone   **Ethisterone**

Progesterone is responsible for the secretory phase of endometrial development. Its effects on the vaginal epithelium and on cervical mucous secretions are the opposite of those of the estrogens. Withdrawal of progesterone results in menstruation. Progesterone is metabolically degraded to pregnanediol, which appears in the urine.

Pharmacological effects of large doses of progesterone include suppression of ovulation, inhibition of the contractility of the uterus, increased sodium excretion, and negative nitrogen balance.

The hormone is assayed in the rabbit on the basis of its progestational effect on the endometrium; the international unit is 1 mg of purified progesterone.

Metabolism   Progesterone is not well absorbed from the gastrointestinal tract following oral administration. It is much more effective when injected intramuscularly or administered sublingually. The intramuscular dose is 10 mg. Similar or even larger doses are used sublingually. Progesterone is metabolically altered in the body, the liver playing an important role in this respect. The urinary excretory products of progesterone are pregnanediol and pregnanolone.

Progesterone and particularly the *progestogens* find applications in numerous   *Clinical uses*
clinical situations. The progestogens are synthetic derivatives of 19-nortestosterone
or progesterone. In contrast with progesterone, they are effective when given orally.
They differ also in that some preparations are androgenic, but others have estrogenic
activity.

Progesterone and the progestogens are used for the cyclic treatment of amenorrhea and dysmenorrhea in addition to antifertility effects. These hormones may
also be useful in the treatment of threatened abortions and as replacement therapy
in infertile women.

Progesterone itself is available in the form of parenteral preparations in water or
oil for intramuscular injection. The drug is ineffective when given by mouth.

The following progestogens are used for purposes other than contraception.

Hydroxyprogesterone caproate (Delalutin) is a progesterone derivative without
estrogenic activity and without masculinizing effect on the fetus. It is available as an
injectable solution in oil, 125 mg/ml, administered intramuscularly.

Dydrogesterone (Duphaston; Gynorest) is a progesterone derivative that is active
by oral administration. The drug has no estrogenic or androgenic activity. It is
available in tablets containing 5 and 10 mg.

Norethindrone (Norlutin) and **norethindrone acetate** (Norlutate) are derivatives
of 19-nortestosterone, having some androgenic activity. They should not be used in
threatened abortion because of masculinizing effect on the fetus. Both drugs are
available in tablets containing 5 mg.

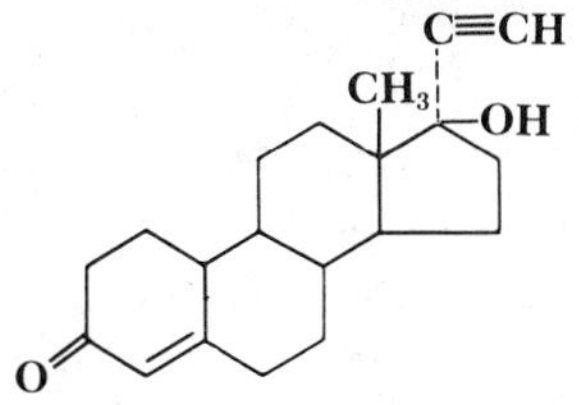

Norethindrone

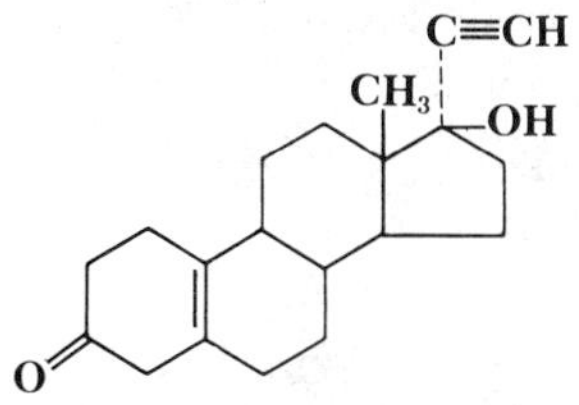

Norethynodrel

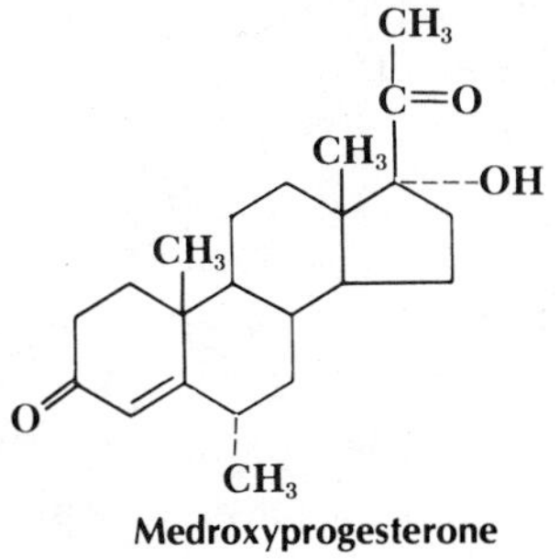

Medroxyprogesterone

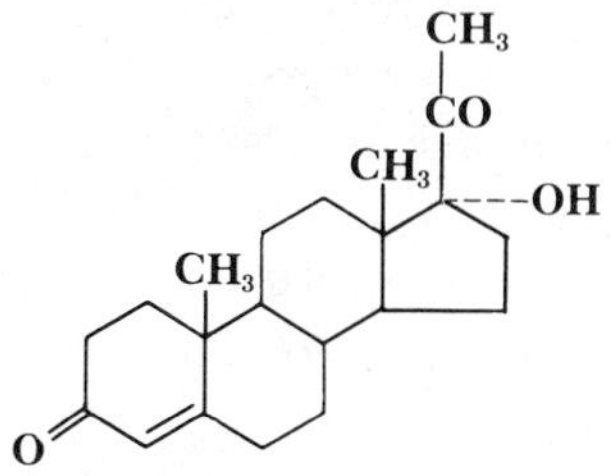

17α-Hydroxyprogesterone

ORAL CONTRACEPTIVES

The first report on the successful inhibition of ovulation by orally administered norethynodrel-mestranol appeared in 1956. Just 10 years later more than 7 million women were taking oral contraceptives. Results indicate that such drugs are the most effective means of controlling fertility, although all the ultimate consequences of such a mass medication are not completely known.

The oral contraceptives contain either a mixture of a synthetic estrogen and progestin or, less frequently, progestin alone ("minipills"). The combination products may contain a "regular" or "low dose" of the estrogen.

Progestogen-estrogen combinations

The mode of action of the combined administration of progestogens and estrogens involves the inhibition of ovulation by an interference with hypothalamic-pituitary mechanisms. They may also have additional sites of action. There is good evidence for an alteration of the characteristics of cervical mucus by the combined treatment. It is possible also that the changes in the endometrium or the secretions of the fallopian tubes are such as to interfere with fertilization.

The progestogen-estrogen combinations are used in the following manner. A single dose a day is taken from the fifth through the twenty-fourth day of the cycle, counting from the first day of menstruation. Withdrawal bleeding occurs within 3 to 4 days after the last dose.

Low-dosage progestogens

Continued low-dosage progestogen is also being tried as an approach to the control of fertility. Chlormadinone, an analog of medroxyprogesterone, has antifertility effects in very small doses. This form of treatment does not prevent ovulation. The mode of action of low-dosage progestogen is not clear. It may put the endometrium out of phase with ovulation or it may alter cervical mucus or tubal physiology.

The "minipills" containing only progestin cause menstrual irregularities and are not popular. They are also less effective than the combination products.

Adverse effects

The major adverse effects of the oral contraceptives are thromboembolic disorders, hypertension, and depression. Minor problems are headache, nausea, weight gain, and mood change. Although the major adverse effects are not as common as in pregnancy, they require caution. Contraindications to the use of the oral contraceptives include estrogen-dependent tumors, liver disease, thrombophlebitis, abnormal uterine bleeding, and pregnancy.

ANDROGENS Testosterone

The principal testicular hormone is testosterone. Its isolation and synthesis from testicular extracts were preceded by the isolation of one of its metabolic products, androsterone.

The orally effective androgens include methyltestosterone, fluoxymesterone, and methandrostenolone. Testosterone propionate is available for parenteral administration. All these compounds are androgenic and anabolic.

The most widely used androgens are testosterone, methyltestosterone propionate, and testosterone cyclopentylpropionate.

Testosterone   Methyltestosterone   Testosterone cyclopentylpropionate

The main effect of the androgens is on the development of secondary sexual **Effects** characteristics in males with stimulation of anabolism, growth, and muscular development. Some synthetic analogs of the androgens may have relatively greater anabolic than androgenic effects, and they are termed anabolic steroids. Despite this claim, they may cause some virilization.

Testosterone is metabolized in the liver and is excreted in the urine as andros- **Metabolism** terone and etiocholanolone. Methyltestosterone and fluoxymesterone are not inactivated readily by the liver because they are substituted in the 17-position. As a consequence, they can be administered orally. Esters of testosterone, such as the propionate are administered parenterally, and they are absorbed slowly from the intramuscular site, having a long duration of action.

Indications for the use of androgens include hypogonadism in the male, metastatic breast carcinoma, and delayed puberty.

After the anabolic effects ot testosterone were recognized, efforts were made to **ANABOLIC** dissociate them from the androgenic effects. This research has resulted in a group **STEROIDS** of drugs known as *anabolic steroids*. Although these steroids have a greater effect on nitrogen retention than their virilizing action would predict, the separation of these effects is not complete. As a consequence, they should be used with great caution in children with growth problems.

Nandrolone phenpropionate   Methandrostenolone

The anabolic steroids are used sometimes in the treatment of osteoporosis and various conditions in which a negative nitrogen balance exists.

Fluoxymesterone

The anabolic steroids available for oral administration are ethylesternol (Maxibolin), methandrostenolone (Dianabol), norethandrolone (Nilevar), oxandrolone (Anavar), oxymetholone (Adroyd; Anadrol), and stanozolol (Winstrol). Anabolic steroids for intramuscular use include nandrolone phenpropionate (Durabolin), nandrolone decanoate (Deca-Durabolin), and norethandrolone injection (Nilevar). Fluoxymesterone (Halotestin; Ora-Testryl; Ultandren) is used not only as an anabolic steroid but also for androgen deficiency.

The anabolic steroids have numerous disadvantages. They may cause sodium retention, masculinization of the fetus if used in pregnant women (a definite contraindication), and aggravation of carcinoma of the prostate. Their use is hazardous in children because of their virilizing effect. In addition, androgens or estrogens may actually lead to premature epiphyseal closure when used in children to stimulate their growth. Another adverse effect caused by anabolic steroids that resemble methyltestosterone (17-alkyl-substituted steroids) is cholestatic jaundice.

REFERENCES

1. Adlercreutz, H.: Hepatic metabolism of estrogens in health and disease, N. Engl. J. Med. **290**:1081, 1974.
2. Brazeau, P., and Guillemin, R.: Somatostatin: newcomer from the hypothalamus, N. Engl. J. Med. **290**:963, 1974.
3. Cassar, J., Mashiter, K., and Joplin, G.F.: Bromocryptine treatment of acromegaly, Metabolism **26**:539, 1977.
4. Chan, L., and O'Malley, B.W.: Mechanism of action of the sex steroid hormones, N. Engl. J. Med. **294**:1322, 1976.
5. Goldgien, A.: Estrogen replacement therapy in postmenopausal women, Ration. Drug Ther. **11**(1):1, 1977.
6. Griffin, J.E., and Wilson, J.D.: The syndromes of androgen resistance, N. Engl. J. Med. **302**:198, 1980.

7. Jensen, E.V., and DeSombre, E.R.: Estrogen-receptor interactions, Science **182**:126, 1973.
8. Kirby, R.W., Kotchen, T.A., and Rees, D.: Hyperprolactinemia—a review of recent clinical advances, Arch. Intern. Med. **139**:1415, 1979.
9. Lipsett, M.B.: Physiology and pathology of the Leydig cell, N. Engl. J. Med. **303**:682, 1980.
10. McGuire, W.L.: Steroid receptors and breast cancer, Hosp. Pract., April 1980, p. 83.
11. Phillips, L.S., and Vassilopoulou-Sellin, R.: Somatomedins, N. Engl. J. Med. **302**:371, 438, 1980.
12. Quigley, M.M., and Hammond, C.B.: Estrogen-replacement therapy—help or hazard, N. Engl. J. Med. **301**:646, 1979.

13. Schally, A.V., Kastin, A.J., and Arimura, A.: Hypothalamic hormones: the link between brain and body, Am. Sci. **65**:712, 1977.

14. Vaisrub, S.: The many faces of bromocriptine (editorial), JAMA **235**:2854, 1976.

15. Van Wyk, J.J., and Underwood, L.E.: Growth hormone, somatomedins and growth failure, Hosp. Pract., Aug. 1978, p. 57.

16. Weindling, H., and Henry, J.B.: Laboratory test results altered by "The Pill", JAMA **229**:1762, 1974.

Chapter 48

Pharmacological approaches to gout

**GENERAL
CONCEPT**

Gout is characterized by hyperuricemia and arthritis. The disease may be *primary*—caused by overproduction or defective renal excretion of uric acid. The *secondary* form develops during some other disease, such as leukemia, or is caused by
drugs such as the thiazide diuretics.

In general, patients with gout may be divided into those who overproduce uric
acid and those who underexcrete it.[6] The overproducers excrete about 1 g of uric
acid daily in the urine and have a large increase in their body pool of uric acid. The
underexcretors have only a moderately increased body pool of uric acid. The daily
urinary excretion of more than 750 mg indicates overproduction.[6]

The pharmacological approach to an acute attack is different from the management
of the chronic disease. The acute attack is a form of acute arthritis that responds best
to *colchicine*, although *phenylbutazone, oxyphenbutazone, indomethacin,* or *adrenal
corticoids* may also be effective. The aim of management of the chronic form of the
disease is to reduce the uric acid content of the body with uricosuric drugs such as
probenecid or *sulfinpyrazone*. The use of *allopurinol*, a xanthine oxidase inhibitor,
may have advantages over the uricosuric drugs in some cases.

COLCHICINE

Colchicine is an alkaloid obtained from *Colchicum autumnale*, or meadow saffron,
a plant belonging to the lily family. Colchicum has been used for centuries for
althralgia that is presumably of gouty origin.

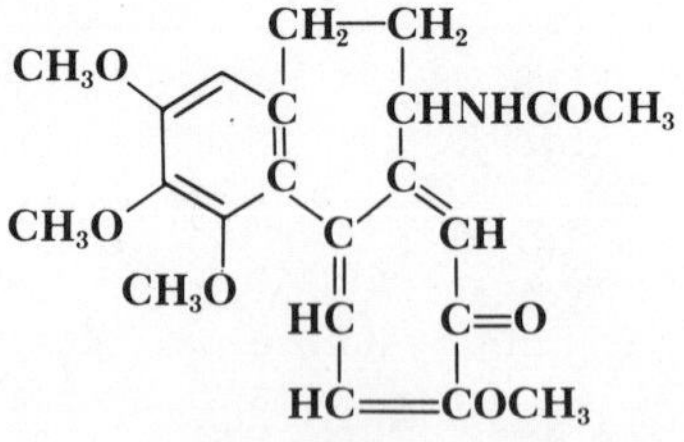

Colchicine

Colchicine is well absorbed from the gastrointestinal tract and has a short half-life in plasma. However, it may remain for a longer period in cells such as the leukocytes. Also, patients with renal disease retain colchicine longer.

When colchicine is given in doses of 0.5 to 1 mg every hour to a patient having an attack of acute gouty arthritis, relief occurs in 2 to 3 hours, but in severe attacks a somewhat longer period is required. It is quite common for gastrointestinal disturbances such as anorexia, nausea, vomiting, diarrhea, and abdominal pain to appear with about the same dosage as the one required for relief. As a consequence, colchicine is administered every hour until relief is obtained or until significant gastrointestinal symptoms develop. In addition to gastrointestinal side effects, colchicine may also cause, although rarely, fever, alopecia, liver damage, and neural and hepatopoietic complications.

Colchicine is known to interfere with the microtubular system in various cells.[7] In the case of gout, it is believed that the effect of colchicine is exerted on leukocytes, which accumulate in the joints and ingest the sharp urate crystals. It is quite possible, however, that the effect of colchicine is also exerted on synovial cells.

In chronic gout the administration of colchicine appears to have prophylactic value with regard to the incidence of acute exacerbations. In addition, it is generally believed that the promotion of uric acid excretion through the use of the uricosuric drugs is beneficial in the gouty patient. The most effective uricosuric agents are probenecid and sulfinpyrazone.

Probenecid (Benemid) was developed for the purpose of inhibiting tubular secretion of penicillin. Although effective, it is seldom used for this purpose because it is simpler to increase the dosage of penicillin rather than to use two drugs to achieve a higher blood level of the antibiotic.

PROBENECID

$$CH_3CH_2CH_2 \diagdown$$
$$NSO_2 - \langle \bigcirc \rangle - COOH$$
$$CH_3CH_2CH_2 \diagup$$

Probenecid

Probenecid causes marked increase in excretion of uric acid in gouty patients. The drug has been given in doses of 0.5 g three or four times daily for years to gouty patients and has produced significant lowering of serum uric acid. In fact, increased urinary concentration of uric acid may lead to the development of urate stones, and therefore alkalinization of the urine may be desirable in the early stages of therapy.

Renal handling of uric acid apparently involves glomerular filtration, tubular reabsorption, and tubular secretion. Organic anions such as salicylates and probenecid cause retention of uric acid at low doses but are uricosuric at high doses. It is likely that in small doses they compete with uric acid for secretion.

The ability of thiazide diuretics and pyrazinamide to cause uric acid retention may be explained also by an interference with uric acid secretion. For the same reason, salicylates should not be used when probenecid is prescribed for a hyperuricemic patient.

In addition to uricosuric effect, probenecid inhibits tubular secretion of penicillin, iodopyracet (Diodrast), and *p*-aminohippurate. It also blocks conjugation of benzoic acid with glycine and increases the blood levels of *p*-aminosalicylate by some unknown mechanism.

Probenecid is rapidly absorbed from the stomach, giving peak plasma concentrations in 4 hours. The urinary excretion of the drug is pH-dependent, being higher at higher pH values. Treatment should begin with small doses, 250 mg twice a day, to decrease the probability of renal stone formation. Dosage must be gradually increased to the 1 or 1.5 g maintenance level, the ultimate dosage being determined by the serum uric acid determinations. Colchicine is often administered concurrently with probenecid to decrease the likelihood of gouty attacks.

During the use of probenecid for chronic gout, adverse effects may occur in a small percentage of patients. The figure generally given is less than 2%, but in some series adverse reactions or side effects have occurred in 8% of patients. Nausea and vomiting, skin rash, and drug fever may occur. Urate stones may cause renal colic.

SULFINPYRAZONE   Sulfinpyrazone (Anturan), which is structurally related to phenylbutazone, is an effective uricosuric agent. This drug prevents tubular reabsorption of uric acid. Its action is antagonized by salicylates but not by probenecid. The marked increase in urate excretion may predispose to urolithiasis. An acute gouty attack may occur at the beginning of treatment, and epigastric distress has been seen. The similarity in structure between sulfinpyrazone and phenylbutazone suggests caution with regard to hematological disturbances. The usual dose is 50 mg four times daily initially, which may be gradually increased until as much as 400 mg is given daily.

Sulfinpyrazone

ALLOPURINOL   An interesting approach to the treatment of gout is the use of an inhibitor of xanthine oxidase. Allopurinol (Zyloprim) was developed originally for the purpose of protecting 6-mercaptopurine against rapid inactivation in the body. The drug causes a marked decrease in plasma uric acid concentration and in urinary uric acid excretion. Although the oxypurines xanthine and hypoxanthine replace uric acid under these circumstances, renal clearance of the oxypurines is much greater than that of uric acid.

Allopurinol is rapidly oxidized in the body to alloxanthine; 90% to 95% of allopurinol administered is excreted as alloxanthine, the remainder as the original allopurinol. The renal clearance of allopurinol is rapid, while that of alloxanthine is slow—only two or three times the clearance of uric acid. Probenecid promotes the excretion of oxypurinol.

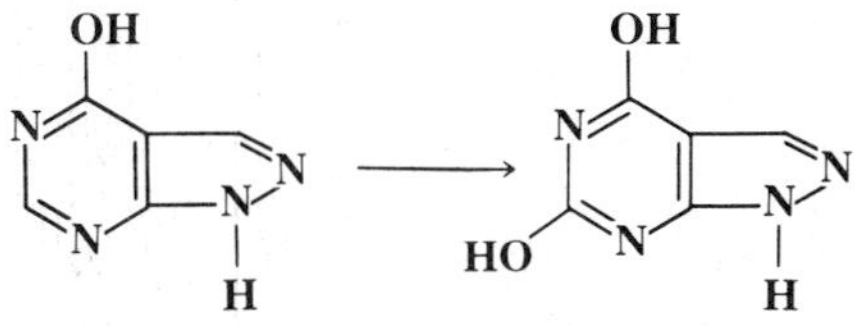

Allopurinol   Oxypurinol

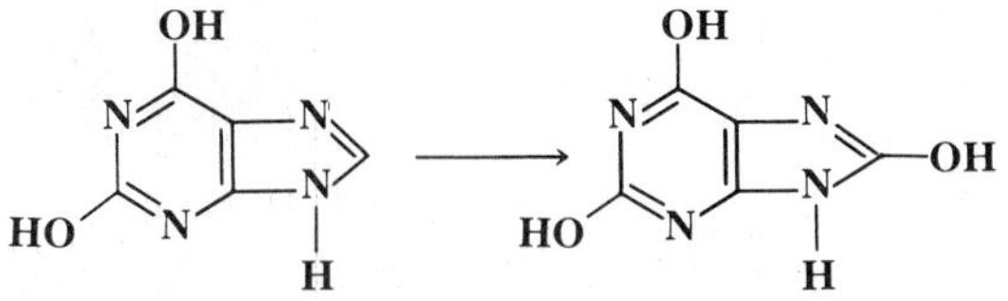

Xanthine   Uric acid

In a series of gouty patients who showed an intolerance to uricosuric agents or failed to respond to them, normal serum urate levels were achieved with doses of 200 to 600 mg/day of allopurinol.

A summary of the present position of allopurinol in the treatment of gout is as follows. Although uricosuric agents are effective in controlling hyperuricemia in most gouty patients, allopurinol may prove to be more useful for a number of reasons. Gouty nephropathy and the formation of urate stones are less likely with allopurinol therapy because the drug *reduces* the amount of uric acid excreted. Colchicine is still the treatment of choice in acute gout and is helpful in the prevention of acute attacks. In severe cases associated with impaired renal function and urate stones, allopurinol appears to be the agent of choice. In addition, the antiinflammatory drugs phenylbutazone and indomethacin may be very useful in the treatment of acute gout.

Reactions to allopurinol have been mild or moderate, although about 3% of patients taking the drug may develop skin eruptions, fever, hepatomegaly, leukopenia, gastrointestinal distress, diarrhea, pruritus, skin rash, headache, and alterations of liver function.

REFERENCES

1. The Anturane Reinfarction Trial Research Group: Sulfinpyrazone in the prevention of cardiac death after myocardial infarction, N. Engl. J. Med. 298:289, 1978.
2. Boss, G.R., and Seegmiller, J.E.: Hyperuricemia and gout, N. Engl. J. Med. 300:1459, 1979.
3. Bryan, J.: Biochemical properties of microtubules, Fed. Proc. 33:152, 1974.
4. Coe, F.L.: Calcium-uric acid nephrolithiasis, Arch. Intern. Med. 138:1090, 1978.
5. Pak, C.Y.C., et al.: Effect of oral purine load and allopurinol on the crystallization of calcium salts in urine of patients with

hyperuricosuric calcium urolithiasis, Am. J. Med. **65:**593, 1978.

6. Rastegar, A., and Thier, S.O.: The treatment of hyperuricemia in gout, Ration. Drug. Ther. **8:**1, 1974.

7. Sorensen, L.B., and Pepe, P.: Hypoxanthine-guanine phosphoribosyltransferase deficiency, Bull. Rheum. Dis. **21:**621, 1970.

8. Steele, T.H., and Boner, G.: Origins of the uricosuric response, J. Clin. Invest. **52:**1368, 1973.

Chapter 49

Antianemic drugs

The maintenance of normal red cell mass and the synthesis of hemoglobin are normally adjusted to take care of the physiological loss of the blood elements. Anemia results when there is excessive loss or diminished replacement of red cells.

GENERAL CONCEPT

Most anemias are deficiency diseases resulting from inadequate tissue concentrations of *iron*, *vitamin* B_{12}, or *folic acid*. Correction of the deficiency is highly successful provided an accurate diagnosis is made. In addition, other drugs, such as *anabolic steroids* and *pyridoxine*, may be useful in some forms of anemia. *Erythropoietin* may be of great importance but is currently only of research interest.

Iron is contained in the body in various forms, principally as hemoglobin. Normal blood contains about 15 g of hemoglobin/100 ml, and each gram of hemoglobin contains 3.4 mg of iron. It may be calculated then that the total normal blood volume contains about 2.6 g of iron, and each milliliter of blood contains 0.5 mg.

IRON Metabolism and effects

In addition to hemoglobin, iron is contained in ferritin, the storage form for iron in the tissues, and in the serum attached to the carrier substance, the globulin transferrin. Minute quantities are also present in the cytochrome enzymes and myoglobin of muscle. Quantitatively, hemoglobin and ferritin contain the bulk of the iron in the body, amounting to a total of about 4 to 5 g.

Under normal circumstances red cells are broken down at a steady rate, their life span being on the order of 120 days. Most of the iron released from the breakdown of hemoglobin is reused. As a consequence, the daily iron requirement in a normal adult is quite low, about 1 mg. Growth, menstruation, and pregnancy increase the iron requirement.

Perhaps the most remarkable fact about the metabolism of iron is the inability of the body to get rid of significant quantities of this element. Only minute quantities are excreted into the feces, and the urinary loss of iron is even less. This is the reason for the very low iron requirement of normal persons.

Absorption and excretion

FIG. 49-1 Metabolism of iron.

Courtesy Lederle Laboratories, American Cyanamid Co., Pearl River, N.Y.

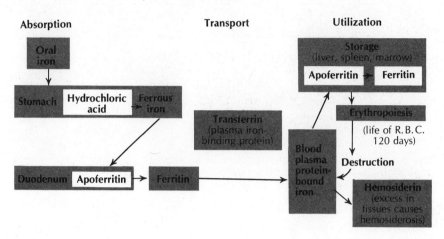

Since the body does not readily eliminate iron, there must be a mechanism that limits its absorption. Otherwise the iron content of the body would steadily increase and hemochromatosis would develop. The mechanism that limits the absorption of iron from the intestine is often referred to as the mucosal block (Fig. 49-1).

Mucosal block   The mucosal cells of the duodenum and proximal jejunum take up iron but transfer only a variable portion of it to the blood. The remainder stays in the cells probably as ferritin and is eventually lost as the cells are sloughed. Iron absorption has the characteristics of a facilitated or active transport. Other metals, such as cobalt and manganese, may cause competitive inhibition.

Iron absorption is altered by various derangements. Increased absorption occurs in iron deficiency and enhanced bone marrow activity. Iron overload and decreased marrow activity may cause lowered rates of iron absorption. The exact mechanism of the control of iron absorption is unknown.

The iron-binding globulin transferrin, or siderophilin, is present in normal blood at such a concentration that when fully saturated it can carry 300 μg of iron/100 ml of blood. Since the normal serum iron level is about 100 μg/100 ml, this means that transferrin is only one-third saturated. The globulin combines with two molecules of iron per protein molecule.

The normal daily diet contains approximately 20 mg of iron. Of this, only about 10% is absorbed, but this quantity is adequate for taking care of the very small daily losses of iron. In iron-deficiency anemia, however, the dietary iron is quite insufficient for reasonably rapid correction of the hemoglobin deficit, even though the mucosal block is greatly diminished.

In addition to the mucosal block, other factors influence the absorption of iron. It is generally believed that ferrous iron is more effectively absorbed than the ferric form. On the other hand, a diet rich in phytate, phosphate (milk), or alkalinizing agents, such as those used for patients with peptic ulcer, tends to decrease absorption of iron.

Dosages of therapeutic iron preparations should be calculated on the basis of their elemental iron content. For the treatment of iron-deficiency anemias in adults a dose of 50 to 100 mg of elemental iron three times daily is recommended.

Iron preparations can be administered both orally and parenterally.

Therapeutic preparations

There are many iron preparations, both organic and inorganic, that may be used in treatment of hypochromic anemias. These drugs differ in absorption from the gastrointestinal tract. It is customary to administer a large excess because not more than 15% of an oral dose is absorbed of even the most effective preparation, ferrous sulfate. The percentage of absorption is considerably less when certain other preparations, such as reduced iron, are administered. The recommended dosages of the various preparations are such that they may be expected to provide absorption of 15 to 25 mg of iron a day in an individual suffering from hypochromic anemia. The following doses are often used:

ORAL

PREPARATION	DOSAGE
Ferrous sulfate tablets	0.3 g three times a day
Ferric ammonium citrate	1.0 g three times a day
Reduced iron	0.5 g three times a day
Ferrous gluconate	0.6 g three times a day
Ferrous fumarate	0.5 g three times a day
Ferrocholinate	0.5 g three times a day

Because of the low degree of efficiency of gastrointestinal absorption of iron, several injectable forms of iron have been introduced.

PARENTERAL

Iron dextran complex (Imferon) is a useful preparation when parenteral administration of iron is mandatory. It was temporarily withdrawn when carcinogenicity in rats and mice and one questionable case in a human being were reported. The preparation contains 50 mg of iron/ml. The dosage is 1 to 4 ml daily intramuscularly. Occasional anaphylactoid and allergic reactions have been reported following its use. Nevertheless, it is less likely to produce severe shocklike states and phlebitis, which may follow the use of the intravenous preparations of iron.

Iron sorbitex (Jectofer) is another intramuscular preparation with characteristics similar to iron dextran.

Dextriferron (Astrafer) is an iron-dextrin complex containing 20 mg/ml of iron. It is replacing saccharated iron oxide (Proferrin) as an intravenous dosage form. The intravenous iron preparations should be used only with the realization of their dangers. They may cause hypotension, vascular collapse, headache, nausea, and ana-phylactoid reactions.

Adverse effects   The oral iron preparations tend to produce nausea and vomiting through a local irritant effect on the stomach. For this reason the preparations are generally admin-istered immediately after meals. Large doses of ferrous sulfate and of ferrous glu-conate have produced poisoning in children. If large amounts of iron are absorbed, it seems that symptoms resembling those of heavy metal poisoning may result.

Parenteral iron should not be used unless oral preparations cannot be tolerated by the patient. Serious reactions may occur, particularly in patients who are also receiving oral iron preparations. Under these circumstances, transferrin is saturated, and the administration of parenteral iron will produce elevated concentrations of unbound metal.

Claims for lower gastrointestinal toxicity of some iron salts are not based on good evidence. It is the amount of ionized iron in a preparation that determines its toxicity.

Chelating agents in   The potent and specific iron chelating agent deferoxamine (Desferal) has been
treatment of iron   used with apparent benefit both in treatment of acute toxic reactions to ferrous
poisoning   gluconate and for removal of iron in patients with overload.

Deferoxamine, also known as desferrioxamine B, is a water-soluble substance of three molecules of trihydroxamic acid. Its molecular weight is 597, and one molecule chelates one molecule of Fe^{+++} ions. The drug is derived from the microbial product ferrioxamine B by removal of iron.

Deferoxamine can bind 8.5 mg iron/100 mg. It removes not only free iron but also iron combined with ferritin and hemosiderin. Transferrin-bound iron is less susceptible to chelation by deferoxamine, and hemoglobin and cytochrome iron are not affected.

Deferoxamine (in combination with iron)

In acute iron poisoning, deferoxamine, 8 to 12 g, is administered by gastic tube. In addition, 1 to 2 g of the drug may be injected intramuscularly or intravenously.

In a small child, repeated doses of deferoxamine (92 mg/kg) have been used with apparent benefit. Smaller doses, 400 to 600 mg daily, are sufficient for promotion of iron excretion in hemochromatosis.

Iron is effective in the treatment of iron-deficiency anemias. In these states the mean corpuscular volume is below 80 μ, and the mean corpuscular hemoglobin concentration is below 30%. These anemic states are generally caused by chronic blood loss or by a deficient dietary supply of iron. The latter is more likely to occur in a growing child.

Use of iron in anemias

In most instances ferrous sulfate is quite adequate for the treatment of iron deficiency. Its main disadvantages are gastric irritation, diarrhea, and constipation. It may be advisable to use small doses at first and to increase the dose gradually over a period of 1 to 2 weeks. In general there is no advantage in the addition of cobalt, other metals, or folic acid to preparations whose purpose is to supply iron.

The effectiveness of therapy with ferrous sulfate manifests itself in a rise of the reticulocyte count within 7 days, an increase in hemoglobin levels by 1 to 2 g/100 ml within 3 weeks, and evidence of clinical improvement in 2 to 3 weeks.

Vitamin B_{12} (cyanocobalamin) is a cobalt-containing compound having a molecular weight of 1400. Its isolation from liver brought to a successful conclusion more than 20 years of investigation aimed at finding the cause of *pernicious anemia*.

VITAMIN B_{12}

Until 1926 pernicious anemia was entirely incurable. At that time the key observation was made that large amounts of liver had a beneficial effect in the treatment of the disease. Subsequent work was aimed at purification of the liver factor responsible for the curative effect. Soon injectable purified liver extracts of great potency were available.

The problem of pernicious anemia appeared more complex, however, than a simple deficiency of a liver factor. Clinical experiments showed that normal gastric juice contained an intrinsic factor that had to interact with a dietary extrinsic factor for the erythrocyte maturation factor present in liver to be obtained.

When folic acid was isolated in 1943, it was believed at first that the compound was in some way related to the cause of pernicious anemia. It was soon found, however, that whereas folic acid could remedy the hematological manifestations of the disease, it either had no effect or aggravated the neurological symptoms. Since liver extract was effective against both these aspects of pernicious anemia, it was clear that folic acid could not represent the liver factor.

The picture became clear when vitamin B_{12} was isolated in 1948. It appears that the absorption of vitamin B_{12} requires the presence of the intrinsic factor of Castle. This is lacking in true addisonian pernicious anemia. Furthermore, injected vitamin B_{12} remedies both hematological and neurological disturbances in pernicious anemia. When reasonable doses of the vitamin are administered by mouth to patients with pernicious anemia, they are ineffective unless some normal gastric juice is given simultaneously. Thus there is little doubt at present that vitamin B_{12} represents both the extrinsic factor and the erythrocyte maturation factor. The function of the intrinsic factor has to do with the absorption of vitamin B_{12}.

Chemistry   The vitamin has been called cyanocobalamin and is only one member of several cobalamins, all of which have vitamin B_{12} activity. The compound has been isolated not only from liver but also from fermentation liquors of *Streptomyces griseus*, the organism that produces streptomycin.

Unlike many other vitamins, vitamin B_{12} is not present in higher plants but can be synthesized by certain microorganisms. Human liver contains at least 400 μg of the vitamin/kg, and beef liver may contain up to 100 μg/kg. Cow's milk contains more than human milk, up to 4 μg/L.

Indication for use   The vitamin is indicated in treatment of megaloblastic states caused by a deficient supply or absorption of vitamin B_{12}. In the majority of cases the deficiency is in the absorption. This is certainly the case in pernicious anemia and following gastrectomy.

Vitamin B_{12}

In *Diphyllobothrium latum* (fish tapeworm) infestation the worm itself may concentrate much of the vitamin supplied in the diet.

There are other megaloblastic states in which a deficiency of folic acid exists, and treatment should be based on correction of the deficiency rather than on administration of vitamin B_{12}. Some of these megaloblastic states are nutritional macrocytic anemia, certain cases of sprue, megaloblastic anemia of pregnancy, megaloblastic anemia of infants, and certain cases of adult scurvy.

When 0.5 µg of labeled vitamin B_{12} was administered orally to normal persons, about 31% was excreted in the feces. In patients with pernicious anemia the fecal excretion averaged 88%. When an intrinsic factor preparation was administered simultaneously, the excretion of the vitamin in patients with pernicious anemia decreased to normal levels. Fecal excretion of the labeled vitamin was also very high in patients following gastrectomy. On the other hand, in megaloblastic anemia of pregnancy there is no deficiency in the absorption of vitamin B_{12}.

Vitamin B_{12} does not appear in urine under normal circumstances, probably because the compound is bound to plasma proteins. However, if a large dose of nonlabeled vitamin B_{12} (1000 µg) is injected intramuscularly following oral administration of the labeled compound, normal individuals excrete as much as 30% of the radioactivity in the urine within 24 hours. Apparently the nonradioactive material displaces the labeled compound from its binding sites. This observation has been adapted to the diagnosis of pernicious anemia, since under similar circumstances a patient suffering from the disease will excrete only insignificant quantities in the urine, usually less than 2.5% of the administered dose.

Following intramuscular injection of large doses, much of vitamin B_{12} is excreted in the urine, both in normal individuals and in patients with pernicious anemia. The percentage of the dose excreted increases with the quantity administered. Thus when 40 µg is injected, 75% appears in the urine, whereas 60% of the dose may be similarly excreted when 100 µg of the vitamin is injected.

Oral administration of very large doses of vitamin B_{12} (such as 3000 µg) may result in some absorption, even in patients with pernicious anemia. This may indicate that the deficiency of intrinsic factor is not absolute or that there is some other mechanism of absorption.

Vitamin B_{12} and folic acid correct megaloblastosis by influencing DNA synthesis. The characteristic delayed nuclear maturation in megaloblastosis results from inadequate DNA synthesis, a consequence of deficiencies of vitamin B_{12} and/or folic acid.

The pathway affected by vitamin B_{12} and folic acid is that leading to the synthesis of DNA thymine from deoxyuridylate (dUMP) through the following steps:

$$\text{Deoxyuridine} \longrightarrow \text{Deoxyuridylate} \longrightarrow \text{Thymidylate} \longrightarrow \text{DNA thymine}$$

The methylation of deoxyuridylate to thymidylate requires 5, 10-methylenetetrahydrofolic acid. This requirement explains the role of folic acid in DNA synthesis.

The role of vitamin B_{12} is in the regeneration of tetrahydrofolic acid from 5-methyltetrahydrofolic acid by homocysteine transmethylation:

$$\text{5-Methyltetrahydrofolic acid} \longrightarrow \text{Tetrahydrofolic acid}$$
$$\text{Vitamin } B_{12}$$
$$\text{Homocysteine} \qquad \text{Methionine}$$

FIG. 49-2   *Pathways for DNA thymine synthesis.*

From Waxman, S., Corcino, J., and Herbert, V.: JAMA *214:101, 1970, copyright 1970, American Medical Association.*

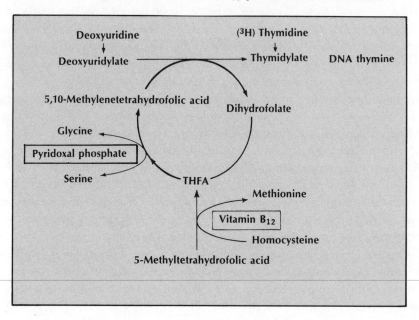

These relationships and the possible role of pyridoxal phosphate are shown in Fig. 49-2.

Preparations and clinical uses

Vitamin B_{12} contains 10 or 15 µg of the vitamin/ml. Injectable liver extracts are now standardized on the basis of their vitamin B_{12} content rather than in terms of USP units, which were based on the hematological response of patients in relapse with pernicious anemia.

In a severely anemic patient, vitamin B_{12} is injected intramuscularly in a dosage of 15 µg. The injection may be repeated every 2 hours for three or four doses. Following this initial treatment, injections of 30 µg of vitamin B_{12} are usually given once a week. In megaloblastic anemias caused by vitamin B_{12} deficiency, a characteristic reticulocyte response appears within 10 days. Some signs of improvement in the general condition of the patient may develop within 48 hours.

FOLIC ACID
Chemistry and nomenclature

Folic acid is pteroylglutamic acid.

The compound may be looked on as a combinaton of pteridine, *p*-aminobenzoic acid, and glutamic acid. In natural materials such as green vegetables the compound occurs in a conjugated form, being attached to six additional glutamic acid residues.

Folic acid is a growth factor for certain microorganisms such as *Streptococcus faecalis*. Its deficiency causes anemia and leukopenia in monkeys and in humans. Folic acid has been synthesized.

Folinic acid (citrovorum factor; Leucovorin) is closely related to folic acid.

Folinic acid

Folic acid is converted in the body to folinic acid. It has been shown that rats fed folic acid excrete some folinic acid in the urine. It has also been demonstrated that rat liver can convert folic acid to folinic acid in vitro, a conversion accelerated by ascorbic acid.

The reactions in which folic acid participates are important in the synthesis of DNA (Fig. 49-2). As a consequence, deficiency of folic acid, whether induced by dietary means or by administration of the folic acid antagonists such as methotrexate, leads to damage in those tissues in which DNA synthesis and turnover are rapid. These include the hematopoietic tissues, the mucosa of the gastrointestinal tract, and the developing embryo.

Functions

Folic acid is available in capsules and tablets containing 5 mg. The vitamin is well absorbed from the gastrointestinal tract, and injectable preparations, although available, are generally unnecessary.

The main use for folic acid is in nutritional macrocytic anemia, certain cases of sprue, megaloblastic anemia of pregnancy, certain cases of megaloblastic anemia in infancy, and scurvy.

It is contraindicated in pernicious anemia. It should not be used in multiple vitamin preparations because it would obscure the diagnosis of unrecognized pernicious anemia. Although it improves the megaloblastic anemia in this instance, it does not protect against the nervous system manifestations of the disease and may even aggravate them.

Preparations and clinical uses

There is evidence for the existence of a circulating erythropoiesis-stimulating factor. This factor, called erythropoietin or hemopoietin, has been detected in the plasma of animals made anemic, exposed to lowered pressures, or treated with cobalt. Such a factor has also been demonstrated in the plasma and urine of anemic human beings. Although this factor is of no therapeutic importance at present, it is of great

ERYTHROPOIETIN

experimental interest and may eventually become important in treatment of certain anemias.

The kidney has been suggested as the site of erythropoietin formation, on the basis of experiments of nephrectomized rats whose response to severe anemia and hypoxia was strikingly reduced. In humans, however, there must be extrarenal sources of erythropoietin, since nephrectomy reduces but does not abolish erythropoiesis. It has also been suggested that the kidney elaborates an erythropoietic factor (REF), the release of which is stimulated by anoxia. This REF acts on a plasma globulin to form erythropoietin.

REFERENCES

1. Propper, R.D., Shurin, S.B., and Nathan, D.G.: Reassessment of the use of desferrioxamine B in iron overload, N. Engl. J. Med. **294**:1421, 1976.

2. Savin, M.A.: A practical approach to the treatment of iron deficiency, Ration. Drug Ther. **11**:1, 1977.

Chapter 50

Vitamins

GENERAL
CONCEPT

The early discoveries of vitamins followed observations on naturally occurring diseases such as scurvy and beriberi. The improvement noted in these diseases when modifications were made in the diet suggested that a deficiency of some sort was the cause of the pathological process. Discoveries came much more rapidly when feeding experiments were performed on experimental animals, and soon the essential nature of many vitamins was recognized.

WATER-SOLUBLE
VITAMINS

Many of the water-soluble vitamins are coenzymes or essential parts of a coenzyme and thus have an essential function in the enzymatic machinery of cells.

Thiamine

Thiamine in the form of thiamine pyrophosphate or cocarboxylase has been shown to play an important role in the decarboxylation of α-keto acids such as pyruvate.

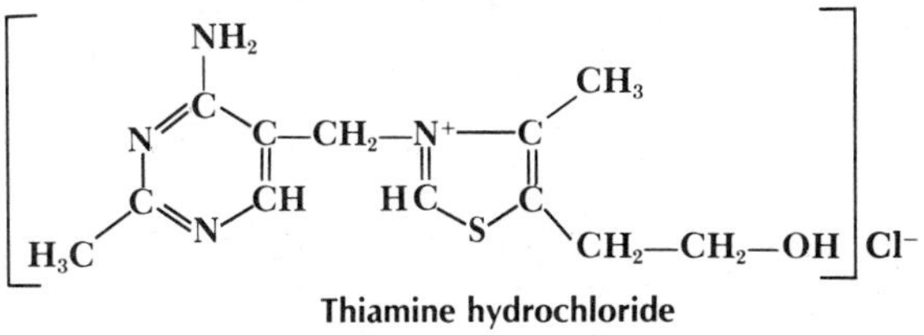

Thiamine hydrochloride

DEFICIENCY

Severe deficiency results in the disease beriberi, characterized by high-output heart failure and peripheral polyneuritis. Other symptoms include anorexia, nausea, intestinal atony, disturbances of peripheral nerves, and mental disorders.

OCCURRENCE

Thiamine is present in sufficient quantities in yeast, wheat germ, and pork. One international or USP unit is equal to 3 μg of thiamine hydrochloride.

Nicotinic acid ·   Nicotinic acid (niacin) is an integral part of at least two important coenzymes, nicotinamide adenine dinucleotide (NAD), formerly called diphosphopyridine nucleotide (DPN), and nicotinamide adenine dinucleotide phosphate (NADP), formerly called triphosphopyridine (TPN).

NAD and NADP can exist in an oxidized or reduced state and can thus act as hydrogen acceptors or donors in many enzymatic reactions of intermediary metabolism. Microsomal enzymes requiring NADP play an important role also in the metabolism of many drugs.

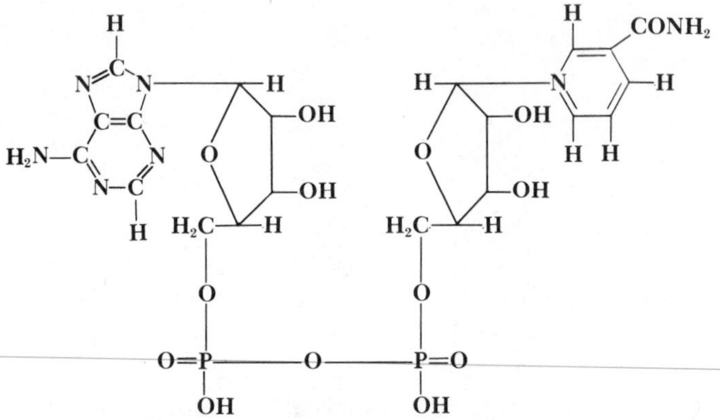

Nicotinamide adenine dinucleotide

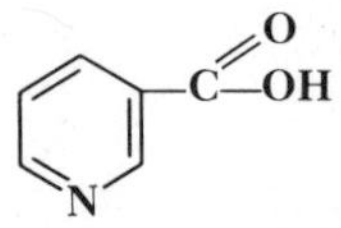

Nicotinic acid 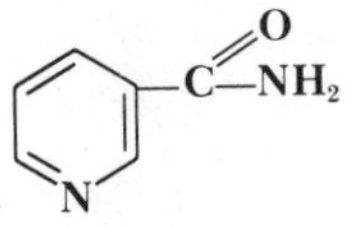   Nicotinamide

---

DEFICIENCY   Pellagra is the disease caused by niacin deficiency. It is characterized by skin lesions, gastrointestinal mucosal changes with diarrhea, and neurological symptoms including mental disorders.

OCCURRENCE   Nicotinic acid is found in significant amounts in yeast, rice, bran, and liver and other meats. Mammals can synthesize nicotinic acid from tryptophan. Pellagra can occur in patients having carcinoid tumor as a consequence of use of tryptophan for serotonin (5-hydroxytryptamine) synthesis.

PHARMACOLOGY   Nicotinic acid, but not nicotinamide, produces marked dilatation of small vessels, an effect that is transient but that may be severe on parenteral administration. On a purely empirical basis, nicotinic acid is used experimentally for lowering serum cholesterol and as a vasodilator, but it is not definitely useful.

Riboflavin is present in flavin adenine dinucleotide (FAD), which is a coenzyme   *Riboflavin*
of flavoprotein enzymes. There is also a flavin mononucleotide (FMN).

A deficiency of riboflavin will cause cheilosis, stomatitis, and keratitis.   *DEFICIENCY*

Riboflavin is present in significant quantities in yeast, green vegetables, liver and   *OCCURRENCE*
other meats, eggs, and milk.

Riboflavin   **Flavin adenine dinucleotide**

Pyridoxine and also pyridoxal and pyridoxamine are various forms of vitamin B_6.   *Pyridoxine*
Pyridoxal phosphate functions as a coenzyme in many reactions such as the decarboxylation of amino acids and transamination reactions between amino acids and keto
acids.

Pyridoxine hydrochloride   **Pyridoxal**   **Pyridoxamine dihydrochloride**

A deficiency of pyridoxine results in dermatitis and convulsions. Thiosemicar-   *DEFICIENCY*
bazide may act as a convulsant by this mechanism. Isoniazid may also cause pyridoxine
deficiency.

Pyridoxine is present in significant amounts in yeast, liver, rice, bran, and wheat   *OCCURRENCE*
germ.

Pantothenic acid   Pantothenic acid is a part of a very important coenzyme known as coenzyme A. Coenzyme A in the form of acetylcoenzyme A is essential for a variety of acetylation reactions such as the formation of acetylcholine from choline and the acetylation of *p*-amino compounds. The coenzyme plays an important role in the Krebs cycle, since citric acid is formed from oxaloacetic acid, acetyl coenzyme A, and water, the reaction regenerating coenzyme A. The coenzyme also plays an important role in fatty acid metabolism.

DEFICIENCY   Pantothenic acid deficiency is not well recognized in humans. In animals it may cause dermatitis, adrenal degeneration, and CNS symptoms.

Coenzyme A

OCCURRENCE   Pantothenic acid is found particularly in yeast, bran, egg yolk, and liver.

Ascorbic acid   Ascorbic acid is a reducing agent whose exact biological function is not understood. It may be a cofactor for the transformation of folic to folinic acid and may be necessary for adrenal cortical function and maintenance of normal connective tissue. The recent claim for ascorbic acid in the prevention of the common cold is not based on convincing evidence, although large-scale, controlled clinical trials are not available for proving or disproving its efficacy.

DEFICIENCY   The classical disease scurvy is characterized by abnormalities in the connective tissue, with capillaries and bone being severely affected.

Ascorbic acid is present in large quantities in citrus fruits, green peppers, to-matoes, and fruits and vegetables in general.

There are several other water-soluble factors essential for experimental animals and presumably for humans. These include biotin, folic acid, choline, and inositol.

The exact biochemical functions of the other water-soluble vitamins are not known, although there is much information available on the clinical consequences of their deficiency.

Vitamin A performs an important function in connection with dark adaptation, being part of the visual purple of the retina. It also maintains the integrity of various epithelial stuctures.

Deficiency of vitamin A produces night blindness, keratinization of the conjunctiva (xerophthalmia), and ulcerations of the cornea (keratomalacia). The skin becomes rough because of hyperkeratosis. Respiratory infections occur in animals deficient in vitamin A, perhaps as a result of changes in the bronchial epithelium, but there is no good evidence to indicate any connection between vitamin A deficiency and respiratory infection in human beings.

Vitamin A

The assay for vitamin A is based on saponification of the oil (palmitate or acetate) by potassium hydroxide, extraction with ethyl ether, and the measurement of the absorbance of ultraviolet light thorugh an isopropanol dilution in a quartz cell at wavelengths of 310, 325, and 334 mμ.

Vitamin A occurs particularly in eggs, milk, vegetables, and fish liver oils.

Vitamin A is stored in the liver. In large quantities the vitamin may cause toxic effects such as anorexia, hepatomegaly, loss of hair, and periosteal thickening of long bones.

Cod liver oil contains 850 IU of vitamin A per gram, a unit being equal to 0.6 μg of β-carotene. Both percomorph liver oil and a water-miscible vitamin A preparation contain 50,000 IU/g. The administration of more than 25,000 IU/day is seldom justified.

Vitamin D   Vitamin D refers to one of several sterols. Vitamin D_2 (calciferol) is obtained by irradiation of ergosterol. The striking developments in relation to vitamin D metabolism are discussed on pp. 549-550.[13]

Vitamin D_3 is present in fish liver oils and is produced in the skin by the action of sunlight on 7-dehydrocholesterol. Dihydrotachysterol has actions resembling those of the parathyroid hormone and was discussed in connection with that subject.

Vitamin D$_2$

Deficiency of vitamin D brings forth the various manifestations of rickets in growing children and animals. There is a disturbance in calcification of bones and teeth. The bones may become soft. Swollen epiphyses and lack of normal calcification are demonstrable by radiological examination.

The main function of vitamin D appears to be exerted on the intestinal absorption of calcium and phosphate. In large quantities the vitamin may exert an effect on bone dissolution similar to the action of the parathyroid hormone.

The daily requirement of vitamin D depends on the calcium needs of the individual. Growing children and pregnant or lactating women require more of the vitamin because their daily calcium absorption must be greater.

Vitamin D preparations are standardized by determining their effect of calcification in rats maintained on a diet deficient in vitamin D. The international unit is 0.025 μg of vitamin D_3.

Adults require 400 units of vitamin D in 24 hours. Infants, children, and also pregnant or lactating women may require as much as twice this amount. It may be administered in the form of fish liver oils, as calciferol (Drisdol), or as synthetic oleovitamin D. Dihydrotachysterol (Hydracalciferol) is used in hypoparathyroidism to raise the serum calcium level.

Vitamin D is hydroxylated in the liver in the 25-position. It is further hydroxylated in the 1 position in the kidney. The implications of the availability of 1,25-hydroxycholecalciferol may be great in therapeutics (p. 550).

TOXICITY   Excessive doses of the D vitamins cause hypercalcemia, with anorexia and metastatic calcifications in the kidney.

Vitamin E is present in wheat-germ oil and in many foods. Its role in animal reproduction has been well established, and the term *tocopherol* implies its importance in childbearing. There are several tocopherols, but α-tocopherol has the highest activity.

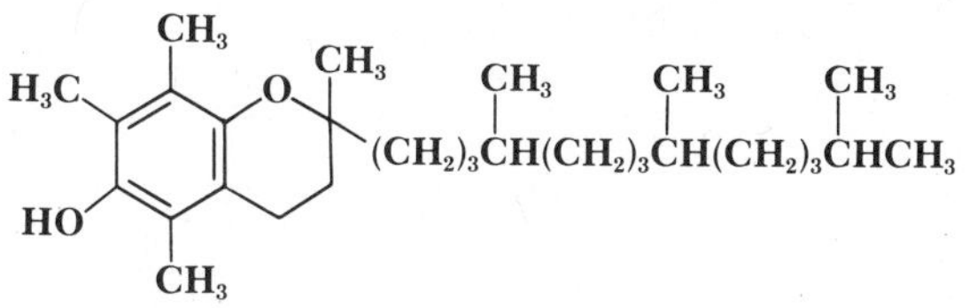

α-**Tocopherol**

Deficiency of vitamin E produces abortion in the female animal and degeneration of the germinal epithelium in the male animal. Muscular dystrophy also develops in animals on a vitamin E–deficient diet. Many other functions have been claimed for α-tocopherol, and many of its therapeutic applications have been suggested largely on the basis of uncritical clinical observations. The exact daily requirements of vitamin E in humans are not known, but quantities of 5 to 30 mg or more have been used in many clinical series.

The feeding of large amounts of unsaturated fats may increase the tocopherol requirements. It has been suggested that tocopherol functions as a biological antioxidant whose function becomes particularly important when tissues contain perioxidizable lipids.

Vitamin K is essential for production of prothrombin by the liver, and in its absence hemorrhagic manifestations occur. Various 1,4-naphthoquinones have vitamin K activity. Vitamin K_1 is 2-methyl-3-phytyl-1,4-naphthoquinone.

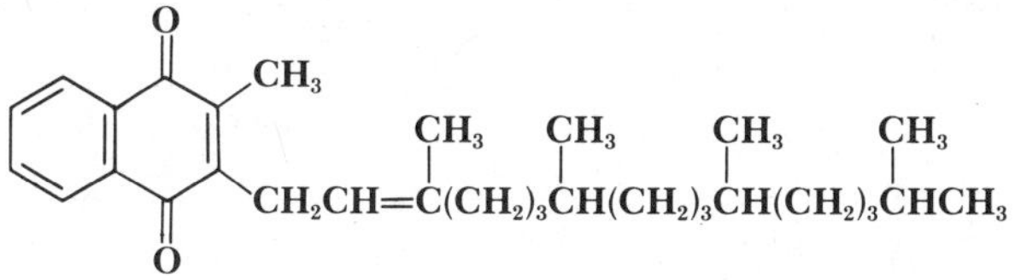

Vitamin K₁

These naphthoquinone compounds are very insoluble in water and are suitable primarily for oral administration. Emulsions of vitamin K_1, however, can be injected intravenously in hemorrhagic emergencies caused by hypoprothrombinemia.

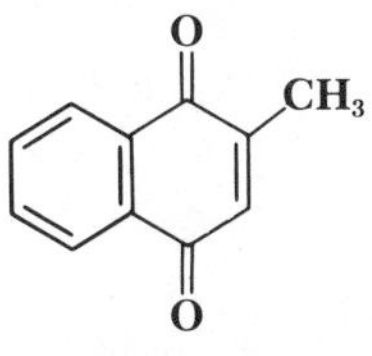

Menadione

Water-soluble derivatives of naphthoquinones have also been prepared. The structural formulas of two such compounds, menadiol sodium diphosphate and menadione sodium bisulfite, are shown below:

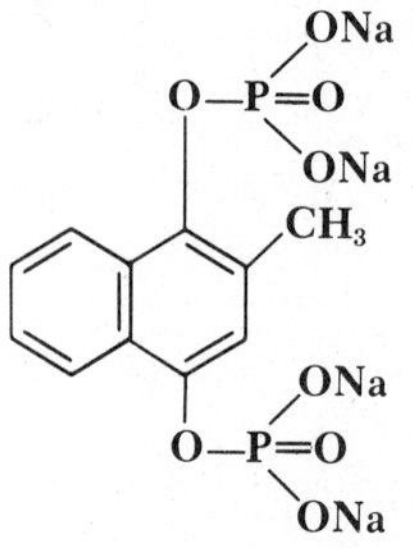

Menadiol sodium diphosphate 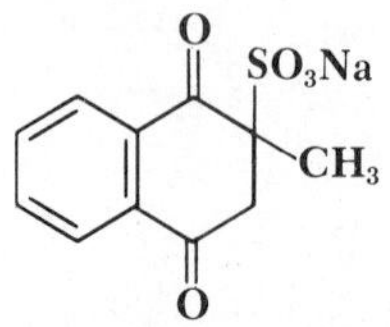   **Menadione sodium bisulfite**

Vitamin K preparations are useful in bleeding caused by hypoprothrombinemia. Causes of hypoprothrombinemia are severe liver disease, biliary obstruction, malabsorption syndromes, coumarin and indanedione drugs, salicylates in large doses, reduction of intestinal flora by chemotherapeutic agents, and hypoprothrombinemia of small infants.

Commonly used preparations are vitamin K_1 (phytonadione; Mephyton) and various forms of vitamin K_3 (menadione; menadiol sodium diphosphate, water soluble, or Synkayvite; and menadione sodium bisulfite or Hykinone, also water soluble).

The daily requirement for vitamin K cannot be stated because considerable quantities are synthesized by the bacterial flora of the intestine. The dosage varies greatly, depending on the nature and severity of prothrombin deficiency. Doses of 1 to 2 mg by mouth or injection may suffice. On the other hand, very large doses may have to be administered in emergency situations when prothrombin levels have been depressed by the anticoagulant drugs. As much as 100 mg or more of vitamin K_1 emulsion has been used in this situation by the intravenous route.

TOXICITY   Individuals who are subject to primaquine-sensitive anemia may react with hemolysis to large doses of vitamin K. Such doses can also aggravate liver disease and produce jaundice, particularly in infants.

MEDICAL USES   Vitamins should be used in medicine in (1) individuals with a poor dietary history, (2) deficiency diseases, (3) special disease states, or (4) hereditary vitamin dependency states[9] (Table 50-1).

Individuals with a poor dietary history include vegetarians who do not consume dairy products, individuals who do not consume fruits and green vegetables, pregnant or lactating women, and infants. Vegetarians develop vitamin B_{12} deficiency and require supplementation with 10 µg daily doses. Ascorbic acid, 50 mg daily, should be given to persons who do not eat fruits and green vegetables. Folate supplementation (0.5 mg) and pyridoxine should be given to pregnant women. Lactating women

TABLE 50-1	Recommended daily dietary allowances and therapeutic doses of vitamins	
Vitamin	Average daily adult requirement	Therapeutic dose
Thiamine	1.5 mg	2-10 mg
Nicotinamide	20 mg	100-300 mg
Riboflavin	2 mg	2-10 mg
Pyridoxine	2 mg	10 mg
Ascorbic acid	60 mg	100-150 mg
Vitamin A	4000 units	25,000 units
Vitamin D	400 units	5000 units or more
Vitamin E	Unknown	30 units

should probably take at least 80 mg of ascorbic acid daily, and their increased thiamine requirements should be met by proper food intake. Infant fed cow's milk should receive about 35 mg ascorbic acid daily, and the newborn should receive a single intramuscular injection of 0.5 to 1 mg of vitamin K, since vitamin K deficiency develops until the intestinal flora is established.[13]

Deficiency diseases include alcoholism, pernicious anemia, total or partial gastrectomy, chronic pancreatitis (fibrocystic disease), celiac disease (nontropical sprue), tropical sprue, short bowel syndrome, and dietary deficiencies.[13] Detailed discussion of the supplementation required in each of these conditions is beyond the scope of this review.

Additional special disease states include infection with *Diphyllobothrium latum*, hypoparathyroidism, and the carcinoid syndrome. The corresponding supplementations are vitamin B_{12}, vitamin D_2, and niacin.

Hereditary vitamin dependency states have been recognized in which the apoenzyme fails to react normally with the coenzyme, the condition being partially overcome by large doses of the corresponding vitamins. For example, an inborn error in the apoenzyme pyruvate carboxylase can produce lactic acidosis and is treated with 20 mg of thiamine daily. There are several rare diseases of this type, which provide some justification for the search for conditions that might be benefited by the megavitamin concept.[13] It should be remembered that the effectiveness of levodopa in parkinsonism would not have been discovered without someone trying unusually large doses of the drug. This, however, should not be considered an endorsement of the megavitamin therapy, which in most cases is ineffective and is not based on sound theory or controlled clinical trials.

Although light excesses of vitamin intake are more wasteful than dangerous, large doses of several of the vitamins can produce adverse effects.   **ADVERSE EFFECTS**

The water-soluble vitamins are generally harmless except in special circumstances. Thiamine injected intravenously has produced a shocklike state, and an anaphylactic-type sensitization to it has been suspected. Nicotinic acid is a fairly potent vasodilator, and for that reason nicotinamide, which does not affect the blood vessels, is preferred. Folic acid may be dangerous in persons who have pernicious anemia, since it may aggravate the neurological manifestations of the disease. For this reason the modern tendency is to eliminate folic acid from multiple vitamin preparations. Ascorbic acid is remarkably nontoxic. When given in large quantities, the vitamin is rapidly cleared by the kidney. Pyridoxine promotes the peripheral decarboxylation of levodopa and thus decreases its effectiveness in the treatment of parkinsonism.

The fat-soluble vitamins are more likely to produce distinct pathological changes when given in excessive quantities.

Hypervitaminosis A has been described as occurring in children when doses of the order of 100,000 units or more are administered for many days. Changes in skeletal development, hepatomegaly, anemia, loss of hair, and other symptoms have been described in these patients.

When used in large quantities, vitamin D can produce hypercalcemia with metastatic calcification in the kidney and blood vessels. This is not likely to happen in the treatment of rickets, but occasionally large amounts of vitamin D_2 are used in other diseases, such as lupus vulgaris, in which there is no reason to suspect a deficiency.

Hemolytic anemia and jaundice have been reported following parenteral use of large doses of the various vitamin K preparations.

The occurrence of these adverse reactions is an additional reason for maintaining a rational attitude toward the use of vitamins in cases in which their indications are not clear.

REFERENCES

1. Axelrod, A.E.: Immune processes in vitamin deficiency states, Am. J. Clin. Nutr. 24:265, 1971.
2. DeLuca, H.F.: Vitamin D endocrinology, Ann. Intern. Med. 85:367, 1976.
3. DeLuca, H.F., and Suttie, J.W.: The fat-soluble vitamins, Madison, 1970, University of Wisconsin Press.
4. Fliss, D.M., and Lamy, P.P.: Trace elements and total parenteral nutrition, Hosp. Formulary 14:698, 1979.
5. Goodman, D.S.: Vitamin A metabolism, Fed. Proc. 39:2716, 1980.
6. Law, D.H.: Current concepts in nutrition: total parenteral nutrition, N. Engl. J. Med. 297:1104, 1977.
7. Rivlin, R.S.: Riboflavin metabolism, N. Engl. J. Med. 283:463, 1970.
8. Rosenberg, L.E.: Vitamin-dependent genetic disease, Hosp. Pract. 5:59, 1970.
9. Schnoes, H.K., and DeLuca, H.F.: Recent progress in vitamin D metabolism and the chemistry of vitamin D metabolites, Fed. Proc. 39:2723, 1980.
10. Scott, M.L.: Advances in our understanding of vitamin E, Fed. Proc. 39:2736, 1980.
11. Suttie, J.W.: Mechanisms of action of vitamin K: demonstration of a liver precursor of prothrombin, Science 179:192, 1973.
12. Suttie, J.W.: The metabolic role of vitamin K, Fed. Proc. 39:2730, 1980.
13. Taylor, K.B.: Uses and abuses of vitamin therapy, Ration. Drug Ther. 9(10):1, 1975.

section nine

Chemotherapy

Chapter 51

Introduction to chemotherapy; mechanisms of antibiotic action

Before 1935 systemic bacterial infections could not be effectively treated with drugs. There were many *antiseptics* and *disinfectants* that could eradicate infections when applied topically, but their systemic use was precluded by their unfavorable therapeutic index. Certain parasitic infections, such as malaria, amebiasis, and spirochetal infections, could be treated effectively. This was an indication that the concept of "chemotherapy" as envisioned by Ehrlich was not unreasonable. Still, systemic bacterial infections, whether seen in patients or produced experimentally in animals, seemed to be hopelessly beyond the reach of existing drugs.

In 1935 a paper appeared in German medical literature claiming that the red azo dye Prontosil was able to protect mice against a systemic streptococcal infection and was curative in patients suffering from such infections. This was a milestone in the history of chemotherapy. In the test tube, Prontosil was ineffective against the bacteria.

It was soon demonstrated that Prontosil was metabolized in the body to *p*-aminobenzenesulfonamide, known later as sulfanilamide. It was also demonstrated that the chemotherapeutic activity of Prontosil was due entirely to the breakdown product sulfanilamide.

These observations initiated a new era in medicine. Numerous derivatives of sulfanilamide were synthesized, and soon a considerable number of systemic infections could be controlled by these drugs. Not only was treatment of many infectious diseases revolutionized, but the study of these drugs led to many great discoveries about bacterial metabolism, opening new fields in pharmacology. The study of biological antagonism and the discovery of the carbonic anhydrase inhibitors, antithyroid drugs, and many other agents were greatly influenced by basic studies on the sulfonamides.

601

Prontosil   **Sulfanilamide**

The successes obtained with the new sulfonamides revived interest in observations on *antibiotics*, or compounds produced by some microorganisms that inhibit the growth of other microorganisms. There were several isolated observations on the phenomenon of antibiosis. One of the most remarkable of these was Fleming's discovery that a mold of the genus *Penicillium* prevented multiplication of staphylococci and that culture filtrates of this mold had similar properties. A concentrate of this antibacterial factor was eventually prepared, and its remarkable activity and lack of toxicity were demonstrated by a team at Oxford led by Florey.

The enormous potency and lack of toxicity of penicillin tuned the attention of many investigators to antibiotics as potential sources of useful chemotherapeutic agents. Soon hundreds of antibiotics were discovered. The great majority of these were too toxic for clinical use, but a few represented welcome additions to therapeutics. Streptomycin, the tetracyclines, chloramphenicol, polymyxin, bacitracin, neomycin, and several newer antibiotics have greatly increased the range of effectiveness of antibacterial chemotherapy.

Currently, interest is centered on the newer penicillins, cephalosporins, newer aminoglycosides, and combinations of sulfamethoxazole with trimethoprim.

GENERAL CONCEPTS   With the availability of large numbers of effective antimicrobial agents, many general principles have evolved that must guide the physician in the selection and dosage of the most appropriate agent to be used in a given patient. Selection and dosage depend not only on the bacteriological diagnosis but on host factors such as renal function, age, and disease states. Thus susceptibility tests do not automatically dictate the kind of antimicrobial agent that must be used.

A number of important concepts have been derived from extensive studies on antibacterial chemotherapy.

Antibacterial spectrum refers to the range of activity of a compound. A broad-spectrum antibacterial agent is one capable of inhibiting a wide variety of microorganisms, usually including both gram-positive and gram-negative bacteria.

Potency, or activity per milligram, of a chemotherapeutic agent is usually expressed on the basis of the lowest concentration at which a chemotherapeutic agent inhibits multiplication of one of the susceptible microorganisms.

Bacteriostatic activity refers to the ability of a compound to inhibit multiplication of microorganisms. *Bactericidal activity* means an actual killing effect, which can only be demonstrated by techniques more complex than the usual plate or tube-dilution methods used for the demonstration of bacteriostatic activity. It is an interesting generalization that those antibacterial substances that disturb the synthesis or function of the microbial cell wall or the cell membrane are usually bactericidal.

The necessity of maintaining *blood levels* varies greatly. This is important in the case of the sulfonamides, but it may be less so in the case of some of the antibiotics such as penicillin.

The terms *antibiotic synergism* and *antibiotic antagonism* usually refer to the magnitude of *bactericidal activity* when combinations of chemotherapeutic agents are used. The *bacteriostatic* activities of such drug combinations are usually additive. For example, if two antibiotics, such as penicillin and streptomycin, exert greater bactericidal activity when given together rather than singly, a phenomenon of *antibiotic synergism* is said to exist. If a bacteriostatic antibiotic interferes with the killing effect of a bactericidal antibiotic, the phenomenon is *antibiotic antagonism*. These concepts are discussed further in connection with penicillin.

Indications for the combined use of antibiotics are to increase the effectiveness of therapy against a resistant organism and to take advantage of a possible synergistic killing effect, to delay the development of resistance, and to broaden the antibacterial spectrum in mixed infections or in cases in which reliable bacteriological diagnosis is unavailable.

There are many disadvantages to the combined use of antibiotics, which may be entirely unnecessary and wasteful. Combinations expose the patient to the adverse effects of the various members, superinfection may develop, and, in rare instances, antibiotic antagonism may be promoted.

RESISTANCE

Resistance to antibiotics may be *genetic* or *nongenetic*. Genetic resistance may be of chromosomal origin or may be transmitted by extrachromosomal *plasmids*. The chromosomal resistance may arise from spontaneous mutations. Nongenetic resistance is usually associated with nonmultiplying bacteria, the so-called persisters.

The way resistant bacteria escape the antibiotic takes many forms. For example, bacteria can (1) synthesize an enzyme that destroys the antibiotic (e.g., β-lactamase capable of cleaving penicillin or cephalosporin β-lactam rings); (2) modify the antibiotic in such a way that the bacterial cell wall is impermeable to the altered drug (e.g., acetylation of chloramphenicol by acetyltransferase); (3) alter macromolecules to which the antibiotic binds (e.g., methylation of large ribosomal subunits by a plasmid-coded RNA methylase affecting binding of erythromycin or change in the β-subunit of bacterial RNA polymerase, preventing binding of rifampin).

Infectious drug resistance

It was recognized in Japan in 1959 that bacterial resistance to several unrelated antibiotics can be transferred to susceptible organisms by cell-to-cell contact or conjugation.

Bacteria contain extrachromosomal genetic elements called R factors that are made up of DNA and act like viruses without coats. Transfer of resistance by RTF, a portion of the R factor, can occur among *Shigella, Salmonella, Klebsiella, Vibrio, Pasteurella,* and *Escherichia coli.* The last-named may be a great reservoir for the transmission of bacterial resistance.

In addition to the gram-negative organisms, staphylococci may also contain extrachromosomal particles called *plasmids,* which may be transferred from cell to cell by phages, a form of *transduction.*

ANTIBACTERIAL
CHEMOTHERA-
PEUTIC AGENTS
Mechanism of action

Most of the commonly used antibacterial chemotherapeutic agents act by one of the following basic mechanisms: competitive antagonism of some metabolite, inhibition of bacterial cell wall synthesis, action on cell membranes, inhibition of protein synthesis, or inhibition of nucleic acid synthesis.

COMPETITIVE
ANTAGONISM

There are a few examples in which antibacterial substances act as antimetabolites. The sulfonamides compete with *p*-aminobenzoic acid for the synthesis of folic acid in bacteria. This concept of competitive antagonism arose from studies on substrates that tended to inhibit the activity of the sulfonamides in vitro. It was shown that the antagonistic effect of yeast extract was probably caused by the presence of *p*-aminobenzoic acid.

It has subsequently been shown that folic acid, a noncompetitive inhibitor of the sulfonamides, contains *p*-aminobenzoic acid. It now appears that certain bacteria require *p*-aminobenzoic acid for the synthesis of folic acid and that the sulfonamides prevent this synthesis by substrate competition.

p-Aminobenzoic acid   Sulfanilamide   Folic acid

Since mammalian organisms do not synthesize folic acid but require it as a vitamin, the sulfonamides are not expected to interfere with the metabolism of mammalian cells. This difference between microorganisms and mammals explains the favorable therapeutic index of the sulfonamides in the treatment of various infections.

There are other examples of competitive antagonism in antibacterial chemotherapy. *p*-Aminosalicylate also competes with *p*-aminobenzoic acid. Interestingly, *p*-aminosalicylate is ineffective against bacteria other than the tubercle bacillus, although these bacteria may require *p*-aminobenzoic acid and are inhibited by the sulfonamides. A reasonable explanation for this invokes a difference in the receptive mechanisms in the two types of microorganisms.

TABLE 51-1	Inhibitors of cell wall synthesis
Antibiotics	Mechanism
Penicillins Cephalosporins	These act at stage 3 in cell wall synthesis. Cross-linking of peptidoglycan strands inactivates the transpeptidase enzyme, specifically blocks binding of the enzyme to the pentapeptide chain of the cell wall, and thus interferes with the formation of the cell wall.
Cycloserine	This acts at stage 1 in cell wall synthesis—formation of nucleotide intermediates. Being a structural analog of D-alanine, it competitively inhibits alanine racemase and D-alanyl-D-alanine synthetase and prevents the formation of the cell wall pentapeptide.
Vancomycin Ristocetin	These act at stage 2 in the cell wall synthesis—formation of linear peptidoglycans.
Bacitracin	This acts at stage 2 in cell wall synthesis and inhibits conversion of phospholipid pyrophosphate to phospholipid, a reaction essential to the regeneration of the lipid carrier involved in cell wall synthesis.

INHIBITION OF BACTERIAL CELL WALL SYNTHESIS

Several antibiotics, including penicillin, the cephalosporins, vancomycin, ristocetin, cycloserine, and bacitracin, act by inhibiting synthesis of the rigid bacterial cell wall (Table 51-1). This cell wall, in contrast to mammalian cell membranes, is rigid, making it possible for bacteria to maintain a very high internal osmotic pressure. If the synthesis of the cell wall is blocked, the high osmotic pressure leads to an extrusion of bacterial protoplasm and eventually to lysis of the cell when exposed to the isosmotic environment present in mammalian tissues.

The structural element of the bacterial cell wall is known as *murein*. The synthesis of murein is divided into three phases: (1) synthesis of nucleotide intermediates, UDP-*N*-acetylglucosamine and UDP-*N*-acetylmuramyl-pentapeptide, terminating in D-alanyl-D-alanine; (2) assembly of the disaccharide intermediate and its incorporation into murein; and (3) the cross-linking of the peptides by transpeptidation with release of D-alanine.

It was known for many years that penicillin is particularly effective against rapidly multiplying bacteria. It was also known that the antibiotic produced morphological changes in bacteria, such as swelling, large body formation, and lysis. Subsequently it was shown by Lederberg that *E. coli* cells were converted to protoplasts in the presence of penicillin and sucrose. Protoplasts are believed to represent cellular units deprived of their rigid cell wall.

ACTION ON CELL MEMBRANES

Some antibiotics act on cell membranes, altering their permeability. This mode of action is sometimes referred to as a detergent-like action. The best examples of this mechanism are provided by the polymyxins and the antifungal polyene antibiotics (Table 51-2).

TABLE 51-2	Inhibitors that act on cell membrane
Antibiotic	**Mechanism**
Amphotericin B Nystatin	Preferentially bind to ergosterol, the principal sterol in fungal cell membrane; show much less affinity for cholesterol, the sterol in animal cell membrane; results in cell disruption
Polymyxin B	Cationic detergent; destroys lipoprotein cell membrane

TABLE 51-3	Inhibitors of protein synthesis
Antibiotic	**Mechanism**
Aminoglycosides	Binds to 30 S ribosomal subunit; details of mechanism of action not elucidated
Tetracyclines	Inhibits binding of aminoacyl-tRNA to 30 S ribosomal subunit; also known to have strong affinity for polycations, which might have bearing in their ability to block protein synthesis
Chloramphenicol Lincomycin Clindamycin	Inhibit peptidyl synthetase on 50 S ribosomal subunit and thus prevent formation of initial dipeptide
Erythromycin	Inhibits translocation of peptidyl tRNA from "A" site to "P" site
Fusidic acid	Inhibits translocation reaction
Cycloheximide Emetine	Interacts directly with enzyme translocase, involved in the translocation reaction

TABLE 51-4	Inhibitors of nucleic acid synthesis pertaining to bacteria and/or virus
Antibiotic	**Mechanism**
Idoxuridine (5 IUdR)	Is converted to IDUTP, which in turn is incorporated into viral DNA, rendering this DNA more susceptible to breakage
Cytarabine (Ara-C)	Ara-CTP competitive with respect to dCTP in DNA polymerizing reaction; potent inhibitor of virally-induced DNA polymerase
Vidarabine (Ara-A)	Ara-ATP competitive with respect to dATP in DNA synthesis; also inhibits polyadenylation of RNA in vitro and in vivo
Acyclovir (acycloguanosine)	Phosphorylated by viral-specific thymidine kinase; viral DNA replication specifically blocked by active triphospate derivative
Nalidixic acid	Inhibits bacterial DNA gyrase, enzyme implicated in DNA replication and transcription
Novobiocin	Inhibits DNA gyrase
Rifamycin	Inhibits prokaryotic DNA-dependent RNA polymerase

Although antibiotics acting on cell membranes have some selective toxicity for microorganisms, they may be quite toxic for mammalian cells also. For example, the polymyxins cause renal tubular damage when administered in doses somewhat larger than therapeutic. They can also cause histamine release from mast cells both in vitro and in vivo.

Polyene antibiotics, such as amphotericin B and nystatin, complex with sterols in the cell wall. They preferentially bind to ergosterol, the principal sterol in fungal membrane; this explains the selective toxicity of the polyenes for fungi.

Most of the commonly used antibiotics inhibit protein synthesis. The list includes the aminoglycosides, tetracyclines, chloramphenicol, lincomycin, clindamycin, erythromycin, and emetine. In addition, the highly toxic experimental tools, such as cycloheximide (Actidione), are potent inhibitors of protein synthesis both in microorganisms and in mammals. Generally, this group of antibiotics can selectively inhibit protein synthesis in microorganisms. However, chloramphenicol is also a potent inhibitor of mitochondrial protein synthesis; this inhibitory property might be responsible for some of its adverse effects. A brief survey of the antibiotics that inhibit protein synthesis is presented in Table 51-3.

INHIBITION OF PROTEIN SYNTHESIS

Most inhibitors of nucleic acid synthesis are used as anticancer agents. Since these drugs inhibit nucleic acid synthesis in normal tissues, they are considered very toxic.

INHIBITION OF NUCLEIC ACID SYNTHESIS

Inhibitors of nucleic acid synthesis that are effective antimicrobial or antiviral agents can be classified as follows: (1) nucleoside analogs, (2) those that bind to RNA polymerase, (3) those that interact directly with DNA, and (4) those that inhibit DNA gyrase (Table 51-4). Although most of these antibiotics are selective inhibitors of nucleic acid synthesis in bacteria or viruses, some of these drugs can also block transcription in the mitochondria of the host cell. For example, rifampin can inhibit RNA synthesis in the mitochondria, which might in part be responsible for its toxicity.

REFERENCES

1. Beneviste, R., and Davies, J.: Mechanism of antibiotic resistance in bacteria, Annu. Rev. Biochem. **42**:471, 1973.
2. Breuer, N.S.: Antimicrobial agents. II. Aminoglycosides, Mayo Clin. Proc. **52**:675, 1977.
3. Goldman, P.: Drug therapy: metronidazole. N. Engl. J. Med. **303**:1212, 1980.
4. Kaufman, H.E.: Antiviral agents, Int. J. Dermatol. **16**:464, 1977.
5. Neu, H.C.: The *in vitro* activity, human pharmacology, and clinical effectiveness of new β-lactam antibiotics, Annu. Rev. Pharmacol. Toxicol. **22**:599, 1982.
6. Nicholas, P.: Erythromycin: clinical review, NY State J. Med. **77**:2088, 2243, 1977.
7. Pratt, W.B.: Chemotherapy of infection, New York, 1977, Oxford University Press.
8. Saral, R., Burns, W.H., Laskin, O.L., Santos, G.W., and Lietman, P.S.: Acyclovir prophylaxis of herpes-simplex-virus infections, N. Engl. J. Med. **305**:63, 1981.

9. Schinazi, R.F., and Prusoff, W.H.: Antiviral drugs: modes of action and strategies for therapy, Hosp. Pract. June 1981, p. 113.
10. Siegel, D.: Tetracyclines: new look at old antibiotic, NY State J. Med. **78**:950, 1115-1120, 1978.
11. Van Scoy, R.E.: Antituberculosis agents, Mayo Clin. Proc. **52**:694, 1977.
12. Young, L.S.: Aminoglycosides, J. Surg. Pract. **7**:22, 1978.

Chapter 52

Sulfonamides

The discovery of the antibacterial action of sulfanilamide and the initial clinical trials in humans in the 1930s are landmarks in the use of pharmacological agents to treat infections in humans. Sulfonamides (sulfas) are true *antimetabolites;* they block a specific step in the biosynthetic pathway of folic acid (see discussion of mode of action). Despite more recent development of many effective antibiotics, sulfonamides still have important therapeutic uses (e.g., for acute urinary tract infections, conjunctivitis, and prevention of infection in burn wounds).

Development of the trimethoprim-sulfamethoxazole combination, which provides sequential blockade in the pathway of folic acid synthesis, extended the usefulness of the sulfonamides (e.g., for shigellosis and *Pneumocystis carinii*). This chapter also discusses nonsulfonamide drugs used for treatment of urinary tract infections.

The initial sulfonamide studied was Prontosil (Table 52-1). Prontosil is active in vivo but not in vitro. It is active only when metabolically cleaved at the diazo bond to yield sulfanilamide. Thus Prontosil is an early example of a *prodrug*. Nearly all currently used sulfonamides are derivatives of sulfanilamide (see Table 52-1). Important structure-activity relationships are: (1) no substitution can occur on the benzene nucleus at position 2, 3, 5, and 6; (2) a free amino group is required in the para position—sulfonamides substituted in this amino group become active only if the substituent is removed in vivo; (3) a sulfur molecule must be attached directly to the benzene ring. Substitution on the R_1 amide group can alter absorption, distribution, and solubility. Table 52-1 gives the structure of the more important and commonly used sulfonamides.

The sulfonamides are effective in vitro against a broad range of microorganisms.[12] Sensitive gram-positive organisms are *Streptococcus pyogenes*, *Streptococcus pneumoniae*, anthrax, *Corynebacterium diphtheriae*, and *Yersinia pestis* (the plague organism). Susceptible gram-negative organisms include some strains of meningococ-

TABLE 52-1 Structures of sulfonamides

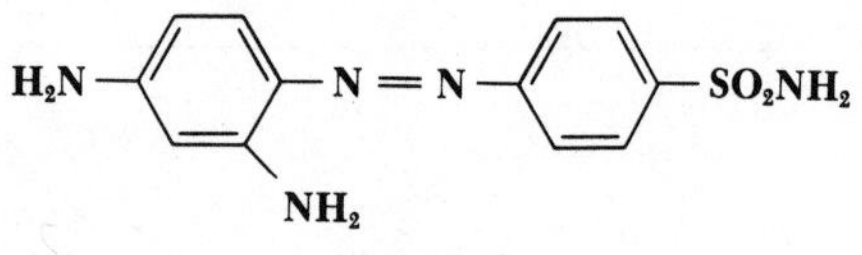

H_2N—(ring)—$N=N$—(ring)—SO_2NH_2
with NH_2 substituent

Prontosil

Sulfanilamide structure with R_1 and R_2 substituents on the amine nitrogens.

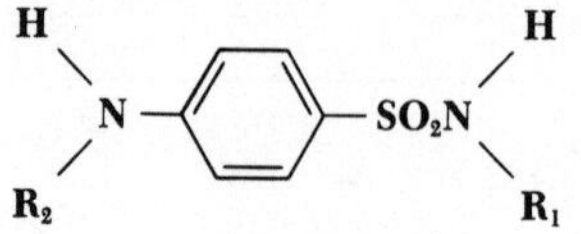

Sulfanilamide

	R_1 substitution	R_2 substitution
Sulfadiazine	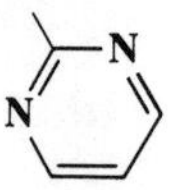 pyrimidine ring	— H
Sulfisoxazole	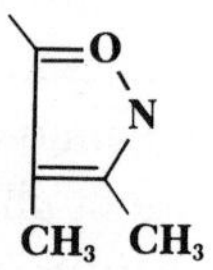 isoxazole ring with CH$_3$ CH$_3$	— H
Sulfamethoxazole (used with trimethoprim)	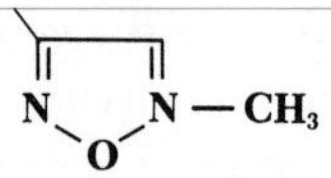 oxadiazole ring $N=N-CH_3$	— H
Succinylsulfathiazole	thiazole ring	— COCH$_2$CH$_2$COOH
Phthalylsulfathiazole	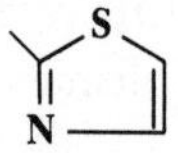 thiazole ring	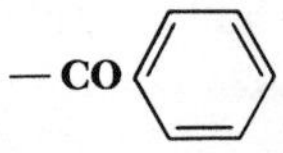 — CO (phenyl)
Dapsone (see chapter on leprosy)	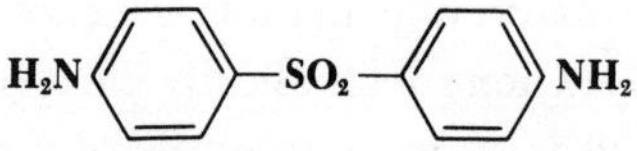 H_2N—(ring)—SO_2—(ring)—NH_2	
Sulfacetamide	— COCH$_3$	— H
Mafenide	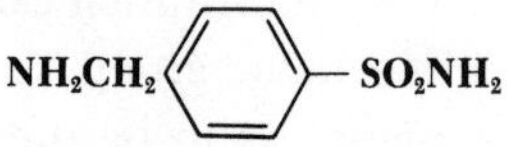 NH_2CH_2—(ring)—SO_2NH_2	
Sulfasalazine (salicylazosulfapyridine)	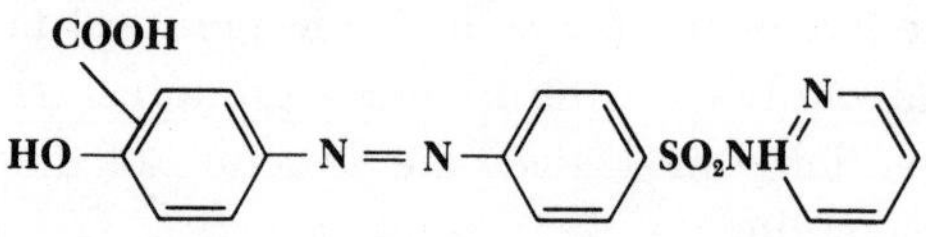 HO—(ring with COOH)—$N=N$—(ring)—SO_2NH—(pyridine)	

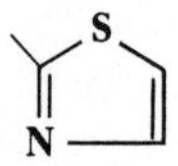

cus, *Hemophilus influenza*, and *Vibrio cholerae*. The sulfonamides are active against *Actinomyces*, *Nocardia*, *Chlamydiae*, and some protozoa. Although efficacious in vitro, the sulfonamides are no longer the drugs of choice for the treatment of certain infections (e.g., *Hemophilus influenza*, *Yersinia pestis*, and *Corynebacterium diphtheriae*). More effective antibiotics are now available for these diseases.

The short-acting sulfonamides (such as sulfisoxazole) are among the drugs of choice for treatment of acute urinary tract infections caused by susceptible bacteria such as *Escherichia coli*. Short-acting sulfonamides are also highly useful in the treatment of nocardiosis, trachoma, and chancroid. Other infections, including otitis media (especially in children) and lower respiratory infections, may respond to sulfonamide treatment, but other antibiotics are usually more effective.

Potency of sulfonamides (activity per milligram) is such that growth inhibition in simple media may be achieved at a concentration of about 0.1 to 1 mg/ml and in blood at concentrations of about 0.1 mg/ml (10 mg/100 ml). Potency as measured in vitro is greatly influenced by the nature of the culture medium. Thus enrichment with yeast extract, pus, or *p*-aminobenzoic acid (PABA) markedly decreases the effectiveness of these drugs. Even in a simple synthetic medium, potency of the sulfonamides is much less than that of other widely used antibiotics. For this reason, when compared with most antibiotics, the sulfonamides must be administered in relatively large doses.

Special comment needs to be made about the combination of trimethoprim-sulfamethoxazole. This combination has expanded the spectrum of the sulfonamides and is used clinically to treat infections caused by *Shigella*, *Salmonella* (resistant to ampicillin and chloramphenicol) or *Pneumocystis carinii*.

A study of the in vitro activity of various sulfonamides and the ionization and electron density of their $-SO_2$ group led to the concept that a relationship exists between this physical property and in vitro activity. Maximum activity appeared around pK_a 6.5 and was less below or above this figure.[2] Since the pK_a of sulfadiazine was close to the optimum figure, it was unlikely that any sulfonamide acting by competition with PABA would have greater antibacterial activity than sulfadiazine. Therefore other sulfonamides are more likely to offer advantages on the basis of increased solubility, less toxicity to the kidney, or reduced sensitizing properties.

Mode of action

The sulfonamides act as competitive inhibitors of the enzyme (dihydropteroate synthase) responsible for the synthesis of dihydropteroic acid, a precurser of folic acid.[4] Sulfonamides are structurally similar to PABA, which combines with a dihydropteridine to form dihydropteroic acid (Fig. 52-1). Only organisms that use PABA to form folic acid are sensitive to sulfonamides. Mammalian cells require preformed folic acid and cannot use PABA. Trimethoprim is a competitive inhibitor of dihydrofolate reductase, another enzyme important in folic acid synthesis.[10] The mammalian enzyme requires 50,000 times the trimethoprim concentration needed for 50% inhibition of the bacterial enzyme.[5] This most likely explains the relative lack of toxicity of trimethoprim observed to date.

FIG. 52-1 *Biosynthetic reactions blocked by sulfonamides and trimethoprim.*

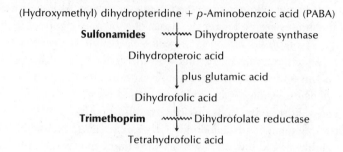

(Hydroxymethyl) dihydropteridine + *p*-Aminobenzoic acid (PABA)

Sulfonamides ⋙ Dihydropteroate synthase

Dihydropteroic acid

plus glutamic acid

Dihydrofolic acid

Trimethoprim ⋙ Dihydrofolate reductase

Tetrahydrofolic acid

Pharmacokinetics   Short-acting sulfonamides (sulfisoxazole and sulfadiazine) are absorbed rapidly from the gastrointestinal tract. These drugs are given in oral doses of 1 to 4 g initially (in adults), followed by 1 g every 4 to 6 hours to maintain blood concentration of approximately 10 mg/100 ml.[12] The pediatric dosage is 150 mg/kg/day. Blood concentrations of sulfonamides are rarely measured today and usually only to monitor serious infections requiring parenteral (intravenous) sulfonamide therapy. The blood half-life of these drugs varies from 4 to 7 hours, with sulfadiazine having a somewhat shorter half-life.

The volume of distribution of most sulfonamides approaches that of total body water, and the drugs penetrate cells. An exception to this is sulfisoxazole, which distributes only in extracellular water. Hence serum sulfisoxazole concentrations are twice as high as those reached after an identical dose of sulfadiazine. Metabolism of these drugs involves acetylation of the free *p*-amino group. The acetylated metabolite has no antimicrobial activity and may be less soluble in the urine, but it retains the capacity to cause toxicity. Genetically controlled differences among subjects in the activity of the acetylase that metabolizes sulfonamides cause large variations in the rates of elimination of these drugs.

Sulfisoxazole is readily excreted in human milk.[6] The milk-plasma ratio is 0.06 for the parent compound and 0.22 for the N^4-acetyl metabolite. Less than 1% of the total maternal dose is excreted in milk, but virtually all that is excreted will be absorbed by the nursing infant. An alternative antibiotic should be used for the lactating mother during the infant's first several weeks of life because of the possibility of displacing bilirubin from albumin.

In plasma sulfonamides are partially bound to proteins. Only the free fraction is considered to possess antibacterial activity. The kidney filters the free fraction through the glomeruli, and the tubules reabsorb a portion of the filtered drug. Urinary concentration of sulfonamides greatly exceeds that in plasma. In fact, urinary concentration may be 25 to 50 times higher, a circumstance that contributes to the usefulness of these drugs as urinary antimicrobials.

The intermediate-acting sulfonamide, sulfamethoxazole, has a longer half-life (up to 12 hours) than the short-acting compounds. Some longer-acting sulfonamides were introduced but later removed from the market when severe and frequently fatal hypersensitivity reactions (Stevens-Johnson syndrome) were found to be associated with their use. These drugs (sulfadimethoxine, sulfamethoxypyridaziner) are rapidly absorbed but slowly excreted; they should not be used clinically.

The relationship between pH and solubility of the various sulfonamides results from the fact that they behave as weak acids because of the dissociation of the sulfamyl group ($-SO_2NH-$). Substitutions of the sulfamyl nitrogens can produce acids considerably stronger than sulfanilamide. Salts (ions) of the sulfonamides are much more soluble than the molecular form; thus the solubility of these drugs increases greatly when the pH exceeds the pK_a of the drug.

The implications of these properties are obvious. The urinary volume must be adequate. Alkalinization with sodium bicarbonate is not usually necessary with adequate hydration.

When several sulfonamides are dissolved in water or urine, the presence of one does not influence the solubility of the others.[8] The antibacterial effects of such mixtures are additive. Such a therapeutic procedure can produce a higher total sulfonamide concentration in the urine with diminished tendency for crystal formation. The high solubility of sulfisoxazole has eliminated the need for the previously widespread use of such mixtures of sulfonamides (e.g., triple sulfas).

Toxicity and hypersensitivity

Virtually every organ system has been involved in toxic reactions to the sulfonamides. Gastrointestinal effects are fairly common (nausea, vomiting, and loss of appetite). Hepatitis and bone marrow depression occur infrequently as do hemolytic anemia and other blood dyscrasias.

Renal toxicity, manifested by nephrosis, crystalluria, and hematuria, is caused by precipitation of the drug within renal tubules. Maintenance of adequate urine output and alkalinization of the urine should prevent this form of toxicity.

Hypersensitivity reactions are of great concern. These include syndromes that resemble arteritis and lupus erythematosus. Skin eruptions may range from a diffuse morbilliform rash or erythema multiforme to exfoliative dermatitis (Stevens-Johnson syndrome). This latter complication is especially dreaded because of its high mortality.

Other serious hypersensitivity reactions include urticaria, serum sickness–like syndrome, and frank anaphylaxis.

Drug interactions

Sulfonamides and methenamines should not be administered simultaneously for the treatment of urinary tract infections, since in acid urine formaldehyde is liberated from methenamine and forms a precipitate with some sulfonamides. Binding of sulfonamides by plasma proteins, especially albumin, leads to displacement of other drugs and may cause increased drug effects. Thus the actions of tolbutamide may be potentiated. Kernicterus in newborns may be caused by sulfonamide administration to the infant in the first few weeks of life or to the mother in the last trimester of pregnancy. The action of coumarins may also be intensified.

Clinical uses   Sulfonamides are most commonly used to treat acute urinary tract infections. In otherwise healthy individuals most of these infections are caused by gram-negative enteric bacteria, especially *E. coli*, usually susceptible to sulfisoxazole. The preferred oral drug is sulfisoxazole (Gantrisin); the parenteral form is the sodium salt of sulfadiazine. Sulfisoxazole has antibacterial properties similar to those of sulfadiazine. Its solubility at pH 6 greatly exceeds that of sulfadiazine. In fact, it is more than 10 times as soluble. At pH 5.5 its solubility in human urine is only about 120 mg/100 ml, which still exceeds by fourfold the solubility of sulfadiazine. But this offers no guarantee against crystal formation in renal tubules. Sulfisoxazole is cleared rapidly from the blood and produces high urinary levels. In pediatric practice, sulfisoxazole in dosages of 500 mg twice daily is used for propylaxis of acute otitis media in children who experience repeated attacks during a short time (recurrent otitis media).[9] Sulfacetamide is available in an ophthalmic preparation (10% and 30%) to treat bacterial conjunctivitis. The pH of its solution is 7.4, thereby producing minimum conjunctival irritation.

Trimethoprim-   The trimethoprim-sulfamethoxazole preparation (co-trimoxazole; Bactrim, Septra)
sulfamethoxazole   exerts a truly synergistic effect on bacteria. The sulfonamide in the combination inhibits PABA utilization in folic acid synthesis, whereas trimethoprim blocks conversion of dihydrofolic acid to tetrahydrofolic acid by dihydrofolate reductase (see Fig. 52-1). Thus the preparation inhibits two consecutive steps in bacterial metabolism. Trimethoprim has much greater affinity for the bacterial than for the mammalian enzyme.

Trimethoprim-sulfamethoxazole is effective against a large variety of gram-positive and gram-negative microorganisms. Acute and chronic urinary tract infections are prime indications. This drug preparation is also effective in the treatment of the following conditions: typhoid and paratyphoid fever (if the organism is resistant to ampicillin), bacterial infections of the lower respiratory tract, (acute exacerbations of chronic infections), otitis media, uncomplicated gonorrhea, vivax and falciparum malaria, *Shigella* and *Pneumocystis carinii*. When seriousness of the infection dictates parenteral therapy, an intravenous form of trimethoprim-sulfamethoxazole is available.

Absorption of trimethoprim-sulfamethoxazole is rapid. Effective concentrations of the drugs may be present in plasma for 6 to 8 hours.[10] Both drugs are excreted mostly unchanged in the urine, although sulfamethoxazole is also excreted in the acetylated form.

All the adverse effects involved in the use of the sulfonamides may occur when trimethoprim-sulfamethoxazole is used. Skin rashes, mild CNS disturbances, and blood dyscrasias have been reported. Crystalluria may occur but is rare. This preparation is contraindicated in patients with blood dyscrasias, hepatic damage, and severe renal impairment. The drug combination should be used cautiously in patients with low folic acid concentrations such as in malnutrition states or as a consequence of the chronic ingestion of phenytoin.

Trimethoprim-sulfamethoxazole (Bactrim, Septra) is available in single-strength tablets containing trimethoprim, 80 mg, and sulfamethoxazole, 400 mg, and a double-strength preparation containing 160 mg trimethoprim and 800 mg sulfamethoxazole. The pediatric suspension contains 40 mg of trimethoprim and 200 mg sulfamethoxazole per 5 ml (1 teaspoon). This ratio (1:5) of these two drugs gives a ratio of blood concentrations of 1:20 trimethoprim/sufamethoxazole.[10]

Topical sulfonamides

Mafenide (Sulfamylon) was widely used as a topical agent in seriously burned patients to prevent wound contamination, especially by *Pseudomonas* species. Three problems occur with this drug: (1) it is painful on application; (2) resistant organisms emerge during treatment; (3) mafenide is a carbonic anhydrase inhibitor and can cause metabolic alkalosis if enough is absorbed through the skin. Mafenide has been replaced by silver sulfadiazine (Silvadene), which is painless and appears to have very low systemic toxicity. Bacterial resistance to silver sulfadiazine has not yet proven to be the problem that it is with mafenide.

Other sulfonamides

Slowly excreted sulfonamides, such as sulfamethoxypyridazine (Kynex) and sulfadimethoxine (Madribon), are no longer used in this country because of the hypersensitivity reactions (Stevens-Johnson syndrome) associated with them. Slow excretion of these drugs is a consequence of their high protein binding.

SULFONAMIDES AS INTESTINAL ANTISEPTICS

Sulfonamides that are poorly absorbed from the intestine have been used for decreasing intestinal bacterial flora.

Succinylsulfathiazole (Sulfasuxidine) and phthalylsulfathiazole (Sulfathalidine) are substituted in the *p*-amino portion of the sulfathiazole molecule. As a consequence, they have no antibacterial activity in the test tube. However, when they are swallowed and reach the large intestine, hydrolysis occurs, and free sulfathiazole reaches high local concentrations. Sulfathiazole is not well absorbed from the large intestine.

When these intestinal antiseptic sulfonamides are administered for several days, coliform and clostridia organisms are markedly decreased in the intestine, and the volume and character of the feces change. Certain organisms, such as *Proteus, Pseudomonas, Salmonella,* and enterococci may be resistant to the action of these drugs. These drugs have been replaced by other nonsulfonamide antibiotics (vancomycin and neomycin) and are no longer available in the United States.

SULFONAMIDES FOR SPECIAL USES	Sulfasalazine (Azulfidine, salicylazosulfapyradine) is used in treating inflammatory bowel disease (such as ulcerative colitis and regional enteritis). Sulfasalazine is a congener of 5-aminosalicylate and sulfapyridine. The parent drug is a *prodrug* and represents a unique delivery system to the lower gastrointestinal tract (site of inflammatory process) in which, after cleavage to sulfapyridine and 5-aminosalicylate, the active drug is the latter.[1] 5-Aminosalicylate cannot be given alone because it is completely absorbed high in the small intestine and rapidly excreted by the kidney.

Dermatitis herpetiformis is the only indication for sulfapyridine. In this instance sulfapyridine acts by a mechanism unrelated to its antibacterial activity.[7] |

Resistance	Bacteria can develop resistance to the sulfonamides. The mechanism of resistance may be related to the ability of the bacteria to produce antagonists to the drug. In some cases the resistant organism increases PABA production.

ANTIBACTERIAL AGENTS FOR URINARY TRACT INFECTIONS	In addition to the sulfonamides, a number of antibacterial agents are used almost exclusively to treat urinary tract infections. Their major characteristics are summarized in Table 52-2.

Nitrofurantoin (Furadantin) is one of a series of nitrofurans that have been introduced as antibacterial agents. |

$$O_2N - \text{furan ring} - CH = NNHC NH_2$$
$$\parallel$$
$$O$$

Nitrofurantoin

The drug is absorbed rapidly, and much of it is excreted unchanged in the urine. Its mechanism of action is unknown. It has a wide antibacterial spectrum; both gram-positive and gram-negative bacteria can be inhibited at concentrations obtained in urine after daily oral administration of 5 to 10 mg/kg. Nitrofurantoin may cause numerous adverse reactions. Nausea and vomiting are common; skin sensitization, peripheral neuritis, and cholestatic jaundice also occur. An acute, dramatic pulmonary reaction (pneumonitis) occurs rarely. An interstitial fibrosis can occur in patients on chronic therapy. A macrocrystalline preparation (such as Macrodantin) may be less nauseating. The sodium salt of nitrofurantoin may be administered intravenously.

Preparations of nitrofurantoin (Furadantin) include tablets, 50 and 100 mg, and a suspension, 25 mg/5 ml. Macrodantin is available in capsules, 25, 50, and 100 mg. Nitrofurantoin sodium (Furadantin sodium) is available for intravenous injection, 180 mg powder in 20 ml sterile vials.

No bacteriostatic blood concentrations are produced following oral administration of nitrofurantoin. Its use in systemic infections is not supported by currently available evidence.[11] Nitrofurazone (Furacin) is used topically for infections of the skin, but it may cause sensitization.

TABLE 52-2   Antibacterial agents used principally for urinary tract infections

Drug	Activity spectrum and characteristics	Dosage	Route	Side effects
Sulfonamides Sulfisoxazole (Gantrisin) Sulfamethoxazole (Gantanol) Trimethoprim-sulfamethoxazole (Bactrim, Septra)	Short-acting sulfonamides best because of high urinary concentration and good solubility at acid pH; more active in alkaline urine; especially effective against *E. coli* and *P. mirabiis;* many strains of *Klebsiella, Aerobacter, Proteus,* and *Pseudomonas* resistant	1 g q.4-6h.	Oral	Allergic reactions; skin rash, drug fever, pruritus, photosensitization; periarteritis nodosa, systemic lupus erythematosus, Stevens-Johnson syndrome, serum sickness syndrome, myocarditis; neurotoxicity (psychosis, neuritis); hepatotoxicity; blood dyscrasias, usually agranulocytosis; crystalluria; nausea and vomiting, headache, dizziness, lassitude, mental depression, acidosis, sulfhemoglobin; hemolytic anemia in G-6-PD-deficient individuals; should not be used in newborn infants or in women near term
Nitrofurantoin (Furadantin)	Many gram-positive and gram-negative organisms; as relates to urinary tract, nitrofurantoin effective against likely pathogens except *Pseudomonas* and some *Klebsiella-Enterobacter* and *Proteus* species; high urinary concentration (ineffective in renal failure); increased activity in acid urine; action much reduced at pH 8 or over	100 mg q.6h. (5-7 mg/ kg)	Oral, intravenous	Nausea and vomiting, hypersensitivity, peripheral neuropathy, pulmonary infiltrate, intrahepatic cholestasis, hemolytic anemia in G-6-PD deficiency; contraindicated in renal failure; should not be used in infants less than 1 month old
Methenamine mandelate (Mandelamine)	Combination effect against most organisms in vitro; methenamine—no action per se but in acid medium is slowly decomposed with liberation of formaldehyde; mandelic acid—also requires acid pH; effective only when acid urine (preferably about pH 5) can be maintained; limited place in therapy; should not be used in tissue infection (pyelonephritis)	1 g q.6h.	Oral	Nausea and vomiting; contraindicated in renal failure because it leads to acidosis; should not be used with sulfonamides
Nalidixic acid (NegGram)	Gram-negative urinary tract pathogens *(Enterobacteriaceae)* except *Pseudomonas;* possible high degree of resistance developing rapidly during therapy	1 g q.6h.	Oral	Gastrointestinal hypersensitivity, fever, eosinophilia, photosensitivity, neurological disturbances (malaise, drowsiness, dizziness, visual disturbances); convulsions, (?); mild leukopenia, thrombocytopenia, hemolytic anemia; can produce false elevations of 17-ketosteroids and 17-ketogenic steroids in urine

Courtesy Dr. Jay P. Sanford, Washington, D.C.

Methenamine mandelate (Mandelamine) is a combination of two old urinary antiseptics, methenamine (Urotropin) and mandelic acid.

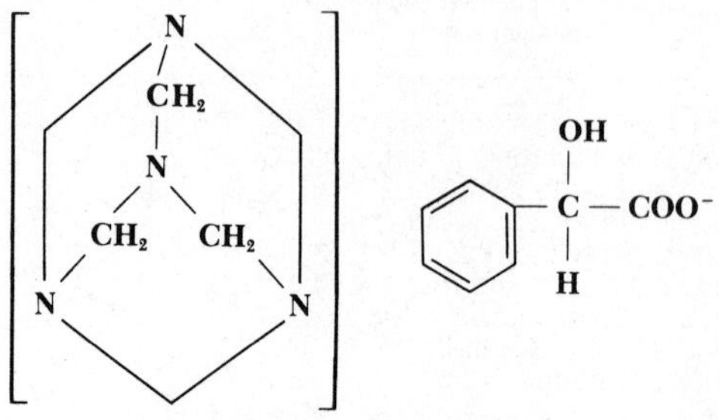

Methenamine mandelate

In acid urine methenamine, or hexamethylenetetramine, liberates formaldehyde. If the pH of the urine is low, mandelic acid is also bactericidal. If the pH of the urine is higher than 6, it is necessary to administer ammonium chloride in amounts of 0.5 to 1 g three or four times daily.

Methenamine mandelate is relatively nontoxic, but gastric irritation may occur following its use. This is probably related to the production of some formaldehyde in the acid gastric juice. For the same reason urinary frequency may also occur. The usual dose of methenamine mandelate is 0.5 to 1 g three times a day.

In addition to methenamine mandelate (Mandelamine), the hippurate salt of methenamine (Hiprex) is also available.

Nalidixic acid (NegGram) is chemically unrelated to other urinary antiseptics.[3] Well absorbed from the gastrointestinal tract, it is excreted in the urine largely unchanged and as an active metabolite, hydroxynalidixic acid. Its mode of action is unusual, since it appears to depend on selective inhibition of bacterial DNA synthesis.

Nalidixic acid is effective only against gram-negative bacteria such as *E. coli*, *Proteus*, and some strains of *Pseudomonas*, *Enterobacter*, and *Klebsiella*. Resistance to the drug develops readily. Nalidixic acid is ineffective against systemic infections because its activity is greatly reduced in the presence of proteins.

Nausea, vomiting, diarrhea, allergic reactions, and neurological disturbances may occur as a consequence of nalidixic acid administration. It may cause increased intracranial pressure in children.

Preparations of nalidixic acid (NegGram) include tablets of 250 and 500 mg and 1 g. A pediatric suspension contains 250 mg/5 ml.

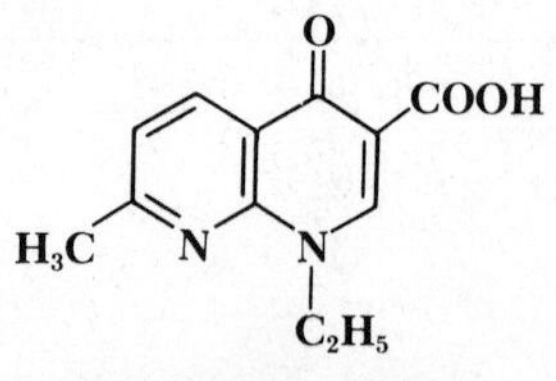

Nalidixic acid

Oxolinic acid (Utibid) is a quinoline derivative, similar in indications and actions to nalidixic acid. It is effective in the treatment of gram-negative urinary tract infections caused by susceptible organisms. The drug may cause CNS side effects. It is no longer manufactured in the United States.

REFERENCES

1. Azad Khan, A.K., Piris, J., and Truelove, S.C.: An experiment to determine the ctive therapeutic moiety of sulphasalazine, Lancet 3:892, 1977.
2. Bell, P.H., and Robin, R.O., Jr.: Studies in chemotherapy: a theory of the relation of structure to activity of sulfanilamide type compounds, J. Am. Chem. Soc. 64:2905, 1942.
3. Carroll, G.: NegGram (nalidixic acid): a new antimicrobial chemotherapeutic agent, J. Urol. 90:476, 1963.
4. De Benedetti, P.G., Rostelli, A., Frassiniti, C., and Cennamo, C.: Structure-activity relationships in dihydropteroate synthesis inhibition by sulfanilamides: comparison with the antibacterial activity, J. Med. Chem. 24:454, 1981.
5. Hansen, I.: The combination trimethoprim-sulphamethoxazole, Antibiot. Chemother. 25:217, 1978.
6. Kauffman, R.E., O'Brien, C., and Gilford, P.: Sulfisoxazole secretion into human milk, J. Pediatr. 97:839, 1980.
7. Lang, P.G., Jr.: Sulfones and sulfonamides in dermatology today, J. Am. Acad. Dermatol. 1:479, 1979.
8. Lehr, D.: Inhibition of drug precipitation in the urinary tract by use of sulfonamide mixtures. I. Sulfathiazole-sulfadiazine, Proc Soc. Exp. Biol. Med. 58:11, 1945.
9. Perrin, J.M., Charney, E., MacWhinney, J.B., Jr., McInerny, T.K., Jr., Miller, R.L., and Nazarian, L.F.: Sulfisoxazole vs chemoprophylaxis for recurrent otitis media, N. Engl. J. Med. 291:664, 1974.
10. Rubin, R., and Swartz, M.N.: Trimethoprim-sulfamethoxazole, N. Engl. J. Med. 303:426, 1980.
11. Sanford, J.P.: Nitrofurantoin in extragenitourinary infection? Curr. Ther. Res. 2:476, 1960.
12. Weinstein, L., Madoff, M.A., and Samet, C.A.: The sulfonamides, N. Engl. J. Med. 263:793, 842, 1960.

Chapter 53

Antibiotic drugs

A. FLEMING, 1929   While working with staphylococcus variants a number of culture-plates were set aside on the laboratory bench and examined from time to time. In the examinations these plates were necessarily exposed to the air and they became contaminated with various microorganisms. It was noticed that around a large colony of contaminating mould the staphylococcus colonies became transparent and were obviously undergoing lysis.

Relatively few of the hundreds of compounds produced by microorganisms with inhibitory action on other microorganisms have a favorable therapeutic index. These few have become the clinically useful antibiotics. This chapter describes and compares the potency, antibacterial spectrum, metabolism, and mode of action of these different antibiotics.

PENICILLIN   Penicillin is a highly effective antibiotic with very low toxicity. If it were not for penicillin allergy, the parent compound, penicillin G, would approach perfection for use against infections caused by susceptible organisms. The story of penicillin's discovery and the subsequent development of its many derivatives has become a scientific classic and a model for the process of biomedical discovery. It exemplifies Pasteur's dictum: "In research chance favors only the prepared mind." After its discovery by Fleming,[6] quoted above, penicillin lay dormant for a decade until Florey and his group in England took Fleming's monumental observation and ushered in the age of chemotherapy.[16]

Penicillin, an organic acid obtained from cultures of the mold *Penicillium chrysogenum*, is commonly administered as the sodium, potassium, and procaine salts. Its antibacterial action results from the inhibition of cell wall synthesis of growing bacteria. If the mold is grown by a deep fermentation process, large amounts of the key intermediate, 6-aminopenicillanic acid, are produced. The newer derivatives are prepared by chemical reactions in which side groups are added at the R position. Consequences of substitution at the R site include: (1) increased gastrointestinal absorption, (2) resistance to destruction by penicillinase, and (3) a widening of the spectrum of organisms susceptible to the compound. Penicillin has been completely synthesized, but at this time synthesis is much too difficult for commercial production.[28]

Penicillin G (benzylpenicillin) is the prototype. Penicillin V, available as the potassium salt, contains a phenoxy group in the R position and has much increased resistance to hydrolysis by gastric acid. It is the preferred oral form of penicillin. Penicillin G remains the intravenous/intramuscular form.

Penicillinase is an enzyme present in those bacteria that are resistant to penicillin G or V. This enzyme breaks the lactam ring (ring A in penicillin structure, p. 622) of penicillin and thus destroys its antibacterial activity. Substitution of bulky chemical groups at the R site protects this lactam ring through steric hindrance. These compounds, frequently referred to as *semisynthetic* penicillins, have been extremely useful against staphylococci resistant to penicillin G. They include methicillin, oxacillin, cloxacillin, dicloxacillin, and nafcillin. These antibiotics are resistant to the action of penicillinase.

Penicillin G and V, as well as the semisynthetic penicillins, are effective only against gram-positive bacteria in usual therapeutic doses. Other penicillins, also synthesized by substitution at the R site, expand the antimicrobial spectrum to include gram-negative organisms.

These "broad-spectrum" penicillins, effective against a wide range of gram-negative organisms, include ampicillin, amoxicillin, carbenicillin, ticarcillin, and piperacillin. All these antibiotics are sensitive to destruction by penicillinase.

For maximum effect against gram-negative organisms difficult to treat, carbenicillin, ticarcillin, and piperacillin are usually used with another antibiotic, especially one of the aminoglycosides.

Potency

Penicillin preparations are standardized on the basis of their capacity to inhibit the growth of test organisms such as *Bacillus subtilis* or sensitive staphylococci. Activity was first expressed in units and measured in comparison with a standard preparation by determining the zone of inhibition of bacterial growth on an inoculated agar plate. The amount of activity represented by 1 unit prevents multiplication of a susceptible organism such as *B. subtilis* or certain staphylococci in as much as 20 to 50 ml of broth. One milligram of penicillin G equals 1667 units. This means that 1 unit is equivalent to 0.6 µg of penicillin G. The dosage of all penicillins is now usually indicated in milligrams (or grams).

The enormous activity of penicillin may be appreciated from the fact that if 1 mg of the antibiotic were placed in about 5 gallons of broth, the growth of several susceptible organisms would be prevented by the resulting minute concentration of the antibiotic. By contrast, it would be necessary to add 2 to 20 g of a sulfonamide to this volume of culture medium to obtain similar growth inhibition.

Microorganisms inhibited by less than 1 µg of penicillin/ml may be considered moderately susceptible. Highly susceptible microorganisms are usually inhibited by less than 0.1 µg/ml. In clinical practice blood concentrations of 0.1 to 1 µg/ml can be achieved without difficulty.

Mode of action

Penicillins are bactericidal drugs that damage the bacterial cell by interfering with the synthesis of the cell wall. The elegant experiments of Park,[21] extended considerably by Strominger,[30] elucidated much of the mechanism of the synthesis of

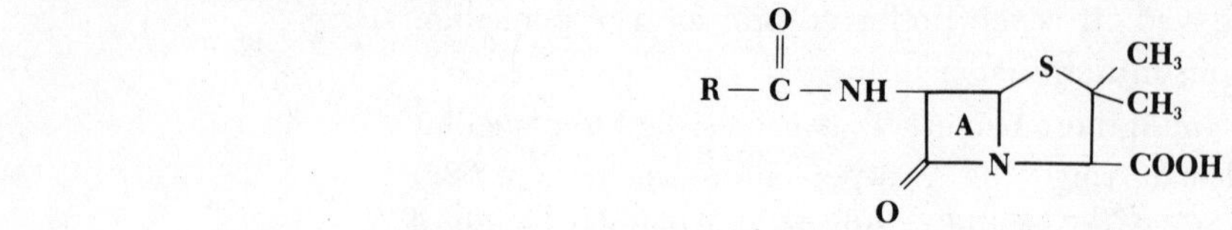

Basic penicillin structure

R side chain

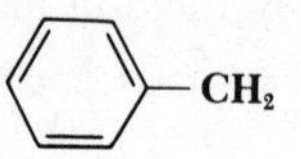

Penicillin G (benzylpenicillin)

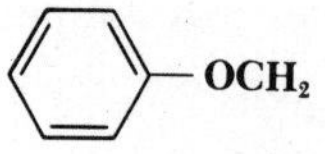

Penicillin V (phenoxymethylpenicillin)

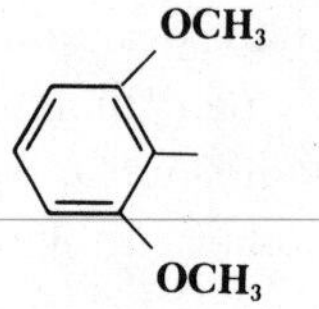

Methicillin (Staphcillin)

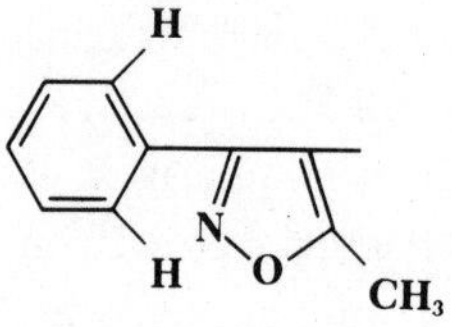

Oxacillin (Prostaphlin)

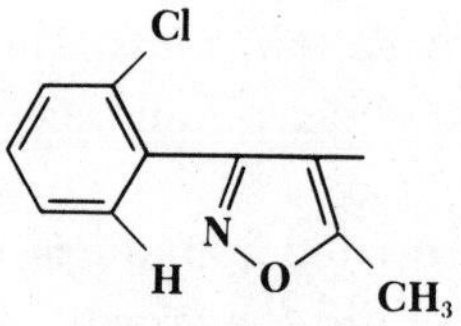

Cloxacillin (Tegopen)

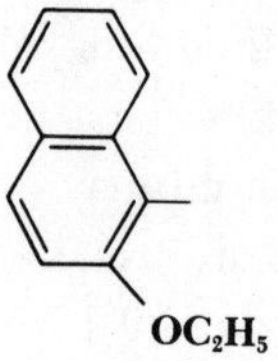

Nafcillin (Unipen)

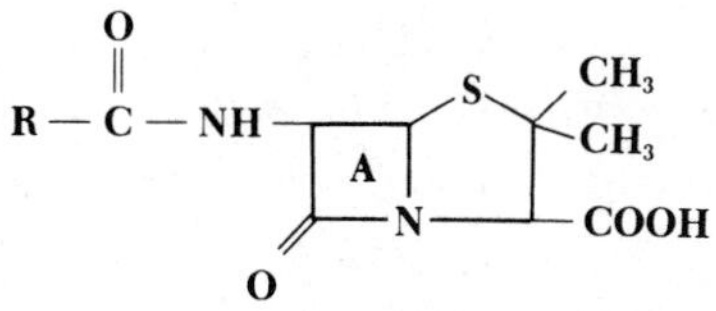

Basic penicillin structure

R side chain

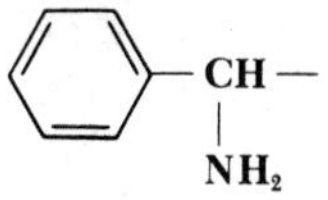

Ampicillin (Polycillin)

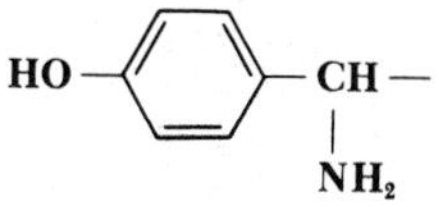

Amoxicillin (Amoxil)

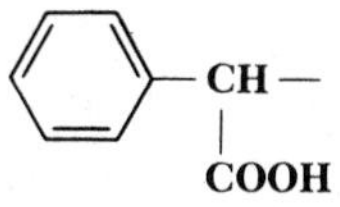

Carbenicillin (Geopen, Pyopen, Geocillin)

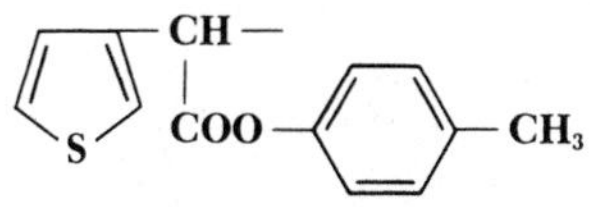

Ticarcillin (Ticar)

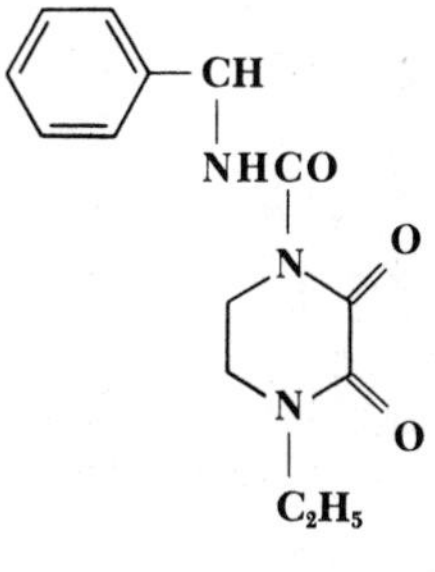

Piperacillin (Pipracil)

the bacterial cell wall. This work was initially done in gram-positive bacteria, but its conclusions apply to gram-negative organisms as well. The following description is simplified to illustrate where penicillin and related antibiotics block cell wall synthesis.

The bacterial cell wall is made of strands of a linear peptidoglycan consisting of alternating building blocks of *N*-acetylglucosamine and *N*-acetylmuramic acid. The latter compound has a "tail" consisting of a pentapeptide ending in D-alanine-D-alanine. These peptidoglycans are cross-linked by a pentaglycine bridge.

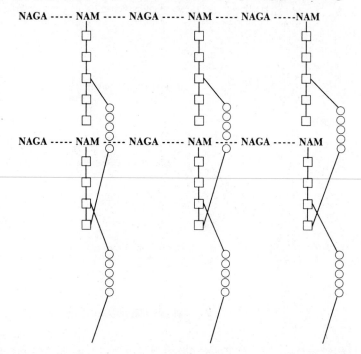

In the early experiments of Park,[21] a nucleotide accumulated in the culture broth of penicillin-treated bacteria. Synthesis of this nucleotide (UDP-*N*-acetylmuramic acid-pentapeptide) is the first step in the building of the cell wall. The second step is the formation of the linear peptidoglycans. The third and last step is the cross-linking of these linear strands. Compounds (several of which are clinically useful antibiotics) are known that inhibit enzymatic reactions at each step in cell wall synthesis.

STEP 1: Synthesis of nucleotide intermediates (requires lipid)

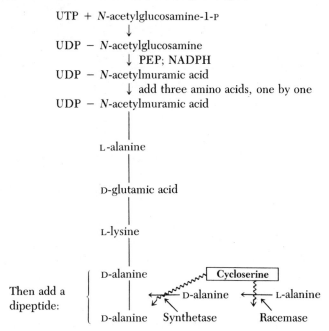

UTP + *N*-acetylglucosamine-1-P
↓
UDP − *N*-acetylglucosamine
↓ PEP; NADPH
UDP − *N*-acetylmuramic acid
↓ add three amino acids, one by one
UDP − *N*-acetylmuramic acid

L-alanine

D-glutamic acid

L-lysine

Then add a
dipeptide:
D-alanine — Cycloserine — D-alanine — L-alanine
D-alanine   Synthetase   Racemase

Cycloserine inhibits both the L-alanine racemase and the D-alanine synthetase by competitive inhibition.

STEP 2: Polymerization to form a linear peptidoglycan (occurs in cell membrane)

UDP − *N*-acetylmuramic acid-pentapeptide
↓ Phospholipid (in cell membrane, a C_{55} isoprenyl alcohol)
Phospholipid − *P*-*N*-acetylmuramic acid-pentapeptide + UMP
↓ UDP − *N*-acetylglucosamine
Phospholipid − *P*-*N*-acetylmuramic acid-pentapeptide-*N*-acetylglucosamine + UDP
↓ 5 glycines (0-0-0-0-0)(need tRNA)
Phospholipid − P-NAM-NAGA (NAM has pentapeptide and five glycines)

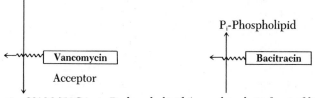

P_i-Phospholipid

Vancomycin   Bacitracin

Acceptor

Acceptor-NAM-NAGA + P-phospholipid (pyrophosphate form of lipid)

Bacitracin blocks the regeneration of the carrier phospholipid.

STEP 3: Cross-linking of the peptidoglycan strands (only two shown for clarity)

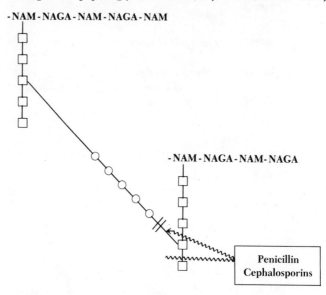

Cross-linking is done by a transpeptidase (which also cleaves a terminal D-alanine). The penicillins and cephalosporins bind to this enzyme and act as competitive inhibitors.

Pharmacokinetics

Absorption of penicillin G from the gastrointestinal tract is incomplete and variable. To obtain comparable blood concentrations it is usually necessary to administer five times as much of the antibotic by the oral route as by intramuscular injection. Incomplete absorption arises from inactivation of the drug by the gastric juice and, once it reaches the large intestine, by bacteria as well. Other penicillins, such as penicillin V, are fairly resistant to an acid environment and have replaced penicillin G as the preferred oral form.

Absorption of penicillin after its oral administration is greatly influenced by the presence of food in the stomach and the rate of gastric emptying. Absorption is best obtained if the drug is taken on an empty stomach.

Blood levels obtained following administration of 100,000 units (60 mg) of penicillin G sodium by various routes are shown in Fig. 53-1. It is clear that very transient high concentrations reaching 2 to 4 units/ml (about 2 to 4 µg/ml) can be obtained by either the intravenous or intramuscular route. The same dose given orally produces a blood concentration of only about 0.4 units/ml (about 0.4 g/ml), but demonstrable activity remains for a longer time. Intramuscular penicillin of any type is quite painful and should be avoided whenever possible. Very ill patients should receive penicillin compounds intravenously; other patients may receive the appropriate oral preparation. Exceptions are intramuscular benzathine penicillin for treatment of streptococcal pharyngitis, syphilis, and for monthly prophylaxis in rheumatic fever. In-

Relative blood serum concentrations of penicillin following intravenous, intramuscular, and **FIG. 53-1**
oral administration of 100,000 units of crystalline sodium penicillin G.

From Welch, H., et al.: *Principles and practice of antibiotic therapy*, New York, 1954, Medical Encyclopedia, Inc.

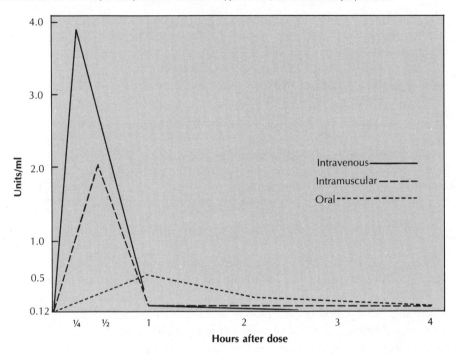

tramuscular procaine penicillin (with oral probenecid) is used to treat sensitive gonococcal infections.

Elimination of penicillin from the body after intravenous administration is entirely
by renal mechanisms; none of the drug is metabolized. Rapid decline of penicillin-
blood concentrations results from rapid renal clearance of the antibiotic. It has been
well established that penicillin is actively secreted by the renal tubules, apparently
by the same mechanism as *p*-aminohippurate or iodopyracet (Diodrast). Drugs have
been developed to block this tubular secretory mechanism. One of these is probenecid (Benemid), which is quite effective. It is not often used in penicillin therapy,
however, since it is easier to use larger doses of penicillin than to administer a second
drug for the purpose of retarding its excretion. A frequent error in the use of penicillin
is administering it at too long intervals. Since penicillin's half-life is approximately
1 hour (Table 53-1), giving a usual dosage interval of every 6 to 8 hours permits
substantial time with low or negligible blood-penicillin concentrations.

Repository preparations are available for the purpose of producing sustained
blood-penicillin concentrations. Procaine penicillin G and benzathine penicillin G

Penicillin	Oral absorption	Elimination half-life (hr)
G	Fair	0.6
V	Good	0.5
Methicillin	Poor (do not use postoperatively)	0.4
Oxacillin	Good	0.4
Dicloxacillin	Good	0.7
Nafcillin	Fair	0.5
Ampicillin	Good	0.8
Amoxicillin	Excellent	1
Carbenicillin (indanyl salt)	Only for urinary tract infections	1
Ticarcillin	Poor	1
Piperacillin	Poor (absent)	0.6

TABLE 53-1 Oral absorption and elimination of various antibiotics

are two such preparations. The latter permits demonstrable penicillin-blood concentrations to be maintained for 20 days or longer. It is important to recognize that demonstrable mean blood concentrations are often defined as 0.03 μg/ml or more. This low concentration may not be sufficient to treat infections, but it may be beneficial in preventing streptococcal infections and hence as prophylaxis against rheumatic fever.

Penicillin is not uniformly distributed in the body. The antibiotic is partially bound to plasma proteins. Under normal circumstances penicillin penetrates poorly into the cerebrospinal fluid, aqueous humor, and joint fluids. Inflammation at these sites greatly increases the permeability to the penicillins.

Cumulative urinary excretion of sodium penicillin G following its oral and intramuscular administration is shown in Fig. 53-2. In less than 4 hours as much as 80% of the intramuscularly administered dose may be recovered in urine. Only about 20% of an oral dose is usually recovered in urine because most of the penicillin is not absorbed. Table 53-1 indicates the extent of oral absorption and the elimination half-life of the penicillins. Penicillin is not used topically or by suppository.

Toxicity and hypersensitivity

The toxicity of penicillin as determined in animal experiments is extremely low. In several animal species the acute toxicity of penicillin is so low that death from overdosage has been attributed to the cation of the salt rather than to penicillin itself.

Unfortunately, a significant percentage of the human population shows hypersensitivity reactions to penicillin. These reactions are diverse, ranging from immediate anaphylactic reactions to late manifestations of the serum sickness type. Several hundred severe anaphylactic reactions have occurred following penicillin injections, many terminating fatally.

Comparison of cumulative urinary excretion of penicillin following intramuscular and oral   **FIG. 53-2**
administration of crystalline sodium penicillin G.

From Welch, H., et al.: *Principles and practice of antibiotic therapy*, New York, 1954, Medical Encyclopedia, Inc.

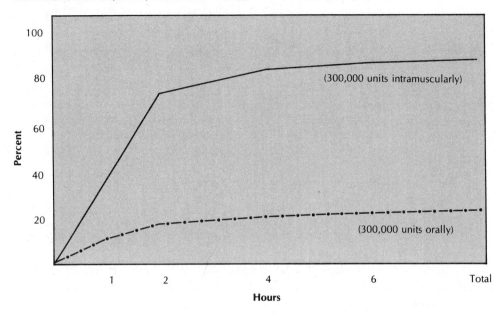

Hypersensitivity reactions are seen most often after topical use of penicillin and most rarely after oral administration. The incidence of such reactions varies from 1% to 8% in the general population.

Skin tests to identify penicillin allergy are unreliable and dangerous when penicillin G itself is injected in small quantities intracutaneously. A skin test is available in which penicilloyl polylysine (PPL; Pre-Pen) is suitable for testing allergy to the major determinant.[9] Patients with a positive reaction to PPL are very likely to also have an allergic reaction to penicillin, but a negative PPL reaction does not ensure absence of allergy to penicillin. Available on an experimental basis is a mixture of penicillin, penicilloate, and other hydrolysis products suitable for testing allergy to the minor determinants. Despite these refinements in diagnosing penicillin allergy, tests are not completely reliable. A history of previous reactions is *very* important. Even in the presence of a negative intradermal test, it is best to be prepared for the possibility of anaphylactic reaction whenever the antibiotic is injected. Patients allergic to one penicillin must be assumed to be allergic to all penicillins.

In addition to hypersensitivity reactions, penicillin can produce other adverse effects. Neural tissue may be susceptible to penicillin, particularly when the drug is injected intrathecally or applied directly to the surface of the brain. Convulsive phenomena have been noted following such exposures. Intrathecal penicillin is no longer used. Seizures may rarely be seen in a patient receiving very high doses intravenously (e.g., bacterial endocarditis requiring 2 million units [1.25 g] every 2 hours).

Other adverse effects have become known with the increasing numbers of new penicillins developed. These reactions include leukopenia (nafcillin), hepatitis (oxacillin), renal damage (methicillin), diarrhea (oral preparations of ampicillin and amoxicillin), and platelet dysfunction (carbenicillin, ticarcillin, and methicillin). Most penicillins are irritating to tissue and care must be taken during intravenous therapy to avoid extravasation.

Broad-spectrum penicillins susceptible to penicillinase	**Ampicillin** (Penbritin, Omnipen, Polycillin) expands the antimicrobial spectrum of penicillin G. It is effective against many gram-negative microorganisms. The drug is more acid resistant and is well absorbed following oral administration. Ampicillin is effective against urinary tract infections caused by *Escherichia coli* and *Proteus mirabilis* (susceptible strains). The antibiotic is also effective in the treatment of respiratory infections and meningitis caused by susceptible strains of *Hemophilus influenzea*. Ampicillin may cause a skin rash, especially if the patient has infectious mononucleosis. This rash produced by ampicillin does not appear to be the type associated with allergies.

Ampicillin (Penbritin, Omnipen, Polycillin) is available in 250 and 500 mg capsules and in a pediatric suspension of 125 or 250 mg/5 ml. The sodium salt is available for parenteral administration.

Amoxicillin trihydrate (Amoxil, Larotid) differs from ampicillin in that it produces higher serum concentrations milligram for milligram. The incidence and severity of diarrhea (especially in children) appear to be less than with ampicillin. Only used orally, amoxicillin is cleaved to ampicillin during intestinal absorption.

Carbenicillin disodium (Geopen) has greater activity than ampicillin against *Pseudomonas aeruginosa* and *Enterobacter*, and *Serratia* organisms. It may also be active against ampicillin-resistant strains of *Proteus* species. A special feature of carbenicillin is its high sodium content. Since 1 g of carbenicillin contains 6 mEq of sodium, large doses may cause sodium overload in renal and cardiac patients. Carbenicillin disodium should not be given orally, since it is not absorbed.

Carbenicillin indanyl sodium (Geocillin) is available in tablets for oral administration but is used only for treatment of urinary tract infections.

Ticarcillin disodium (Ticar) is closely related to carbenicillin and is available for intramuscular and intravenous use. It has greater potency than carbenicillin against the difficult gram-negative bacilli (e.g., *Pseudomonas* organisms). Carbenicillin and ticarcillin are usually used in combination with an aminoglycoside in treating these serious gram-negative infections.

Piperacillin (Pipracil), like carbenicillin and ticarcillin, is used for parenteral treatment of certain gram-negative organisms. Its spectrum is broader and includes *Pseudomonas*, *Serratia*, *Enterobacter*, and *Klebsiella* species and *Bacteroides fragilis*. It is also used in combination with an aminoglycoside.

Mezlocillin (Mezlin) resembles piperacillin in its clinical activity and use.

Penicillinase-resistant penicillins are very useful against infections caused by organisms resistant to penicillin G, especially staphylococcal infections. Although these penicillins are resistant to staphylococcal penicillinase, strains are appearing with "methicillin resistance" not based on drug inactivation by penicillinase. Sensitivities should be done by the laboratory to determine the most appropriate antibiotic. Most staphylococcal infections, whether hospital or community acquired, are resistant to treatment by penicillin G or V.

Penicillins resistant to penicillinase

Methicillin sodium (Staphcillin) is administered intramuscularly or intravenously and is unstable in solution. Its only advantage is in infections caused by staphylococci that are resistant to penicillin G. The antibiotic may be nephrotoxic.

Nafcillin sodium (Unipen, Nafcil) can be administered orally, intramuscularly, or intravenously. More potent than methicillin, nafcillin may penetrate the spinal fluid better and is largely excreted in the bile.

Oxacillin sodium (Prostaphlin, Bactocill) is very similar to nafcillin in actions and indications. It may be given orally or parenterally. Cloxacillin sodium (Tegopen, Cloxapen) and dicloxacillin sodium (Dynapen, Dycill) resemble oxacillin and are available for oral administration in capsules and suspensions. Table 53-2 summarizes the clinical uses of the penicillins.

The cephalosporins are β-lactam antibiotics obtained originally from a *Cephalosporium* mold. These antibiotics have the same mechanism of action as the penicillins but differ in antibacterial spectrum, resistance to β-lactamase, and pharmacokinetics. Whereas penicillins are derivatives of 6-aminopenicillanic acid, the cephalosporins are derivatives of 7-aminocephalosporanic acid. The related cephamycins have a 7-methoxy group, which may increase their resistance to β-lactamases. Development of cephalosporins is proceeding at a rapid rate. It is expected that newer compounds will continue to offer advantages in broader spectrum, pharmacokinetics, and penetration to body cavities.[19]

CEPHALOSPORINS

The antibacterial spectrum of the original cephalosporins (cephalothin, cephapirin, cephalexin, and cefazolin) is similar to that of the penicillinase-resistant penicillins. Cefaclor and cefamandole are active against *H. influenzae*, an important pathogen in the pediatric age group. The most recently developed cephalosporins, moxalactam, cefadroxil, and cefotaxime, are active against a wide spectrum of gramnegative organisms, including *E. coli*, species of *Proteus, Klebsiella, Serratia*, and *Enterobacter*, and *B. fragilis*. Moxalactam and cefotaxime are the only cephalosporins at the present time with sufficient penetration into cerebrospinal fluid to justify their use in treating meningitis. They may well become drugs of choice in treating neonatal meningitis caused by gram-negative organisms. Development of newer cephalosporins with wider spectrums, higher potency, and greater penetration into body cavities can be expected in the future.[19]

Cephalosporins are eliminated both by glomerular filtration and tubular secretion. Probenecid prolongs the half-life of these drugs, as does renal impairment. Elimi-

TABLE 53-2   Summary of current usage of penicillins

Agent generic name (trade name)	Spectrum of activity	Usual adult dosage (gastrointestinal absorption)	Route	Mode of action (cidal or static)	Side Effects
Penicillin G	Gram positive, β-hemolytic streptococcus, pneumococci, gonococcus	Usual dose: 600,000-1 million U Large dose: 10-12 million U	Intramuscular Intravenous	Cidal Cidal	Anaphylactoid reactions, drug fever, skin rashes, Coombs positive hemolytic anemia Skin rashes, convulsions, (high dose, especially in renal failure)
		Usual dose: 1 million U (1 g) before meals	Oral (Use penicillin V.)	Cidal	Gastrointestinal (uncommon)
Benzathine penicillin G (Bicillin)	β-Hemolytic streptococcus, gonococcus	600,000-1 million U	Intramuscular	Cidal	Same as above, local inflammatory reactions
Ampicillin (Penbritin, Omnipen, Polycillin)	Gram positive (not resistant staphylococci), gram negative (*H. influenzae*)	0.25-0.5 g q.6h. 150-200 mg/kg/day	Oral, intramuscular, intravenous	Cidal	Gastrointestinal, skin rash (especially in patients with infectious mononucleosis), fever, rate ↑SGOT, anaphylactoid reactions, convulsions (with excessively rapid intravenous administration)
Carbenicillin (Pyopen, Geopen)	Gram positive (not resistant staphylococci), gram negative (especially *E. coli*, species of *Pseudomonas, Proteus, Enterobacter*, not *Klebsiella*)	5 g q.4h. given over 2-hr period (non-absorbed orally)	Intravenous	Cidal	Similar to other penicillins, ↑SGOT, nausea, neutropenia, hemolytic anemia, convulsions (high dose in patients with renal failure), possible abnormalities in coagulation tests (high dose in patients with uremia), NOTE: 4.7 mEq (108 mg) Na$^+$/g, possible hypokalemia

Drug	Spectrum	Dosage	Route	Type	Side effects
Piperacillin (Pipracil)	Gram positive (not resistant staphylococci), gram negative (especially *E. coli*, species of *Pseudomonas, Proteus, Enterobacter, Klebsiella), B. fragilis*	4 g q.4h.	Intravenous	Cidal	Similar to other penicillins, ↑ SGOT, nausea, neutropenia, hemolytic anemia, convulsions (high dose in patients with renal failure), possible abnormalities in coagulation tests (high dose in patients with uremia). NOTE: 4.7 mEq (108 mg) Na$^+$/g, possible hypokalemia
Methicillin (Staphcillin, Dimocillin)	Gram positive, especially staphylococci	1-2 g q.6h.	Intramuscular, intravenous	Cidal	Similar to penicillin G, eosinophilia, leukopenia, nephrotoxicity, Coombs positive hemolytic anemia
Nafcillin (Unipen)	Gram positive, especially staphylococci	0.25-1 g q.6h. a.c. 0.5-1 g q.5-6h.	Oral, intramuscular, intravenous	Cidal	Gastrointestinal, fever, skin rash, asymptomatic > SGOT
Oxacillin (Prostaphlin, Resistopen)	Gram positive, especially staphylococci	0.5-1 g q.4-6h.	Oral, intramuscular	Cidal	Occasional gastrointestinal, fever, skin rash, asymptomatic ↑ SGOT, ↓ hemoglobin, neutropenia, transient hematuria (infants)
Dicloxacillin (Dynapen, Pathocil, Veracillin)	Gram positive, especially staphylococci	0.125-0.5 g q.6h. a.c.	Oral	Cidal	Gastrointestinal bleeding

Courtesy Dr. Jay P. Sanford, Washington, D.C.

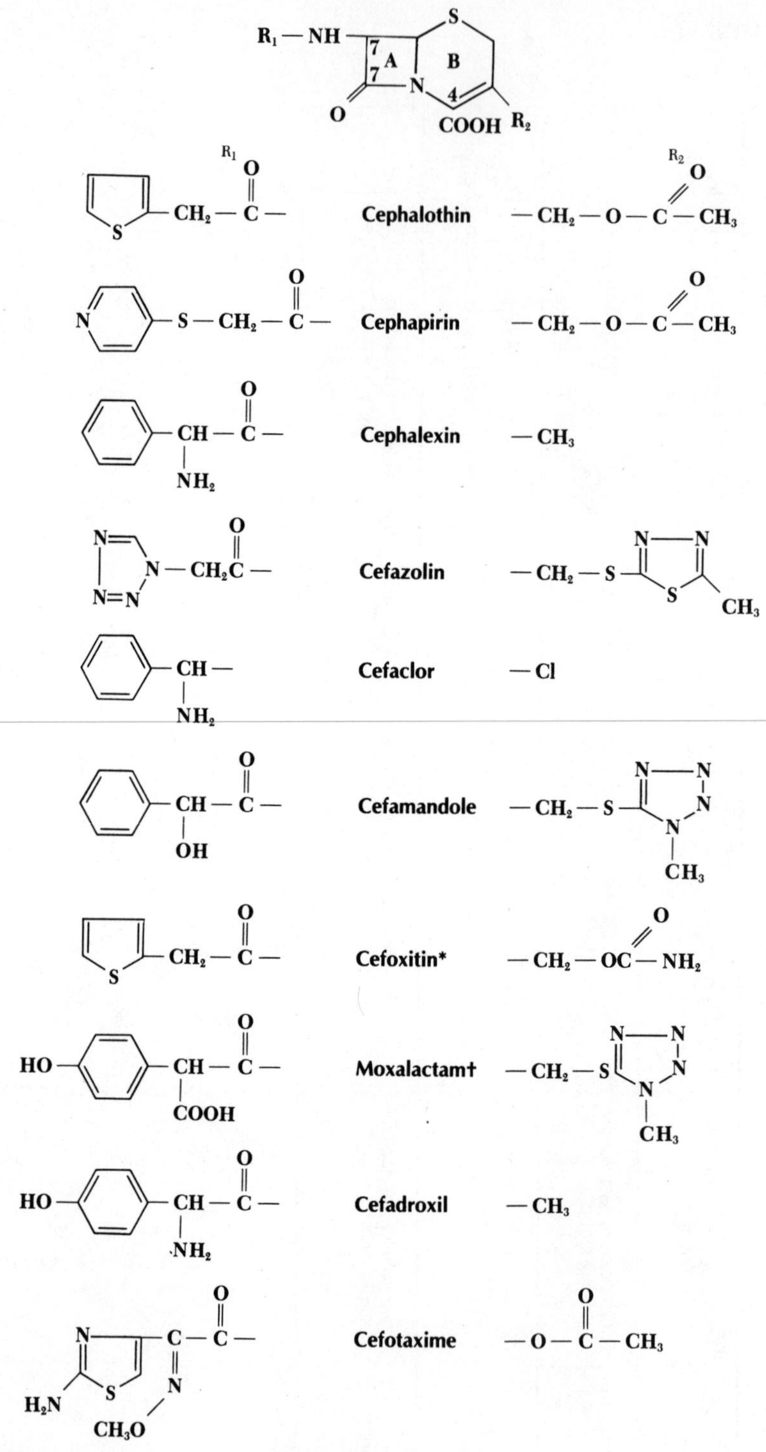

The core structure:

R_1—NH—[7A] [7] A B ring with S, N at position 4, COOH, R_2
O

	R_1	Name	R_2
	(thiophene)—CH_2—C(=O)—	**Cephalothin**	—CH_2—O—C(=O)—CH_3
	(pyridine)N—S—CH_2—C(=O)—	**Cephapirin**	—CH_2—O—C(=O)—CH_3
	(phenyl)—CH(NH$_2$)—C(=O)—	**Cephalexin**	—CH_3
	(tetrazole)N—CH_2C(=O)—	**Cefazolin**	—CH_2—S—(thiadiazole)—CH_3
	(phenyl)—CH(NH$_2$)—	**Cefaclor**	—Cl
	(phenyl)—CH(OH)—C(=O)—	**Cefamandole**	—CH_2—S—(tetrazole)—CH_3
	(thiophene)—CH_2—C(=O)—	**Cefoxitin***	—CH_2—OC(=O)—NH_2
	HO—(phenyl)—CH(COOH)—C(=O)—	**Moxalactam†**	—CH_2—S—(tetrazole)—CH_3
	HO—(phenyl)—CH(NH$_2$)—C(=O)—	**Cefadroxil**	—CH_3
	H_2N—(thiazole)—C(=N—O—CH_3)—C(=O)—	**Cefotaxime**	—O—C(=O)—CH_3

---

*Cefoxitin has a methoxy group at position 7 of the β-lactam ring.

†Moxalactam has a methoxy group at position 7 of the β-lactam ring. The sulfur atom in ring B is replaced by an oxygen atom.

nation half-lives of the cephalosporins in patients with normal renal function are two to four times larger than those of the penicillins.

$T_{\frac{1}{2}}$ 2-4 x PGN

The cephalosporins share all of the toxicities of the penicillins. The most frequent side effect is an allergic reaction: hives, serum sickness, and anaphylaxis. Special toxic reactions should be recognized when using certain cephalosporins; for example, a disulfiram-like reaction can occur with moxalactam (Table 53-3).

Toxicity

Cephalosporins can be classified according to their mode of administration. The orally administered members of the group include cephalexin monohydrate (Keflex), cefaclor (Ceclor), and cefadroxil (Duricef). Parenteral forms are cephapirin sodium (Cefadyl), cefazolin sodium (Ancef, Kefzol), cefamandole nafate (Mandol), the cephamycin cefoxitin sodium (Mefoxin), cefotaxime (Claforan), and moxalactam (Moxam).

These drugs are generally overused in many clinical situations in which other antibiotics (especially one of the penicillins) would be just as effective and considerably less costly. There are five major categories of use:

Uses of cephalosporins

1. In persons allergic to penicillin (Many patients allergic to penicillin may also be allergic to cephalosporins.[10] One must proceed with caution in this situation.)

2. For certain gram-negative infections, especially *Klebsiella* species

3. For therapy of mixed infections or initial treatment of infections of unknown causes

4. For prophylaxis before surgery, especially gastrointestinal, pelvic, or orthopedic surgery (the latter involving plastic or metal implants)

5. For meningitis caused by gram-negative organisms (cefotaxime and moxalactam only)—may become drug of choice

Use of these antibiotics should be guarded by sensitivity testing of the microorganism isolated from the patient. See Table 53-3 for comments on usage of individual groups.

Clycloserine inhibits both the racemase and synthetase enzymes responsible for the synthesis of the dipeptide D-alanine-D-alanine in the first stage of cell wall synthesis. Cycloserine is easily absorbed, giving peak blood concentrations in 3 to 4 hours after an oral dose. It is highly diffusable even to cerebrospinal fluid. In 12 hours 50% of a dose is excreted unchanged by the kidney. The remaining fraction is metabolized. Adverse reactions involve the CNS: headaches, psychosis, and seizures. Cycloserine is used only in the treatment of tuberculosis, especially when the mycobacteria are resistant to other drugs.

OTHER ANTIBIOTICS THAT INHIBIT CELL WALL SYNTHESIS
Cycloserine

TABLE 53-3 Summary of current usage of cephalosporins

Agent generic name (trade name)	Spectrum of activity	Usual adult dosage	Route	Mode of action (Cidal or static)	Side effects
Cephalothin (Keflin)	Gram positive, gram negative (especially *E. coli*, *P. mirabilis*), not enterococci, indole positive *Proteus*, *Pseudomonas* species	0.5-3 g q.6h.	Intramuscular, intravenous	Cidal	Rash, fever, eosinophila, ↑ SGOT, neutropenia, anaphylactoid reactions, convulsions, (high dose in patients with renal failure), positive Coombs test, thrombocytopenia, false positive "Clinitest," phlebitis, local pain on injection
Cephapirin (Cetadyl)	See Cephalothin				
Cephalexin (Keflex)	Gram positive (not enterococci, variable against resistant staphylococci and neisseriae), gram negative (urinary infections caused by most *E. coli*, *P. mirabilis*, and some *Klebsiella* organisms; variable against *Salmonella* and *Shigella* species)	0.25-0.5 g q.6h.	Oral	Cidal	Similar to other cephalosporins, gastrointestinal

Cefazolin (Ancef, Kefzol)	Similar to cephalothin	0.25 g q.8h.–1 g q.6h.	Intramuscular, intravenous	Cidal	Rash (uncommon), ↑ SGOT, ↑ alkaline phosphatase
Cefaclor (Ceclor)	Same as for cephalothin, *H. influenzae*	0.5 g q.8h.	Oral	Cidal	
Cefamandole (Mandol)	Same as for cephalothin, *H. influenzae*	0.5–4 g q.4–8h.	Intramuscular, intravenous	Cidal	See cephalothin, also disulfiram reaction, bleeding
Cefoxitin (Mefoxin)	Same as for cephalothin, penicillinase producing gonococcus	0.5–4 g q.4–8h.	Intramuscular, intravenous	Cidal	See cephalothin
Moxalactam (Moxam)	Same as for cephalothin, *Klebsiella, Serratia, Enterobacter, Bacteroides* species	0.5–4 g q.4–8h.	Intramuscular, intravenous	Cidal	See cefamandole, superinfection with enterococci; *Pseudomonas* and *Candida* species
Cefadroxil (Duricef, Ultracef)	See cephalexin	0.5–1 g q.12–24h.	Oral	Cidal	See cephalexin
Cefotaxime (Claforan)	See moxalactam	1–3 g q.4–6h.	Intramuscular, intravenous	Cidal	See moxalactam

Courtesy Dr. Jay P. Sanford, Washington, D.C.

Cycloserine

Vancomycin	Vancomycin is a complex glycopeptide obtained from an actinomycete. It inhibits the second stage of cell wall formation—polymerization of the peptidoglycan polymer. Bactericidal against gram-positive bacteria, vancomycin is poorly absorbed when administered via the oral route; advantage of this is taken in treating enterocolitis caused by staphylococci and *Clostridium difficile* (pseudomembranous colitis). This drug is used intravenously to treat serious systemic infections caused by staphylococci resistant to other drugs. It is also used in patients allergic to both penicillins and cephalosporins. Its half-life is about 6 hours. Most of the drug is eliminated through renal mechanisms. Vancomycin is quite irritating to tissues and can cause ototoxicity and nephrotoxicity.
Bacitracin	Bacitracin is a polypeptide that inhibits the second stage of cell wall synthesis. It is now only used topically for skin infections caused by gram-positive organisms.
Polymyxin B	The polymyxins are basic peptides that act as cationic detergents and cause lysis of the lipoprotein cell membrane. Polymyxin B is particularly active against gram-negative bacteria. Serious nephrotoxicity has limited its parenteral use. It is used chiefly for treatment of local infections: external otitis, eye infections, and skin infections with organisms sensitive to polymyxin. Colistin is a very similar compound.
AMINOGLY-COSIDES	The aminoglycoside antibiotics (aminocyclitols) are bactericidal drugs commonly used to treat serious infections caused by many gram-negative bacilli and some gram-positive organisms. Streptococci, pneumococci, clostridia, anaerobes, and fungi are resistant. Aminoglycosides inhibit bacterial protein synthesis by interfering with binding of bacterial aminoacyl tRNAs to the 30 S ribosomal subunit (see Chapter 51). Distinguishing characterstics of the major aminoglycosides are summarized in Table 53-4.
General features	The aminoglycosides, including streptomycin, neomycin, kanamycin, gentamicin, tobramycin, amikacin, and spectinomycin, are important antibiotics for serious, usually systemic, infections caused by gram-negative organisms.[23] The most commonly used antibiotic in this group is gentamicin.

The aminoglycosides, being polar cations, are poorly absorbed following oral administration and do not reach the CNS. For that reason they are usually administered intramuscularly or intravenously, except neomycin, which has some usefulness in decreasing intestinal flora when given orally. The aminoglycosides are not highly bound to serum proteins. They are well distributed in the body, except in

TABLE 53-4   Summary of characteristics of aminoglycosides

Agent generic name (trade name)	Spectrum of activity	Usual dosage	Route	Mode of action (cidal or static)	Side effects
Streptomycin	Enterococcus, mycobacterium tuberculosis, *Brucella* species, tularemia, *Yersinia pestis* (plague),	0.5-2 g/day q.12h. Children: 20-30 mg/kg/day	Intramuscular	Cidal	Vestibular damage, auditory damage, drug fever, neuromuscular blockade, skin rash, circumoral paresthesias with flushing
Neomycin	Used only for alterations in bowel flora (see p. 641)				Same as for kanamycin, malabsorption with oral use
Kanamycin (Kantrex)	Gram-negative bacilli, TBC (rarely)	15 mg/kg/day q.8h. Children: 15-20 mg/kg/day	Intramuscular, intravenous	Cidal	Ototoxicity (auditory) nephrotoxicity, neuromuscular blockade, skin rash (rare)
Gentamicin (Garamycin)	Gram-negative bacilli (*Proteus, Pseudomonas, Serratia* species)	3-5 mg/kg/day q.8h. Children: 3-7.5 mg/kg/day	Intramuscular, intravenous	Cidal	Nephrotoxicity (protein ↑ blood urea nitrogen), vestibular toxicity, fever, skin rash—avoid concurrent use with ethacrynic acid
Tobramycin (Hebcin)	Same as gentamicin	Same as gentamicin	Intramuscular, intravenous	Cidal	Same as gentamicin
Amakacin (Amikin)	Same as gentamicin; may be more effective against some strains of *Pseudomonas*	15 mg/kg/day q.8-12h. Children: 15 mg/kg/day q.8-12h.	Intramuscular, intravenous	Cidal	Same as gentamicin
Spectinomycin (Trobicin)	Gonorrhea (penicillin-resistant infection)	2 g (single injection) Children: 40 mg/kg (single injection)	Intramuscular	Cidal	Chills, fever, urticaria

Courtesy Dr. Jay P. Sanford, Washington, D.C.

the CNS, and are excreted by glomerular filtration without tubular resorption. Renal elimination is rapid. Plasma half-lives are 2 to 3 hours.

The aminoglycosides are ototoxic, nephrotoxic, and may cause neuromuscular blockade. Ototoxicity reflects itself in vestibular and auditory disturbances by damage to the sensory receptors such as the hair cells in the cochlea. Whereas streptomycin and neomycin primarily affect vestibular function, kanamycin has relatively greater auditory toxicity. These drugs may cause dose-related changes in vestibular and auditory function, ranging from disturbances in equilibration and tinnitus to permanent deafness. The risk of ototoxicity may be greater in patients with decreased renal function. Ototoxicity is minimized if trough plasma concentrations are maintained below 2 μg/ml.

Manifestations of nephrotoxicity, which is usually reversible, may range from only mild proteinuria to severe azotemia. Since the aminoglycosides are excreted by the kidney, preexisting renal damage calls for caution and readjustment of dosage schedules.[4]

The neuromuscular blocking effect of the aminoglycosides may lead to apnea, particularly in myasthenia gravis or with certain general anesthetics and neuromuscular blocking agents. Neuromuscular blockade is most likely to occur with large intravenous doses given rapidly or with instillation into the peritoneal cavity. Intravenous calcium gluconate is effective in antagonizing neuromuscular effects of the aminoglycosides (except kanamycin), and neostigmine may be useful.

Resistance develops rapidly to the antibacterial action of streptomycin and more slowly to the other aminoglycosides. Resistance is acquired by (1) a single mutational step (streptomycin), (2) the inability to transport the drug to an intracellular site, or (3) the induction of enzymes that metabolize the drug and render it inactive. The latter form of resistance is carried by R factors (plasmids), which may also confer resistance to several other nonaminoglycoside antibiotics. Resistance to one aminoglycoside does not necessarily mean resistance to all. The plasmids induce production of enzymes that acetylate or phosphorylate the aminoglycoside. These enzymes may be specific for some but not all aminoglycosides. For example, some organisms, such as *Pseudomonas*, may be resistant to gentamicin but susceptible to amikacin.

Streptomycin   Streptomycin, discovered in 1944, differs from penicillin in being an organic base rather than an acid.[25] It is not absorbed from the gastrointestinal tract, has a much broader antibacterial spectrum (although a generally lower potency), and causes direct toxic effects in mammals. At present the main usefulness of this antibiotic is in the treatment of tuberculosis (see Chapter 54) and in combination with penicillin for treatment of endocarditis caused by the enterococcus. It is useful in tularemia, plague, and brucellosis. Resistance may emerge rapidly (induced by R factors), especially when streptomycin is used as a single agent.

Streptomycin

Neomycin is too toxic for parenteral administration. Topical use should be avoided *Neomycin* because of the possibility of sensitization. With application to large areas of abraided skin, significant absorption may occur and result in systemic toxicity. Currently oral neomycin is used mainly for prophylaxis for bowel surgery, for decreasing urea production by gut flora in patients with hepatic insufficiency, and for treatment of infants with enterocolitis resulting from pathogenic strains of *E. coli*. Neomycin is available in 500 mg tablets for oral use.

Kanamycin (Kantrex, Klebcil) is used parenterally against gram-negative bacilli *Kanamycin* causing serious systemic disease. Renal damage and ototoxicity may occur, especially in patients with preexisting renal disease.

Gentamicin sulfate (Garamycin) and tobramycin sulfate (Nebcin) are very similar *Gentamicin and* chemically and pharmacologically. Their main difference is the greater potency of *tobramycin* tobramycin against *P. aeruginosa*.

The major usefulness of gentamicin and tobramycin is in the treatment of systemic infections caused by susceptible gram-negative bacteria, especially *Pseudomonas, Klebsiella,* and *Serratia* species. Streptococci, pneumococci, anaerobic bacteria, and fungi are resistant. Some staphylococci, resistant to the semisynthetic penicillins, may be sensitive to gentamicin. In the clinical use of these drugs, renal elimination, nephrotoxicity, ototoxicity, and neuromuscular dysfunction should be taken into consideration. Plasma concentrations of these aminoglycosides should be monitored whenever possible; trough concentrations should not exceed 2 μg/ml. In addition, gentamicin should not be mixed with carbenicillin or heparin. Tobramycin is usually more active than gentamicin against *Pseudomonas* species.

Gentamicin sulfate (Garamycin) is available in solutions containing 20 mg/ml and in disposable syringes. Tobramycin sulfate (Nebcin) is available in solutions containing 10 or 40 mg/ml and in disposable syringes. The dosage of either drug for adults with normal renal function is 3 to 5 mg/kg daily. Doses are divided and administered intramuscularly or intravenously.

Amikacin sulfate

A derivative of kanamycin, amikacin sulfate (Amikin) is a chemically modified semisynthetic aminoglycoside. The chemical modification confers resistance to the inactivating effect of enzymes capable of destroying the activity of gentamicin and tobramycin. The drug is used to treat infections caused by gram-negative bacteria. It is available for intramuscular and intravenous administration in solutions containing 50 and 250 mg/ml.

Spectinomycin

Spectinomycin (Trobicin), used only for penicillin-resistant gonorrheal infections, is given as a single 2 g intramuscular injection. This drug is *not* effective against syphilis.

TETRACYCLINES

The tetracyclines are broad-spectrum bacteriostatic antibiotics. They inhibit protein synthesis in bacteria by blocking the binding of aminoacyl transfer ribonucleic acid (tRNA) to the 30 S ribosomal subunit. Although largely replaced by better, less toxic antibiotics, the tetacyclines are sill highly effective in the treatment of brucellosis, *Mycoplasma pneumoniae,* cholera, rickettsial disease, and chlamydiae. They may also be useful as alternatives in the treatment of infections resistant to the drug of choice, such as in gonorrhea and certain urinary tract infections. Tetracycline in low doses has been an important agent in the treatment of acne, although the new synthetic retinoid, isotretinoin, has just been successfully introduced. Being bacteriostatic, the tetracyclines occasionally interfere with the killing effect of a bactericidal antibiotic such as penicillin.

The three tetracyline antibiotics, chlortetracycline (Aureomycin), oxytetracycline (Terramycin), and tetracycline, were discovered as a result of extensive screening experiments on antibiotics produced by soil organisms. Essentially bacteriostatic drugs, except in very high concentrations, tetracyclines may in some cases modify an infection rather than eradicate it. Their characteristics are summarized in Table

53-5. Because these compounds have significant side effects, they should not be used in pregnant women nor in infants and children under 8 years of age.

Tetracycline is a true broad-spectrum antibiotic. For that reason it has been overused. Such excessive use led to development of many resistant strains of bacteria and to superinfections, whose incidence in some series has been as high as 20% of patients. In general, broad-spectrum agents are more conducive to superinfections than antibiotics with a narrow spectrum.

Tetracycline hydrochloride is widely used in the treatment of infections with *M. pneumoniae*, chlamydiae, cholera, and rickettsiae. Lower doses than used for these infections are employed in the management of pustular acne.

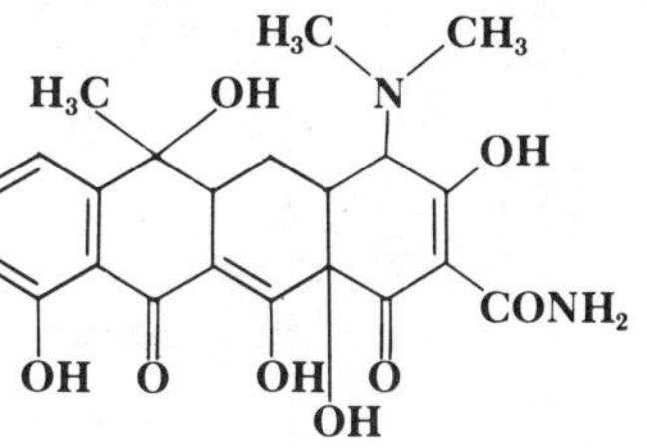

Tetracycline

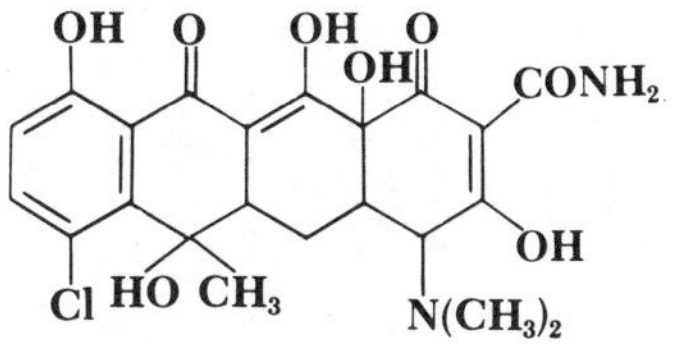

Chlortetracycline

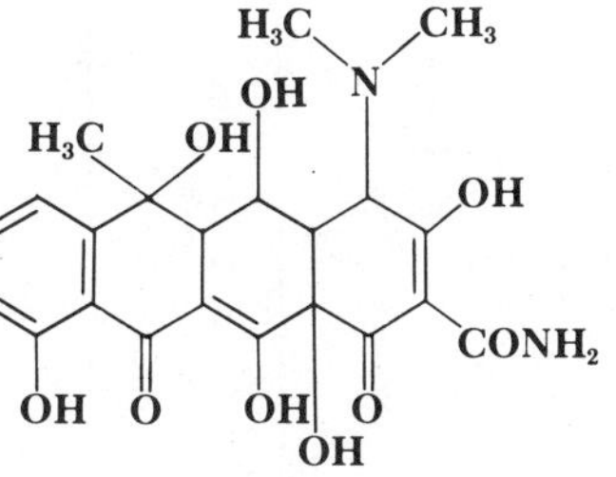

Oxytetracycline

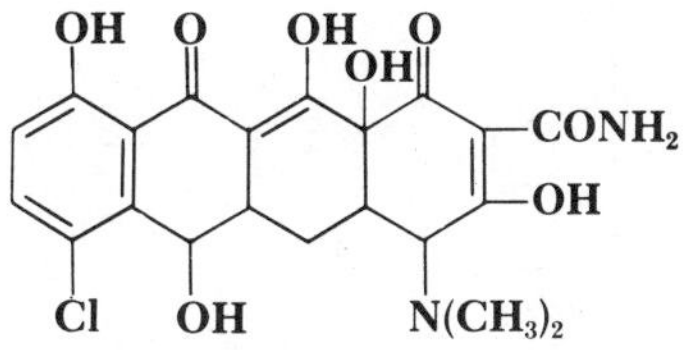

Demeclocycline

In addition to the three well-known tetracycline antibiotics, other derivatives have been introduced. Demeclocycline (Declomycin) may cause severe photosensitization. Doxycycline monohydrate (Vibramycin) differs from other tetracyclines in requiring less frequent administration because of slower elimination. It may also cause phototoxicity. Rolitetracycline (Syntetrin), a very soluble derivative of tetracycline, is suitable for parenteral administration. It may be injected intravenously or intramuscularly.

Another slowly excreted member of the tetracycline family, minocycline (Minocin), may cause severe vertigo and nausea. The slowly excreted tetracyclines may accumulate in the body and produce toxicity when renal function is impaired. Doxycycline is slowly excreted also but appears to be safer in renal failure.

PROBLEM 53-1. *The causative agent in a stubborn urinary tract infection was found to be most susceptible to the tetracyclines. The physician selected doxycycline because of the convenience of twice-daily administration. Was this a good choice? No, because doxycycline is not excreted in the urine to the same extent as some other tetracyclines.*

TABLE 53-5 Summary of characteristics of tetracyclines

Agent generic name (trade name)	Spectrum of activity	Usual dosage	Route	Mode of action (cidal or static)	Side effects
Tetracycline Chlortetracycline Oxytetracycline	Gram positive, gram negative, *Bacteroides* species, chlamydiae (LGV), *M. pneumoniae, rickettsiae*, oxytetracycline-tuberculosis	0.25-0.5 g q.6h. 0.2-0.6 g/day 0.5-1 g q.12h.	Oral, intramuscular, intravenous	Static	Gastrointestinal, skin rash, anaphylactoid reactions (rare), deposition in teeth and bone, negative nitrogen balance, hepatotoxicity, enamel agenesis, benign ↑ cerebrospinal fluid pressure
Demeclocycline (Declomycin)	Gram positive, gram negative, *M. pneumoniae*, chlamydiae	0.15-0.3 g q.6h.	Oral	Static	Gastrointestinal, skin rash, deposition in teeth and bone, negative nitrogen balance, phototoxicity, benign ↑ cerebrospinal fluid pressure, onycholysis, anaphylactoid reactions
Minocycline (Minocin)	Gram positive, gram negative, chlamydiae	100 mg q.12h.	Oral	Static	Similar to other tetracyclines
Doxycycline (Vibramycin)	Gram positive, gram negative, *M. pneumoniae*, chlamydiae	0.1 g q.12h. on first day, then 0.1 g/ day	Oral	Static	Similar to other tetracyclines, phototoxicity less than demeclocycline, probably greater than tetracycline

Courtesy Dr. Jay P. Sanford, Washington, D.C.

Average serum concentration following oral administration of 0.25 g of tetracycline.　　FIG. 53-3

From Welch, H., et al.: Principles and practice of antibiotic therapy, New York, 1954, Medical Encyclopedia, Inc.

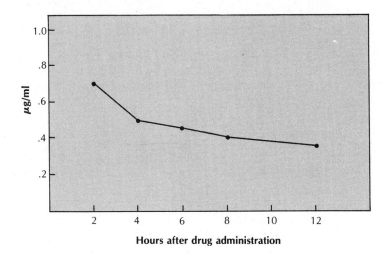

Pharmacokinetics

All these drugs are absorbed rapidly but incompletely from the gastrointestinal tract.[12,13] Calcium salts and gastric antacids prevent their absorption. Variable amounts may remain in the large intestine, and the bacterial flora of the intestinal contents may be altered considerably. The development of serious staphylococcal gastroenteritis during tetracycline therapy has been attributed to the phenomenon of superinfection with staphylococci that produce exotoxin.

Oral administration of a 250 mg dose of tetracycline will produce a serum concentration of about 0.7 μg/ml in less than 2 hours (Fig. 53-3). This concentration declines gradually to about half this value in approximately 12 hours. The slow decline may be explained by low renal clearance of the drug. During the first 12 hours, only about 10% to 20% of the dose appears in urine.

Widely distributed in most tissues, tetracycline probably enters cells, but in the cerebrospinal fluid its concentration is less than in plasma. As a consequence of its chelating properties, tetracycline tends to localize in bones and teeth, where it may be detected by its fluorescence.[20] Tetracycline fluorescence is widespread but tends to disappear from normal tissues, except from bones and teeth, in about 24 hours. Tetracycline remains in inflammatory tissue somewhat longer and clings to neoplastic tissue for a surprisingly long time.

PROBLEM 53-2. *Inhibition of gastrointestinal absorption of tetracycline by gastric antacids is generally attributed to chelation. Would sodium bicarbonate interfere with the absorption of the antibiotic, and if so, by what mechanism? In an experimental study of this problem, it was found that sodium bicarbonate interferes with the dissolution of tetracycline contained in capsules and thus interferes with absorption.*

Adverse effects

Adverse effects caused by tetracyclines include nausea, vomiting, enterocolitis, stomatitis, and superinfections. Phototoxicity may occur after the administration of demeclocycline.

Administration of the tetracyclines in large doses has produced liver damage, as proved by liver biopsy. Recent evidence suggests that tetracycline is large doses produces a negative nitrogen balance and probably exerts an antianabolic action. Interference with protein synthesis may be the basis of these effects and the mechanism of its action against bacteria.

CHLORAM-PHENICOL

Chloramphenicol (Chloromycetin) is a broad-spectrum antibiotic with an antibacterial spectrum very similar to that of the tetracyclines.[12,18] Ineffective against *Entamoeba histolytica*, it is more useful than the tetracyclines in the treatment of typhoid fever.

It may be seen from the structural formula of chloramphenicol that this antibiotic is a derivative of nitrobenzene.

$$O_2N\!\!-\!\!\langle\rangle\!\!-\!\!\overset{\displaystyle OH}{\underset{\displaystyle |}{CH}}\!\!-\!\!\overset{\displaystyle CH_2OH}{\underset{\displaystyle |}{CH}}\!\!-\!\!NH\!\!-\!\!\overset{\displaystyle O}{\overset{\displaystyle \|}{C}}\!\!-\!\!CHCl_2$$

Chloramphenicol

Chloramphenicol binds exclusively to the 50 S ribosomal subunit, thereby interferring with protein synthesis (see Chapter 51).

The drug is largely bacteriostatic. Considerable evidence indicates that it also interferes with protein synthesis in human protein-synthesizing systems, at least as demonstrated with human bone marrow cells in tissue culture.

Significant plasma concentrations occur in 30 minutes; peak concentrations occur in 2 hours. Since chloramphenicol is poorly absorbed after intramuscular administration, it is used intravenously if the parenteral route is required.

Toxicity

The acute toxicity of chloramphenicol in experimental animals is about the same as that of the tetracyclines. In clinical usage many side effects, such as gastrointestinal disturbances, glossitis, skin rash, and superinfection, may occur. Optic neuritis and encephalopathy are rare. These are similar to the effects produced by the tetracyclines. On the other hand, it is generally recognized that chloramphenicol has a much greater tendency than commonly used antibiotics to produce blood dyscrasias, including reversible marrow suppression and aplastic anemia.[15] Although the incidence of this latter serious toxic effect is low, it is sufficient to make physicians very cautious in the use of chloramphenicol. Chloramphenicol is metabolized chiefly (90%) by conjugation to the ineffective monoglucuronide (also nontoxic). Failure to perform this metabolic function results in elevated plasma concentrations of free drug, which can cause the "gray baby" syndrome in newborns and toxicity in older patients with significant hepatic disease.[18,32]

The "gray baby" syndrome occurs chiefly in premature and newborn infants. Symptoms consist of cyanosis and vascular collapse. Plasma chloramphenicol concentration is elevated. The syndrome apparently results from lack of development of hepatic glucuronyl transferase, which normally detoxifies the antibiotic by changing it to the inactive glucuronide.[32] Because this syndrome has now been described in infants beyond the neonatal age range, therapy with this drug should be monitored with daily determinations of free chloramphenicol plasma concentrations. Concentrations should be maintained between 10 and 20 μg/ml.[18]

Chloramphenicol, when used wisely, is an excellent antibiotic. Major indications include rickettsial disease, typhoid fever (not *Salmonella* organism infections confined to the intestinal tract with no septicemia), and invasive *H. influenzae* infections (sepsis, meningitis, pneumonia, epiglottitis, arthritis, and cellulitis). Many strains of *H. influenzae* are now resistant to ampicillin derivatives. Some anaerobic infections respond to chloramphenicol.

Since penicillin and the previously mentioned broad-spectrum antibiotics became available, several important additional discoveries have been made in the fight against gram-positive organisms, such as the introduction of erythromycin, the discovery of antibiotics effective against resistant staphylococci, and the development of the newer penicillins.

NEWER ANTIBIOTICS AGAINST GRAM-POSITIVE ORGANISMS

Erythromycin (Ilotycin, Erythrocin), a macrolide antibiotic isolated from a strain of *Streptomyces*, is an organic base having a molecular weight of about 700. Used mainly to treat susceptible infections in patients allergic to penicillin,[12] erythromycin is particularly effective against gram-positive microorganisms. However, gonococci, *H. influenzae*, the large viruses of the lymphogranuloma venereum group, and mycoplasmae are to varying extents affected by it. The antibacterial spectrum of erythromycin is between that of penicillin and the tetracyclines, but the gram-negative bacilli, such as *E. coli* and *Salmonella* organisms, are not inhibited by it. Erythromycin is the drug of choice for Legionnaire's disease *(Legionella)* and can eliminate the carrier state for diphtheria and pertussis. Its mode of action appears to be largely bacteriostatic; a true killing effect is exerted only at very high concentrations. Erythromycins should not be used in serious staphylococcal infections or in the treatment of gonococcal infections; better drugs are available. Erythromycins are among the safest antibiotics.

Erythromycin

Gastric juice tends to destroy erythromycin, but enteric-coated preparations and erythromycin stearate are well absorbed. Given in doses of 0.5 g every 6 hours, erythromycin can attain blood concentrations of 2 μg/ml or more. Many gram-positive organisms are inhibited by concentrations below this amount. Erythromycin diffuses rapidly into tissues and distributes in total body water, although penetration to cerebrospinal fluid is poor. Plasma elimination half-life of erythromycin is 1.5 to 2.5 hours. Its excretion is mostly gastrointestinal, with only 5% to 15% eliminated in urine.

Erythromycin estolate   Erythromycin estolate (Ilosone) is stable in acid, well absorbed, and excreted in lesser amounts in bile. Thus when taken with food, it gives faster, higher, and longer lasting blood concentrations than comparable doses of erythromycin base. Cholestatic jaundice has been reported following the use of this form of the drug and other esters of erythromycin. Although this occurs rarely, caution is necessary in its use.

In addition to erythromycin estolate (Ilosone), the antibiotic is also available as erythromycin base (Ilotycin), the stearate, erythromycin ethylsuccinate (Pediamycin), erythromycin gluceptate (Ilotycin Gluceptate), and erythromycin lactobionate (Erythrocin Lactobionate). In general, the erythromycin base is rapidly destroyed by gastric juice, and the stearate is more stable but not absorbed as well as the esters. Gastrointestinal upset is the most common side effect. Allergic reactions are very rare.

Lincomycin   Lincomycin (Lincocin) is structurally unrelated to previously discussed antibiotics. Its antibacterial spectrum resembles that of erythromycin. It is effective against certain gram-positive organisms and *Bacteroides* species. Administered by mouth, intramuscularly, or intravenously, the usual adult dose is 0.5 g every 6 to 8 hours. Side effects include gastrointestinal irritation, skin rashes, and anaphylactic reactions. Lincomycin has been replaced by clindamycin.

Lincomycin

Clindamycin   Clindamycin (Cleocin) is closely related to lincomycin structurally; it differs only in a chlorine substitution of the 7-hydroxyl group. The spectrum of activity of the drug includes certain gram-positive organisms, *Actinomyces* species, and *B. fragilis*. Clindamycin is administered by mouth; the usual adult dose is 150 to 450 mg every 6 hours (children: 1 to 25 mg/kg/day). The intravenous dose is 250 to 750 mg every 6 hours (children: 10 to 40 mg/kg/day). The drug may be either bactericidal or bacteriostatic and acts by inhibiting bacterial protein synthesis in the 50 S subunit of the ribosome. Adverse effects caused by clindamycin include gastrointestinal irritation, neutropenia, eosinophilia, rashes, and elevated serum glutamic-oxaloacetic transaminase (SGOT).

Although clindamycin has produced excellent results in the treatment of anaerobic infections,[1] severe pseudomembranous colitis has occurred in some patients. This serious complication limits the usefulness of clindamycin.

Clindamycin hydrochloride (Cleocin hydrochloride) is available in capsules of 75 and 150 mg. Clindamycin palmitate is available in granules for suspension, 75 mg/ 5 ml. Clindamycin phosphate (Cleocin phosphate) is available in injectable solutions containing 150 mg/ml.

Bacitracin, polymyxin, colistin, and vancomycin are discussed as a group for two reasons. First, they all have significant toxicity when administered systemically in large enough doses. Second, they are used mostly for special purposes and only rarely as systemic chemotherapeutic agents. All four interfere with bacterial cell wall structure. *POLYPEPTIDE ANTIBIOTICS*

Bacitracin, a mixture of polypeptides, was first isolated from cultures of a gram-positive bacillus. It was named for Tracy, the patient from whom the bacillus was isolated. *Bacitracin*

The antibacterial spectrum of bacitracin is remarkably similar to that of penicillin. It is particularly effective against staphylococci resistant to penicillin G.

The main usefulness of bacitracin is in treating infections of the skin and mucous membranes, where it can be applied topically. When used parenterally, renal tubular damage regularly occurs in patients if large enough doses are used.

The activity of bacitracin is expressed in a unit that represents 26 µg of a standard preparation. For topical use, ointments containing 500 units/g of base are available.

Bacitracin is valuable for topical application and, compared to penicillin, has the great advantage of seldom causing sensitivity reactions. The drug is not absorbed from the gastrointestinal tract.

Polymyxin B is one of a series of polypeptide antibiotics produced by *Bacillus polymyxa*, a soil bacillus. This antibiotic has a potent bactericidal effect on gram-negative bacilli. Unfortunately, when administered parenterally to patients in daily doses exceeding 4 mg/kg, it is likely to cause renal tubular damage. This appears to be a direct toxic effect, readily demonstrable in experimental animals. *Polymyxins*

The main usefulness of polymyxin is for topical application. Many preparations are available for this purpose, and the drug is generally combined with either bac-itracin or neomycin to widen the antibacterial spectrum. The polymyxins are useful in the treatment of severe urinary tract infections (catheter irrigation) and topically for infected wounds and otitis externa.

The systemic use of polymyxin is hazardous. In addition to nephrotoxicity, systemic use of polymyxin can produce CNS effects such as vertigo and paresthesia. It is rarely used systemically since the development of safer antibiotics of the semi-synthetic penicillin type and aminoglycosides.

Polymyxin B is not absorbed significantly from the gastrointestinal tract and may occasionally be used by mouth for intestinal chemotherapy. When the drug is applied to open wounds, absorption may take place and the total quantity applied in a day should not exceed 3 to 4 mg/kg.

Colistin	Colistin (polymyxin E) is a polypeptide antibiotic very similar in antibacterial spectrum and toxicity to polymyxin B. Although some investigators believe that colistin is less neurotoxic and less likely to produce paresthesia, others question the superiority of colistin over polymyxin B.[22] Colistin is available as sodium colistimethate (Coly-Mycin), used in daily doses of 2 to 5 mg/kg by intramuscular injection.

Vancomycin hydrochloride	Vancomycin hydrochloride (Vancocin hydrochloride) is a glycopeptide that is highly toxic but bactericidal against gram-positive cocci. It should only be used orally to treat staphylococcal enteritis and pseudomembranous colitis associated with *C. difficile* and parenterally in severe infections caused by gram-positive cocci when other antibiotics may be ineffective or the patient is allergic to them.[12] Vancomycin can cause permanent deafness and fatal uremia.

ANTIFUNGAL ANTIBIOTICS	The antifungal drugs and their side effects are shown in Table 53-6.

Nystatin	Nystatin (Mycostatin) and amphotericin B (Fungizone) are also called *polyene* antibiotics because they contain a large ring with a conjugated double-bond system. The polyene antibiotics injure fungal membranes, perhaps by complexing with sterols in these membranes.[17] Thus sterols protect yeasts against these antibiotics. Bacterial membranes are not injured by polyenes. However, hemolytic anemia, sometimes caused by polyene antibiotics, may arise from injury of the red cell membrane, known to contain cholesterol.

Nystatin is effective against *Candida albicans* and some other fungi. It appears to be useful only against candidal infections that can be reached by topical application. Since the drug is inactivated by gastric juice, no systemic effects can be expected after its oral administration.

Amphotericin B, an effective antibiotic against deep-seated mycotic infections,[3] has been demonstrated to be useful against aspergillosis, mucormycosis, histoplasmosis, cryptococcosis, blastomycosis, and coccidioidomycosis. It has also proved effective in systemic infections caused by *C. albicans*.

The drug is administered intravenously but can cause thrombophlebitis at the site of injection and may also produe renal damage, skin rash, gastrointestinal upset, fever, and chills. Test doses of 1 to 5 mg are injected first. If no untoward reaction occurs, daily doses of 20 to 50 mg may be tried cautiously. Although amphotericin B is obviously a dangerous drug, its use may be justified in severe systemic fungal infections. It may be used topically for candidiasis of skin, nails, and mucous membranes.

The drug is poorly absorbed from the intestine. Its very slow metabolism accounts for its very long biological half-life of about 15 days.

TABLE 53-6 Summary of antifungal drugs and their side effects*

Type of infecting fungi	Site of infection	Antifungal agent	Route of administration	Dosage	Side effects and comments
Candida species	Superficial	Amphotericin B or nystatin	Topical	Not applicable	Applied three or four times daily for 7 to 14 days; with vaginitis, daily or twice daily for 14 days (side effects: essentially none)
	Intestinal	Nystatin (Myco-statin)	Oral	500,000 U three times daily for 7 to 14 days	Side effects: essentially none; large doses, occasional gastrointestinal distress and diarrhea
	Chronic muco-cutaneous candidiasis	Ketoconazole	Oral	200 mg/day in one dose	May also require amphotericin B (side effects: nausea, skin rashes, hepatitis)
	Systemic—not endocarditis	Amphotericin B (Fungizone)	Intravenous	Initial dose 0.25 mg/kg intravenously over 6 hr (suspended in 5% glucose solution, *not* saline), then increased stepwise to 1 mg/kg administration daily or 3 times a week; Total dose 0.5-1 g 50-500 mg kg/day	If administered rapidly, convulsions, anaphylaxis, hypotension, ventricular fibrillation, or cardiac arrest; phlebitis, fever, nausea, vomiting, anorexia, metallic taste, abdominal pain, nephrotoxicity, anemia, hypokalemia, decreased urinary 17 OH corticoids
		Flucytosine (Ancobon)	Oral		Gastrointestinal distress (nausea, vomiting, diarrhea), leukopenia
	Systemic endocarditis	Amphotericin B	Intravenous	Same as above	Removal of prosthesis or primary surgery usually required
Dermatophytes	Intradermal and hair	Griseofulvin (Fulvicin, Grifulvin, Grisactin)	Oral	12.5 mg/kg or 500 mg/day in adults	Photosensitivity, urticaria, gastrointestinal upset, fatigue, leukopenia (rare); interferes with coumarin drugs; increases blood and urine prophyrins, therefore should not be used in patients with porphyria Adjunct treatment: tolnaftate (Tinactin) or Desenex two or three times daily
	Onychomy-cosis	Griseofulvin	Oral	12.5 mg/kg or 500 mg/day in adults for 6-12 months	

Continued.

Courtesy Dr. Jay P. Sanford, Washington, D.C.
*See also reference 3.

TABLE 53-6 Summary of antifungal drugs and their side effects—cont'd

Type of infecting fungi	Site of infection	Antifungal agent	Route of administration	Dosage	Side effects and comments
Fungi causing deep mycoses, actinomycosis		Penicillin G, ampicillin, or tetracycline	Intravenous	10,000-20,000 U/kg 50 mg/kg 25 mg/kg	Usual side effects of the penicillin
Nocardia species		Rapid-acting sulfonamide and/or cycloserine (Seromycin), sulfamethoxazole-trimethoprim	 Oral	1 g q.4h. 15 mg/kg	Usual side effects of sulfonamides and cycloserine
Sporotrichosis	Cutaneous and lymphatic	Potassium, iodide, iodide saturated solution (1 g/ml)	Oral	10 drops q.8h. after meals	Skin rash, fever, lymphadenopathy
Histoplasmosis, coccidioidomycosis, systemic sporotrichosis, aspergillosis, mucormycosis, chromoblastomycosis	Systemic	Amphotericin B	See *Candida*, systemic, not endocarditis		Total dosage variable, but usually 2.5 g or more
Blastomycosis	Systemic	Amphotericin B or 2-hydroxystilbamidine	See *Candida*, systemic, not endocarditis		
Cryptococcosis	Systemic	Amphotericin B or flucytosine	See *Candida*, systemic, not endocarditis		

Griseofulvin (Fulvicin, Grifulvin V, Grisactin), produced from a *Penicillium* mold, *Griseofulvin* represents a novel approach to treatment of certain dermatomycoses. When given orally for long periods of time, griseofulvin is apparently incorporated into the skin, hair, and nails and exerts a fungistatic activity against various species of *Microsporum*, *Trichophyton*, and *Epidermophyton*. Prolonged administration is necessary because ringworm of the skin may require several weeks for improvement. In fungal infections of the nails, treatment may have to be continued for several months. The most common side effects are gastric discomfort, diarrhea, and headache. Urticaria and skin rash may also occur. This drug also has some antiinflammatory activity.

Griseofulvin

Griseofulvin (Fulvicin, Grifulvin V, Grisactin) is available in tablet form containing 125, 250, or 500 mg.

Several other antifungal agents are available, mostly for topical application. These include candicidin, miconazole, clotrimazole, flucytosine, ketoconazole, natamycin, haloprogin, tolnaftate, iodochlorhydroxyquin, and undecylenic acid.

Candicidin (Candeptin, Vanobid) is a polyene antibiotic available in ointments and capsules or tablets to be inserted in the vagina.

Miconazole nitrate (Monistat, Micatin) is an imidazole derivative, which may act on the fungal plasma membrane. Although the drug can be given intravenously for treatment of infections caused by *C. albicans* and *Cryptococcus* and *Aspergillus* organisms, its main use is topically for dermatophytosis and candidal infections. It may cause intense pruritus.

Clotrimazole (Lotrimin), related structurally to miconazole, is used primarily as a topical fungicide in the form of creams, solution, or vaginal tablets.

Flucytosine (Ancobon) is a fluorinated compound available for the treatment of systemic infections caused by *C. albicans* or *Cryptococcus neoformans*. Although less toxic than amphotericin B, flucytosine may cause blood dyscrasias and CNS toxicity. It is used synergistically with amphotericin B.

Ketoconazole (Nizoral), an alternative to amphotericin B, produces less toxicity. Very effective in chronic mucocutaneous candidiasis, ketoconazole is used orally for prolonged periods (6 to 12 months).

Natamycin (Natacyn) is a polyene antibiotic used for fungal keratitis, blepharitis, and conjunctivitis. It is available in an ophthalmic preparation.

Haloprogin (Halotex) is a synthetic topical antifungal agent used for treatment of skin infections caused by various fungi.

Tolnaftate (Tinactin) is a synthetic, topical, somewhat selective antifungal agent. Although effective in epidermophytosis, tolnaftate does not eliminate candidal organisms and is inadequate for fungal infections of the nails, scalp, and soles of the feet.

Iodochlorhydroxyquin (clioquinol; Vioform) is useful in epidermophytosis and also has antibacterial effects. It should be used topically on the skin, avoiding areas around the eyes.

Undecylenic acid is a harmless topical agent for mild epidermophytosis.

ANTIVIRAL AGENTS

Several recent advances have occurred in the chemotherapy of viral diseases (Table 53-7). An inhibitor of nucleic acid synthesis, idoxuridine, produced spectacular results after topical application in herpetic keratitis, and amantadine has provided a new approach to the prevention and amelioration of influenza A infections (A$_2$ most susceptible). Amantadine blocks penetration of virus into host cells.[5,29] In addition to these approaches, there is great interest in the stimulation of endogenous interferon production by synthetic polyanions of defined composition, such as pyran copolymer.

Idoxuridine

Idoxuridine (5-iodo-2′-deoxyuridine, IDU; Stoxil) is a pyrimidine analog that blocks the synthesis of nucleic acids. It is applied topically in a 0.1% solution to the conjunctiva every 1 to 2 hours in the treatment of herpetic keratitis caused by the herpes simplex virus. This is an important therapeutic advance because herpetic keratitis can lead to blindness. No effective treatment existed before the introduction of idoxuridine. Unfortunately, the drug is ineffective by systemic administration, probably because of rapid destruction. Toxic effects of idoxuridine include bone marrow depression, alopecia, gastric ulcers, loss of fingernails, and hepatotoxicity. These seldom occur with conjunctival use.

Idoxuridine   Amantadine

Amantadine

Amantadine (Symmetrel), a synthetic drug of unusual structure, inhibits penetration of certain viruses into host cells. In vitro it is effective against influenza and rubella viruses. In humans its effectiveness as a chemoprophylactic measure against influenza A$_2$ (Asian) virus has been demonstrated. Amantadine reduced the number of clinical illnesses and also diminished the serological response to influenza infection. Mice could be protected against several strains of influenza A$_2$ virus even when treatment was delayed as much as 72 hours after viral inoculation.[5]

TABLE 53-7 Summary of currently used antiviral drugs

Drug	Indication	Usual adult dosage	Route	Side effects	Comments
Amantadine (Symmetrel)	Prophylaxis of influenza A, possible therapy of influenza A in elderly or chronically ill patients if seen less than 20 hr after onset of illness	100 mg b.i.d.	Oral	Jitteriness, inability to concentrate, insomnia, tremors, confusion, depression, hallucinations; incidence generally at low level and dose-related	Primary reliance on prevention of influenza A infections remains with immunization
Adenine arabinoside (vidarabine; Ara-A)	Severe herpes simplex infections and mucocutaneous infections	10-15 mg/kg/day	Intravenous	Nausea, vomiting, diarrhea, CNS disturbances, anemia (mild)	

Courtesy Dr. Jay P. Sanford, Washington, D.C.

Amantadine (Symmetrel) is available in 100 mg capsules and also as a syrup (50 mg/5 ml). The adult daily dose is 200 mg.

Although amantadine appears to be nontoxic on the basis of animal experiments, it can in large doses produce CNS stimulation and even convulsions. Nervousness, dizziness, hallucinations, and even grand mal convulsions have been associated with amantadine use in humans. These adverse reactions are uncommon, however, and are more likely to occur following administration of large doses.

Amantadine represents a new approach to viral diseases. Its ultimate place in chemoprophylaxis and treatment in comparison with immunization procedures is a matter of debate.[11,26] Amantadine has some therapeutic effect in parkinsonism (see Chapter 12).

Vidarabine

Vidarabine (Vira-A) or adenine arabinoside inhibits DNA viruses such as herpes simplex and varicella. Topically, vidarabine may be used for treatment of ocular herpes simplex, although results in genital herpes infections have been poor. Vidarabine may be administered intravenously for treatment of herpes encephalitis and systemic herpes in neonates and immune compromised patients.[33] For intravenous infusion, vidarabine (Vira-A) is available as a suspension containing 200 mg/ml. Systemic use may cause many adverse effects and should be undertaken only in grave illnesses.

Trifluridine

Trifluridine (Viroptic) is a trifluoro analog of thymidine, available as a 1% solution for instillation into the eye to treat herpes simplex keratitis and keratoconjunctivitis.

Acyclovir

Acyclovir, a nucleoside analog, 9-(2-hydroxymethyl) guanine, is an important investigational agent active against herpesvirus infections.[27] Cells infected with herpes simplex phosphorylate the drug much faster than uninfected cells. This phosphorylation yields acycloguanosine triphosphate, which preferentially inhibits virus-specified DNA polymerase.

Investigational antiviral agents include immunopotentiating compounds, such as levamisole and methisoprinol (Isoprinosine), and other antimetabolites such as 2-deoxyglucose or purine and pyrimidine analogs.

Interferon inducers

Inducers of endogenous interferon represent a novel approach to antiviral chemotherapy. Interferons are antiviral proteins that exist in multiple molecular forms in different cells where they arise as a consequence of viral infections. Not only viruses but also bacteria and their products are capable of inducing the formation of interferons by host cells. More recently, it has been shown that chemically defined substances, such as a polyanionic pyran copolymer or double-stranded RNA from a synthetic source, can also induce interferons. Early trials in humans and animals indicate that these synthetic materials can induce demonstrable serum interferon levels.

Metronidazole (Flagyl), originally developed as an agent against *Trichomonas* organisms, is also effective in the treatment of amebiasis and giardiasis. The antimicrobial properties of metronidazole appear to be mediated by a partially reduced intermediate that binds to critical sites in susceptible cells. DNA breakage may be its mechanism of action. An intravenous form of metronidazole is available for treatment of serious anaerobic bacterial infections (especially *B. fragilis*).[1] The drug diffuses well to all tissues, including the CNS. Toxicity includes gastrointestinal disturbances, thrombophlebitis, seizures, peripheral neuropathy, and a disulfiram-like reaction to ethyl alcohol. It may be a potential mutagen and carcinogen.

METRONIDAZOLE

Clinical experience with chemotherapeutic agents in a wide variety of infections allows certain generalizations regarding the best drug choice.[31] More common infections and the indicated drugs are summarized in Table 53-8, based on extensive experience.[2] There may be exceptions to these recommendations in individual cases in which susceptibility tests reveal resistance of the causative agent to a drug that ordinarily would be a good choice (Table 53-8). It is imperative that the physician avoid indiscriminate prescription of antibiotics for undocumented infections.[14]

CLINICAL PHARMACOLOGY OF ANTIBACTERIAL AGENTS

Availability of effective drugs against most infections makes it difficult to explain the occasional failure to cure a theoretically amenable infection.[7] Some causes of failure with antiinfective therapy are unavoidable. Others, however, of an iatrogenic nature, could and should have been avoided.

Causes of therapeutic failure include:

Incorrect clinical or bacteriological diagnosis
Improper selection of drugs
Improper method of drug administration or inadequate dose
Poor patient compliance (not taking drug as prescribed)
Alteration in bacterial flora during drug administration and superinfection with a resistant organism
Infection in a location inaccessible to the drug administered
Failure to use indicated surgical drainage
Development of drug resistance by mutant forms of the infecting organism
Deficiency in host defenses
Drug toxicity and hypersensitivity

Effects of certain antibiotics on the gastrointestinal tract are of two general types. They may alter the bacterial flora, or they may have direct toxic effects unrelated to the bacterial flora.

Alteration of the bacterial flora is deliberately sought when antibiotics are used before bowel surgery. Nonabsorbable antibiotics, such as neomycin, kanamycin, and certain sulfonamides, have often been employed for this purpose. Despite enthusiastic proponents of such prophylaxis, many investigators believe that it has no advantage over preoperative cleansing of the bowel. Staphylococcal enterocolitis has occurred in patients who received oxytetracycline, neomycin, multiple antibiotics,

TABLE 53-8   Drugs of choice for various infections

Causative agent	Drugs
Gram positive	
Streptococcus pyogenes	Penicillin; erythromycin; a cephalosporin
*Streptococcus viridans**	Penicillin with streptomycin; ampicillin; vancomycin
*Enterococcus**	Penicillin with streptomycin; vancomycin with streptomycin
Pneumococcus	Penicillin; erythromycin; a cephalosporin
Staphylococcus aureus (penicillinase-producing)	Oxacillin; nafcillin; cloxacillin; others based on susceptibility such as a cephalosporin; erythromycin; lincomycin
Clostridium	Penicillin; erythromycin; tetracycline
Corynebacterium diphtheriae	Penicillin; erythromycin; tetracycline
Actinomyces	Penicillin with tetracycline; sulfonamides
Gram negative	
Neisseria meningitidis	Penicillin; chloramphenicol; sulfonamides
Neisseria gonorrhoeae	Penicillin; tetracycline; spectinomycin
Salmonella	Chloramphenicol; ampicillin
Shigella	Trimethoprim-sulfamethoxazole; tetracycline; ampicillin; chloramphenicol
*E. coli**	Gentamicin; tobramycin; ampicillin; tetracycline
*Enterobacter**	Gentamicin; tobramycin; tetracycline; a cephalosporin
*Klebsiella**	A cephalosporin; chloramphenicol; gentamicin; tobramycin
Brucella	Tetracycline; chloramphenicol; streptomycin
H. influenzae	Ampicillin; chloramphenicol
Hemophilus ducreyi	Trimethoprim-sulfamethoxaole; tetracycline; erythromycin
Bordetella pertussis	Erythromycin; trimethoprim-sulfamethoxazole
*Pseudomonas**	Gentamicin; tobramycin; amikacin; polymyxin B
*Proteus**	Gentamicin; chloramphenicol; ampicillin for *Proteus mirabilis;* a cephalosporin
Bacteroides	Penicillin; clindamycin; chloramphenicol; tetracycline; metronidazole
Legionella	Erythromycin; rifampin
Miscellaneous	
Fusobacterium (Vincent's angina)	Penicillin; erythromycin; tetracycline
Treponema pallidum	Penicillin; erythromycin; tetracycline
Leptospira	Penicillin; tetracycline
Rickettsia	Tetracycline; chloramphenicol
Psittacosis (lymphogranuloma group)	Tetracycline; chloramphenicol
Histoplasma capsulatum	Amphotericin B
Candida	Amphotericin B; nystatin
Cryptococcus	Amphotericin B
Coccidioides	Amphotericin B
Blastomyces	Amphotericin B
Microsporum and *Trichophyton*	Griseofulvin

*Susceptibility tests may be essential.

or preoperative bowel antisepsis. A recent assessment of antimicrobial prophylaxis may be found in *Medical Letter*.[24]

Candidiasis occurs commonly in patients who receive long-term treatment with broad-spectrum antibiotics. The number of yeasts in stools can be diminished by simultaneous use of nystatin, but it is not certain that the gastrointestinal symptoms are caused by yeasts. The condition improves if the antibiotic is discontinued.

Prevention of incipient hepatic coma is an indication for the prophylactic use of oral neomycin. The mode of action of this antibiotic in prevention of hepatic coma is its inhibitory effect on ammonia production by intestinal bacteria.

Malabsorption syndrome may result from the continued oral administration of neomycin. Changes in the jejunal mucosa and interference with the absorption of fat, glucose, D-xylose, iron, and vitamin B_{12} have been demonstrated.

Liver disease may be induced by some antibiotics. Large doses of intravenously administered tetracycline are hepatotoxic. Erythromycin estolate can produce obstructive hepatitis.

Effectiveness and safety of antibiotic therapy depend on several host factors discussed in the following summary. Elimination routes and dose intervals are shown in Table 53-9.

Host factors in antibiotic therapy

Defense mechanisms of the host greatly influence success or failure of any treatment. Debilitating diseases, poor nutrition, or administration of large doses of corticosteroids or immunosuppressant drugs may interfere with antibiotic therapy.

The age of the patient influences both the effectiveness and safety of antibiotic therapy. Infants in the first month of life excrete penicillin more slowly, presumably because of less developed tubular secretory mechanisms. Older infants and children require larger doses of penicillin than adults. Tetracycline may be deposited in tooth enamel and dentin and perhaps also in the bones of children. When given to infants during the first month of life, chloramphenicol can cause the "gray baby" syndrome. Underdeveloped hepatic capacity to conjugate drugs by glucuronidation (because of age or hepatic disease) makes chloramphenicol more hazardous.

Pregnancy is a contraindication to the use of several antibiotics. Tetracyclines can cause dental defects in the fetus. Pregnant women are more sensitive to the hepatotoxicity of tetracyclines.

Liver disease may be aggravated by chloramphenicol, the tetracyclines, and erythromycin. Defective renal function causes accumulation of sulfonamides, tetracyclines, and other antibiotics largely cleared by the kidney.

Obstructions in any part of the urinary tract are a most important host factor in making eradication of infection very difficult.

Pharmacogenetic defects, such as G-6-PD deficiency, may predispose an individual to hemolytic anemia from various antimicrobial drugs such as the sulfonamides, nitrofurantoin, and chloramphenicol.

TABLE 53-9   Elimination and dose intervals of antimicrobial agents

Drug	Route of elimination	Normal half-life (hr)	Dose intervals	
			Normal	Moderate renal failure
Cephalothin	Renal, hepatic	0.5-0.85	q.6h.	q.6h.
Chloramphenicol	Hepatic (renal)	2.5	q.6h.	q.6h.
Erythromycin	Hepatic	1.5	q.6h.	q.6h.
Gentamicin	Renal	2.5	q.8h.	q.12-14h.
Isoniazid	Renal, hepatic	2-4	q.8h.	q.12h.
Kanamycin	Renal	3-4	q.8h.	q.24-72h.
Lincomycin	Hepatic	4.5	q.6h.	q.6h.
Nitrofurantoin	Renal	0.5	q.8h.	Avoid
Aminosalicylic acid	Renal, hepatic	1	q.8h.	Avoid
Ampicillin	Renal, hepatic	1.5	q.6h.	q.6h.
Carbenicillin	Renal, hepatic	1.5	q.6h.	q.6h.
Methicillin	Renal, hepatic	0.5	q.4h.	q.4h.
Oxacillin	Renal, hepatic	0.5	q.6h.	q.6h.
Penicillin G	Renal (hepatic)	0.5	q.8h.	q.8h.
Streptomycin	Renal	2.5	q.12h.	q.24h.
Sulfisoxazole	Renal	3-4	q.6h.	q.8-12h.
Tetracycline	Renal, hepatic	6-8	q.6h.	q.24-48h.

Modified from Bennett, W.M., et al.: Ann. Intern. Med. **86**:754, 1977.

REFERENCES

1. Bartlett, J.G.: Anti-anaerobic antibacterial agents, Lancet **2**:478, 1982.
2. The choice of antimicrobial drugs, Med. Lett. **24**:21, 1982.
3. Cohen, J.: Antifungal chemotherapy, Lancet **2**:532, 1982.
4. Cutler, R.E., Gyselynck, A.M., Fleet, W.P., and Forrey, A.W.: Correlation of serum creatinine concentration and gentamicin half-life, JAMA **219**:1037, 1972.
5. Eggers, H.J., and Tamm, I.: Antiviral chemotherapy, Annu. Rev. Pharmacol. **6**:231, 1966.
6. Fleming, A.: On the antibacterial action of cultures of a penicillium, with special reference to their use in the isolation of *B. influenzae*, Br. J. Exp. Pathol. **10**:226, 1929.
7. Gardner, P.: Reasons for "antibiotic failures," Hosp. Pract. **11**:41, 1976.
8. Geddes, A.M.: A framework for prescribing, Lancet **2**:537, 1982.
9. Green, G.R., Rosenblum, A.H., and Sweet, L.C.: Evaluation of penicillin hypersensitivity: value of clinical history and skin testing with penicilloyl-polylysine and penicillin G, J. Allergy Clin. Immunol. **60**:339, 1977.
10. Grieco, M.H.: Cross-allergenicity of the penicillins and cephalosporins, Arch. Intern. Med. **119**:141, 1967.
11. Hirsch, M.S., and Swartz, M.N.: Drug therapy: antiviral agents, N. Engl. J. Med. **302**:903, 949, 953, 1980.
12. Kucers, A.: Chloramphenicol, erythromycin, vancomycin, tetracyclines, Lancet **2**:425, 1982.
13. Kunin, C.M., and Finland, M.: Clinical pharmacology of the tetracycline antibiotics, Clin. Pharmacol. Ther. **2**:51, 1961.

14. Kunin, C.M., Tupasi, T., and Craig, W.A.: Use of antibiotics; a brief exposition of the problem and some tentative solutions, Ann. Intern. Med. **79**:555, 1982.

15. Lewis, C.N., Putnam, L.E., Hendricks, F.D., Kerlan, I., and Welch, H.: Chloramphenicol (Chloromycetin) in relation to blood dyscrasias, with observations on other drugs, Antibiot. Chemother. **2**:601, 1952.

16. Macfarlane, G.: Howard Florey: the making of a great scientist, Oxford, 1979, Oxford University Press.

17. Medoff, G., and Kobayashi, G.S.: Strategies in the treatment of systemic fungal infections, N. Engl. J. Med. **302**:145, 1980.

18. Meissner, H.C., and Smith, A.L.: The current status of chloramphenicol, Pediatr. **64**:348, 1979.

19. Neu, H.C.: Clinical uses of cephalosporins, Lancet **1**:252, 1982.

20. Owen, L.N.: Flourescence of tetracyclines in bone tumors, normal bone, and teeth, Nature **190**:500, 1961.

21. Park, J.T.: Uridine-5'-pyrophosphate derivatives. 1. Isolation from *Staphylococcus aureus*, J. Biol. Chem. **194**:877, 885, 897, 1952.

22. Petersdorf, R.G.: Colistin: a reappraisal, JAMA **183**:123, 1963.

23. Phillips, I.: Aminoglycosides, Lancet **2**:311, 1982.

24. Prevention of wound infections and sepsis in surgical patients, Med. Lett. **23**:77, 1981.

25. Schatz, A., Bugie, E., and Waksman, S.A.: Streptomycin: a substance exhibiting antibiotic activity against gram-positive and gram-negative bacteria, Proc. Soc. Exp. Biol. Med. **5**:66, 1944.

26. Schinazi, R.F., and Prusoff, W.H.: Antiviral drugs: modes of action and strategies for therapy, Hosp. Pract. **16**:113, 1981.

27. Serota, F.T., Starr, S.E., Bryan, C.K., Koch, P.A., Plotkin, S.A., and August, C.S.: Acyclovir treatment of herpes zoster infections, JAMA **247**:2132, 1982.

28. Sheehan, J.C., and Henery-Logan, K.R.: A general synthesis of the penicillins, J. Am. Chem. Soc. **81**:5838, 1959.

29. Smith, R.A., Sidwell, R.W., and Robins, R.K.: Antiviral mechanisms of action, Ann. Rev. Pharmacol. Toxicol. **20**:259, 1980.

30. Strominger, J.L.: The actions of penicillin and other antibiotics on bacterial cell wall synthesis, Johns Hopkins Med. J. **133**:63, 1973.

31. Weinstein, L.: Some principles of antimicrobial therapy, Ration. Drug Ther. **11**(3):1, 1977.

32. Weiss, C.F., Glazko, A.J., and Weston, J.K.: Chloramphenicol in the newborn infant: a physiological explanation of its toxicity when given in excessive doses, N. Engl. J. Med. **262**:787, 1960.

33. Whitley, R.J., Soong, S-J, Rolin, R., Galasso, G.J., Ch'ien, L.T., Alford, C.A., and the Collaborative Study Group: Adenine arabinoside therapy of biopsy-proven herpes simplex encephalitis, N. Engl. J. Med. **297**:289-294, 1977.

Chapter 54

Drugs used in treatment of tuberculosis

Tuberculosis remains a frequently occurring disease. The advent of effective chemotherapy in the late 1940s markedly decreased the incidence of serious forms of the disease, especially miliary and bone tuberculosis. The protean nature of this disease remains a fact of medicine; this disease should be included in the differential diagnosis of a patient with fever of unknown origin, indolent meningitis, or chronic infection at any site.

The slow multiplication of the tubercle bacillus *(Mycobacterium tuberculosis)*, its relatively protected intracellular location, and its propensity to become drug resistant make chemotherapy difficult.

The primary drugs used in the treatment are isoniazid, ethambutol hydrochloride, and rifampin. Secondary drugs include streptomycin, *p*-aminosalicylic acid, ethionamide, capreomycin, kanamycin, and pyrazinamide.

Isoniazid and rifampin are the most effective drugs. Streptomycin is used infrequently because it must be administered parenterally, toxicity is considerable, and resistance may develop rapidly. *p*-Aminosalicylic acid is still used in children, but it has considerable gastrointestinal toxicity, and patient compliance is poor. The secondary drugs are generally more toxic than members of the primary group but may be indicated in selected cases (Table 54-1), especially with organisms resistant to the primary drugs.

Combinations of drugs are necessary in the treatment of tuberculosis but not for prophylaxis. The purpose of combinations is to prevent the development of resistant tubercle bacilli.

PRIMARY AGENTS
Isoniazid

The potent effect of isoniazid (INH) on the tubercle bacillus was discovered accidentally during routine screening of chemical intermediates in the synthesis of thiosemicarbazones of nicotinamide (a known inhibitor of tubercle bacilli in vitro).

Isoniazid is remarkably potent against the tubercle bacillus. It inhibits growth in the test tube at concentrations of less than 1 μg/ml. Its mechanism of action is

TABLE 54-1	Current antituberculous agents and side effects*		
	Usual dosage	Route	Side effects, toxicity, and precautions
Primary agents			
Isoniazid (INH)	Adults: 3-5 mg/kg/day, usually 300 mg/day Children: 10-20 mg/kg/day, up to 300 mg/day	Oral (intravenous and intramuscular rarely used)	Peripheral neuropathy (less than 1%); pyridoxine 10 to 50 mg daily will reduce this incidence; other neurological sequelae include convulsions, optic neuritis, toxic encephalopathy, psychosis, muscle twitching, dizziness, and alterations of sensorium (all rare); allergic skin rashes, fever, hepatitis (less than 1%); blood dyscrasias (rare)
Ethambutol	Adults: 25 mg/kg/day for 2 months, then 15 mg/kg/day Children: 15 mg/kg/day, up to 1500 mg/day	Oral (intravenous available)	Optic neuritis with decreased visual acuity, central scotomas, and loss of green and red perception; peripheral neuropathy and headache (rare); rashes (rare); monthly evaluation of visual acuity, with greater than 10% loss considered significant, usually reversible if drug is discontinued
Rifampin	Adults: 600 mg/day (single dose) Children: 10-20 mg/kg/day, up to 600 mg/day	Oral	Although toxicity is uncommon, the following have been reported: gastrointestinal irritation, drug fever, skin rash, mental confusion, thrombocytopenia, leukopenia, transient abnormalities in liver function (SGOT, alkaline phosphatase); interferes with some chemical determinations of bilirubin (false evaluation); eosinophilia (rare); avoid in first trimester of pregnancy; discolors urine, tears, and sweat an orange color; increases requirements for coumarin-type anticoagulants
Secondary agents			
p-Aminosalicylic acid (PAS) (Na+ or K+ salt)	Adults: 10-12 g/day (200 mg/kg/day) Children: 200 mg/kg/day, up to 12 mg daily divided into 3 doses	Oral	Gastrointestinal irritation (10% to 15%); goitrogenic action (rare); depressed prothrombin activity (rare); G6PD-mediated anemia (rare), drug fever, rashes, hepatitis, myalgia, arthralgia; Na+ or K+ must be taken into account in those with heart failure or renal insufficiency; give medication with meals or antacids
Ethionamide	Adults: 500-750 mg/day (10-15 mg/kg/day) Children: 10-20 mg/kg/day in 3 doses up to 1000 mg/day	Oral	Gastrointestinal irritation (up to 50% on large dose); goiter; peripheral neuropathy (rare); convulsions (rare); changes in affect (rare); difficulty in diabetes control; rashes, hepatitis, purpura; stomatitis; give drug with meals or antacids; 50 to 100 mg pyridoxine/day concomitantly; SGOT monthly

Courtesy Dr. Jay P. Sanford, Washington, D.C.

*See also references 2, 3, 5, 7, 10, and 12.

Continued.

TABLE 54-1	Current antituberculous agents and side effects—cont'd		
	Usual dosage	Route	Side effects, toxicity, and precautions
Secondary agents—cont'd			
Pyrazinamide (PZA)	Adults: 25 mg/kg/day (maximum 2.5 g/day) Children: 15-30 mg/kg/day, up to 2000 mg/day	Oral	Hyperuricemia (with or without symptoms); hepatitis (not over 2% if recommended dose not exceeded); gastric irritation; photosensitivity (rare); SGOT monthly; serum uric acid periodically or if symptomatic gouty attack occurs
Cycloserine	Adults: 750-1000 mg/day (15 mg/kg/day)	Oral	Convulsions, psychoses (5% to 10% of those receiving 1.0 g/day); headache, somnolence; hyperreflexia; increased CSF protein and pressure; contraindicated in epileptics; 100 mg pyridoxine (or more) daily should be given concomitantly
Kanamycin	Adults: 1.0 g 3 or 4 times/wk (or 0.5 g daily)	Intramuscular	Ototoxicity (largely hearing loss); vertigo less common; nephrotoxicity; neuromuscular blockade; paresthesias; eosinophilia; drug fever; rashes; anaphylactoid reactions (rare); periodic renal functional assessments; audiograms when indicated
Experimental agent			
Capreomycin	Adults: 1.0 g/day (15 mg/kg/day)	Intramuscular	Similar to kanamycin

unknown, but it is of interest that pyridoxine (B_6) antagonizes its neurotoxic effect without preventing its antibacterial action. Possibly the drug is incorporated into nicotinamide-containing coenzymes in mycobacteria. Some adverse CNS effects of isoniazid have been attributed to interference with enzymes that require pyridoxine.

Isoniazid

Isoniazid is rapidly absorbed from the gastrointestinal tract, is widely distributed in the body, and penetrates efficiently into the cerebrospinal fluid. It is metabolized by acetylation to acetylisoniazid and by hydrolysis to isonicotinic acid. Acetylisoniazid can be further metabolized to acetylhydrazine, which may be the mediator of the hepatotoxicity that can be observed with this compound.[11,17] These metabolites, as well as unchanged drug, are cleared by the kidney.

Genetically transmitted differences in the rate of isoniazid acetylation are classic examples of pharmacogenetics. Persons with slow acetylating ability maintain higher blood concentrations of isoniazid and are more subject to the drug's toxic effects.[14] In the United States approximately 50% of patients are slow acetylators, and neurotoxicity may be more common in this group.

Isoniazid is administered in doses of 3 to 5 mg/kg once a day. Larger doses have been used in tuberculous meningitis. Oral administration is preferred, but parenteral routes of administration can be used in seriously ill patients.

Adverse effects caused by isoniazid include peripheral neuritis, sensory disturbances, hepatic necrosis, arthritic reactions, and hematological disturbances.[4,11] Neurotoxicity is treated with pyridoxine (10 mg of pyridoxine for every 100 mg isoniazid). Neurotoxicity has not been described in prepubertal children; hence vitamin B_6 supplementation is not necessary in this group. Liver toxicity is also very rare in preadolescents.

Drug interactions may be significant. Rifampin increases the hepatic toxicity of isoniazid. Isoniazid increases phenytoin toxicity by interfering with the metabolism of the antiepileptic drug. Adjustments of phenytoin dosage are usually necessary.

Resistance of tuberculosis organisms to isoniazid develops rapidly. Combination of isoniazid with another effective drug delays or prevents development of resistance.

Although administration of vitamin B_6 may prevent neurotoxicity that may occur after chronic dosage with isoniazid, there is no reason to believe that the antitubercular effect of the drug involves this vitamin, since mycobacteria can synthesize B_6. Furthermore, pyridoxal phosphate does not prevent the effect of isoniazid on the tubercle bacillus.[14]

Isoniazid is available in 50, 100, and 300 mg tablets, as well as a syrup containing 10 mg/ml and a solution (100 mg/ml) for intramuscular administration.

Ethambutol hydrochloride (Myambutol) is highly effective in combination with other drugs in the treatment of tuberculosis. Its mechanism of action is unknown. It has largely replaced *p*-aminosalicylic acid therapy in adults.

Ethambutol hydrchloride

Ethambutol is absorbed rapidly from the gastrointestinal tract and is excreted mostly unchanged by the kidney. The drug does not normally cross the blood-brain barrier but may do so in meningitis.

The major adverse effect of ethambutol is optic neuritis, which is dose dependent. Optic neuritis manifests itself in loss of visual acuity and alterations in color perception. These manifestations are reversible and are uncommonly experienced if dosage is limited to a single 15 to 25 mg/kg dose each day. It is believed that zinc deficiency may increase the ocular toxicity of ethambutol. Patients receiving ethambutol should have visual screening and color perception tests before institution of therapy and during therapy. Because cooperation is necessary in visual testing, proper monitoring for toxicity cannot be done in small children.

Ethambutol hydrochloride (Myambutol) is available in 100 and 400 mg tablets.

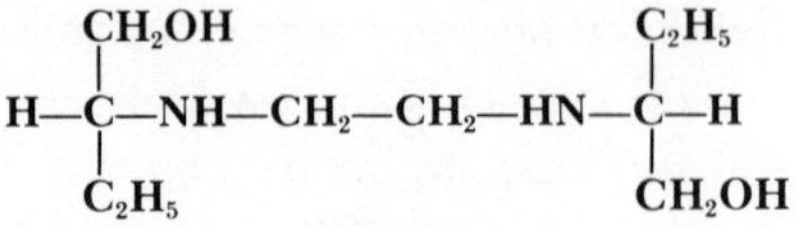

Ethambutol

Rifampin   Rifampin, a semisynthetic derivative of rifamycin B produced by *Streptomyces mediterranei*, is highly effective in the treatment of tuberculosis.[7,18,19] The antibacterial spectrum of rifampin is broad, including both gram-positive and gram-negative organisms. Its therapeutic efficacy in the elimination of the carrier state for meningococci and *Hemophilus influenzae* has been demonstrated.[5,6] Rifampin inhibits deoxyribonucleic acid (DNA)–dependent RNA polymerase,[8] the bacterial enzyme being more susceptible than its mammalian counterpart. This mechanism is discussed in more detail in Chapter 51. Oral administration of 600 mg of rifampin produces blood concentrations of 8 µg/ml in less than 2 hours.[6] Serum antibacterial activity is often present 12 hours after a dose.[18] Combinations of isoniazid and rifampin are highly effective in the treatment of tuberculosis.[18]

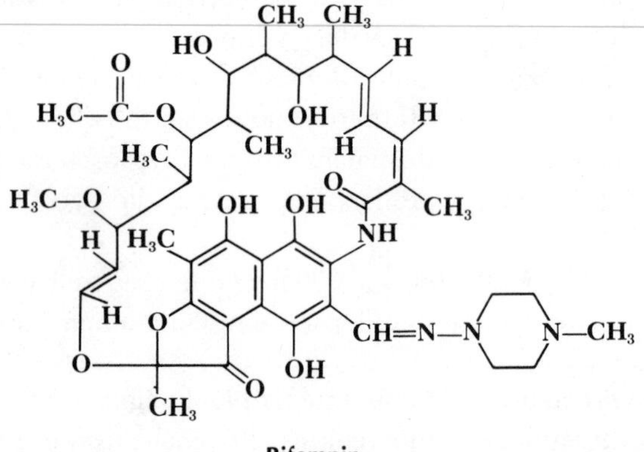

Rifampin

Rifampin, whose development represents a major advance in antituberculosis chemotherapy, is of great value in patients with drug-resistant infections. Since resistance to rifampin develops, it is imperative to use rifampin in combination with another antituberculosis agent, usually isoniazid.

Absorbed well from the gastrointestinal tract and widely distributed through the body fluids, including the cerebrospinal fluid, rifampin is metabolized in the liver and excreted mostly in the bile. Rifampin and its metabolites may stain body fluids (urine, sweat, tears) orange, which may be alarming to patients who are not forewarned.

Although most patients tolerate rifampin well, it may cause adverse effects and drug interactions. Adverse effects include abdominal symptoms, leg cramps, hepatotoxicity, and hypersensitivity with an influenza-like disease. Drug interactions are numerous. Rifampin increases the hepatotoxicity of isoniazid and decreases the effectiveness of oral anticoagulants and oral contraceptives.[16] Aminosalicylic acid may interfere with the absorption of rifampin. Rifampin may increase rates of hepatic drug metabolism through induction.

Rifampin acts on many bacteria and viruses in addition to being tuberculocidal. Since resistance to rifampin develops rapidly, rifampin is not recommended for infections other than tuberculosis.

Rifampin (Rifadin; Rimactane) is available in 300 mg capsules. It is administered in a single daily dose of 10 to 20 mg/kg.

A number of drugs are viewed as alternatives to the previously discussed agents in the treatment of tuberculosis. Because of their frequent and serious side effects, their use should be limited to severe infections in which the aforementioned less hazardous primary agents may be ineffective.

Streptomycin was the first effective drug in the treatment of tuberculosis. Because it must be administered intramuscularly and because of its numerous toxic effects and the development of resistance, the drug is rarely used in adults. It may still be used in children for serious tuberculosis infections (miliary, endobronchial, CNS). It is used in combination with other drugs in the early months of therapy. The dose of streptomycin is 20 mg/kg once daily (20 to 40 mg/kg/day up to 1000 mg/day) for 4 weeks. Streptomycin sulfate is available as a sterile powder and in solution for injection containing 400 mg/ml or 500 mg/ml.

The discovery of the usefulness of *p-aminosalicylic acid* (PAS) in the treatment of tuberculosis was a consequence of fundamental studies on the effect of various substances, including salicylic acid, on oxygen uptake by the tubercle bacillus.[1] Salicylic acid was found to increase the oxygen consumption of virulent tubercle bacilli, and it became of interest to study the effect of related drugs.

p-Aminosalicylic acid at concentrations as low as 1 µg/ml inhibits growth of virulent tubercle bacilli. It has no effect in virulent saprophytic mycobacteria. The drug must be administered in very large doses of up to 15 to 20 g/day. The great value of the drug results from the fact that it delays development of resistance to other tuberculostatic drugs. It is well absorbed and distributed throughout total body water.

SECONDARY AGENTS

Salicylic acid   *p*-Aminosalicylic acid

Adverse effects of *p*-aminosalicylic acid include gastrointestinal disturbances (which may be so severe as to warrant termination of therapy), occasional skin rash, and, rarely, hepatic damage and interference with thyroid function.

The inhibitory effect of *p*-aminosalicylic acid on the tubercle bacillus is antagonized by *p*-aminobenzoic acid, a finding that suggests a mode of action related to antagonism of this growth factor.

This drug has been largely replaced by ethambutol.

Ethionamide (Trecator) is, like isoniazid, a pyridine derivative. It is usually used in the treatment of drug-resistant cases of tuberculosis in doses of 0.5 to 1 g/day. It is less effective than isoniazid.

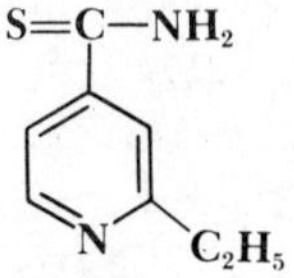

Ethionamide

Cycloserine (Seromycin) has been effective in treatment of some cases of tuberculosis in combination with other drugs. Unfortunately, it is neurotoxic. Cycloserine is administered by mouth in doses of 250 mg daily. Frequent side effects such as nausea, vomiting, hypotension, mental changes, and peripheral neuritis limit its usefulness.

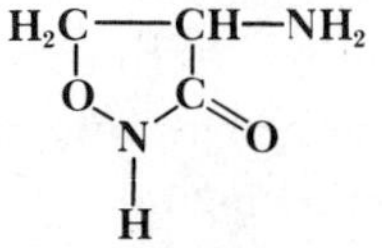

Cycloserine

The mechanism of action of cycloserine involves competition for D-alanine as a precursor of some bacterial cell wall component.[9] As a consequence, the drug induces protoplast formation. Despite its neurotoxicity, cycloserine has some usefulness as a second-line drug in the treatment of tuberculosis and also some urinary infections.

Cycloserine is well absorbed from the gastrointestinal tract, is widely distributed in the body, and penetrates well into the spinal fluid. It is excreted mostly unchanged in urine.

Pyrazinamide (pyrazinoic acid amine), an analog of nicotinamide, is inhibitory to the tubercle bacillus when administered in large doses. It can cause hepatic damage and retention of uric acid.

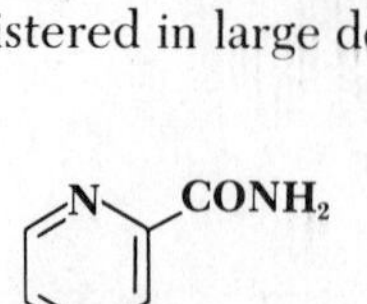

Pyrazinamide

Capreomycin sulfate (Capastat Sulfate) is a polypeptide antibiotic related to viomycin. Renal damage and ototoxicity limit the usefulness of this drug. **Kanamycin sulfate** (Kantrex) is not very useful in the treatment of tuberculosis. It must be administered parenterally and can cause severe eighth nerve damage.

Mycobacteria other than *Mycobacteria tuberculosis* may be responsible for some forms of granulomatous disease. These organisms are referred to as atypical mycobacteria. Infections caused by these bacilli are more difficult to treat than infections caused by *Mycobacteria tuberculosis*. The most common atypical mycobacteria are susceptible to a combination of rifampin, isoniazid, and ethambutol; severe disease may require a five-drug regimen, the two other drugs being selected from streptomycin, ethionamide, kanamycin, and oxacillin.

REFERENCES

1. Bernheim, F.: The effect of various substances on the oxygen uptake of the tubercle bacillus, J. Bacteriol. **41**:387, 1941.

2. British Thoracic and Tuberculosis Association: Short-course chemotherapy in pulmonary tuberculosis, Lancet **2**:1102, 1976.

3. Buechner, H.A.: The medical management of tuberculosis, Ration Drug·Ther. **14**:1, Oct. 1980.

4. Byrd, R.B., Horn, B.R., Soloman, D.A., and Griggs, G.A.: Toxic effects of isoniazid in tuberculosis chemoprophylaxis, JAMA **241**:1239, 1979.

5. Committee on Infectious Diseases, American Academy of Pediatrics: Report of the Committee on Infectious Diseases (Red Book), ed. 19, Evanston, Ill., 1982, American Academy of Pediatrics.

6. Deal, W.B., and Sanders, E.: Efficacy of rifampin in treatment of meningococcal carriers, N. Engl. J. Med. **281**:641, 1969.

7. Glassroth, J., Robins, A.G., and Snider, D.E.: Tuberculosis in the 1980's, N. Engl. J. Med. **302**:1441, 1980.

8. Hartman, G., Honikel, K.O., Knusel, F., and Neusch, J.: The specific inhibition of DNA-directed RNA synthesis by rifamycin, Biochem. Biophys. Acta **145**:843, 1967.

9. Hoeprich, P.D.: Alanine: cycloserine antagonism, Arch. Intern. Med. **112**:405, 1963.

10. Kagan, B.M.: Antimicrobial therapy, ed. 2, Philadelphia, 1974, W.B. Saunders Co.

11. Mitchell, J.R., Zimmerman, H.J., Ishak, K.G., Thorgeirsson, U.P., Timbrell, J.A., Snodgrass, W.R., and Nelson, S.D.: Isoniazid liver injury: clinical spectrum, pathology, and probable pathogenesis, Ann. Intern. Med. **84**:181, 1976.

12. Mitchell, R.S.: Control of tuberculosis, N. Engl. J. Med. **276**:842, 905, 1967.

13. Rifampin—a major new chemotherapeutic agent for the treatment of tuberculosis (editorial), N. Engl. J. Med. **280**:615, 1969.

14. Robson, J.M., and Sullivan, F.M.: Antituberculosis drugs, Pharmacol. Rev. **15**:169, 1963.

15. Ruiz, R.C.: D-Cycloserine in the treatment of tuberculosis resistant to standard drugs, study of 116 cases, Dis. Chest **45**:181, 1964.

16. Skolnick, J.L., Stoler, B.C., Katz, D.B., and Anderson, W.H.: Rifampin, oral contraceptives and pregnancy, JAMA **236**:1382, 1976.

17. Timbrell, J.A., Wright, J.M., and Baillie, T.A.: Monoacetylhydrazine as a metabolite of isoniazid in man, Clin. Pharm. Ther. **22**:602, 1977.

18. Vall-Spinosa, A., Lester, W., Moulding, T., Davidson, P.T., and McClatchy, J.K.: Rifampin in the treatment of drug-resistant *Mycobacterium tuberculosis* infections, N. Engl. J. Med. **283**:616, 1970.

19. Verbist, L., and Gyselen, A.: Antituberculosis activity of rifampin in vitro and in vivo and the concentrations obtained in human blood, Am. Rev. Respir. Dis. **98**:923, 1968.

Chapter 55

Drugs used in treatment of leprosy

Leprosy (Hansen's disease) is a complex, destructive, and widespread disease afflicting between 12 to 15 million individuals worldwide.[1] Multiple clinical presentations and an extremely long latent period (5 to 40 years) between exposure and clinical presentation make diagnosis difficult.[1,2] Currently the disease is classified by both clinical presentation and the degree of evidence for cell-mediated immune response to the etiological agent. This latter response is determined by the patient's reaction to intradermal inoculation of sterilized lepromatous tissue (lepromin reaction). Anergic patients have lepromatous leprosy; hyperergic patients have tuberculoid leprosy. Diagnoses between these two extremes are borderline-tuberculoid, borderline, and borderline-lepromatous leprosy. There is also an indeterminant group. Drug therapy is dictated by the diagnostic classification (Table 55-1).

$$H_2N-\langle\text{—}\rangle-SO_2-\langle\text{—}\rangle-NH_2$$

4,4′-Diaminodiphenylsulfone

The first effective drug against leprosy was found to be a sulfone, 4,4′-diaminodiphenylsulfone (dapsone). Dapsone remains the principal drug used, but resistance to it occurs. Development of more effective chemotherapy has been hampered by inability to grow the causative organism, *Mycobacterium leprae*, in vitro. The precise mechanism of action of dapsone is unknown; numerous processes involved in inflammation are affected.[3] Other sulfonamides are ineffective in leprosy; thus it is not known whether dapsone actually acts by inhibiting bacterial metabolism of *p*-aminobenzoic acid. Dapsone is administered on a once-daily basis (50 to 100 mg) and must be given for years. Toxicity from dapsone is similar to that for sulfonamides, with added risk of hemolysis (production of methemoglobinemia), leukopenia, and agranulocytosis.[3] Dapsone must be used with caution in individuals with glucose-6-phosphate dehydrogenase deficiency.

TABLE 55-1	Diagnostic classification and drug therapy for leprosy
Diagnostic classification	Drug therapy
Tuberculoid	Dapsone (rifampin may be added)
Borderline-tuberculoid	Dapsone and rifampin
Borderline	Dapsone, rifampin, and clofazimine
Borderline-lepromatous	Rifampin, dapsone, and clofazimine
Lepromatous	Rifampin, dapsone, and clofazimine
Indeterminate	Dapsone and rifampin

A syndrome resulting from dapsone toxicity occurs consisting of severe skin lesions, hepatomegaly, and psychosis.

Antitubercular drugs, including rifampin, ethionamide, and prothionamide, may be active against the organism that causes leprosy. A new drug, clofazimine, is effective in patients with borderline-lepromatous and lepromatous leprosy. Its major side effect is darkening of the skin. This increased pigmentation may clear when the drug is discontinued. The drugs mentioned in this paragraph are of investigational status in the United States for use in leprosy.

Clofazimine

Complications in the course of leprosy include reversal reactions and erythema nodosum leprosum. In the reversal reaction, the patient experiences increasing intensity of cell-mediated immunity. This may present as an acute neuritis, which is responsive to therapy with corticosteroids. Erythema nodosum leprosum is an inflammatory complication with acute onset of skin nodules (painful) and iridocyclitis. Thalidomide, corticosteroids, and clofaximine are effective for this condition. Thalidomide (investigational use only) cannot be used in women of childbearing age because of its well-known teratogenic properties.

Leprosy is an exceedingly complex disease whose successful management often requires precise diagnostic classification (including histopathology), frequent drug monitoring, surgical consultation, and continuous rehabilitation management. Chemotherapy should be guided by consultation with physicians experienced in treating this disease.

REFERENCES

1. Binford, C.H., Meyers, W.M., and Walsh, G.P.: Leprosy, JAMA **247**:2283, 1982.
2. Lewis, W.R., Schuman, J.S., Friedman, S.M., and Newfield, S.A.: An epidemiologic evaluation of leprosy in New York City, JAMA **247**:3221, 1982.
3. Millikan, L.E.: Sulfones: a review of approved and investigational indications, Hosp. Formulary **17**:102, 1982.

Chapter 56

Antiseptics and disinfectants

There are many drugs that are useful in decreasing the bacterial flora when applied directly to the skin, infected wounds, instruments, or excreta. These locally effective drugs have a low enough therapeutic index to make them unsuited as systemic chemotherapeutic agents.

Antiseptics are drugs that are applied to living tissues for the purpose of killing bacteria or inhibiting their growth. *Disinfectants* are bactericidal drugs that are applied to nonliving materials. Other terms related to antiseptics and disinfectants that are commonly misused are as follows:

germicide Anything that destroys bacteria but not necessarily spores.
fungicide Anything that destroys fungi.
sporicide Anything that destroys spores.
sanitizer An agent that reduces the number of bacterial contaminants to a safe level, as may be judged by public health requirements.
preservative An agent or process that prevents decomposition by either chemical or physical means.

Disinfectants were used long before the discovery of bacteria. The first germicides used were deodorants, since foul odors were associated with disease. Chlorinated soda was used on infected wounds as early as 1825 (Labarraque), and its use was recommended at about the same time for the purification of drinking water.

Phenol was used also as a deodorant and later as an antiseptic for infected wounds. Lister (1867) is usually credited with the introduction of phenol into surgery, but it was actually used long before the nature of infections was understood.

The use of alcohol was delayed for many years because Koch (1881) had reported that it did not kill anthrax spores. The superior germicidal properties of 70% alcohol were established by Beyer (1912).

Tincture of iodine was introduced into the *United States Pharmacopeia* in 1830, but it was not used extensively until the Civil War.

The importance of cleansing the hands with chlorine-containing solutions for the prevention of puerperal fever was clearly demonstrated by Semmelweis. This clinician, while working as an assistant at the Lying-in Hospital in Vienna, made some shrewd observations on the cause of puerperal fever. The ward where he worked was used for the training of medical students. Semmelweis noted that the mortality on the ward was lower when the medical students were on vacation. This observation by itself could have had many different explanations. He also noted, however, the odor from the autopsy room whenever the students were present. He suspected that the students were carrying "decomposing organic matter" from the autopsy room to the delivery room. He proved his hypothesis when cleansing of the students' hands with a solution of chloride and lime resulted in a marked reduction in mortality from puerperal sepsis (For a detailed history see Reddish.[3])

POTENCY OF ANTISEPTICS

Before the discovery of chemotherapeutic agents there was much preoccupation with the development of more and more potent antiseptics. Much effort was expended in synthesizing new compounds that could kill bacteria rapidly at high dilutions. The new antiseptics were generally compared with phenol, and the ratio of the dilutions necessary for killing test organisms in vitro was called the *phenol coefficient*. These efforts were so successful that antiseptics were synthesized that were hundreds of times more potent than phenol in killing bacteria in less than 10 minutes.

In retrospect, much of this effort was misdirected. Any drug that can kill bacteria in a few minutes is bound to have toxic effects on mammalian tissues. It is not surprising that even the most potent antiseptics were completely incapable of curing a systemic bacterial infection because the testing method used for their development was designed for *potency* and not for a favorable *therapeutic index*. The discoverers of Prontosil decided to test every compound against a systemic infection in mice. The sulfonamides and penicillin would never have been discovered by testing methods such as the use of the phenol coefficient. Not only the phenol coefficient but all tools for the evaluation of antiseptics are poor. It is not surprising that the field is dominated by empiricism and greatly influenced by fashion.

COMMONLY USED ANTISEPTICS AND DISINFECTANTS
Phenols

Phenol is a caustic substance that precipitates proteins. In a 1:90 dilution it can kill many bacteria in less than 10 minutes. Phenol has considerable systemic toxicity and is absorbed from denuded surfaces or burned areas. It can cause convulsions and renal damage.

Many derivatives of phenol find application as antiseptics or disinfectants. Saponated solutions of cresol (Lysol), resorcinol, and thymol have some medicinal uses, but the most widely used phenol derivative is hexachlorophene, which is incorporated into soaps and creams. In a 3% solution, hexachlorophene causes a marked reduction of bacterial counts on the skin without being irritating. Soaps containing hexachlorophene are generally used for preoperative scrubbing of the surgeon's hands and for antisepsis of the patient's skin.

The safety of hexachlorophene preparations, particularly for bathing newborn infants, has been seriously questioned. Such infants absorb some of the drug through the skin when the bath contains 3% of the antiseptic. Although no obvious toxicity has been demonstrated in human infants, newborn monkeys washed daily for 90 days with 3% solutions of hexachlorophene showed mean plasma levels of 2 to 3 μg/ml and developed brain lesions.[2] The Food and Drug Administration now advises against the use of 3% hexachlorophene for total body bathing. Such a product is still considered effective as a bacteriostatic skin cleanser and possibly effective in the treatment of staphylococcal skin infection. Evidence is lacking for the effectiveness and safety of hexachlorophene as an "aid to personal hygiene."

Tincture of iodine containing 2% iodine is often used for the preoperative preparation of the skin. The tincture stains the skin and is irritating to some individuals.

Halogen compounds

Povidone-iodine is a complex of polyvinylpyrrolidone and iodine. It releases iodine slowly and is claimed to be less irritating than tincture of iodine.

Sodium hypochlorite and chloramine T release chlorine. They were popular at one time for the cleansing of infected wounds.

Sodium hypochlorite and chloramine T

Halazone, tetraglycine hydroperiodide (Globaline), and aluminum hexaurea sulfate triiodide (Hexadine S) are among the compounds that are used for water disinfection by means of halogen release.

Hydrogen peroxide, 3%, releases "nascent" oxygen in the presence of catalase in the tissues. Probably its only value lies in its ability to remove foreign material by means of the oxygen bubbles it forms. Other oxidizing antiseptics are potassium permanganate, zinc peroxide, and sodium perborate.

Oxidizing agents

Ethyl alcohol is most bactericidal at 70% concentration by weight (78% by volume). It is commonly used as a skin antiseptic.

Alcohols and aldehydes

Isopropyl alcohol is at least as good an antiseptic as ethyl alcohol. It may be used as a 50% solution, but it is quite active when concentrated.

Formaldehyde in 40% concentration in formalin is used for the disinfection of instruments and excreta. It probably kills bacteria by combining with their proteins.

Surface-active compounds have both hydrophilic and hydrophobic groups. They tend to accumulate in interfaces and probably disturb bacterial cell membranes that contain lipids. The surface-active antiseptics are of two types: anionic and cationic.

Surface-active compounds

Anionic antiseptics. Various soaps and detergents such as sodium lauryl sulfate and sodium ethasulfate are antibacterial largely against gram-positive organisms. They are not nearly as important as the cationic antiseptics.

Cationic antiseptics. The hydrophilic group is usually a quaternary ammonium. Common representatives are benzalkonium (Zephiran), cetylpyridinium (Ceepryn), and benzethonium (Phemerol).

The cationic surface-active antiseptics are more potent at a higher pH. Their activity is decreased by soaps. In general they kill both gram-positive and gram-negative organisms, with some exceptions in the latter category.

The cationic antiseptics such as benzalkonium are commonly used for antisepsis of the skin and disinfection of instruments. The phenol coefficient of these compounds is very high, up to 500, but is reduced in the presence of pus and organic matter in general.

Metal-containing antiseptics	Mercuric chloride in a 1:1000 solution has been used widely as a skin antiseptic. It undoubtedly combines with SH groups in bacteria. Yellow mercuric oxide ointment, 1%, is used in the treatment of conjunctivitis.

Metal-containing antiseptics

Mercuric chloride in a 1:1000 solution has been used widely as a skin antiseptic. It undoubtedly combines with SH groups in bacteria. Yellow mercuric oxide ointment, 1%, is used in the treatment of conjunctivitis.

The organic derivatives of mercury have been widely used as skin antiseptics. Some popular preparations are thimerosal (Merthiolate), nitromersol (Metaphen), and merbromin (Mercurochrome). These antiseptics are largely bacteriostatic.

Silver nitrate in a 1% solution has been traditionally applied to the eyes of newborn infants to prevent ophthalmia neonatorum caused by gonococci. This practice is being replaced by the application of penicillin in the conjunctival sac of the newborn infant.

Zinc salts are mild antiseptics and also astringents. Zinc sulfate ointment is used in some types of conjunctivitis, and zinc oxide ointment is a traditional remedy in the treatment of a variety of skin diseases. Calamine lotion USP contains mostly zinc oxide with a small amount of ferric oxide. Phenolated calamine lotion USP also contains 1% phenol.

Nitrofurans

Nitrofurazone (Furacin) has been used in the form of ointments and solutions at a concentration of 0.2%. Although quite effective against both gram-positive and gram-negative organisms, it can cause skin sensitization in many patients.

Acids

Benzoic acid and salicylic acid have been used for many years as fungistatic agents. Whitfield's ointment is a mixture of 6% benzoic acid and 3% salicylic acid. It is commonly used for the treatment of fungal infections of the feet. Undecylenic acid (Desenex) is widely used in the treatment of "athlete's foot" and other fungal infections of the skin.

Mandelic acid and methenamine, used as urinary antiseptics, are discussed on p. 618.

Phenol   Hexachlorophene   Benzalkonium chloride

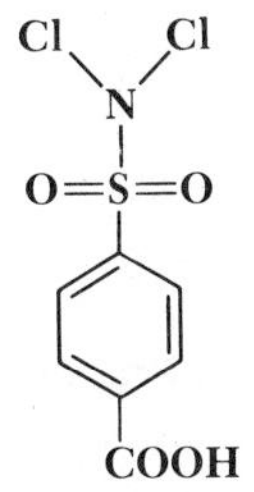

Halazone

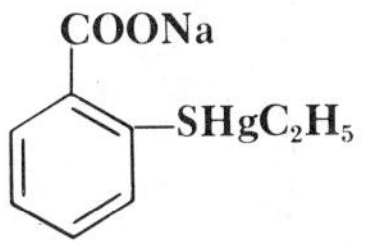

Thimerosal

INDICATIONS AND USES OF ANTISEPTICS

With the development of powerful chemotherapeutic agents, the indications for the use of antiseptics have declined. They are unquestionably useful for reducing the bacterial counts on the skin, both on the surgeon's hands and on the patient. They generally have no place in the treatment of fresh wounds or infected wounds, where cleansing with saline is most important. Deeply infected wounds call for systemic chemotherapy.

There is no general agreement on the most effective antiseptics. Some authorities consider the iodophors and chlorhexidine (Hibiclens) most effective. The iodophors release iodine slowly and are not as irritating as tincture of iodine. Chlorhexidine (Hibiclens) in a 4% solution is highly effective as a surgical scrub. Ethyl alcohol as a 70% aqueous solution is an efficient bactericidal agent. Isopropyl alcohol is somewhat more bactericidal than ethyl alcohol. Benzalkonium chloride (Zephiran) is an effective antiseptic, but some gram-negative bacteria resist its action. Hexachlorophene (pHisoHex) has several disadvantages. Its action is delayed, it is ineffective against several gram-negative organisms, and its absorption in infants can cause systemic toxicity.

Experimental studies indicate that alcohol is an excellent rapidly acting skin antiseptic. Hexachlorophene does not kill bacteria as rapidly. Much of the benefit of hexachlorophene is attributed to the film it leaves on the skin after repeated applications.

The skin cannot be completely sterilized. Cleansing, facilitated by surface-active agents such as the anionic or cationic surfactants, removes the superficial bacterial flora, which probably contains most of the pathogenic organisms. Alcohol is also excellent for preoperative preparations of the skin, but mild tincture of iodine and organic mercurials still have some advocates.

REFERENCES

1. Dineen, P.: Local antiseptics. In Modell, W., editor: Drugs of choice 1982-1983, St. Louis, 1982, The C.V. Mosby Co.
2. FDA Drug Bulletin, Dec., 1971.
3. Reddish, G.F., editor: Antiseptics, disinfectants, fungicides and chemical and physical sterilization, Philadelphia, 1957, Lea & Febiger.

Chapter 57

Drugs used in treatment of amebiasis

Amebiasis is caused by the protozoon *Entamoeba histolytica*. It occurs sporadically or in epidemics, the latter often following contamination of a water supply with sewage.

Entamoeba histolytica has two principal phases in its life cycle: the *trophozoite* and the *cystic*. The trophozoite is motile and can penetrate into the intestine, eventually reaching the liver. Ingested cysts liberate trophozoites in the intestine and cause the intestinal and extraintestinal forms of amebiasis.

From a therapeutic standpoint the amebicides can be divided into intestinal and extraintestinal drugs. The former are often poorly absorbed from the intestine and are used primarily for eradicating the infection at that site. Most antiamebic drugs belong to this category and cannot be relied on for eradication of the trophozoites in the liver or lungs. On the other hand, metronidazole, emetine, and chloroquine are effective in the extraintestinal forms of the disease.

Drugs useful in the treatment of intestinal amebiasis include, in addition to metronidazole and emetine, the antibiotics tetracycline and paromomycin, iodoquinol, and the obsolete arsenicals such as carbarsone.

Paromomycin is amebicidal, whereas tetracycline alters the bacterial flora with an indirect effect on the amebae. Antiamebic and other antiprotozoal drugs are shown in Table 57-1.

ALKALOIDS OF
IPECAC
Emetine

Emetine is obtained from the dried root of *Cephaelis ipecacuanha*, or ipecac. The crude preparation has been used for centuries in treatment of dysentery, although it is only effective against amebic and not bacillary enteric infections. As early as 1912, emetine was used by intramuscular injection in treatment of amebiasis. The drug is still useful in efforts at eradication of the extraintestinal trophozoites. Emetine is useful also in controlling symptoms in acute amebiasis but is not curative.

The alkaloid is directly amebicidal at high dilutions in vitro. It exerts similar effects on trophozoites localized in tissues. It has a marked symptomatic effect in acute amebic dysentery but cannot be relied on for eradication of *Entamoeba his-*

TABLE 57-1	Antiamebic and some other antiprotozoal drugs of choice			
Infecting organism	Drug of choice	Usual dosage	Route	Side effects and alternative agents
Entamoeba histolytica Intestinal (nondysenteric)	Iodoquinol (diiodo-hydroxyquin; Diodoquin)	650 mg t.i.d.—21 days	Oral	Nausea, abdominal cramps, rash
Intestinal (dysenteric)	Metronidazole (Flagyl)	750 mg t.i.d.—10 days	Oral	Local pain, electrocardiographic changes, arrhythmias, peripheral neuropathy
Extraintestinal	Metronidazole (Flagyl)	750 mg t.i.d.—10 days	Oral	Nausea, headache, diarrhea; alternatives: emetine or chloroquine
Giardia lamblia	Quinacrine hydro-chloride	100 mg t.i.d.—5 days	Oral	CNS effects, yellow staining of skin and sclerae, urticaria, blood dyscrasias; alternative: metronidazole
Balantidium coli	Tetracycline	500 mg t.i.d.—7 days	Oral	
Trichomonas vaginalis	Metronidazole (Flagyl)	250 mg t.i.d.—10 days	Oral	Nausea, headache, diarrhea, rash, paresthesias

tolytica within the intestinal contents. As a consequence, if used alone, it would convert the acute form of the disease into the chronic or carrier phase.

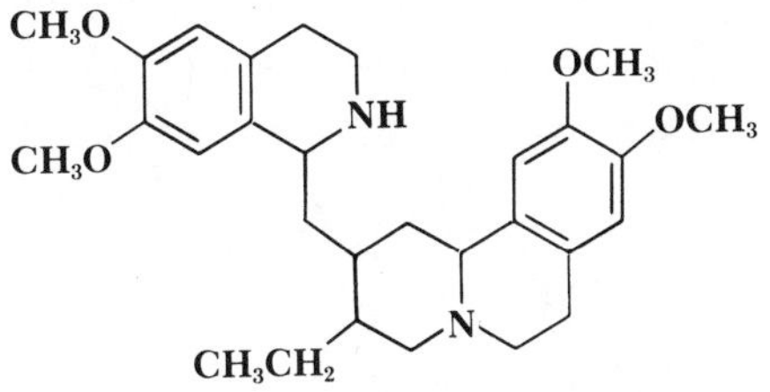

Emetine

The mechanism of action of emetine involves inhibition of protein synthesis in the parasites and in mammalian cells but not in bacteria. The related dihydroemetine dihydrochloride is available only from the Centers for Disease Control, Atlanta, Ga. It may be somewhat less cardiotoxic than emetine.

Emetine is a toxic drug. Its main toxic action is manifest on cardiac and skeletal muscle. A dosage schedule of 65 mg/day for 10 days can be tolerated by most adults, but even on this dosage there may occur electrocardiographic changes such as T-wave inversion. Emetine is a cumulative drug, and its administration should not be continued beyond 10 days.

IODOQUINOL

Iodoquinol (diiodohydroxyquin; Yodoxin) is an intestinal amebicide that may be useful in combination with other drugs in the treatment of various forms of amebiasis. It may be used alone in asymptomatic carriers. The related drug, iodochlorhydroxyquin, has caused an epidemic of subacute myelooptic neuropathy (SMON) in

Japan and is not used in the United States. In rare cases iodoquinol can also cause SMON, but its most common adverse effects are related to gastrointestinal symptoms.

Iodoquinol (Yodoxin) is available in 210 mg tablets. The drug is also available generically. The usual dosage for adults is 650 mg three times daily for up to 3 weeks.

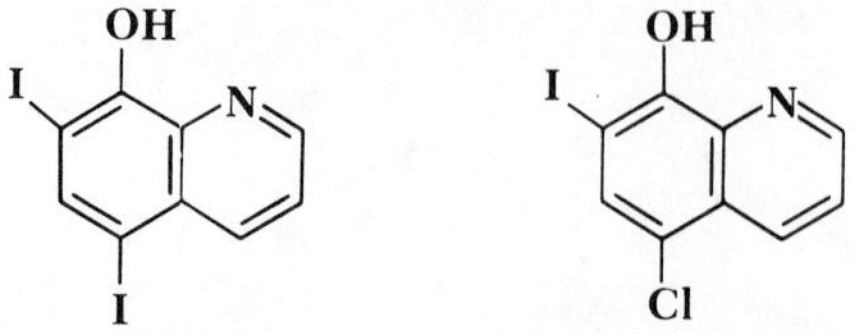

Diiodohydroxyquin   **Iodochlorhydroxyquin**

ARSENICALS   The organic arsenicals carbarsone and glycobiarsol are intestinal amebicides, which have become obsolete because more effective and less toxic drugs are available.

Carbarsone, or *p*-ureidobenzenearsonic acid, is a pentavalent arsenical that has been used in the treatment of amebiasis for many years. Its effectiveness is comparable to that of the iodoquinolines. Since the drug is absorbed from the gastrointestinal tract, arsenic poisoning may occur, and most experts advise against its use in the presence of liver damage.

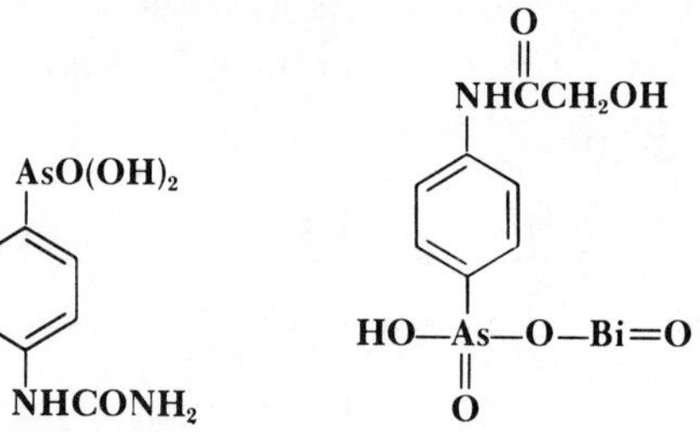

Carbarsone   **Glycobiarsol**

Another arsenical, **glycobiarsol** (Milibis), contains both arsenic and bismuth. It is not well absorbed from the gastrointestinal tract and is very effective against the intestinal ameba, although no action can be expected against trophozoites in the tissues. Thus in hepatic amebiasis, additional amebicides such as chloroquine or emetine are necessary.

AMINO-
QUINOLINES:
CHLOROQUINE

Chloroquine (Aralen) is a well-known antimalarial compound that is highly concentrated in the liver[5] and is highly effective in treatment of amebic hepatitis and amebic abscess of the liver. Its introduction as an extraintestinal amebicide was a most important therapeutic development in view of the many side effects and cardiotoxicity encountered with emetine, the only other effective extraintestinal antiamebic compound.

Chloroquine cannot be expected to eradicate the intestinal form of *Entamoeba histolytica*, and concomitant medication with an intestinal amebicide such as iodoquinol is mandatory.

The recommended dosage of chloroquine is 0.25 g four times daily for 2 days, followed by 0.25 g twice daily for 2 weeks. Other dosage schedules have also been recommended. Additional information on chloroquine is included in Chapter 59.

ANTIBIOTICS

Early work with the antibacterial drugs has shown that patients with intestinal amebiasis improve more rapidly when these drugs are added to the usual antiamebic regimen. Later the tetracyclines, erythromycin, bacitracin, and paromomycin were found to be quite effective against intestinal forms of the disease.

The antibiotics may be useful as therapeutic adjuncts in amebiasis but are not effective enough to be used without some other amebicide. Paromomycin (Humatin) and erythromycin are directly amebicidal, whereas the tetracyclines act by modifying the bacterial flora and influence the amebae indirectly.

DRUGS USED IN TREATMENT OF TRICHOMONIASIS

Many amebicidal drugs have a killing effect on *Trichomonas vaginalis* also. Most of them such as carbarsone, glycobiarsol, and iodochlorhydroxyquin are effective only when applied topically.

Metronidazole (Flagyl) is effective against all forms of amebiasis. Its toxicity is minor, but it may cause an antabuse-like reaction if alcohol is ingested. The drug is administered in doses of 250 mg two or three times a day by mouth. The drug is contraindicated in pregnant women. Metronidazole is also effective in the treatment of *Giardia* infections.

Metronidazole

REFERENCES

1. Anderson, H.H.: Newer drugs in amebiasis, Clin. Pharmacol. Ther. **1**:78, 1960.
2. Balamuth, W., and Lasslo, A.: Comparative amoebicidal activity in some compounds related to emetine, Proc. Soc. Exp. Biol. Med. **80**:705, 1982.
3. Berberian, D.A., Dennis, E.W., and Pipkin, C.A.: The effectiveness of bismuthoxy *p*-N-glycolylarsanilate (Milibis) in the treatment of the intestinal amebiasis, Am. J. Trop. Med. **30**:613, 1950.
4. Clark, D., Solomons, E., and Siegal, S.: Drugs for vaginal trichomoniasis, Obstet. Gynecol. **20**:615, 1962.
5. Conan, N.J., Jr.: The treatment of hepatic amebiasis with chloroquine, Am. J. Med. **6**:309, 1949.
6. Kean, B.H.: The treatment of amebiasis, a recurrent agony, JAMA **235**:501, 1976.
7. Most, H.: Treatment of common parasitic infections of man encountered in the United States (second of two parts), N. Engl. J. Med. **287**:698, 1972.
8. Most, H., and Van Assendelft, F.: Laboratory and clinical observations of the effect of terramycin in treatment of amebiasis, Ann. N.Y. Acad. Sci. **53**:427, 1950.
9. Powell, J.S.: Therapy of amebiasis, Bull. N.Y. Acad. Med. **47**:469, 1971.
10. Sikat, P., Heemstra, J., Brooks, R., and Yankton, S.D.: Metronidazole chemotherapy for Trichomonas vaginalis infections, JAMA **182**:904, 1962.
11. Wittner, M., and Rosenbaum, R.M.: Role of bacteria in modifying virulence of *Entamoeba histolytica*, Am. J. Trop. Med. Hyg. **19**:755, 1970.

Chapter 58

Anthelmintic drugs

GENERAL CONCEPT   Drugs that rid the body of parasitic worms are called anthelmintics. Several billion people are infected with worms. *Ascaris* alone is thought to infect about a quarter of the world's population. The fairly prevalent notion that helminthiasis is only a problem in "third world" nations is false. Many types of worms have always resided in the populations of the United States and Europe. Moreover, public health workers in developed countries now encounter unfamiliar parasites with increasing regularity because of emigrations from tropical or semitropical regions and unprecedented international travel.

The life cycles of many parasitic worms are exceedingly complex and beyond the scope of this chapter. Most helminths are transmitted by the oral route through contaminated foods or hands. However, hookworms, schistosomes, and *Strongyloides* organisms enter the body percutaneously.

In addition to undergoing maturation in various vectors, most worms also migrate in the human host before settling in a preferred tissue or body space. Pinworms and whipworms are nonmigrators. Many of the more common worms spend their adult lives in the gastrointestinal tract (Fig. 58-1). Others, such as flukes and *Trichinella spiralis*, lodge elsewhere in the body.

Applications for various anthelmintics are summarized in Table 58-1. Several choice compounds are recent developments not released as yet by the U.S. Food and Drug Administration for general use. Of the drugs listed, bithionol, metrifonate, niclosamide, niridazole, and suramin can be obtained from the Centers for Disease Control in Atlanta, Ga. Praziquantel (Biltricide), until recently available only on an investigational basis, was cleared in 1983 for general use. For mass applications, cost per unit course of treatment (not per dose) is at least as important as efficacy in determining which anthelmintic gets distributed.

INDIVIDUAL ANTHELMINTICS
Thiabendazole   The first imidazole anthelmintic in general use was thiabendazole (Mintezol). The drug is absorbed rapidly after oral administration, inactivated in the liver by hydroxylation, and excreted in urine and feces as a conjugate. Thiabendazole inhibits

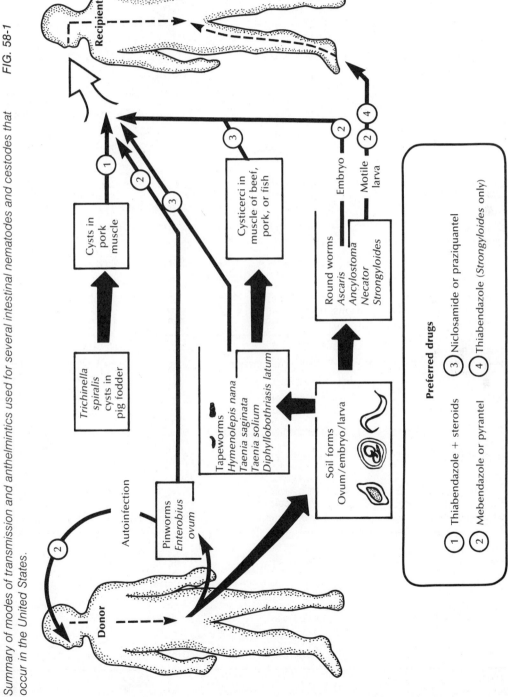

Summary of modes of transmission and anthelmintics used for several intestinal nematodes and cestodes that occur in the United States.

FIG. 58-1

TABLE 58-1   Anthelmintic drug applications

Organism	Drugs of choice	Usual adult dose*
Nematodes—intestinal		
Trichuris trichiura (whipworm)	Mebendazole	200 mg/day for 3 days
	or	
	Thiabendazole	25 mg/kg/day for 3 days
Enterobius vermicularis (pinworm)	Mebendazole	100 mg single dose, repeat in 2 weeks
	or	
	Pyrantel	11 mg/kg single dose, repeat in 2 weeks
	or	
	Pyrvinium	5 mg/kg single dose, repeat in 2 weeks
Ascaris lumbricoides (roundworm)	Mebendazole	See *Trichuris trichiura*
	or	
	Pyrantel	11 mg/kg single dose
Necator americanus and *Ancylostoma duodenale* (hookworms)	Mebendazole	See *Trichuris trichiura*
	or	
	Pyrantel	11 mg/kg single dose
	or	
	Bephenium	5 g/day for 3 days
Trichostrongylus spp.	Pyrantel	See *Ascaris lumbricoides*
	or	
	Levamisole	2.5-3 mg/kg single dose
	or	
	Mebendazole	See *Trichuris trichiura*
Strongyloides stercoralis (threadworm)	Thiabendazole	25-50 mg/kg/day for 3-5 days
	or	
	Mebendazole	200 mg/day for 4 days
Nematodes—extraintestinal		
Wuchereria bancrofti, W. malayi, Loa loa, Acanthocheilonema perstans (filariasis)	Diethylcarbamazine	50 mg first day, then 150 mg second day, then 300 mg third day, then 6 mg/kg/day × 18 days
Onchocerca volvulus	Diethylcarbamazine followed by	25 mg/day for 3 days, then 50 mg/day for 5 days, then 100 mg/day for 3 days, then 150 mg/day for 12 days
	Suramin	100-200 mg IV, then 1 g/week for 5 weeks
Dracunculus medinensis (guinea worm)	Niridazole	25 mg/kg/day for 15 days
	or	
	Metronidazole	750 mg/day for 10 days
Trichinella spiralis (trichinosis)	Thiabendazole (plus corticosteroids)	50 mg/kg/day for 5 days
Larva migrans (creeping erupticn)	Thiabendazole	50 mg/kg/day for 5 days
Trematodes		
Schistosoma haematobium	Metrifonate	10 mg/kg every 14 days for 3 doses
	or	
	Praziquantel	40 mg/kg single dose
S. japonicum	Praziquantel	30 mg/kg twice in 1 day
	Niridazole	25 mg/kg/day for 10 days
S. mansoni	Oxamniquine	15 mg/kg single dose
	or	
	Praziquantel	40 mg/kg single dose

*Divided doses by oral route unless otherwise specified.

TABLE 58-1	Anthelmintic drug applications—cont'd	
Organism	Drugs of choice	Usual adult dose
S. mekongi	Praziquantel	20 mg/kg 3 times in 1 day
Clonorchis sinesis, Fasciola hepatica, Paragonimus westermani (flukes)	Praziquantel or Bithionol	25 mg/kg 3 times in 1 day
		30-50 mg/kg alternate days for 10-15 doses
Cestodes		
Diphyllobothrium latum, Taenia saginata, T. solium, Dipylidium caninum (tapeworms)	Niclosamide or Paromomycin	2 g single dose
		1 g every 15 min for 4 doses
Hymenolepis nana (dwarf tapeworm)	Niclosamide or Praziquantel	2 g once daily for 5 days
		15-20 mg/kg single dose

fumarate reductase, a key enzyme in ATP production under anaerobic conditions. Vermicidal actions of the drug could be due to negative effects on energy metabolism or to microtubular disruption as a consequence of colchicine-like binding to tubulin dimers.

Thiabendazole has a wide spectrum of anthelmintic activity, but side effects (nausea, chills, vertigo, hypotension, hallucinosis, leukopenia, crystalluria) have limited its use. It remains a first-line drug for strongyloidiasis and trichinosis. The drug is ovicidal and larvicidal. It will kill both adult *Trichinella* in the small bowel during the initial phase of infection and migrating larvae of the same parasite. Claims that thiabendazole also destroys *Trichinella* cysts in human skeletal muscle are receiving careful scrutiny. Steroids are sometimes needed in trichinosis to suppress inflammatory reactions to the cysts.

Thiabendazole is dispensed as chewable tablets (500 mg) and oral suspensions (500 mg/5 ml). The dose for adults and children is 25 mg/kg twice daily after meals to a maximum of 3 g. The duration of treatment is usually 1 to 5 days, depending on the helminth.

Thiabendazole   Mebendazole

Mebendazole   Interest in benzimidazole derivatives as anthelmintics was spurred by success with thiabendazole. Mebendazole (Vermox) is one of several congeners that retain the broad spectrum of activity but have fewer untoward reactions. Mebendazole is a first-line drug against all common intestinal nematodes. In ascariasis, the cure rate exceeds 90% with a single dose. The drug is also anticestodal, especially in the treatment of invasive larvae as in cysticercosis. Mebendazole, like thiabendazole, depletes helminth energy stores and disrupts the capacity for cytoskeletal transport by binding to tubulin. Unlike thiabendazole, mebendazole is poorly absorbed, so that colonic concentrations are high. This restriction in distribution may be the reason why the drug has only limited vermicidal actions against invasive larvae but also has fewer side effects. Since it is teratogenic in animals, it should not be given to women who are, or may become, pregnant.

For most infections, a 100 mg tablet is chewed twice daily for several days. Pinworms can be eradicated with a single dose, but reinfection may necessitate periodic readministration. Filariasis (for which mebendazole is a second-line drug) requires daily therapy for a month.

Pyrantel   Pyrantel pamoate (Antiminth) is useful against intestinal nematodes (Table 58-1) with the exception of *Trichuris*. Intestinal worms depend heavily on their muscular systems to maintain the necessary degree of proximity to host tissues to which they are adapted. Several anthelmintics, pyrantel being an example, are neuromuscular blockers. Muscle regulation in worms is complicated and seems to require serotonin and γ-aminobutyric acid as transmitters in addition to acetylcholine. Atropine and *d*-tubocurarine have no effects on parasites, but pyrantel depolarizes worm muscle. The persistent nicotinic activation by pyrantel paralyzes worms so that they are expelled by host peristalsis.

Pyrantel is poorly absorbed so that intestinal parasites are exposed to high concentrations after oral administration. The small fraction that is absorbed causes minimal side effects (dizziness, headache, rash, fever). Pyrantel pamoate is marketed as an oral suspension, 250 mg/5 ml.

Pyrantel   Diethylcarbamazine   Piperazine hexahydrate

Piperazine   Piperazine citrate (Antepar) is converted in vivo to the hexahydrate. It is now considered alternative therapy for *Ascaris* and *Enterobius* infections. Piperazine can cause gastrointestinal and allergic reactions, since it is readily absorbed from the intestine. Some individuals taking piperazine develop an ataxia that has been given the soubriquet "worm wobble". Between 15% and 75% of a dose may be recovered unchanged in the urine. Piperazine paralyzes worms by hyperpolarizing their skeletal muscles. Since pyrantel and piperazine have opposing actions on the membrane potentials of muscle fibers, they are never coadministered.

In persons very heavily infected with *Ascaris*, mebendazole has been reported to cause aberrant migration of worms into the bile duct and nasopharyngeal cavities. A suggested preventive measure is to give a single dose of piperazine, which paralyzes the worms, before giving mebenazole to kill them.

DIETHYL-CARBAMAZINE

The drug of choice for filariasis and *Onchocerca* infections is diethylcarbamazine citrate (Hetrazan), a piperazine derivative. The mode of action is unclear, but piperazine alone is ineffective in filariasis. In humans, the drug causes microfilariae to disappear from the circulation. Diethylcarbamazine is believed to kill or sterilize adult worms. Microfilariae of *O. volvulus* killed by the drug cause fairly predictable and often violent allergic manifestations. Reversible allergic reactions to the drug itself are less frequent if the dose is increased slowly to the desired level (see regimens in Table 58-1). Diethylcarbamazine is dispensed as 50 mg tablets.

Niclosamide

Tapeworm infections are treated with niclosamide (Niclocide). The drug inhibits sugar phosphorylation, which reduces ATP synthesis by depressing glucose uptake. Tapeworms exposed to the drug become susceptible very quickly to host digestive enzymes. Worm segments and the scolex appear in the feces severely damaged, but mature eggs will still be viable. *Taenia solium* ova are of special concern, since the larvae of the pig tapeworm (a parasite also in many game animals) may become invasive. Treatment of *T. solium* with niclosamide should be followed in an hour or two by a cathartic purge. The drug should not be used if there is intestinal obstruction.

Niclosamide is available as 500 mg tablets. Adults and children over 8 take two doses of 1 g each 1 hour apart. The drug is not absorbed by the host, and the incidence of side effects (nausea, abdominal pain) is very low.

Niclosamide   Praziquantel

Praziquantel

The dwarf tapeworm, *Hymenolepis nana*, is the most frequently encountered cestode in developed countries. It is more refractory than other tapeworms to niclosamide therapy, probably beause its ova, although noninvasive, are immediately infective through autotransmission. Praziquantel (Biltricide), a compound now available after extensive clinical trials, seems to have a better cure rate against *H. nana* than other anthelmintics. Moreover, it is effective against schistosomes that infect humans. Traditionally, schistosomiasis has been one of the more difficult infections to treat.

Praziquantel is readily absorbed from the gut. It is metabolized rapidly by the host but not by the worms, which seem to concentrate the drug. The mode of action appears to involve changes in integument permeability to monovalent and divalent cations. In the tapeworm, influx of calcium is thought to be responsible for muscular spasticities that dislocate the worm from the intestinal wall. Side effects thus far are mild (sedation, headache, nausea, rash), transient (few minutes to an hour), and infrequent (less than 5% of patients).

OTHER USEFUL ANTHELMINTICS

Some of the other drugs listed in Table 58-1 are discussed very briefly here.

Pyrvinium pamoate (Povan) is a cyanine dye that inhibits tissue respiration and glycolysis in intestinal nematodes. It is used mostly in pinworm infections.

Biphenium hydroxynapthoate (Alcopar), used widely for hookworm in many parts of the world, was never available for routine use in the United States. Its quaternary ammonium structure suggests possible actions at parasite neuromuscular junctions.

Suramin (Germanin) is used consequent to a course of diethylcarbamazine for onchocerciasis. Suramin is given intravenously at weekly intervals to kill circulating microfilariae that persist after diethylcarbamazine administration.

Niridazole (Ambilhar) kills certain extraintestinal worms, specifically *Schistosoma haematobium*, *S. japonicum*, and *Dracunculus medinensis*. The initial effect of the drug is to damage female reproductive tissues and decrease egg production. Affected liver trematodes undergo autolysis in situ.

Metronidazole (Flagyl) has pronounced amebicidal and trichomonocidal activities. It has a limited range of utility against parasitic worms *(Dracunculus)*. Enthusiasm for the drug has been tempered by revelations that it is carcinogenic in rodents and mutagenic in bacteria.

Metrifonate (Bilarcil) is an organophosphorous inhibitor of trematode cholinesterase. It is a drug of choice for *S. haematobium*. In East Africa, where this parasite is endemic, large segments of the population are treated periodically with the drug.

Oxamniquine (Vansil) is employed for infections with *S. mansoni*. African strains of the parasite are more resistant to the drug than South American strains.

Bithionol (Bitin) can be used for lung flukes but seems to be less effective than praziquantel. Side effects include photosensitivity and urticaria.

Paromomycin (Humatin) is an antibiotic that is not absorbed from the gut. It is amebicidal, antibacterial, and cestodicidal. Its main uses as a vermicide are for infections with *T. saginata* and *T. solium*.

Compounds containing antimony (tartar emetic, stibophen) are effective against some schistosomes but cause frequent and often severe untoward effects. Similarly, tetrachloroethylene (for hookworm) and hexylresorcinol (for *Trichuris*) have been superseded by more effective, less toxic drugs.

REFERENCES

1. Drugs for parasitic infections, Med. Lett. **24:**5, 1982.
2. Mansour, T. E.: Chemotherapy of parasitic worms: new biochemical strategies, Science **205:**462, 1979.
3. Sheth, U. K.: Mechanisms of anthelmintic action, Prog. Drug Res. **19:**147, 1975.
4. Stürchler, D.: Chemotherapy of human intestinal helminthiasis: a review, with particular reference to community treatment, Adv. Pharmacol. Chemother. **19:** 129, 1982.
5. Wang, C. C.: Current problems in antiparasite chemotherapy, Trends Biochem. Sci. **7:**354, 1982.

Chapter 59

Antimalarial drugs

For centuries malaria was treated with cinchona bark, and until fairly recently the cinchona alkaloid, quinine, was the most generally employed antimalarial drug. Since World War II, very important developments have taken place in this field. Much more effective drugs have been developed, and new concepts concerning antimalarial therapy have evolved.

PRESENT
CONCEPTS OF
MALARIA

The malarial parasite is a protozoan organism of the genus *Plasmodium*. Of four species of *Plasmodium* that infect human beings, three are important. These are *Plasmodium falciparum*, *Plasmodium vivax*, and *Plasmodium malariae*. The fourth, *Plasmodium ovale*, is numerically unimportant. Other plasmodia also occur in animals, and some of these have been important in antimalarial screening studies.

The insect vector is the female *Anopheles* mosquito. Public health measures directed at eradication of the mosquito are of great importance. It is unlikely, however, that such efforts will be completely successful. The other approach to the problem of malaria is chemotherapy.

The life cycle of the malarial parasite has been divided into several phases: (1) sporozoite phase, (2) primary tissue phase, (3) asexual blood phase, (4) sexual phase, and (5) secondary tissue phase, which, however, does not occur in *P. falciparum* infections.

The major new concept of great importance in therapy is recognition of the importance of the primary and secondary tissue phases, which are commonly referred to as the exoerythrocytic cycle of the malarial parasite. The liver is the only organ in which exoerythrocytic stages have been demonstrated.

The *Anopheles* mosquito inoculates *sporozoites* into the bitten person. The various antimalarial agents have no effect on sporozoites, which remain in the bloodstream for a very short time and are localized in various tissues such as the liver.

From this primary tissue localization the parasite penetrates into red cells, where it is first seen as a *trophozoite*, which develops into the mature *schizont*. When the parasitized red cell bursts, it releases *merozoites*, and a malarial chill occurs. Certain modified trophozoites develop into *gametocytes*. These sexual forms represent the link between the human being and the mosquito and are important in the perpetuation of the disease in an area. Fertilization takes place in the mosquito, and sporozoites eventually appear in its salivary glands, ready for the next person who may be bitten.

TREATMENT OF MALARIA

The classification of antimalarial drugs is based on the various stages of the life cycle of the *Plasmodium*. Drugs that cure a clinical attack by eliminating the asexual forms are known as *schizonticides*. They include chloroquine (Aralen), amodiaquine hydrochloride (Camoquin), quinine sulfate (Quine), hydroxychloroquine (Plaquenil), and pyrimethamine (Daraprim). Tetracycline and combinations of a sulfonamide with pyrimethamine are effective also.

Radical cure implies the elimination of both the asexual forms and the exoerythrocytic forms of the malarial parasite from the body. In falciparum malaria the usual schizonticides may be sufficient to achieve radical cure, since no exoerythrocytic forms are left after treatment. In vivax malaria primaquine must be added to the treatment to obtain a radical cure.

Clinical prophylaxis can be achieved by the schizonticide chloroquine administered in a 300 mg dose once a week. Individuals receiving clinical prophylaxis may have to take primaquine after returning from an area where malaria is prevalent. *Causal prophylaxis* involves the use of primaquine, and because of the toxicity of this drug, there is no general agreement on the need for causal prophylaxis (Table 59-1).

Chloroquine

Chloroquine (Aralen), a 4-aminoquinoline derivative, was first synthesized in Germany in 1934. It was considered too toxic on the basis of a few tests in human beings and was discarded. A closely related compound was used by the French in North Africa in World War II and appeared quite effective and well tolerated. Subsequently a larger series of related compounds was synthesized in the United States, and extensive studies soon showed that chloroquine was the most satisfactory in the group.

Chloroquine

ANTIMALARIAL ACTIVITY

Chloroquine is highly effective against erythrocytic parasites. It is a suppressive drug that can produce radical cure in susceptible falciparum malaria but will not eliminate the exoerythrocytic forms of *P. vivax*. Consequently, relapses occur in vivax

TABLE 59-1 Summary of drugs used in the treatment of malaria

Infecting organism	Drug of choice	Usual dosage	Route	Side effects and comments
Malaria				
Acute attack due to *P. vivax, P. malariae, P. ovale,* "chloroquine-sensitive" *P. falciparum*	Chloroquine phosphate (Aralen, Resochin) plus	1 g (600 mg base), then 0.5 g in 6 hours, then 0.5 g daily for 2 days. (Total dose 2.5 g)	Oral	Pruritus, vomiting, headache, skin eruption, depigmentation of hair, partial alopecia, hemolytic anemia, leukopenia, thrombocytopenia, rare deafness, retinal damage
	Primaquine phosphate	26.3 mg (15 mg base) daily for 14 days	Oral	Hemolytic anemia in G6PD defect, neutropenia, GI, rare CNS symptoms, hypertension, arrhythmias
Acute attack due to *P. falciparum* (chloroquine-resistant strains—S.E. Asia, S. America)	Quinine sulfate plus	650 mg t.i.d.—10 days	Oral	Arrhythmias, tinnitus, hypotension, headache, nausea, abdominal pain, visual disturbance, blood dyscrasia
	Pyrimethamine (Daraprim) plus	25 mg every 12 hours for 3 days	Oral	Megaloblastic anemia, blood dyscrasia, rare rash, convulsions, shock
	Sulfadiazine	500 mg q.i.d.—5 days	Oral	*Alternative:* Dapsone (Avlosulfon), 25 mg daily for 28 days
Prophylaxis and suppression	Chloroquine phosphate plus	500 mg (300 mg base) once weekly, continued for 6 weeks after last exposure	Oral	As above
	Primaquine phosphate	26.3 mg (15 mg base) daily for 14 days after last exposure in endemic area	Oral	As above

Courtesy Dr. Jay P. Sanford, Washington, D.C.

malaria treated with chloroquine, although the drug can terminate the clinical attacks very efficiently.

METABOLISM Chloroquine is rapidly and almost completely absorbed from the gastrointestinal tract. Its distribution is such that some tissues such as liver may contain more than 500 times as much of the drug as does plasma. This affinity for the liver suggested its use in hepatic amebiasis.

Chloroquine may occasionally be injected by the intramuscular route. However, this is seldom necessary. For intramuscular injection, chloroquine hydrochloride is given in a dose of 250 mg. For other uses see p. 680.

TOXICITY Studies in human volunteers have shown that the toxicity of chloroquine is quite low when suppressive doses are employed. In larger doses dizziness, blurring of vision, headache, diarrhea, and epigastric distress have been reported. These symptoms disappear when the dosage is decreased. Retinopathy and corneal deposits may also occur and may result in blindness.

RESISTANCE TO CHLOROQUINE

Chloroquine-resistant *P. falciparum* has been encountered with increasing frequency in South America, Southeast Asia, and Africa. Such strains have created a serious problem in South Vietnam since 1965. While combined chloroquine-quinine therapy was usually effective, a very high percentage of patients, more than 40%, had relapses within 2 weeks. Several new drug combinations have been introduced to meet this problem.

One of these combinations is quinine with tetracycline. Also, quinine with pyrimethamine and a sulfonamide are effective in the treatment of chloroquine-resistant falciparum malaria. This may be the only use for quinine in malaria.

Amodiaquin

Amodiaquin (Camoquin) is similar to chloroquine as an antimalarial. It is given by mouth in doses of 0.6 g daily as a suppressive antimalarial or 1.8 g in divided doses the first day, followed by 0.6 g/day for 2 or 3 days for clinical control.

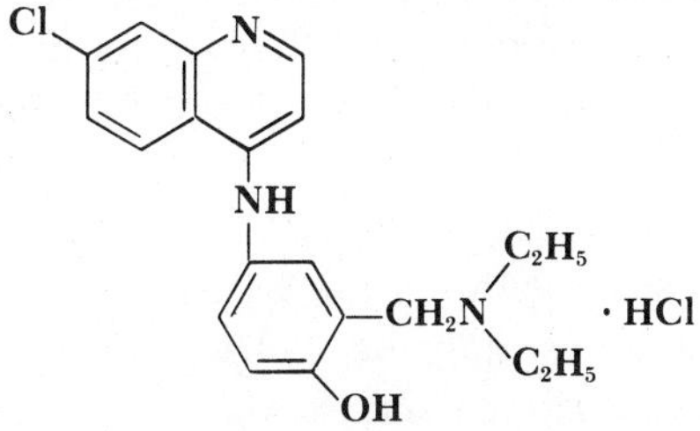

Amodiaquin hydrochloride

Hydroxychloroquine

Hydroxychloroquine sulfate (Plaquenil) is a 4-aminoquinoline, which is very similar to chloroquine without significant advantages over the parent drug.

Primaquine

Certain 8-aminoquinolines have the ability to destroy exoerythrocytic malarial parasites. Primaquine is at present considered to be the most effective representative of this group of antimalarial drugs.

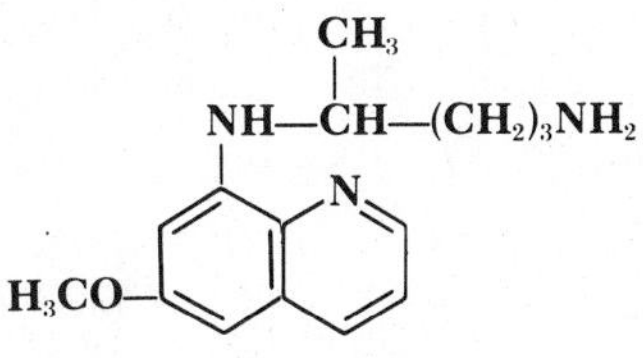

Primaquine

The development of primaquine is a late consequence of studies on the synthetic antimalarial drug pamaquine (Plasmochin). It was shown as early as 1925 that this drug was lethal to gametocytes, although it was not safe enough for complete elimination of the asexual forms from the blood. The drug was tried in some areas in combination with quinine for the purpose of controlling malaria by eliminating the gametocytes. There was an indication during these trials that the relapse rate in vivax malaria was reduced. This finding suggested an important property of the 8-amino-quinolines. Pamaquine was fairly toxic and did not appear promising. On the other hand, when related 8-aminoquinolines were synthesized during World War II, several were found to be safer than pamaquine. Pentaquine was first used as a curative antimalarial drug but was superseded by primaquine because the latter was found to be less toxic.

ANTIMALARIAL ACTIVITY
: Primaquine is useful in producing radical cure in *P. vivax* infections because of its effect on the exoerythrocytic stages. It is also effective against the exoerythrocytic forms of *P. falciparum*. It has some activity against the asexual forms of these parasites, but this activity is not high enough to make it an efficient suppressive as well as curative drug. For this reason primaquine is usually given in combination with a suppressive antimalarial drug.

Clinical trials in vivax malaria have shown that concomitant administraton of chloroquine as a suppressive, coupled with 15 mg primaquine/day for 14 days, will often achieve a radical cure. In a comparable group rceiving chloroquine alone, the relapse rate was 39%.

METABOLISM
: Primaquine is rapidly absorbed from the gastrointestinal tract. In contrast with chloroquine, however, it is also rapidly metabolized and excreted. Its tissue fixation is very slight, and the drug is altered and excreted in less than 24 hours.

TOXICITY
: Although primaquine is generally well tolerated at the recommended therapeutic dosages, some patients may complain of anorexia, nausea, abdominal cramps, and other vague symptoms. There may be depression of the activity of the bone marrow, with leukopenia and anemia. The effects on the blood, including some methemo-globinemia, are aggravated by concomitant use of quinacrine.

Hemolytic anemia that follows primaquine therapy is related to an interesting genetic abnormality. It is more likely to occur in dark-skinned races. The red cells of susceptible persons show a defect in the mechanisms that protect hemoglobin against denaturation. The reduced glutathione (GSH) content of such cells was as low as 50 mg/100 ml as compared with 75 mg/100 ml in normal cells. The metabolic error in primaquine-sensitive red cells appears to be a deficiency of glucose-6-phos-phate dehydrogenase. These GSH-deficient red cells are also sensitive to acetanilid, sulfanilamide, phenylhydrazine, sulfoxone, and acetophenetidin (p. 60).

Pyrimethamine is an inhibitor of dihydrofolate reductase of malarial parasites. *Pyrimethamine*
Resistance to its action develops rapidly, and for this reason the drug is only used
for prophylaxis and for the treatment of *P. falciparum* malaria, which is resistant to
chloroquine.

The discovery of the potent antimalarial drug pyrimethamine (Daraprim) was the
result of observations on the similarities between the antimalarial drug chlorguanide
and certain folic acid antagonists such as the 2,4-diamino-5-substituted pyrimidines.
One of these antimetabolites was found to have antimalarial activity in animals, and
soon many others were tested. Pyrimethamine is a member of this series.

Pyrimethamine

Pyrimethamine appears to be quite safe when administered in doses of 25 to 50 *TOXICITY*
mg once or twice a week. Megaloblastic anemia of a transient nature has occurred
in some persons following the use of pyrimethamine. This action may be related to
metabolic antagonism to folic acid or folinic acid. Pyrimethamine blocks the enzyme
dihydrofolic acid reductase.

Pyrimethamine is related to trimethoprim; however, the latter has a greater
affinity for bacterial dihydrofolic acid reductase.

The drug is not recommended for treatment of the acute attack because it is slow-
acting. Although it has remarkable gametocidal activity against some strains of *P.
falciparum*, it is ineffective against others. Resistant strains have become common.

Trimethoprim is a synthetic diaminopyrimidine compound related to pyrimeth- *Trimethoprim*
amine. Both inhibit dihydrofolate reductase. Trimethoprim is synergistic with sulfonamides, which is to be expected since it acts sequentially with the latter in blocking
the synthesis of folic acid in bacteria. For the same reason pyrimethamine and
sulfonamides may be synergistic in the treatment of malaria. Trimethoprim in combination with sulfamethoxazole is being used in the treatment of some bacterial
infections (p. 614).

Quinine has been the traditional antimalarial remedy that has been gradually *Other antimalarial*
replaced by newer drugs. It is a suppressive drug and will not cure vivax malaria. *drugs*
Even as a suppressive, it is not nearly as efficient as chloroquine or other newer
antimalarial drugs. The drug has become very important again in the treatment of
chloroquine-resistant falciparum malaria.

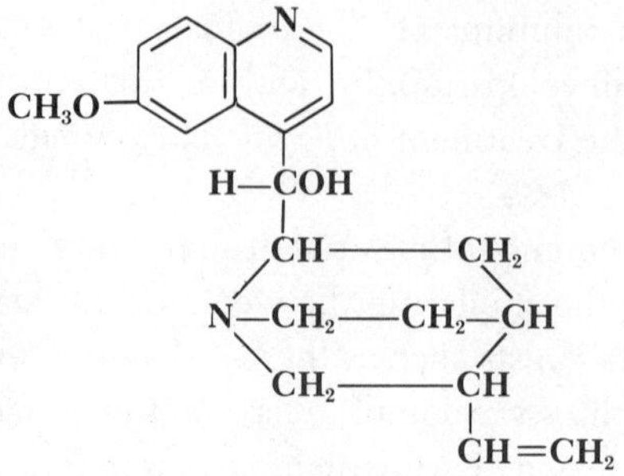

Quinine

The adult dose of quinine sulfate is 1 g three times daily. The drug is rapidly absorbed, and most of it is metabolized, about 10% being excreted unchanged in the urine and the remainder in the form of metabolic products. Metabolism and excretion are both rapid, and no cumulation occurs when quinine sulfate is given daily for long periods of time. In a patient who cannot take or tolerate oral quinine, the drug may be injected as the dihydrochloride by slow intravenous drip. For this purpose 650 mg of quinine is dissolved in 300 ml of saline solution.

Quinine can produce a variety of toxic effects, some of which are known by the collective name *cinchonism*. Headache, nausea, tinnitus, and visual disturbances can occur. Allergic skin rashes and asthmatic attacks have also been reported.

Quinine has other uses in medicine. It is given occasionally for the relief of leg cramps, as a diagnostic test for myasthenia gravis, in the treatment of myotonia congenita, and as a sclerosing agent.

Quinacrine (Atabrine) is a yellow acridine derivative. It was at one time an important antimalarial, but chloroquine has so many advantages over quinacrine that the latter is gradually being abandoned in treatment of malaria.

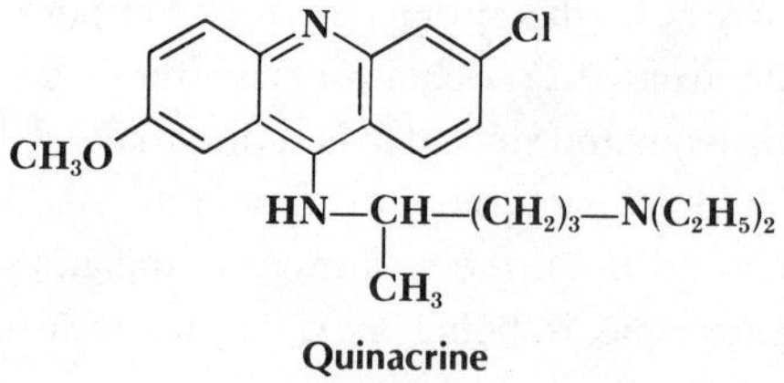

Quinacrine

Quinacrine is probably more valuable at present for purposes other than antimalarial therapy. It is important in the treatment of certain tapeworm infestations.

Chlorguanide (Paludrine) was synthesized in England during World War II. It is a suppressive antimalarial drug. Its action may be related to metabolic antagonism to folic acid, perhaps because of a metabolic product of this compound. The suppressive effect of chlorguanide is somewhat slow in onset.

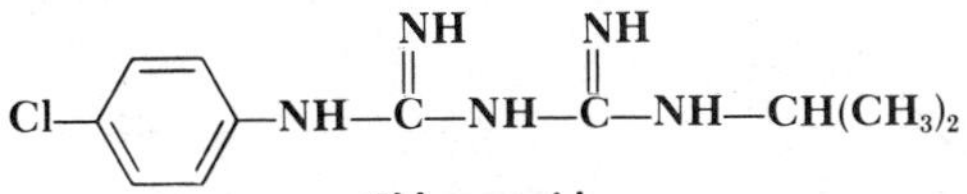

NH   NH
‖   ‖
Cl—⟨benzene ring⟩—NH—C—NH—C—NH—CH(CH₃)₂

Chlorguanide

Perhaps the greatest disadvantage of this drug has to do with development of resistance by plasmodia. Studies on the chemical relationship between chlorguanide and folic acid antagonists are directly responsible for the development of pyrimethamine. A chlorguanide derivative appears promising as a long-term suppressant when injected as pamoate salt.

Cycloguanide pamoate (Camolar), an insoluble salt of a chlorguanide derivative, is remarkable in that a single intramuscular injection exerts a protective effect for several months. This prolonged effect is a consequence of its extremely slow absorption from muscle. Cycloguanide pamoate may play an important role in eradication of malaria in some parts of the world, provided that its continued use does not reveal serious adverse effects. The drug is not yet generally available.

REFERENCES

1. Drugs for parasitic infections, Med. Lett. **20**:17, 1978.
2. Drugs for parasitic infections, Med. Lett. **24**:5, 1982.
3. Most, H.: Treatment of common parasitic infections of man encountered in the United States (second of two parts), N. Engl. J. Med. **287**:698, 1972.

Drugs used in chemotherapy
of neoplastic disease

GENERAL
CONCEPT

The search for pharmacological approaches to neoplastic disease has made some impressive gains. Drugs can cure patients having choriocarcinoma, Hodgkin's disease, and acute lymphatic and myelogenous leukemia. In combination with surgery and radiation, drugs have prolonged life in many other forms of cancer, although the quality of life is often impaired.

The current emphasis in cancer chemotherapy is on combinations. Such combinations take into account the phase of the cell cycle affected by the drug, synergistic effects, and prevention of drug resistance.

The cell cycle is divided into several portions. The resting phase is designated as G_0. The G_1 phase ends with a sudden increase in RNA synthesis, which signals the beginning of the S phase. During the S phase there is a marked increase in DNA synthesis, which ceases when the cells enter the short G_2 phase that ends with the mitotic process.

The cancer chemotherapeutic agents may be *cell cycle–specific* or *cell cycle–nonspecific*. Cells that are in a resting state do not respond to cell cycle–specific agents. However, they may respond to alkylating agents or to other drugs that combine directly with DNA.

DEVELOPMENT OF
ANTINEOPLASTIC
CHEMOTHERAPY

The antileukemic activity of the nitrogen mustards was discovered during World War II. The discovery was an outgrowth of earlier observations on the leukopenic effect of mustard gas (bis[2-chloroethyl]sulfide). As a result of this discovery, the less toxic nitrogen mustards (bis[chloroethyl]amines) and eventually many other alkylating agents were introduced into chemotherapy of neoplastic diseases.

The development of folic acid antagonists and other antimetabolites as potential antitumor agents originated from observations on the role of folic acid in white cell production. It seemed reasonable that compounds structurally related to folic acid could inhibit white cell production, and this was indeed demonstrated.

These observations stimulated interest in other metabolic antagonists as possible chemotherapeutic agents, and eventually several purine, pyrimidine, and amino acid antagonists were discovered. Nucleic acid biosynthesis has been the chief target of the chemotherapeutic approach.

The drugs currently employed in the management of malignant diseases fall into the following categories:

CLASSIFICATION

Alkylating agents
  Mechlorethamine hydrochloride
    (Mustargen)
  Chlorambucil (Leukeran)
  Cyclophosphamide (Cytoxan)
  Melphalan (Alkeran)
  Thiotepa
  Busulfan (Myleran)
  Carmustine (BCNU)
  Lomustine (CCNU)
Antimetabolites
  Methotrexate
  Cytarabine (Cytosar)
  Fluorouracil (Adrucil)
  Mercaptopurine (Purinethol)
  Thioguanine

Hormones
  Adrenal corticostroids
  Estrogens
  Antiestrogens
  Androgens
Antibiotics
  Bleomycin sulfate (Blenoxane)
  Dactinomycin (Cosmegen)
  Doxorubicin hydrochloride (Adriamycin)
  Mithramycin (Mithracin)
  Mitomycin (Mutamycin)
Miscellaneous
  Vinblastine sulfate (Velban)
  Vincristine sulfate (Oncovin)
  Hydroxyurea (Hydrea)
  Procarbazine hydrochloride (Matulane)
  Cisplatin (Platinol)
  Mitotane (Lysodren)
  Vindesin (Eldisine)

The mechanism of action of the various cancer chemotherapeutic agents is shown in Fig. 60-1.

The alkylating agents are highly reactive agents that transfer alkyl groups to important cell constituents by combining with amino, sulfhydryl, carboxyl, and phosphate groups. They are *cell cycle–nonspecific*, being capable of combining with cells at any phase of their cycle. It is believed that they alkylate DNA and, more specifically, guanine. This basic action may explain the preferential toxicity of these compounds for rapidly multiplying cells (Table 60-1).

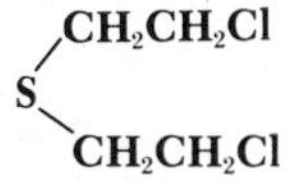

ALKYLATING AGENTS

$$S \begin{cases} CH_2CH_2Cl \\ \\ CH_2CH_2Cl \end{cases}$$

Sulfur mustard

$$CH_3N \begin{cases} CH_2CH_2Cl \\ \\ CH_2CH_2Cl \end{cases}$$

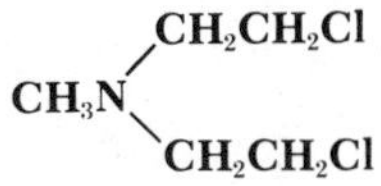

Nitrogen mustard

Mechlorethamine hydrochloride (nitrogen mustard; Mustargen) must be injected intravenously because the compound is highly reactive. More recently, attempts have been made to inject the drug intraarterially close to the tumor. It is believed that the action of mechlorethamine hydrochloride lasts only a few minutes and that it disappears from the blood very rapidly.

700

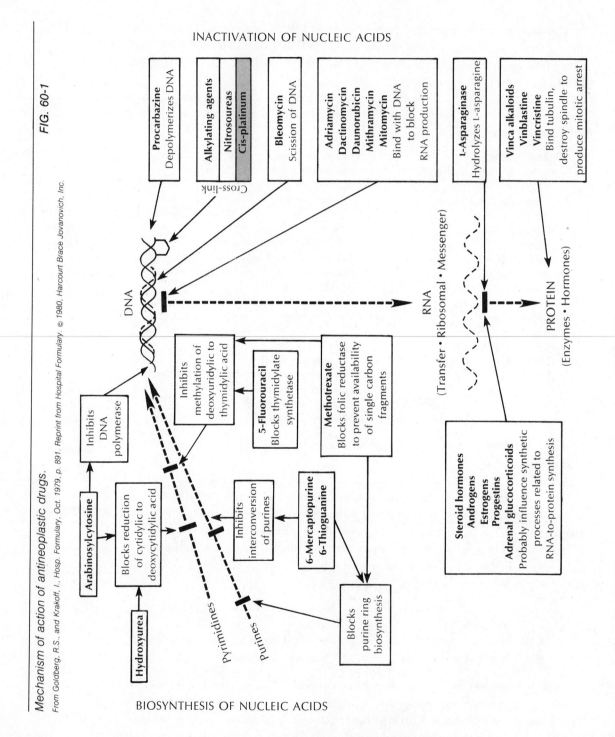

INACTIVATION OF NUCLEIC ACIDS

FIG. 60-1

Mechanism of action of antineoplastic drugs.

From Goldberg, R.S., and Krakoff, I., Hosp. Formulary, Oct. 1979, p. 891. Reprint from Hospital Formulary. © 1980, Harcourt Brace Jovanovich, Inc.

BIOSYNTHESIS OF NUCLEIC ACIDS

TABLE 60-1   Dosage and toxicity of alkylating agents

Drug	Route of administration	Usual dose	Toxic effects
Mechlorethamine hydrochloride	Intravenous	0.1 mg/kg/day	Nausea and vomiting; bone marrow depression and bleeding; venous thrombosis
Chlorambucil	Oral	0.1-0.2 mg/kg/day	Bone marrow depression and bleeding
Cyclophosphamide	Intravenous Oral (maintenance)	4 mg/kg/day 1-3 mg/kg/day	Nausea and vomiting; bone marrow depression and bleeding; alopecia may occur
Thiotepa	Oral Intravenous	5-10 mg/day 0.2 mg/kg	Bone marrow depression and bleeding Nausea and vomiting; bone marrow depression and bleeding
Busulfan	Oral	2-8 mg/day	Bone marrow depression and bleeding

The dose of mechlorethamine hydrochloride is 0.1 to 0.2 mg/kg/day for 4 days, injected intravenously. The drug can cause venous thrombosis, severe vomiting, and delayed depression of the bone marrow. In toxic doses mechlorethamine hydrochloride can cause involution of lymphatic tissues and the thymus, ulcerations of gastrointestinal mucosa, convulsions, and death.

Nitrogen mustard   Ethyleneimmonium intermediate   Cyclophosphamide

Busulfan   Melphalan

The main indication for mechlorethamine hydrochloride (Mustargen) is in the treatment of Hodgkin's disease and lymphomas, but the drug may be useful in other malignancies also.

Other alkylating agents have the advantage over mechlorethamine in that they can be administered orally.

Chlorambucil (Leukeran) is used primarily in chronic lymphocytic leukemia, Hodgkin's disease, multiple myeloma, and primary macroglobulinemia. **Cyclophos-**

phamide (Cytoxan) is a widely used cytotoxic drug, which is metabolically activated in the liver. The drug is generally useful in the treatment of lymphomas, acute lymphocytic leukemia in children, multiple myeloma, and some solid tumors, such as those of the ovary and breast, neuroblastoma, and others. Cyclophosphamide is commonly used as an immunosuppressive agent in a variety of diseases. Hemorrhagic cystitis is a characteristic toxic effect of cyclophosphamide. **Melphalan** (Alkeran) is a phenylalanine derivative of nitrogen mustard. It has been used in the treatment of multiple myeloma and some solid tumors, such as those of the ovary, testis, and breast. Occasionally the drug is infused intraarterially for the regional treatment of certain tumors. **Thiotepa** is used parenterally in the treatment of carcinoma of the ovary and breast. **Busulfan** (Myleran) is used mainly in the treatment of chronic myelocytic leukemia, since the drug has a selective effect on granulocytes.

Carmustine (BCNU) and **lomustine** (CCNU) are nitrosoureas that alkylate DNA and RNA.

$$\underset{\text{Carmustine}}{\text{ClCH}_2\text{CH}_2\text{N}\overset{\overset{\displaystyle\text{NO}}{|}}{-}\text{C}\overset{\overset{\displaystyle\text{O}}{\|}}{-}\text{NHCH}_2\text{CH}_2\text{Cl}}$$

Carmustine

Lomustine

Lomustine may have additional effects on DNA synthesis. An important characteristic of the nitrosoureas is their lipid solubility, which allows them to cross the blood-brain barrier and exert an effect on brain tumors.

ANTIMETABOLITES

Folic acid antagonists

The folic acid antagonists inhibit nucleic acid synthesis by blocking the enzyme dihydrofolate reductase. **Methotrexate,** formerly known as amethopterin, is effective in the treatment of acute leukemias of children and lymphomas and may be curative in women with choriocarcinoma. In combination with other agents, methotrexate may be useful in the treatment of some solid tumors such as carcinoma of the breast, ovary, and colon. Methotrexate produces many toxic effects such as nausea, vomiting, diarrhea, alopecia, aphthous stomatitis, skin rash, and bone marrow depression. Leucovorin calcium, within a few hours after overdosage, may serve as an antidote. Methotrexate is available in tablets containing 2.5 mg, and methotrexate sodium in a powder for injection, 5 and 50 mg.

Folic acid (pteroylglutamic acid)

Methotrexate

The most important purine antagonist, mercaptopurine, acts by several mechanisms. First, it is converted to the ribonucleotide. As such it competes with enzymes that convert hypoxanthine ribonucleotide (inosinic acid) to adenine and xanthine ribonucleotides. In addition, mercaptopurine is converted into 6-methyl mercaptopurine and its ribonucleotide. This metabolite ties up the enzyme that synthesizes phosphoribosylamine, which is required for RNA and DNA synthesis.

Thioguanine is also metabolized to the ribonucleotide, which enters the pathway of nucleic acid synthesis by substituting for guanine. Thus "fraudulent" polynucleotides that block nucleic acid synthesis are produced.

Mercaptopurine is effective in the treatment of acute lymphocytic and chronic myelocytic leukemias. Its toxic manifestations include bone marrow depression, gastrointestinal disturbances, and jaundice. Allopurinol was originally developed for the purpose of blocking the metabolism of mercaptopurine by xanthine oxidase. Mercaptopurine (Purinethol) is obtainable in tablets containing 50 mg.

Thioguanine is an antimetabolite similar to mercaptopurine with essentially the same indications and adverse effects.

Azathioprine, a derivative of mercaptopurine, has become widely used as an immunosuppressive drug in organ transplantation. Bone marrow depression, oral lesions, gastrointestinal disturbances, alopecia, and intercurrent infections are some of the toxic effects of azathioprine. Azathioprine (Imuran) is available in tablets containing 50 mg. Azathioprine is much more useful as an immunosuppressant than in cancer chemotherapy. It splits in the body to 6-mercaptopurine.

Purine antagonists

Mercaptopurine   **Azathioprine**

Fluorouracil is a pyrimidine antimetabolite of some usefulness in the treatment of carcinoma of the colon, breast, ovary, pancreas, and liver. It is a highly toxic drug, producing the same sort of disturbances as mercaptopurine and also hyperpigmentation and photosensitization. The drug is available as a solution, 50 mg/ml, for intravenous injection. Fluorouracil is also available for topical application as Efudex solution or cream. The solution contains 2% or 5% fluorouracil, the cream 5%.

Pyrimidine antagonists

Fluorouracil is converted to the ribonucleotide, which may be reduced to 5-fluoro-2′-deoxyuridine-5′-phosphate (F-dUMP). This enzymatic product inhibits thymidylate synthetase, which is involved in the production of deoxyuridylic acid (dUMP).

Cytarabine (cytosine arabinoside; Cytosar) is a pyrimidine antagonist that differs from deoxycytidine (cytosine deoxyriboside) in containing arabinose rather than deoxyribose. It is converted to the nucleotide, which then blocks the conversion of cytidine nucleotide to deoxycytidine nucleotide. It also prevents the formation of DNA by blocking the incorporation of deoxycytidine triphosphate.

Cytarabine

Cytarabine must be injected intravenously, since it is not effective after oral administration. It finds some usefulness in the treatment of acute lymphocytic and acute myelocytic leukemias. It is also of interest as a possible antiviral agent (p. 655).

HORMONAL AGENTS

Steroid hormones such as estrogens, androgens, and corticosteroids are useful in some neoplastic diseases. The estrogens include diethylstilbestrol and ethinyl estradiol. Androgens that are widely used particularly in the treatment of carcinoma of the breast, include testosterone propionate, fluoxymesterone, and the recently introduced calusterone (Methosarb). The most widely used corticosteroid is prednisone, which is effective in various lymphomas and some other malignancies.

The progestogens include medroxyprogesterone (Provera), hydroxyprogesterone (Delalutin), and megestrol acetate (Megace). The progestogens are sometimes effective in renal and endometrial carcinomas.

Estrogens, alone with castration and other measures, are used in treatment of prostatic carcinoma. Both androgens and estrogens have been employed in management of advanced mammary carcinoma. The choice depends on the age of the patient. Estrogens are used in women well past the menopause, whereas androgens may be helpful in patients who are still menstruating. The main benefit obtained from this treatment is reduction of pain related to metastatic lesions in the bones.

The *rationale* for the use of the estrogens and androgens is the belief that prostatic and mammary carcinoma are to some extent "hormone dependent."

The adverse effects of the estrogens (diethylstilbestrol) are gastrointestinal symptoms, hypercalcemia, edema, uterine bleeding, and feminization in males. The adverse effects expected from large doses of androgens (testosterone propionate) in the treatment of advanced mammary carcinoma are virilization, edema, and hypercalcemia.

Tamoxifen citrate (Nolvadex) is an antiestrogen, which apparently competes with estradiol for the estrogen receptor. The drug is not a steroid. Its main usefulness is in carcinoma of the breast in postmenopausal and also premenopausal women. Carcinoma of the breast is also being treated with this antiestrogen.

Radioactive phosphorus (^{32}P) is used in the treatment of polycythemia vera and also in chronic leukemias. It has a biological half-life of about 8 days in humans. It is handled just like normal phosphorus, being incorporated into nucleic acids and deposited in bone. It emits β rays that exert a destructive effect on the rapidly multiplying cells in which it is concentrated. ^{32}P is administered in doses of about 1 mCi daily for 5 days. Either the oral or intravenous route may be used, and the doses are not greatly different.

Radioactive iodine (^{131}I), radioactive gold (^{198}Au), and other isotopes are not as useful as ^{32}P. Nevertheless, ^{131}I has some limited application in metastatic thyroid carcinoma. Colloidal ^{198}Au has been tried in the treatment of lymphomas and in neoplastic diseases involving serous cavities. Its uses are largely experimental.

RADIOACTIVE ISOTOPES

Bleomycin sulfate (Blenoxane) binds to DNA and has been found useful in the treatment of squamous cell carcinomas of the head and neck. Also, this drug has some usefulness in treatment of testicular tumors and malignant lymphomas. Although bleomycin is not a depressant of the bone marrow, it can cause an unusual toxic manifestation—pulmonary fibrosis.

ANTIBIOTICS

Dactinomycin (actinomycin D; Cosmegen) is a toxic antibiotic that combines with DNA and blocks RNA production. It is effective in the treatment of choriocarcinoma of women, Wilms' tumor, and testicular carcinoma. The drug causes bone marrow depression and gastrointestinal toxicity.

Doxorubicin hydrochloride (Adriamycin) is an anthracycline antibiotic that combines with DNA and is cell cycle–specific, inhibiting the S phase preferentially. Doxorubicin is useful in the treatment of a variety of acute leukemias such as Hodgkin's disease and neuroblastoma. The drug is combined with cisplatin in the treatment of tumors of the bladder and testicular and ovarian carcinoma. Bone marrow depression is common and a characteristic toxic effect is cardiotoxicity. Tissue necrosis is severe in case of extravasation.

Mithramycin (Mithracin) is a toxic antibiotic that inhibits DNA-dependent RNA synthesis. In addition to its effect in testicular tumors, the drug has an effect on calcium metabolism, probably by acting on osteoclasts. Among numerous toxic effects, thrombocytopenia, bleeding, and gastrointestinal manifestations are most common.

Mitomycin (Mutamycin) is a toxic antibiotic, which is an alkylating agent that combines with DNA. The drug is used occasionally when other alkylating agents are ineffective. It causes severe bone marrow depression, gastrointestinal toxicity, and renal toxicity.

Vinblastine (Velban) is an alkaloid obtained from the periwinkle plant *(Vinca)*. It has antineoplastic activity, presumably as a consequence of mitotic arrest. Its toxic effects, commonly seen also with other antimetabolites, include nausea and vomiting, leukopenia, and alopecia. It is administered intravenously in doses of 0.1 to 0.15 mg/kg daily. Other alkaloids related to vinblastine are also being investigated. It is quite effective in the treatment of Hodgkin's disease and choriocarcinoma.

Vincristine (Oncovin) is a *Vinca* alkaloid that is particularly effective in the treatment of acute leukemia in children and Wilms' tumor. Nausea, vomiting, leukopenia, neurotoxic effects, and alopecia are toxic effects of the *Vinca* alkaloids. Vincristine is a spindle toxin.

L-Asparaginase is an enzyme that is effective in the treatment of human leukemia. Apparently some malignant cells require exogenous asparagine, but normal cells synthesize their own. The discovery of L-asparaginase as an antineoplastic agent resulted from observations on the suppressive effect of guinea pig serum, now known to contain L-asparaginase, on experimental leukemias. The drug is still experimental but is of great interest because it exploits a basic metabolic difference between normal and malignant cells.

Procarbazine (Matulane) is a synthetic methylhydrazine derivative that finds some usefulness in the treatment of generalized Hodgkin's disease. The drug has numerous adverse effects ranging from gastrointestinal symptoms, bone marrow depression, monoamine oxidase (MAO)–inhibitory action, and disulfiram-like effects. Procarbazine is available in capsules, 50 mg.

Hydroxyurea (Hydrea) may be useful in patients with chronic myelocytic leukemia when there is no response to busulfan. Bone marrow depression is its most serious adverse effect. The drug is available in capsules, 500 mg.

Mitotane (Lysodren) is a synthetic compound related to DDT that has specific toxicity for the adrenal gland. The drug is available in 500 mg tablets.

In addition to the use of surgery and radiation, various drugs may be effective in the treatment of malignancies. In fact, chemotherapy is considered the primary method of treatment in the following conditions: choriocarcinoma of the female, Wilms' tumor, acute and chronic leukemias, multiple myeloma, and polycythemia vera. Dosage and toxicity of various antineoplastic drugs are shown in Table 60-2.

As a general rule, the drugs of choice for various malignancies change rapidly in the light of statistics accumulated by cancer chemotherapy study groups. This is particularly true for possible synergistic combinations.

Chronic myelocytic leukemia responds to a number of drugs. In order of preference they are busulfan, chlorambucil, and mercaptopurine. It is believed that the drugs are as effective as irradiation and can be substituted for each other as resistance develops.

TABLE 60-2 Dosage and toxicity of some antimetabolites, antibiotics, hormones, and *Vinca* alkaloids

Drug	Route of administration	Usual dose	Toxic effects
Antimetabolites			
Methotrexate	Oral and intravenous	2.5 mg daily for leukemia 10-30 mg daily for choriocarcinoma	Stomatitis, enteritis, bone marrow depression, alopecia, skin rash; leucovorin is a useful antidote if given within a few hours after methotrexate
Fluorouracil	Intravenous	15 mg/kg daily for 4 days	Stomatitis, enteritis, leukopenia, hemorrhages
Mercaptopurine	Oral	2.5 mg/kg daily	Stomatitis, enteritis, jaundice, bone marrow depression
Antibiotic			
Actinomycin D	Intravenous	75 μg/kg total dose in 5 days	Vomiting, stomatitis, enteritis, leukopenia, alopecia
Hormones			
Diethylstilbestrol	Oral	1-5 mg three times/day	Nausea, vomiting, feminization, hypercalcemia
Fluoxymesterone	Oral	10 mg three times/day	Masculinization, hirsutism, fluid retention, hypercalcemia
Prednisone	Oral	1 mg/kg daily	Cushing-type effects
Vinca alkaloids			
Vinblastine	Intravenous	0.10-0.15 mg/kg weekly	Nausea, vomiting, stomatitis, leukopenia, alopecia
Vincristine	Intravenous	0.02-0.05 mg/kg weekly	Nausea, vomiting, neurotoxic effects, leukopenia, alopecia

Based on data from several sources.

Chronic lymphocytic leukemia may be treated with irradiation or drugs when the disease becomes progressive. Chlorambucil is preferred by many experts. In resistance cases, corticosteroids may be useful, and among these prednisone in large doses is favored by many.

Acute leukemias in children respond well to antimetabolites such as methotrexate. The acute lymphoblastic leukemias are also responsive to corticosteroids and vincristine. Other drugs are being used also, but nitrogen mustards are ineffective. In acute myeloblastic and monocytic leukemias, mercaptopurine has been found useful; cytarabine has been effective in causing remissions in acute granulocytic leukemias of adults.

Hodgkin's disease and *lymphosarcoma* are often treated with chlorambucil, mechlorethamine hydrochloride, methotrexate, vinblastine, and corticosteroids. Occasional favorable response is obtained but no definite prolongation of life.

Multiple myeloma responds to the alkylating agents such as cyclophosphamide or melphalan. Prednisone is useful also, as is vincristine.

Choriocarcinoma is most effectively treated with methotrexate or in resistant cases with actinomycin D. Vinblastine may be useful when the two preferred agents become ineffective.

Regional cancer chemotherapy by means of intraarterial nitrogen mustards or methotrexate with folinic acid is being used with some favorable results in selected patients.

Malignant effusions are often treated with mechlorethamine instillations, although quinacrine solutions may also be effective.

Drug combinations

Certain combinations of chemotherapeutic agents have shown distinct advantages, particularly in the treatment of Hodgkin's disease and lymphomas. The combination designated as MOPP consists of mechlorethamine, Oncovin (vincristine sulfate), procarbazine, and prednisone. COP refers to the combined use of cyclophosphamide, Oncovin, and prednisone. There is every reason to believe that other drugs, such as adriamycin and the nitrosoureas, may become important in combination chemotherapy. Another combination that has been used widely is known as CAM. It consists of cyclophosphamide, cytarabine, and methotrexate.

REFERENCES

1. Busch, H., and Lane, M.: Chemotherapy, Chicago, 1967, Year Book Medical Publishers, Inc.
2. Cancer chemotherapy, Med. Lett. **20**:81, 1978.
3. Cancer chemotherapy, Med. Lett. **25**:1, 1983.
4. Chabner, B.A., Myers, C.E., Coleman, N., and Johns, D.G.: The clinical pharmacology of antineoplastic agents, N. Engl. J. Med. **292**:1159, 1975.
5. Cortes, E.P., Holland, J.F., Wang, J.J., and Sinks, L.F.: Doxorubicin in disseminated osteosarcoma, JAMA **221**:1132, 1972.
6. DeVita, V.T., and Schein, P.S.: The use of drugs in combination for the treatment of cancer, N. Engl. J. Med. **288**:998, 1973.
7. Folkman, J.: Tumor angiogenesis: therapeutic implications, N. Engl. J. Med. **285**:1182, 1971.
8. Haskell, C.M., and Cline, M.J.: The treatment of acute leukemia, Ration. Drug Ther. **8**:1, 1974.
9. Hersh, E.M., Whitecar, J.P., McCredie, K.B., Bodey, G.P., and Freireich, E.J.: Chemotherapy, immunocompetence, immunosuppression and prognosis in acute leukemia, N. Engl. J. Med. **285**:1211, 1971.
10. Hoover, R., Gray, L.A., Cole, P., and MacMahon, B.: Menopausal estrogens and breast cancer, N. Engl. J. Med. **295**:401, 1976.
11. Krakoff, I.H.: Cancer chemotherapeutic agents, CA **23**:208, 1973.
12. Leyland-Jones, B.: Hormones in cancer, Ration. Drug Ther. **16**:1, 1982.
13. Lokich, J.J.: Managing chemotherapy-induced bone marrow suppression in cancer, Hosp. Pract., Aug 1976, p. 61.
14. Marsh, J.C., and Mitchell, M.S.: Chemotherapy of cancer, Drug Therapy, Jan. 1974.
15. Miller, E.: The metabolism and pharmacology of 5-fluorouracil, J. Surg. Oncol. **3**:309, 1971.
16. Oswalt, C.E., and Cruz, A.B.: Cancer chemotherapeutic agents, Tex. Med. **73**:57, 1977.
17. Stone, M.J.: Recent advances in oncology, Dallas Med. J., Sept. 1978, p. 406.

section ten

Principles of
immunopharmacology

Chapter 61

Principles of immunopharmacology

The control of disease by immunological means has two objectives: the production of *desired immunity* and the elimination of *undesired immune reactions*. The first of these objectives is achieved by *immunization procedures* rather than drugs. For this reason, discussions of immunopharmacology are more concerned with the chemical basis of *undesired* immune reactions and their possible elimination by means of drugs.

The impressive developments in clinical immunology with emphasis on various classes of lymphocytes have not been matched by corresponding advances in the pharmacological approach. In treating immunological disorders, physicians rely largely on corticosteroids, immunosuppressive agents, and replacement of deficiencies.

The basic mechanisms of immunological injury are anaphylactic mechanisms, cytolytic mechanisms, immune complex disorders, and delayed hypersensitivity reactions. In actual practice, physicians deal with autoimmune diseases, allograft rejections, immune complex problems, and erythroblastosis fetalis. There are other immunological disorders that are difficult to classify.

Several groups of drugs have been used clinically for the purpose of suppressing the immune response. Following are the most important:

1. Corticosteroids
2. Cytotoxic drugs
    a. Antimetabolites: mercaptopurine and azathioprine (Imuran)
    b. Alkylating agents: cyclophosphamide (Cytoxan) and nitrogen mustard
    c. Folic acid antagonists: methotrexate

In addition to these drugs, radiation and antilymphocytic serum (ALS) are also potent immunosuppressive agents.

IMMUNO-SUPPRESSIVE AGENTS

711

Mode of action

There is general agreement on certain features of the mode of action of the immunosuppressive drugs,[29] which can be summarized as follows:

1. The cytotoxic drugs tend to destroy replicating cells. They have been classified as *cell cycle drugs* and *noncycle drugs*. The cell cycle drugs destroy *only* rapidly multiplying cells, whereas the noncycle drugs are injurious to nonreplicating cells as well. The antimetabolites and folic acid antagonists act only on dividing cells; the alkylating agents, being noncycle drugs, cause depletion in the total number of small lymphocytes.

2. Immunosuppressive agents inhibit the primary immune response more readily than an established immune state or an anamnestic response. Their main effect on antibody synthesis is exerted during the time when the antigen converts its clone of lymphocytes to antibody-producing cells.

3. Various components of the immune response are not equally affected by all suppressive drugs. Delayed hypersensitivity and IgG synthesis can be inhibited selectively. For example, mercaptopurine and antilymphocyte serum can inhibit the development of delayed hypersensitivity without blocking IgG synthesis.[1]

4. The goal of immunosuppressive therapy is the development of drug-induced immune tolerance to specific antigens, with conservation of other immunological capabilities.

5. Immunosuppressive drugs have many adverse effects. These are not unexpected because immune processes are important defenses against infections and may play a role in protecting the individual against neoplastic cells as well.

EFFECTOR
MECHANISMS AND
MEDIATORS IN
IMMUNE INJURY

Several types of immune injury are recognized, each having characteristic effector mechanisms. Some of the latter are (1) anaphylaxis, (2) cytolysis, (3) immune-complex reactions, and (4) delayed hypersensitivity.

Anaphylactic
mechanisms

The antibody in anaphylactic reactions is largely of the IgE type, which attaches itself to cells such as mast cells and leukocytes. When exposed to the antigen, the sensitized mast cells release vasoactive mediators, among which histamine appears the most important. The slow-reacting substance (SRS), an acidic lipid, may not originate from mast cells. In the rat[15] it is released by polymorphonuclear leukocytes. Serotonin is probably not present in human mast cells.

The release of histamine from human basophils or mast cells does not require complement when these cells are sensitized by IgE antibodies. On the other hand, if antibodies are prepared against mast cells, they will attack these cells and cause histamine release by a cytolytic mechanism that requires complement.

Cytolytic
mechanisms

Cytolytic mechanisms are involved in the pathogenesis of various types of hemolytic anemia, thrombocytopenia, and leukopenia. The antigen may be a constituent of the cell, such as the Rh factor, or drug attached to the cell. The antibodies are of

Schema of mediator release caused by interaction of cell-bound IgE antibody and antigen.　FIG. 61-1

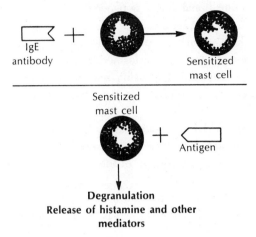

the IgE variety except for the cold hemagglutinins (IgM). Complement is not required for cytolysis except when cold agglutinins are involved.

Immune-complex mechanisms are most clearly seen in acute and chronic glomerulonephritis and in serum sickness. Soluble antigen-antibody complexes may be deposited in the glomerular basement membranes where they activate the complement system. Leukotactic factors are generated, which attract polymorphonuclear leukocytes. The release of lytic enzymes from leukocytic lysosomes leads to digestion of the basement membrane.[2] There are variations on this theme. The antibodies may be directed against the basement membrane. In other instances the continued deposit formation leads to membranous glomerulonephritis.

The antibodies involved in immune-complex disease are of the IgG and IgM type, and complement plays an important role in the immunological injury.

Immune-complex mechanisms

The clinical condition that is a prime example of delayed hypersensitivity is *contact dermatitis*. Similar mechanisms are involved also in the rejection of grafts and in the tuberculin reaction.

No humoral antibodies are involved in this type of reaction. Instead, sensitized small lymphocytes are responsible for recognizing the antigen. In addition, large numbers of nonsensitized mononuclear cells that accumulate at the site over a period of 24 to 48 hours act as the "inflammatory cells." The slow accumulation of these cells explains the delayed nature of the reaction. The mechanism of their accumulation may be related to the observation that sensitized lymphocytes exposed to the antigen in vitro release a factor (migration-inhibition factor) that causes macrophages to stick to capillary tubes, thus preventing their migration. There are other mediators of

Delayed hypersensitivity mechanisms

delayed hypersensitivity, such as lymphotoxin.[7] The role of the so-called lymph node–permeability factor is questionable and nonspecific.

Anaphylactic mechanisms are not susceptible to cytotoxic drugs for a number of reasons. These reactions depend on preformed antibodies, and the reactions are of the immediate type. Although it is possible that long-continued administration of cytotoxic drugs would have some effect, the toxicity of these agents precludes their prolonged administration.

The therapeutic approaches to anaphylactic injury are aimed at (1) the development of blocking antibodies by hyposensitization, (2) inhibition of the release of vasoactive mediators, and (3) prevention of the effect of the mediators such as histamine.

The widely employed hyposensitization procedures are believed to increase the formation of blocking antibodies (IgG) that may bind the allergen. It is possible that other mechanisms are also involved. In the rapid desensitization to an antigen such as a serum in an individual known to be hypersensitive to it, there must clearly be other mechanisms involved than the production of blocking antibodies.

Disodium cromoglycate (Intal) is a chroman derivative that is claimed to inhibit the release of vasoactive mediators caused by interaction of antigen with reaginic antibodies.[15] When administered by inhalation, it exerts some therapeutic effect in asthma, which is demonstrable statistically in controlled series. That it is not a powerful therapeutic agent is indicated by some conflict of opinion about its efficacy.

Disodium cromoglycate

Of great interest are observations indicating that histamine release from human leukocytes and animal mast cells is inhibited by drugs that are expected to raise intracellular cyclic AMP levels. Isoproterenol and theophylline, widely used in the treatment of asthma, have an inhibitory activity on histamine release by allergens from human leukocytes.[6] Although the relative importance of their action on release processes in relation to their bronchodilator action is impossible to state under clinical conditions, these observations have stimulated much research on the role of the β-adrenergic system in the allergic diathesis.[23]

There is not much known about drug effects on cytolysis. On the other hand, drugs may act at several sites in immune-complex disease. Immunosuppressive drugs may reduce the antibody levels and lower the number of granulocytes. It is of great interest that agranulocytic animals do not develop glomerulonephritis despite the

Inhibitory effect of cyclic 3',5'-AMP on mediator release and the influence of some drugs. **FIG. 61-2**
Broken arrow indicates an inhibitory effect.

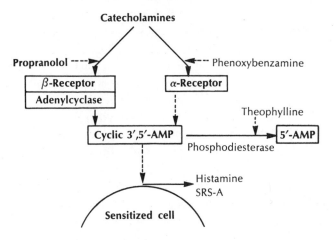

presence of complexes in the circulation. Corticosteroids are employed in the treatment of glomerulonephritis. Their action is attributed to stabilization of granulocytic lysosomes, which are believed to play an important role in damaging the basement membrane of the glomeruli. Theoretic approaches to immune-complex disease include also the use of decomplementing agents. A glycoprotein extracted from cobra venom depletes the third component of complement[11] a finding of great experimental interest.

Delayed hypersensitivity is susceptible to several drugs. The immunosuppressive drugs such as the antimetabolites have important effects on the nonsensitized inflammatory cells. This is understandable, since the inflammatory cells are short-lived and have very active nucleic acid metabolism.[21]

IMMUNOSUPPRESSIVE AND ANTIINFLAMMATORY DRUG ACTIONS

There is commonly an overlap in the antiinflammatory and immunosuppressive effects of various drugs. For example, the corticosteroids have both actions. Mercaptopurine treatment reduces the number of mononuclear cells at inflammatory sites[17] in animal experiments.

The simplest way to explain the overlap is to consider that the immune injury leads to inflammation as a consequence of the activity of "inflammatory" cells. Drugs that reduce the number of these cells or inhibit their activities may exert both antiinflammatory and apparent immunosuppressive effects. The cytotoxic drugs inhibit the multiplication of cells, whereas the milder antiinflammatory drugs may exert more subtle effects on the inflammatory cells or may block the actions of their products. *Theoretically,* the antiinflammatory drugs may block the effects of leukotactic factor on inflammatory cells, or they may inhibit the elaboration of mediators by these cells. They may also block the action of the mediators. No simple theory such as that of lysosomal stabilization[27] is sufficient to account for the vast differences in the spectrum of activity of the various types of antiinflammatory drugs (p. 532).

CLINICAL APPLICATIONS

From the foregoing discussion it should be clear that some types of immune injury may be ameliorated by drug therapy. Some of the examples are discussed briefly.

Rh hemolytic disease of the newborn is prevented very successfully by Rh_0 (D) immune globulin (RhoGAM). It is used for the passive immunization of the mother to prevent the formation of antibodies. It is injected within 72 hours after birth of an RH_0-positive (D-positive or D^u-positive) baby to a mother who is negative with respect to these factors.

Acute glomerulonephritis is often treated with corticosteroids (prednisone) and occasionally with other immunosuppressive agents. The same is true for idiopathic thrombocytopenic purpura and autoimmune hemolytic anemia.

Renal transplantation has been greatly aided by the availability of azathioprine (Imuran), prednisone, and antilymphocytic serum (ALS). These drugs are used also in the transplantation of other organs. The fungal metabolite cyclosporin A is currently undergoing clinical trials. This immunosuppressive agent selectively inhibits the immune response at the level of the T lymphocyte and offers great promise as a useful agent in organ transplants.[12]

The usefulness of drugs in the management of allergic and rheumatic diseases is discussed in Chapters 20 and 31.

IMMUNOTOXINS

In the past decade, advances in molecular biology have revolutionized the field of immunology. Although these developments have not yet reached the clinical level, they serve as harbingers for the use of immunological reagents as true pharmaceuticals.

The first development involves the construction of immunotoxins, which are pharmaceutical agents composed of toxic substances covalently linked to antibodies. In general terms, the antibody can be any cell-binding immunoglobulin and the toxin can be any antibiotic. The cell-binding antibody serves to direct the toxin to the target cells, and the toxin of course functions to destroy that cell. For this combination to be of practical use it is necessary that only target cells are affected. One way this can be brought about is through the use of antibodies directed against defined antigenic determinants. The availability of hybridoma technology permits the production of such antibodies.

The in vitro fusion of antibody-producing cells with myeloma cells yields hybrid cells (hybridomas) that have the ability to grow indefinitely. After identification of cells that produce antibodies of appropriate specificity, a genetically homogeneous population of cells can be propagated, and unlimited quantities of antibodies directed toward a single antigenic site can be obtained. If hybridoma cells are selected that secrete antibody against a cell-surface antigen unique to a certain cell type (e.g., a particular type of tumor), then an infinite supply of molecules capable of seeking out particular cells will be available. If these cell-specific antibodies are combined with a potent toxin, they are then capable of destroying specific cells among a milieu of other cells.

The toxin that has most promise for immunotoxin therapy is ricin, a plant toxin consisting of two polypeptide chains. One (the B chain) is a lectin capable of binding to cell surfaces. The other (the A chain) is able to inhibit protein synthesis. Since immunotherapy requires binding to specific cells rather than the generalized cellular binding exhibited by the B chain, only the A chain is used in preparation of the immunotoxin. Hence, ricin A chain is covalently linked to cell surface–specific antibody. Because the A chain is not active outside of the cytoplasm, it will exert its effect only on those cells to which it becomes bound via the antibody. Immunotoxins containing ricin A chain have been used successfully to kill mouse and human tumor cells in vitro as well as leukemic cells in mice.[25] Ricin is not the only deleterious agent under consideration as an immunotoxin. Other inhibitors of cellular processes including diphtheria toxin, abrin (another plant toxin), daunorubicin, and methotrexate are also under study.

Although historically discussions of vaccines are usually confined to microbiology texts, the development of synthetic vaccines brings this subject into the realm of pharmacology. Synthetic vaccines use chemically synthesized antigens (usually peptides) as the immunizing agent. The success of these vaccines relies on the ability of an antibody elicited in response to a small, defined peptide to recognize (and bind to) that peptide as part of a larger molecule. For example, if the sequence of only a few amino acid residues of a viral protein is known, this small peptide can be synthesized and used to immunize a population against the virus. Advantages of synthetic vaccines are twofold. First, since they do not rely on live or attenuated virus, they are quite safe. Second, the peptides can be easily synthesized on a large scale. In practical terms the amino acid sequences of proteins of interest are often most easily discernible from the nucleotide sequence of the gene. From the amino acid sequence a variety of peptides can be synthesized. These peptides can then be used to immunize a test population (e.g., guinea pigs) subsequently challenged with virus to determine which peptide provided protection. Preliminary studies indicated that synthetic vaccines can offer animals protection against foot and mouth disease virus.[22] It can also be speculated that in addition to their usefulness in protecting against viral agents, synthetic vaccines may have some application in immunization against tumor antigens.

SYNTHETIC
VACCINES

REFERENCES

1. Borel, Y., and Schwartz, R.S.: Inhibition of immediate and delayed hypersensitivity by 6-mercaptopurine, J. Immunol. 92:754, 1965.
2. Dixon, F.J.: The pathogenesis of glomerulonephritis, Am. J. Med. 44:493, 1968.
3. Gowans, J.L., and McGregor, D.D.: Immunological activities of lymphocytes, Prog. Allergy 9:1, 1965.
4. Ishizaka, K.: The identification and significance of gamma E, Hosp. Pract. 4:70, 1969.
5. Johnson, A.R., and Moran, N.C.: Inhibition of the release of histamine from rat mast cells: the effect of cold and adrenergic drugs on release of histamine by compound 48/80 and antigen, J. Pharmacol. Exp. Ther. 175:632, 1970.
6. Lichtenstein, L.M.: Mechanism of allergic histamine release from human leukocytes. In Austen, K.F., and Becker, E.L., editors: Biochemistry of the acute allergic reactions, Philadelphia, 1967, F.A. Davis Co.
7. Mackaness, G.B., and Blanden, R.V.: Cellular immunity, Prog. Allergy 11:89, 1967.
8. Makinodan, T., Santos, G.W., and Quinn, R.P.: Immunosuppressive drugs, Pharmacol. Rev. 22:189, 1971.
9. Medawar, P.: Antilymphocyte serum: its properties and potentials, Hosp. Pract. 4:26, 1969.
10. Mota, I.: The mechanism of anaphylaxis. I. Production and biological properties of "mast cell sensitizing" antibody, Immunology 7:681, 1964.
11. Muller-Eberhard, H.J.: Chemistry and reaction mechanisms of complement, Adv. Immunol. 8:1, 1968.
12. Najarian, J.S.: Immunologic aspects of organ transplantation, Hosp. Pract. Oct. 1982, p. 61.
13. Norman, P.S.: The clinical significance of IgE, Hosp. Pract. Aug., 1975, p. 41.
14. Novack, S.N., and Pearson, C.M.: Cyclophosphamide therapy in Wegener's granulomatosis, N. Engl. J. Med. 284:938, 1971.
15. Orange, R.P., and Austen, K.F.: Pharmacologic dissociation of immunologic release of histamine and slow-reacting substance of anaphylaxis in rats, Proc. Soc. Exp. Biol. Med. 129:836, 1968.
16. Orange, R.P., Valentine, M.D., and Austen, K.F.: Antigen-induced release of slow-reacting substance of anaphylaxis in rats prepared with homologous antibody, J. Exp. Med. 127:767, 1968.
17. Page, A.R., Condie, R.M., and Good, R.A.: Effect of 6-mercaptopurine on inflammation, Am. J. Pathol. 40:519, 1962.
18. Parker, C.W.: Control of lymphocyte function, N. Engl. J. Med. 295:1180, 1976.
19. Piper, P.J., and Vane, J.R.: Release of additional factors in anaphylaxis and its antagonism by anti-inflammatory drugs, Nature 223:29, 1969.
20. Reinherz, E.L.: Current concepts in immunology, N. Engl. J. Med. 303:370, 1980.
21. Schwartz, R.S.: Therapeutic strategy in clinical immunology, N. Engl. J. Med. 280:367, 1969.
22. Sutcliffe, J.G., Shinnick, T.M., Green, N., and Lerner, R.A.: Antibodies that react with predetermined sites on proteins, Science 219:660, 1983.
23. Szentivanyi, A.: The beta adrenergic theory of the atopic abnormality in bronchial asthma, J. Allerg. 42:203, 1968.
24. Uhr, J.W., and Moller, G.: Regulatory effects of antibody on antibody formation, Adv. Immunol. 8:81, 1968.
25. Vitetta, E.S., Krolick, K.A., Miyama-Inaba, M., Cushley, W., and Uhr, J.W.: Immunotoxins: a new approach to cancer therapy, Science 219:644, 1983.
26. Ward, P.A., and Zwaifler, M.J.: Complement-derived leukotactic factors in inflammatory synovial fluids of humans, J. Clin. Invest. 50:606, 1971.
27. Weissmann, G.: Structure and function of lysosomes, Rheumatology 1:1, 1967.
28. Weissmann, G.: Lysosomal mechanisms of tissue injury in arthritis, N. Engl. J. Med. 286:141, 1972.
29. Winkelstein, A.: Principles of immunosuppressive therapy, Bull. Rheum. Dis. 21:627, 1971.

section eleven

Poisons and antidotes

Chapter 62

Poisons and antidotes

A poison may be defined as any substance causing death, disease, or injury. Poisons arise from various sources, including industrial pollutants, burning of fossil fuels (carbon monoxide radionuclides), or the bacterial toxins. Drugs fit this definition of a poison and are commonly classified as such. Poisoning resulting from drugs is usually a matter of degree; a small quantity may produce a desired (therapeutic) effect, whereas a larger amount may produce an untoward or toxic effect.

Toxicology is defined as the science of poisons and poisonings. It includes the diagnosis, treatment, mechanisms of action, and identification of poisons. Individuals skilled in this area of endeavor are classified as clinical, forensic, or industrial toxicologists. Chemical analysis is central to the diagnosis of drug intoxication.

DIAGNOSIS OF POISONING

The diagnosis of poisoning can be difficult. The victim is often unconscious. Recognition of the cause and severity of poisoning depends largely on physical examination, past history, and chemical identification and quantification of the compound responsible. Some victims of poisoning are admitted to a hospital with an incorrect diagnosis. The conscious patient may not admit to self-poisoning, and this possibility may not enter the physician's mind. A suspicious mind is essential to detect these cases, and poisoning should be included much more frequently in the differential diagnosis. Poisoning should be suspected when a person who is ill does not respond to treatment with time. There are many misdiagnosed cases of self-poisoning where the initial diagnosis of some particular disease turned out to be caused by drug ingestion. Symptoms and pathological changes can be quite characteristic for certain types of poisoning. The victim's family should be encouraged to produce bottles of medication, particularly empty or partially empty ones, to which the patient had access.

Since more poisons exist than diseases and since almost all medical training is focused on the diseases, physicians may consider themselves less equipped to handle poisoning than other problems. Physicians in this predicament should consult experts in clinical toxicology at major regional poison centers.

PRINCIPLES OF
TREATMENT

Overtreatment of the poisoned patient with large doses of antidote, sedatives, or stimulants can cause more damage than the poison itself.[2] The judicious use of drugs and other therapeutic measures is a requirement of utmost importance.

General principles of poison treatment include (1) removal of the poison from the stomach, except where contraindicated; (2) administration of an antidote; (3) symptomatic and supportive therapy, and (4) identification of the chemical responsible as soon as possible.

The importance of emptying the stomach cannot be overemphasized; this mainstay of treatment in any ingested poison can be lifesaving. Exceptions to this principle are when the patient is having a seizure, is comatose, or has ingested a petroleum distillate or corrosive or if too much time has elapsed since the poison was ingested. If vomiting has not occurred, the conscious patient should be made to vomit, since vomiting is more effective than the most intensive gastric lavage.[1] If vomiting has not occurred or cannot be induced, gastric lavage should be performed at once. Most poisons are themselves emetics, but if vomiting does not occur spontaneously, it should be induced. This can be accomplished by gagging (stimulation of pharynx) with a finger after having the victim drink a glass of milk or water or by use of drugs that induce vomiting.

Emetics

Two drugs recommended for the induction of vomiting in poisoning are apomorphine hydrochloride and syrup of ipecac (not the fluid extracts). For best results fluids should be given before the administration of emetics, since emesis does not readily occur if the stomach is empty.

Injection of **apomorphine hydrochloride** (6 mg/kg for adult, 0.066 mg/kg for child) subcutaneously produces prompt emesis. To terminate the narcotic effects of apomorphine (rarely necessary), the narcotic antagonists, are administered, preferably naloxone hydrochloride (NARCAN), 0.01 mg/kg intravenously, intramuscularly, or subcutaneously. Apomorpine has the advantages of producing rapid vomiting (within 5 minutes) with emptying of all gastric contents and of promoting the reflux of contents from the upper intestinal tract into the stomach. The drug should not be used if the patient is deeply depressed or comatose.

Ipecac is an effective emetic. It results in rapid emesis, can be kept at home for use at the time of ingestion, and is inexpensive and safe. The average time before emesis with a dosage of 15 to 20 ml of ipecac is 15 minutes. If one dose does not induce emesis in 20 minutes, another 15 ml dose may be administered. If two doses of ipecac fail to induce vomiting, gastric lavage becomes imperative, since ipecac is an irritant, and, when absorbed, is a cardiotoxin. Syrup of ipecac should never be given simultaneously with charcoal because charcoal absorbs the ipecac, thereby preventing its emetic effect. Charcoal should be given after vomiting has stopped.

Cupric sulfate (0.25 g in 1% solution) induces vomiting more rapidly and in a larger number of cases than ipecac. If vomiting does not occur within 15 minutes after administration of cupric sulfate, 0.15 g of potassium ferrocyanide in 1% solution is administered, followed by aspiration and gastric lavage. Cupric sulfate as an emetic is corrosive to the gastrointestinal tract and damages the liver and kidney; it should be replaced in the management of poisoning by safer agents (ipecac, apomorphine). The lethal dose of this nephrotoxic, hepatotoxic, and hemolytic agent has been as low as 1 g.

One gram of activated charcoal has a surface area that exceeds 3000 m². It is a potent absorbent for many organic and inorganic poisons except cyanide and lithium. The adsorbed material is rigidly retained throughout its passage through the gastrointestinal tract. About 15 g (5 to 6 teaspoons) in a glass of milk or water is given after emesis.[10]

Tannic acid forms insoluble salts with many alkaloids and heavy metals. Approximately 30 to 50 g/L of water is an effective concentration. Larger amounts than those recommended should be avoided because of its hepatotoxicity.

Magnesium oxide is used as a neutralizing agent for acids and has the added advantage of not forming gas. In this regard it differs from sodium bicarbonate. The recommended concentration is approximately 25 g/L.

A universal antidote consisting of these three substances in combination has been recommended in the past. The modern trend is to avoid this practice, since the three together can render each other ineffective.[9] Furthermore, it produces a gastric pH of 9 to 9.5, which could favor the absorption of some drugs. Other locally acting antidotes against unabsorbed poisons include vinegar, potassium permanganate, milk, egg white, sodium sulfate, sodium bicarbonate (aerosol), soap, calcium, ammonia water, starch, vegetable oil, and normal saline (lavage).

ANTIDOTES
Nonsystemic antidotes

Some antidotes are effective after they have been absorbed. Dimercaprol (2,3-dimercapto-propanol or BAL) is a drug routinely used in the treatment of mercury, gold, and arsenic poisoning. It was developed during World War II as an antidote to vesicant arsenicals. It had been known that arsenicals combine with sulfhydryl groups. After several such compounds were synthesized, it was found that dimercaprol was most effective in this binding, most likely due to a pair of vicinal sulfhydryl groups that enable it to form a stable ring structure with the metal.

Systemic antidotes
DIMERCAPROL

$$CH_2-SH$$
$$CH-SH$$
$$CH_2-OH$$
Dimercaprol

Therapeutic objectives. There are two major objectives in the use of dimercaprol. The first objective is inactivation of the poison by forming a chelate or a complex with it, thus preventing it from combining with the sulfhydryl groups of essential enzyme systems. The second objective is to promote excretion of the drug complex from the body, since it is water soluble at pH 7.5 and readily excreted.

Metabolism. Detoxification of dimercaprol is catalyzed by a microsomal enzyme through S-methylation. Its use is contraindicated in the presence of liver disease, in severe renal disease, and in iron poisoning.

Toxicity and adverse effects. Dimercaprol is potentially dangerous. Some of its unpleasant side effects are flushing, myalgia, nausea and vomiting, nephrotoxic effects, hypotension, pulmonary edema, salivation, lacrimation, and fever. Despite its side effects, it has been in use over 30 years and has not been replaced by a better antidote.

Preparations. Dimercaprol (BAL), USP is available as a 10% solution (100 mg/ml) in peanut oil. Dosage varies from 2.5 to 3 mg/kg intramuscularly repeated from one to four times a day, depending on the severity of the intoxication.

CALCIUM DISODIUM EDETATE AND DISODIUM EDETATE

Ethylenediamine tetraacetic acid and its salt, disodium edetate, are powerful chelating agents that form a highly stable complex with calcium. Despite the stability of the chelate, calcium is displaced from it by lead, zinc, chromium, copper, cadmium, manganese, and nickel. This exchange of calcium for lead occurs because of their relative positions in the atomic table. Calcium disodium edetate, also called calcium disodium versenate, is used in combination with BAL in the treatment of lead poisoning associated with encephalopathy.

Edetate calcium disodium   Disodium lead edetate

The calcium derivative should be used, since the disodium salt will chelate calcium, producing hypocalcemia. Although the older literature states that the intravenous route of administration is preferred for edetate administration, recent drug schedules for these agents use deep intramuscular injections of BAL and edetate. More severe reactions have been observed with intravenous administration. Oral administration of edetate is unsatisfactory and may be harmful because absorbable edetate-lead complexes can form in the gastrointestinal tract. The rate of urinary lead excretion is enhanced by combined BAL-edetate treatment.

Disodium edetate

Toxicity and adverse effects. The toxicity of edetate is probably due to binding of essential metal ions. Large doses are nephrotoxic in humans. Edetate is not metabolized. It is excreted by the kidney and hence contraindicated in the presence of anuria, proteinuria, or microscopic hematuria.

Preparations. Edetate calcium disodium, USP for parenteral use is a 20% solution. The total daily dose should not exceed 50 mg/kg of body weight in order to avoid toxic symptoms. It is also marketed as 500 mg tablets (not usually given orally).

Edetate disodium is marketed in 20 ml ampules that contain 150 mg/ml or 15 ml ampules containing 200 mg/ml. It is used to treat hypercalcemia and to control arrhythmias associated with digitalis toxicity.

Therapeutic objectives. Penicillamine (Cuprimine) and its acetyl derivative, *N*-acetyl-penicillamine, can chelate copper and other metals. It is used presently to remove copper in hepatolenticular degeneration (Wilson's disease). Penicillamine chelates not only copper but other metals such as mercury, lead, and iron. Since other drugs are more effective, the drug is recommended only for removal of copper. Penicillamine is of value in the treatment of cystinuria and the associated nephrolithiasis. It is useful in the treatment of rheumatoid arthritis.

Toxicity and adverse effects. Adverse effects of penicillamine are acute allergic reactions, leukopenia, eosinophilia, and thrombocytopenia. D-Penicillamine is relatively nontoxic. It is the preferred form. Much of the drug's toxicity was due to the former use of the L or D,L forms.

D-Penicillamine, USP is marketed as 125 or 250 mg capsules and is administered orally, 1 to 4 g/day, in four divided doses.

$$CH_3-\underset{\underset{SH}{|}}{\overset{\overset{CH_3}{|}}{C}}-\underset{\underset{NH_2}{|}}{CH}-COOH$$

Penicillamine

$$CH_3-\underset{\underset{SH}{|}}{\overset{\overset{CH_3}{|}}{C}}-\underset{\underset{N}{\diagdown}}{CH}\underset{\overset{H}{\diagup}}{\overset{}{}}COOH$$

N-Acetylpenicillamine

Deferoxamine mesylate is isolated from *Streptomyces pilosus* and has high affinity for ferric iron and low affinity for calcium. This chelating agent is used in the treatment of iron poisoning and hemochromatosis. It is metabolized by plasma enzymes and also excreted unchanged in the urine. Reactions to the drug include diarrhea, hypotension, and cataract formation. The drug is toxic and should be used only if the severity of the poisoning justifies it. Deferoxamine mesylate, USP (Desferal) is available in ampules containing 500 mg. The recommended dose in iron poisoning is 1 g intramuscularly or intravenously, repeated if necessary every 4 to 12 hours. The total amount of drug given should not exceed 6 g in 24 hours.

LIFE-SUSTAINING MEASURES	Certain patients with severe drug intoxication or underlying systemic diseases in whom the complications of drug overdose are more hazardous may require special modalities to enhance drug removal from the body. Currently available modalities include forced diuresis, peritoneal dialysis, hemodialysis, lipid dialysis, hemoperfusion, or exchange transfusion.

Forced diuresis	Forced diuresis depends on the kidney's ability to excrete the drug and its metabolites. Many substances diffuse across tubular cells and are reabsorbed, leading to low clearance rates. There are two types of diffusion. One type is pH independent: here the way to change the excretion rate of a drug is to increase the volume of urine passing through the renal tubule to minimize the time for renal reabsorption of the drug (osmotic forced diuresis). The other type of diffusion is pH dependent: here, by changing the urine pH, an increase in excretion rate of the drug is obtained. Drugs that are weak acids are excreted faster in alkaline urine, whereas drugs that are weak bases are excreted faster if the urine is acidic. The reason is that under these conditions the drugs are in their ionized form and are thus unavailable for reabsorption across the lipid tubular cell membrane.

Peritoneal dialysis	For peritoneal dialysis to be effective the drug or poison should be freely permeable through the peritoneal membrane. Larger molecular weight compounds will not diffuse through. Neither will those with a high degree of protein or lipid binding.

Hemodialysis	Hemodialysis can enhance removal of some drugs from the body. A single 6-hour hemodialysis can remove as much barbiturate as a 24-hour diuresis or peritoneal dialysis. Long-acting barbiturates can be removed in greater quantity than short-acting ones. The latter are better removed by lipid dialysis. In this procedure soybean oil is circulated on the dialysate side of the membrane.

Hemoperfusion	Hemodialysis for the treatment of drug intoxication has waned in recent years as a result of poor clearance of many drugs with standard procedures.[11] Hemoperfusion, on the other hand, is being promoted for treatment of numerous exogenous poisons. This procedure has been shown to achieve high clearance rates for most common intoxicants, and its application has been, on occasion, lifesaving. Clearance values obtained by this procedure are substantially higher than those by hemodialysis.

ESSENTIAL FEATURES OF CERTAIN POISONINGS	Toxic effects of the most common poisonings in the adult are summarized in Table 62-1. The essential features of some other poisonings are discussed in this section.

Scopolamine and atropine intoxication	Scopolamine intoxication is not uncommon, since the drug is contained in some proprietary hypnotic preparations (Sominex). The symptoms produced by scopolamine and other atropinic drugs develop rapidly after ingestion. These include dry

TABLE 62-1   Essential features of common poisons

Drug	Oral fatal dose (estimated)	Lethal blood levels (estimated)	Effects	Therapy
Barbiturates			Respiratory depression, hypotension, renal shutdown, hypothermia, pneumonia	Respiratory assistance, diuresis, hemoperfusion
Short acting	3 g	3.5 mg/100 ml		
Long acting	5 g	8.0 mg/100 ml		
Glutethimide	10-20 g	3.0 mg/100 ml	Apnea, mydriasis, hypotension, flaccid paralysis	Gastric lavage, respiratory assistance, diuresis, hemoperfusion
Salicylates	10-20 g	50 mg/100 ml	Hyperventilation, respiratory alkalosis, metabolic acidosis (later), hypoprothrombinemia	Alkaline diuresis, vitamin K, dialysis
Phenothiazines	50 mg/kg of chlorpromazine or equivalent	Unknown	Miosis, irritability	Supportive control of convulsions
Meprobamate	12 g	Unknown	Hypotension, respiratory depression, coma	Respiratory assistance, dialysis
Acetaminophen	5-10 g	30 mg/100 ml; 4 hr 12 mg/100 ml; 12 hr	Liver and kidney damage, jaundice oliguria or anuria	*N*-acetylcysteine inactivates toxic metabolites, hemoperfusion, supportive until liver function returns
Methaqualone	8 g	2-3 mg/100 ml	Excessive central depression, delerium, convulsions, hyperreflexia	Respiratory assistance, supportive therapy, hemoperfusion

mouth, blurred vision, fever, tachycardia, hypotension, widely dilated pupils, mental symptoms, urinary retention, and hot, dry, and flushed skin. Infants and young children are more susceptible to the toxic effects of these drugs. The antidote to atropine poisoning is physostigmine given as a slow intravenous injection of 1 to 4 mg (0.5 to 1.0 mg in children). In the presence of marked excitement and to control convulsions, diazepam is the drug of choice. Phenothiazines should never be used, since they aggravate the anticholinergic or atropine-like effects of scopolamine. Ice packs may be needed to help control hyperthermia. Urinary retention may require catheterization.

Bromide intoxication

The toxic dose is about 30 g or a serum bromide level that exceeds 19 mEq/L. Chronic administration of bromide results in its accumulation in the body. Many over-the-counter preparations contain bromide. Small doses cause sedation and drowsiness. Large doses lead to mental depression, respiratory depression, hypotension, and loss of consciousness. Bromide replaces chloride in the extracellular fluid. It is removed slowly from the body when bromide ingestion stops. The treatment of bromide poisoning should include gastric lavage and osmotic diuresis with added chloride. Severe cases may require peritoneal dialysis or hemodialysis.

Ethylene glycol and diethylene glycol intoxication

Ethylene glycol is contained in antifreeze preparations. The lethal dose is about 100 ml. Ethylene glycol is metabolized via alcohol dehydrogenase to oxalate, which is nephrotoxic.

Striking oxalate formation is present throughout the renal tubules. Crystals may even appear in the brain. Ethylene glycol produces CNS depression, which can progress to narcosis, coma, and death. It produces severe renal injury and failure. The metabolic acidosis that results from ingestion of ethylene glycol is caused by formic acid production.

Gastric lavage should be performed to remove the offending substance. Specific treatment is aimed at correcting the metabolic acidosis with sodium bicarbonate. Ethanol markedly inhibits the metabolism of ethylene glycol and protects against the acute toxicity resulting from ethylene glycol metabolism, since ethanol is a potent competitive inhibitor of and a much better substrate for alcohol dehydrogenase. Renal dialysis is effective in reducing the body load of ethylene glycol, as it is with all alcohols. Calcium lactate should be administered for the relief of muscle spasms resulting from calcium chelation by the oxalate formed.

Diethylene glycol has many industrial uses; however, its ingestion can cause hepatic and renal damage and death. It was used as a solvent in an elixir of sulfanilamide and caused 105 fatalities among 353 people taking the preparation. From this catastrophe it was estimated that the oral lethal dose is approximately 1 ml/kg.

Carbon monoxide poisoning

Carbon monoxide is a highly poisonous, odorless, colorless, flammable gas. Since carbon monoxide is not an irritant and does not cause irritation of air passages, its effects are insidious, and a dangerous state of intoxication can arise before the victim becomes aware of it. Carbon monoxide competes with oxygen for ferrous sites on hemoglobin and can displace oxygen from hemoglobin. Tissue hypoxia and acidosis follow.

Symptoms of carbon monoxide poisoning consist of headache, dizziness, weakness, nausea, vomiting, loss of muscular control, collapse, unconsciousness, and death. Carbon monoxide affects the cardiac and respiratory systems as a result of hypoxia. Cardiac arrhythmias are common, and myocardial infarction usually occurs.[8]

Coma and death occur when about 60% of the hemoglobin is in the form of carboxyhemoglobin; in cardiac patients lower levels may be fatal. The skin shows a cherry-red color, which can be detected when as little as 25% of the hemoglobin is saturated with carbon monoxide. Retinal hemorrhages have been observed in individuals with subacute carbon monoxide poisoning.

Oxygen containing 5% to 7% carbon dioxide is used in the treatment of carbon monoxide poisoning. Carbon dioxide increases both ventilatory exchange and hastens dissociation of carbon monoxide from hemoglobin. The use of two atmospheres of oxygen will result in faster conversion of carboxyhemoglobin to oxyhemoglobin than will breathing 100% oxygen at sea level. Treatment with two atmospheres for 1 hour is usually sufficient. Hyperbaric oxygen reduces the carboxyhemoglobin level by one-half in 40 minutes. The same effect would not occur for over 4 hours if ordinary air were breathed.

Cyanide inhibits cellular respiration by reacting with cytochrome oxidase. Cytotoxic hypoxia results. Cyanide reacts only with iron in the ferric state. Thus it reacts with cytochrome oxidase to form a cytochrome oxidase-cyanide complex and with methemoglobin to form cyanmethemoglobin.[14] The minimal lethal dose of cyanide is about 0.5 mg/kg; autopsy data indicate that death usually results at about 1.4 mg/kg body weight.

Cyanide poisoning

Symptoms of poisoning appear very quickly after cyanide ingestion. They consist of giddiness, headache, palpitations, unconsciousness, convulsions, and death. Diagnosis is usually made by the characteristic odor of oil of bitter almond associated with asphyxia. Death sometimes can be delayed; therefore prompt treatment can be lifesaving, since effective antidotes are available.[13]

Treatment of cyanide poisoning is specific and must be given rapidly to be effective. The objective is to produce a high concentration of methemoglobin ($HbFe^{+++}$) by administering nitrite.

$$HbFe^{++} + NaNO_2 \rightleftarrows HbFe^{+++}$$

Methemoglobin competes with cytochrome oxidase ($Cyto\text{-}Fe^{+++}$) for the cyanide ion. The concentration gradient favors methemoglobin. Cyanmethemoglobin is formed, and cytochrome oxidase activity is restored. Actual detoxification is achieved by administration of thiosulfate, which reacts with cyanide to form thiocyanate (SCN^-). Thiocyanate is excreted in the urine.

$$Na_2S_2O_3 + CN^- \rightleftarrows SCN^- + Na_2SO_3$$

This reaction is reversible, and symptoms can return following initial treatment. A solution of 0.5 g of $NaNO_2$ in 15 ml of water is injected intravenously over a 3-minute period, followed by 12.5 g of $Na_2S_2O_3$ in 50 ml of water in a slow intravenous injection over a 10-minute period. If symptoms reappear, the aforementioned procedure is repeated with half the doses. Amyl nitrite should be given while one is waiting for the solutions to be made up. It is inhaled for 30 seconds every 2 minutes. Hydroxycobalamin can also prevent toxicity from cyanide by combining with it to form vitamin B_{12}. Hypoxia resulting from methemoglobinemia should be treated by oxygen inhalation.

Various metals may produce vastly different symptoms, but one characteristic they share is their tendency to accumulate to produce chronic as well as acute poisoning.[12]

Heavy metal poisoning

Lead poisoning was a recognized disease even in colonial times, and in 1723 Massachusetts passed a law preventing the distillation of rum and liquors in retorts or pipes containing lead. In 1975 the Centers for Disease Control reported that more than 28,000 young children suffered from increased lead absorption. Ingestion is unsafe if it exceeds 0.5 mg/day; 3 months of daily ingestion at this rate is required to reach dangerous levels. A few small chips of old paint may contain more than 100 mg of lead.

Early symptoms of lead poisoning include anorexia, apathy, irritability, and perhaps sporadic vomiting. After the early symptoms, acute encephalopathy characterized by ataxia, persistent vomiting, lethargy, stupor, convulsions, and coma can occur rapidly. Children are at greater risk than adults of developing encephalopathy. Twenty-five percent of children who survive encephalopathy suffer severe permanant brain damage. Organic lead produces symptoms predominantly of the CNS, whereas inorganic lead poisoning is accompanied by disturbances in hemoglobin synthesis.

The primary screening procedure for lead toxicity is the free erythrocyte protoporphyrin (FEP) test. It is used to detect metabolic evidence of toxicity. Measurements of urinary δ-aminolevulinic acid and coproporphyrin III are also useful in assessing lead poisoning. All values obtained from these tests are elevated in increased lead absorption and lead poisoning. The toxic concentration of lead in whole blood is above 50 μg/100 ml whereas concentrations of FEP above 110 μg/100 ml are consistent with lead intoxication. Urine lead concentrations above 200 μg/L, urine coproporphyrin concentrations larger than 800 μg/L, and urinary δ-aminolevulinic acid concentrations higher than 19 mg/L indicate dangerous amounts of lead absorption.

Chelation therapy is started in patients with encephalopathy using BAL and calcium disodium edetate for 5 to 7 days depending on severity. Patients with seizures should be controlled with diazepam. If the patient is symptomatic but without encephalopathy, BAL may be omitted. Patients should be separated from the source of lead, since calcium disodium edetate increases the absorption of lead from the intestine.

The half-life of lead in blood and soft tissue is about 15 days; in bone it is about 15 years. After absorption, 80% to 90% of blood lead is in the erythrocytes. Over 90% of lead is in bone. Chelating agents remove lead from blood and soft tissue but will not remove lead tightly bound to bone. Only the ionic form of lead is dangerous because only the ionic form binds sulfhydryl groups.

Mercury has disappeared from antisyphilitic therapy. Mercury contaminates the atmosphere as a result of burning fossil fuels and enters the food chain via fish from water contaminated with mercury compounds. Such a mercury cycle was illustrated by the tragic deaths of those eating mercury-contaminated fish from Minamata Bay in Japan. Mercury wastes from insecticide manufacture were poured into the Bay from industrial plants on its shores. Another deplorable event was the death of 459 victims in Iraq who ate bread prepared from wheat treated with a methylmercury fungicide.

The approximate lethal dose of $HgCl_2$ is 1 g, and symptoms of mercury poisoning are first observed at whole blood concentrations of 100 μg/100 ml. Symptoms of *chronic* mercury poisoning most frequently involve the CNS and manifest themselves as tremor and psychotic behavior. Other symptoms include gingivitis, stomatitis, excessive salivation, dermatitis, anorexia, anemia, and weight loss.[4] Acute poisoning produces acute gastroenteritis with severe abdominal pain and bloody diarrhea. Proteinuria may occur. Anuria and uremia are common. Methyl mercury is a subtle, difficult to detect, long-lasting poison that easily passes into the CNS. The half-life of methyl mercury is 65 days; therefore repeated exposure leads to accumulation.

The antidote for mercury poisoning is BAL, which forms a chelate or complex with mercury depending on the molar ratio of antidote to poison. The complex is water soluble at pH 7.5, binds mercury more tightly than does the chelate, and is rapidly exceted.

$$H_2C - S \diagdown \atop HC - S \diagup Hg \qquad CH_2 - S - Hg - S - CH_2$$

Mercury chelate   Mercury complex

Thallium was used to a greater extent than arsenic in antiquity for poisoning. Acute poisoning has been caused by rodenticides and depilatory preparations. Cases of chronic industrial poisoning have involved metal alloys, jewelry, optical lenses, thermometers, electronic equipment, and pigment making. The average acute lethal dose of thallium sulfate is about 1 g. Among the most lethal of metal poisons, thallium produces one of the highest incidences of long-term neurological sequelae.

Manifestations of poisoning involve mainly the gastrointestinal tract and the CNS. They include hematemesis, bloody diarrhea, mental changes, tremors, choreiform movements, ataxia, convulsions, cyanosis, and death.

Diagnosis is usually late if it depends only on the thallium alopecia that occurs about 3 weeks after exposure. Hair loss is complete, including hair in the axillary and pubic regions. Black pigmentation around hair roots can be seen as early as 3 days after exposure. Lunula stripes develop as a result of transient disturbances in nail growth. Marked tachycardia appears 1 to 4 weeks after contact.

Gastric lavage or emesis should be instituted promptly. BAL is used in maximum doses. Activated charcoal is given in a dose of 0.5 g/kg twice daily for 5 days along with 3 to 5 g of potassium chloride daily for 5 to 10 days.

Gold in the form of soluble salts has been given intramuscularly for treatment of rheumatoid arthritis for half a century. Its use is empirical and its mode of action is not understood, but it does induce remissions and occasionally cures the disease. Dermatitis and stomatitis with fever are the most common toxic manifestations of gold. Gold also causes a nephritis with albuminuria, gastritis, colitis, and hepatitis. Other organ systems affected are the hematopoietic system, where gold may produce agranulocytosis or aplastic anemia, and the respiratory system, where it initiates a rare pneumonitis marked by diffuse interstitial inflammation, fibrosis, and lymphocyte and plasma cell infiltration.

BAL is an effective antidote when given early. Penicillamine used as an oral chelating agent has also been reported to be effective.

Arsenic, a protoplasmic poison, is found in many herbicides, fungicides, and pesticides. Fortunately, its emetic effect can be lifesaving.[6] Other effects of its toxicity are erosion of the gastrointestinal tract, intense diarrhea, and anuria, whereas inhalation of arsine gas leads to rapid hemolysis and jaundice with the released hemoglobin blocking renal tubules. Even though it passes the blood-brain barrier slowly and brain levels are among the lowest in the body, it induces encephalopathy.

BAL is the antidote of choice.[7] Organic and inorganic trivalent arsenicals have a high affinity for adjacent thiol groups with formation of stable five-membered rings:

$$
\begin{array}{ccccc}
& \text{O} & \text{HS} - \text{CH}_2 & & \text{S} - \text{CH}_2 \\
& \diagup & | & & \diagup \quad | \\
\text{R-As} & + & \text{HS} - \text{CH} & \rightarrow \quad \text{R-As} & | \qquad + \ \text{H}_2\text{O} \\
& \diagdown & | & & \diagdown \quad | \\
& \text{O} & \text{HO} - \text{CH}_2 & & \text{S} - \text{CH} \\
& & & & | \\
& & & & \text{HO} - \text{CH}_2
\end{array}
$$

Trivalent arsenical   **BAL**   **BAL-arsenic complex**

Iron in the ferrous form has proven fatal to children. Symptoms include vomiting, erosion of the gastrointestinal tract, hemorrhage, cyanosis, coma, respiratory depression, and shock.

Gastric lavage must be instituted immediately. In severe intoxication calcium disodium edetate is administered orally; if an intravenous dose is used shortly thereafter, the size of the dose must be appropriately reduced. Deferoxamine (Desferal), also effective in the treatment of severe acute poisoning, can be given orally or intravenously but may produce systemic toxicity. Acidosis and shock occur in severe iron poisoning and demand prompt treatment.

Aluminum compounds are widely distributed in nature. Despite an oral intake of 10 to 100 mg daily, little aluminum is absorbed. This barrier may be broken, however, in uremic patients maintained on long-term hemodialysis receiving aluminum-containing antacids to decrease phosphate absorption. A few such patients develop a peculiar neurological syndrome characterized by speech abnormalities, dyspraxia, asterixis, myoclonus, personality changes, disordered EEGs, dementia and psychosis, all progressing to death. Lung damage caused by inhalation of fumes containing Al_2O_3 results in shortness of breath, cyanosis, substernal pain, and often spontaneous pneumothorax (Shaver's disease). The use of calcium disodium edetate may be unnecessary, since effects of the metal are self-limited. Its source should be found and eliminated.

Insecticides   Although humans developed pesticides for the deliberate killing of animals, as fate would have it, they in turn kill humans. All of the organochlorine compounds are CNS stimulants, promote convulsions, and are absorbed through the skin as well as the gastrointestinal tract.

The **cyclodiene** insecticides (e.g., dieldrin and chlordane) cause seizures similar to epilepsy along with tremor, nausea, vomiting, and ataxia. Endrin is the most toxic compound in this group.

The **chlorinated ethane derivatives** are related to DDT. Since its ban, DDT has been largely replaced by methoxychlor, which is less toxic and less effective as an insecticide. Sudden death from ventricular fibrillation has been reported following ingestion of these substances due to sensitization of the myocardium to endogenous epinephrine. In DDT poisoning, death may also result from respiratory failure secondary to medullary paralysis. These compounds tend to accumulate in fat and induce the microsomal enzyme system.[3]

The **chlorocyclohexanes** are represented by benzene hexachloride and its γ isomer, lindane, which is used in the treatment of pediculosis. In addition to producing severe convulsions, they also induce pulmonary edema, liver, and kidney damage as well as agranulocytosis. These substances also can sensitize the myocardium, as seen with DDT. If renal and hepatic damage should occur from the organochlorine compounds, their treatments are the same as for these injuries arising from other causes.

Other types of insecticides are thiocyanates, phosphate esters, organophosphate compounds (anticholinesterases), fluorides, and the botanicals such as nicotine, pyrethrins, and rotenoids. For symptoms and treatment of organophosphate poisoning refer to Chapter 11.

Rodenticides

In contrast to the insecticides, the rodenticides are designed to kill animals with essentially the same major biochemical pathways as humans. These include the anticoagulants such as coumarins and indandiones; heavy metals such as the arsenicals, thallium, and copper and lead salts; botanicals such as squill and strychnine; and miscellaneous substances such as fluoracetate, phosphorus and zinc phosphide. The treatment for rodenticide poisoning varies with the poison because the substances are extremely varied in their composition.

Solvents

A significant number of poisonings occcur from solvents used at home and in industrial settings. Since these are fat solvents, they cross the lipid cellular membranes quite easily; the brain is a principal target organ because of its high lipid content. In the brain these solvents exert narcotic or convulsant effects depending on the molecule. In general, solvents that are aliphatic hydrocarbons induce coma. Reflexes are weak or absent. Aromatic solvents are associated with motor unrest, tremors, jactitations and hyperactive reflexes.

Toluene represents in many ways the typical solvent, since it is extensively used in industrial and household products. Essentially replacing benzene because of its reduced toxicity,[5] toluene (glue-sniffing) is a psychotropic and neurotoxic agent. Neurological symptoms are its most frequently cited effects. It can produce sudden death, addictive-like behavior, renal abnormalities, hepatic and hematological illness, and an acute brain syndrome with EEG changes, visual hallucinations, confusion, and seizures. Since it accumulates in bone marrow and has a slow rate of elimination from this tissue, toluene exposure can cause alterations in the hematopoietic system (blood dyscrasias).

The distribution rate of toluene into various tissues is faster after inhalation than after oral administration. Exercise enhances blood levels and total uptake of inhaled toluene, largely by increasing respiration and cardiac output.

Toluene is sometimes contaminated with benzene, a highly toxic substance. Industrial grade toluene contains as much as 25% benzene. Toluene in combination with other solvents is more toxic than would be predicted on the basis of the additive toxic action of each component by itself.

REFERENCES

1. Arena, J.M.: Poisoning, Emerg. Med. 8:171, April 1976.
2. Arena, J.M.: Poisoning: toxicology, symtoms, treatments, Springfield, Ill., 1978, Charles C Thomas, Publisher.
3. Bayer, M.J., and Rumack, B.H.: Poisoning and overdose, Rockville, Md., 1983, Aspen Systems Corp.
4. Burston, G.R.: Self-poisoning, London, 1970, Lloyd-Luke, Ltd.
5. Doull, J., Klaassen, C.D., and Amdur, M.O.: Toxicology: the basic science of poisons, ed. 2, New York, 1980, MacMillan Publishing Co., Inc.
6. Dreisbach, R.H.: Handbook of poisoning, ed. 10, Los Altos, Calif., 1980, Lange Medical Publications.
7. Loomis, T.A.: Essentials of toxicology, ed. 3, Philadelphia, 1978, Lea & Febiger.
8. Matthew, H., and Lawson, A.A.H.: Treatment of common acute poisoning, ed. 2, Edinburgh, 1970, E. & S. Livingstone.
9. Moeschlin, S.: Poisoning: diagnosis and treatment, New York, 1965, Grune & Stratton, Inc.
10. Neuvonen, P.J.: Clinical pharmacokinetics of oral activated charcoal in acute intoxications, Clin. Pharmacokinet. 7:465, 1982.
11. Okonek, S.: Hemoperfusion in toxicology: basic considerations of its effectiveness, Clin. Toxicol. 18:1185, 1981.
12. Polson, C.J., and Tattersall, R.N.: Clinical toxicology, ed. 2, Philadelphia, 1969, J.B. Lippincott Co.
13. Thienes, C.L., and Haley, T.J.: Clinical toxicology, ed. 5, Philadelphia, 1972, Lea & Febiger.
14. Vennesland, B., Castric, P.A., Conn, E.E., Solomonson, L.P., Violini, M., and Westley, J.: Cyanide metabolism, Fed. Proc. 41:2639, 1982.

section twelve

Drug interactions

Chapter 63

Drug interactions

When several drugs are administered concurrently, they may influence each other favorably or unfavorably. The adverse drug interactions may be of great clinical importance when the margin of safety of the drugs is small. Most adverse drug interactions listed in extensive tables are not significant and are often based on animal experiments or anecdotal reports.

The clinically significant drug interactions can be minimized by avoiding combinations of drugs known to be incompatible according to the current pharmacological literature and tables of drug interactions such as the one presented in this chapter. It should be possible to develop systems in hospital pharmacies that would prevent the dispensing of incompatible drugs. Ultimately, however, it is the physician's familiarity with the current clinical literature and understanding of the mechanisms underlying drug interactions that are more likely to prevent their occurrence.

Adverse drug reactions based on drug interactions are not always iatrogenic. Self-medication with over-the-counter drugs may be a contributing factor. In addition, environmental contaminants such as the chlorinated insecticides (DDT) may stimulate drug metabolism by hepatic microsomal enzymes and could conceivably contribute to unusual reactions to drugs.

Adverse drug interactions may be divided into *pharmacokinetic* and *pharmacodynamic* interactions. The pharmacokinetic interactions may be at the level of (1) absorption, (2) distribution, (3) metabolism, or (4) excretion. The pharmacodynamic interactions are usually at the receptor site.

MECHANISMS UNDERLYING ADVERSE EFFECTS OF DRUG INTERACTIONS

Antacids that contain calcium, magnesium, or aluminum interfere with the absorption of tetracycline, which forms a chelate with the metals. Antacids containing aluminum interfere with the absorption of phosphate. Carbonates and phytates (cereals) prevent the absorption of iron. Cholestyramine may interfere with the absorption of phenylbutazone, warfarin, and thyroxine.

Intestinal absorption

Antacids may influence drug absorption also by changing the lipid-soluble non-ionized moiety of weak acids and bases in the gastrointestinal tract. It should be recalled (p. 19) that the lipid-soluble, nonionized fraction is much better absorbed. Because of this, antacids would be expected to diminish the absorption of weak acids such as phenylbutazone, nitrofurantoin, sulfonamides, and some barbiturates and oral anticoagulants.

Other gastrointestinal drug interactions may be of clinical significance. Antibiotics that alter the bacterial flora in the intestine may decrease the formation of vitamin K and thus increase the anticoagulant action of the coumarins. Folate deficiency may result from the use of drugs that inhibit the intestinal conjugase that breaks down the polyglutamate portion of the naturally occurring folic acid. By this mechanism, megaloblastic anemia may result in some patients after the use of phenytoin or triamterene. Mineral oil may interfere with the absorption of vitamin D.

Direct chemical interactions may occur not only in the gastrointestinal tract but also when drugs are mixed for intravenous infusions. Unstable drugs, such as methicillin or levarterenol, should not be mixed with other drugs without consideration of possible direct drug interactions. Carbenicillin inactivates gentamicin when mixed for intravenous infusion.

Distribution The most important adverse drug interactions caused by displacement from plasma proteins occur with the coumarin anticoagulants. Although in general the increase in the concentration of the free drug is expected to increase its elimination, in many instances the displacer inhibits drug metabolism as well. Phenylbutazone displaces warfarin from its binding sites and also inhibits its metabolism and may cause bleeding.

Competition for plasma protein binding Many drugs are bound to plasma proteins to varying degrees, and the bound fraction fails to exert pharmacological effects. For example, two antibiotics having the same potency in a protein-free culture medium will have vastly different clinical effectiveness if their affinities for plasma proteins differ greatly.

Tolbutamide can be displaced from its plasma binding by dicumarol, resulting in severe hypoglycemia. Chloral hydrate increases the anticoagulant action of warfarin because its metabolite, trichloracetic acid, competes with the anticoagulant for plasma protein binding.

Metabolism or biotransformation The inhibition of the metabolism of one drug by another is a well-established mechanism of enhanced drug effect. By their enzyme-inhibiting action, the anticholinesterases enhance the actions of acetylcholine, succinylcholine, and some other choline esters. Allopurinol inhibits xanthine oxidase and thus increases the plasma levels of mercaptopurine and azathioprine. The monoamine oxidase (MAO) inhibitors have caused severe reactions by preventing the destruction of tyramine in the body.

Many drugs can accelerate their metabolism and also that of other drugs by induction of hepatic microsomal enzymes (p. 36). Phenobarbital accelerates the metabolism of coumarin anticoagulants, phenytoin, griseofulvin, cortisol, estrogens, androgens, and progesterone. In addition to the barbiturates, glutethimide, phenytoin, and the chlorinated hydrocarbon insecticides, such as DDT, are enhancers of drug metabolism (p. 36).

Enzyme induction by phenobarbital and other drugs leads to a decreased effectiveness of drugs and may also result in catastrophes when the inducer is discontinued without changing the dose of the second drug. For example, if phenobarbital is suddenly discontinued without lowering the dosage of a coumarin anticoagulant, severe hemorrhagic episodes may develop (see Fig. 4-2).

Phenobarbital combined with phenytoin greatly increases the clearance of quinidine, probably as a consequence of enzyme induction. Rifampin is a potent inducer also.

In some instances a drug may alter hepatic blood flow and inhibit drug metabolism by that mechanism. The β-adrenergic blocking agents, such as propranolol and metoprolol, raise lidocaine concentrations by this mechanism. Cimetidine has important effects also and may decrease clearance of theophylline very significantly.

An important drug interaction involves digoxin and quinidine. Quinidine decreases the distal tubular secretion of digoxin, thus causing often dangerous concentrations of digoxin in the plasma. In addition, quinidine decreases the volume of distribution of digoxin, probably by decreasing the binding of digoxin in muscle.

Renal excretion

There are several interesting examples of drug interactions resulting from an influence on renal tubular resorption. The best example, of course, is the inhibition of penicillin excretion by probenecid. Interference in the uricosuric action of probenecid by small doses of salicylates and the promotion of phenobarbital clearance after sodium bicarbonate administration are other examples of one drug influencing the renal excretion of another.

Acidification of the urine after the oral administration of ammonium chloride or alkalinization following sodium bicabonate may have a demonstrable effect on the renal clearance of several drugs, but the quantitative importance of such knowledge in therapeutics is not great except in phenobarbital poisoning.

Pharmacodynamic interactions

The numerous pharmacodynamic interactions usually take place at the receptor level. The innumerable synergisms and antagonisms discussed throughout the text are examples of pharmacodynamic interactions. These interactions may be at the same receptor or at different receptors.

INTERACTIONS IN VARIOUS DRUG CATEGORIES

Most drug interactions present themselves in therapeutics as either an enhanced or diminished drug effect. The enhanced drug effects may manifest themselves as idiosyncratic responses that may occasionally have catastrophic consequences (Table 63-1).

Diminished responses resulting from drug interactions are generally not very dramatic. It can happen, however, that manipulations of dosage necessitated by drug

TABLE 63-1   Clinically observed adverse effects based on drug
interactions

Major symptoms	Drugs involved
Hypertensive crisis	MAO inhibitors + Tyramine (cheese) MAO inhibitors + Methamphetamine
Hemorrhagic episodes	Warfarin + Phenylbutazone Warfarin + Phenyramidol
Respiratory paralysis	Neomycin + Succinylcholine Neomycin + Ether
Hypoglycemic reaction	Tolbutamide + Phenylbutazone Tolbutamide + Sulfisoxazole
Cardiac arrhythmias	Digitalis + Chlorothiazide Digitalis + Reserpine

interactions may have serious consequences when one of the drugs is discontinued without simultaneous adjustment of the dosage of the other drug. For example, chloral hydrate stimulates the metabolism of several coumarin anticoagulants. If the dosage of the coumarin is increased over a period of several days and then chloral hydrate is suddenly discontinued, the anticoagulant effect may become excessive and bleeding will follow. But the interactions of chloral hydrate with the oral anticoagulants may be more complex than previously thought. The metabolic product of chloral hydrate, trichloracetic acid, interferes with the binding of warfarin to plasma proteins. Increased anticoagulation may result, which is the opposite of the interaction resulting from increased metabolism of dicumarol just described.

The clinically significant drug interactions are listed in Table 63-2 along with their probable mechanisms. The table is only a quick survey; for details the original references should be consulted.

Significance of adverse drug reactions   Some drug interactions, such as those in Table 63-1, may be life-threatening, whereas others are unimportant and require only a simple adjustment in the dosage. An important determinant of the seriousness of an interaction is the therapeutic margin of the drugs involved. With anticoagulants, oral hypoglycemic drugs, digitalis, and antiarrhythmic drugs, the margin of safety is not great, and relatively small changes in plasma concentration resulting from drug interactions could have catastrophic effects. On the other hand, drugs with great margins of safety do not cause serious problems as a consequence of drug interactions. This principle should be kept in mind when examining large tables of drug interactions.

TABLE 63-2	Clinically significant drug interactions		
First drug	Second drug(s)	Possible result	Mechanism*
β-Adrenergic blocking drugs	Hypoglycemic drugs	Increased hypoglycemia, masking of signs of hypoglycemia	7
Analgesics			
Aspirin	Anticoagulant	Enhanced anticoagulation	2
	Sulfonylureas	Enhanced hypoglycemia	2
	p-Aminosalicylate	PAS toxicity	2
	Probenecid	Decreased uricosuria	8
Phenylbutazone	Anticoagulant	Enhanced anticoagulation	2
	Sulfonylurea	Enhanced hypoglycemia	2,3
	Estrogen, androgen	Decreased hormonal effects	3
Phenyramidol	Anticoagulant	Enhanced anticoagulation	3
Morphine	Phenothiazine	Enhanced analgesia	7
Meperidine	Atropine	Enhanced atropine effect	7
Propoxyphene	Amphetamine	Enhanced amphetamine effect	7
Anticoagulants			
Coumarin drugs	Aspirin, acetaminophen, clofibrate, phenylbutazone, indomethacin, methyldopa, methylphenidate, quinidine	Enhanced anticoagulation	2
	Barbiturates, glutethimide, griseofulvin, meprobamate	Decreased anticoagulant effect	3
	Chloral hydrate	Increased or decreased anticoagulant effect	2,3
	Vitamin K	Decreased anticoagulant effect	7
Heparin	Polymyxin	Incompatibility in intravenous solution	10
Antimicrobials			
Aminoglycosides	d-Tubocurarine	Enhanced tubocurarine effect	7
Cephalothin	Barbiturates, erythromycin, tetracycline	Incompatibility in intravenous solution	10
Chloramphenicol	Barbiturates, phenytoin	Enhanced sedation	3
	Anticoagulants	Enhanced anticoagulation	3
	Penicillin	Antibiotic antagonism (some infections)	7
	Diphtheria or tetanus toxoid	Decreased immune response	11
Furazolidone	Amphetamine, methyldopa, sympathomimetics, tyramine	Hypertension, excitement	3
Griseofulvin	Phenobarbital	Decreased phenobarbital effect	3
Penicillin G	Sulfonamides, tetracycline	Antibiotic antagonism (some infections)	7
Polymyxin B	d-Tubocurarine, succinylcholine	Muscle paralysis	7
Sulfonamides	Aspirin, phenylbutazone	Sulfonamide toxicity	2
	Anticoagulants	Enhanced anticoagulation	2
	Sulfonylureas	Enhanced hypoglycemia	2
			1
Tetracycline	Antacids	Decreased absorption	1
Antihistamines			
Antihistaminic drugs	Alcohol, reserpine, phenothiazines	Enhanced sedation	7
	Atropine	Enhanced atropine effects	7

*Mechanisms: 1, interference with gastrointestinal absorption; 2, plasma protein binding competition; 3, metabolism or biotransformation; 4, enzyme induction; 5, adrenergic neuronal uptake; 6, depletion of catecholamines at adrenergic neuron; 7, action at receptor site or related to end-organ response; 8, renal excretion; 9, alteration of electrolyte balance; 10, direct combination; 11, inhibition of protein synthesis. *Continued.*

TABLE 63-2   Clinically significant drug interactions—cont'd

First drug	Second drug(s)	Possible result	Mechanism
Anticonvulsants			
Phenytoin	Dicumarol, chloramphenicol, methylphenidate, phenyramidol	Enhanced phenytoin effect	3
	Phenobarbital	Decreased phenytoin effect	3
Antidepressants			
MAO inhibitors	Tyramine, amphetamine, levodopa, methyldopa, sympathomimetics	Hypertension, excitement	3
Tricyclic drugs	Guanethidine	Decreased guanethidine effect	5
	MAO inhibitor	Enhanced MAO inhibitor toxicity	7
	Phenothiazines, antianxiety drugs	Additive effect	7
Antihypertensives			
Guanethidine	Sympathomimetics, amphetamine	Hypertensive crisis	5
	Levarterenol	Enhanced levarterenol effect	5
	Tricyclic antidepressants	Decreased guanethidine effect	5
Methyldopa	Sympathomimetics	Decreased methyldopa effect	7
Pargyline (same as MAO inhibitors)	MAO inhibitors	Decreased methyldopa effect	3
Reserpine	Sympathomimetics, tricyclic drugs	Decreased reserpine effect	7
	Indirect sympathomimetics, metaraminol	Decreased metaraminol effect	6
	Anesthetic	Hypotension	
	Levarterenol	Enhanced levarterenol effect	6
			7
Antineoplastic agents			
Mercaptopurine	Allopurinol	Enhanced mercaptopurine effect	3
Methotrexate	Aspirin, sulfonamides	Enhanced methotrexate toxicity	2
Digitalis			
Digitalis preparations	Thiazides, calcium	Digitalis toxicity	9
	Reserpine	Arrhythmias	7
	Phenobarbital	Decreased digitalis effect	4
Diuretics			
Thiazides	Digitalis	Digitalis toxicity	9
	Antihypertensive drugs	Enhanced antihypertensive effect	7
	Sulfonylureas	Antagonism of hypoglycemia	7
	Curare drugs	Enhanced curare effects	9
Mercurials	Ammonium chloride	Enhanced diuresis	9
	Alkalinizing agents	Decreased diuresis	9
Ethacrynic acid	Aminoglycosides	Ototoxicity	7
Antianxiety and antipsychotic drugs			
Benzodiazepines	Alcohol, hypnotics, phenothiazines, tricyclic antidepressants	Enhanced sedation	7
Phenothiazines	Alcohol, hypnotics, narcotics, antihistamines, tricyclic antidepressants	Enhanced sedation	7
	Antihypertensives	Enhanced antihypertensive effect	7
	Convulsants	Lowered convulsive threshold	7

TABLE 63-2   Clinically significant drug interactions—cont'd

First drug	Second drug(s)	Possible result	Mechanism
Hormones			
Insulin	Oral hypoglycemics, propranolol, MAO inhibitors	Enhanced hypoglycemic effect	7
Corticosteroids	Barbiturates, phenytoin, antihistamines	Decreased corticosteroid effect	4
Estrogens, progestogens	Androgens	Antagonism of androgen anticancer effect	7
	Clofibrate	Decreased hypocholesterolemic effect	3
Hypnotics			
Phenobarbital	Anticoagulants, phenytoin, griseofulvin, hypnotics, corticosteroids	Decreased drug effects	4
	Alcohol, phenothiazines, antianxiety drugs	Enhanced sedation	7
Chloral hydrate	Alcohol	Enhanced sedation	7
	Anticoagulant	Increased or decreased anticoagulant effect	2,3
Uricosuric agents			
Probenecid	Aspirin, ethacrynic acid	Decreased uricosuria	7
	Penicillin	Enhanced penicillin levels	7

REFERENCES

1. Brater, D.C., and Morelli, H.F.: Cardiovascular drug interactions, Annu. Rev. Pharmacol. Toxicol. **17:**293, 1977.

2. Hansten, P.D.: Drug interactions, Philadelphia, 1979, Lea & Febiger.

section thirteen

Prescription writing and drug compendia

Chapter 64

Prescription writing and drug compendia

A prescription is a written order given by a physician to a pharmacist. In addition to the name of the patient and that of the physician, the prescription should contain the name or names of the drugs ordered and their quantities, instructions to the pharmacist, and directions to the patient.

The art of prescription writing has been declining in modern medicine as a result of several developments. Most of the preparations are compounded today by pharmaceutical companies, and the pharmacist's role in most cases consists only of dispensing. Also, the practice of writing long, complicated prescriptions containing many active ingredients, adjuvants, correctives, and various vehicles has been abandoned in favor of using single pure compounds. Even when combinations of several active ingredients are desirable, the pharmaceutical companies often have available several forms of suitable combinations. It may be said that this practice deprives the physician of the opportunity to adjust the various components of a mixture to the individual requirements of the patient. The custom of prescribing trademarked mixtures also has other disadvantages. The physician may be so accustomed to prescribing a mixture of drugs by a trade name that he may not be quite certain about the individual components of it, some of which may be unnecessary or undesirable in a given case.

Drugs may be prescribed by their official names, which are listed in the *United States Pharmacopeia* (USP) or *National Formulary* (NF); by their nonofficial generic names, or *United States Adopted Name* (USAN); or by a manufacturer's trade name. The designation USAN has been recently coined for generic or nonproprietary names adopted by the American Medical Association–United States Pharmacopeia Nomenclature Committee in cooperation with the respective manufacturers. Adoption of USAN names does not imply endorsement of the product by the American Medical Association Council on Drugs or by the United States Pharmacopeia.

There is considerable advantage to prescribing drugs by their official or generic names. This often allows the pharmacist to dispense a more economical product than a trademarked preparation of one company. It would also eliminate the expense of each pharmacy's maintaining a multiplicity of very similar preparations, a saving that could ultimately benefit the patient.

On the other hand, the physician may have reasons for prescribing one manufacturer's product. This is often the only way to be certain that the preparation given to the patient will be exactly what is intended, not only in its active ingredients but even to the point of its appearance and taste. A child who is accustomed to the flavor of a certain vitamin mixture may refuse to swallow a similar product if its taste is different. Also, there are some childlike adults who pay much attention to the physical properties and taste of products to which they are accustomed.

Although it is not generally appreciated by physicians, absorption of a drug from the gastrointestinal tract may vary greatly, depending on the manufacturing process used in the preparation of a tablet or capsule. For example, chloramphenicol capsules made by various manufacturers may produce quite different blood levels. The whole problem of generic equivalence needs to be reexamined.

On the whole, the use of generic names is more common in teaching hospitals than in general practice. There is much discussion at present concerning the relative advantages of prescribing by generic names rather than by trade names. The outcome of this debate should be of great interest in medical economics.

Parts of prescription

Traditionally a prescription is written in a certain order and consists of four basic parts:

1. *Superscription*—This is simply ℞, the abbreviation for *recipe*, the imperative of *recipere*, meaning "take thou."

2. *Inscription*—This represents the ingredients and their amounts. If a prescription contains several ingredients in a mixture, it is customary to write them in the following order: (1) basis or principal ingredient, (2) adjuvant, which may contribute to the action of the basis, and (3) corrective, which may eliminate some undesirable property of the active drug or the vehicle, which is the substance used for dilution.

3. *Subscription*—This contains directions for dispensing. Often it consists only of *M*., the abbreviation for *misce*, meaning "mix."

4. *Signature*—This is often abbreviated as *Sig*. and contains the directions to the patient, such as "Take one teaspoonful three times a day before meals." The signature should indicate whether the medicine is intended for external application and whether it has some special poisonous properties. Wherever possible, instructions of a general nature, such as "take as directed," should be avoided since the patient may misunderstand verbal directions given by the physician.

In addition to the basic parts of a prescription, it should have the patient's name and the physician's signature, followed by the abbreviation *M.D*.

Modern trends in prescription writing

The parts of the prescription described in the previous paragraphs represent a tradition that is undergoing considerable change. Latin, even in the form of abbreviations, is not really necessary. Its main purpose in the past was to conceal from the patient the nature (and often worthlessness) of a drug. At the present time, prescriptions are written in English. Even such abbreviations as *M.* or *Sig.* may be avoided. It is also advisable to avoid as much as possible the use of the decimal point and state the number of milligrams in a dose instead of using the decimal fraction of a gram.

There are other interesting trends in prescription writing.[2] Much confusion results from the fact that the name of a drug is not spelled out on the label, and therefore the patient knows only that he is taking some sort of pills having certain physical characteristics. The busy physician wastes much time trying to identify medications given to his patients by other physicians. It may not be an exaggeration to say that drug treatment in some instances may be truly double-blind.

To avoid this unsatisfactory development, some physicians ask the pharmacist to name the drug on the label, indicating their wish by checking an appropriate box on the prescription form. They also indicate in another box the number of allowable refills.

Until recently, prescriptions for narcotic drugs were regulated by the Harrison Anti-Narcotic Act and the drug abuse control amendments of 1965. These regulations have been replaced by the Federal Controlled Substances Act of 1970 and the regulations issued by the Director of the Federal Bureau of Narcotics and Dangerous Drugs. The new regulations became effective May 1, 1971. The drugs controlled by the Act are placed in five categories, or schedules:

Prescriptions and the Federal Controlled Substances Act

Schedule I. Hallucinogenic substances and some opiates for which there is no current accepted medical use.

Schedule II. Drugs of high abuse potential, such as most narcotics of the former Class A group, amphetamines, some closely related compounds, and some barbiturates.

Schedule III. Depressants such as some barbiturates, nalorphine, straight paregoric, certain amphetamine combination drugs, and narcotics of former class B group.

Schedule IV. Chloral hydrate, meprobamate, paraldehyde, and some long-acting barbiturates. (Generally, the abuse potential for drugs in this schedule is lower than for the representatives of the previous schedules.)

Schedule V. Paregoric combination preparations and other drugs and compounds for which the abuse potential is lower than for members of schedule IV.

All prescriptions for controlled drugs (schedules II to V) must contain the full name and address of the patient, full name, address, and DEA (Drug Enforcement Administration) number of the prescribing doctor, signature of the prescribing doctor, and date. Prescriptions for schedule II drugs are not refillable. Schedules III and IV drugs may be refilled up to five times within 6 months of initial issuance if so authorized by the prescribing physician. Prescriptions for schedule V drugs may be refilled as authorized by the prescribing physician.

Two examples of prescriptions are shown below.

John Doe, M.D.
555 Medical Arts Building
City
Telephone: 361-4282

Name   David Smith   Date   May 9, 1981

Address   201 Hall Street   Age   37

℞

     Tetracycline USP, 250 mg
     Dispense twenty capsules
     Label: Take one capsule four times a day

Reg. No. _____   John Doe, M.D.

John Doe, M.D.
555 Medical Arts Building
City
Telephone: 361-4282

Name   David Smith   Date   May 9, 1981

Address   201 Hall Street   Age   37

℞

                                       g or ml
     Ammonium chloride   12
     Terpin hydrate elixir, to make   120
     M.
     Label: Take one teaspoonful in half glass
              of water for cough every 4 hours if
              necessary

Reg. No. _____   John Doe, M.D.

DRUG COMPENDIA   Authoritative information on drugs can be found in the *United States Pharmacopeia* and the *National Formulary* as well as in many textbooks of pharmacology. The *United States Pharmacopeia* and the *National Formulary* are referred to as official publications. The official position of these compendia is based on the Federal Food, Drug and Cosmetic Act of 1938, which recognizes them as "official compendia."

The *United States Pharmacopeia* was first published in 1820. It and the *National Formulary* became official in 1906, when they were so designated by the first Food and Drug Act. The *United States Pharmacopeia* is revised by physicians, pharmacists, and medical scientists who are elected by delegates to the United States Pharmacopeial Convention. The delegates originate from schools of medicine and pharmacy, from medical and pharmaceutical societies, and from some departments of the government.

The *United States Pharmacopeia* is published every 5 years. For a drug to be included there must be good evidence for its therapeutic merit or its pharmaceutical necessity.

The *National Formulary* is compiled by a board of the American Pharmaceutical Association. It is published every 5 years, and only drugs of demonstrated therapeutic value are included.

AMA Drug Evaluations 1983 is a valuable source of information on most drugs that are available in the United States. It is particularly useful in checking on currently accepted therapeutic practices and available preparations.

If physicians could limit their use of drugs to those that are listed in the *United States Pharmacopeia* or those that have been recommended by *AMA Drug Evaluations 1983*, they would be protected against unfounded claims or the power of advertising. When a new drug represents a great therapeutic advance, physicians may be unable to wait for such authoritative reviews. They must often rely on the written or verbal statements of recognized experts in the field. In any case, they should not depend solely on the advertising literature or drug circulars and package inserts.

1. Cutting, W.: A note on names, Clin. Pharmacol. Ther. **5**:569, 1963.
2. Friend, D.G.: Principles and practices of prescription writing, Clin. Pharmacol. Ther. **6**:411, 1965.
3. Ingelfinger, F.J., and Elia, J.J.: Prescription and proscription, N. Engl. J. Med. **285**:1199, 1971.

REFERENCES

appendixes

Appendix A

Drug blood concentrations

The concentration of drugs in the blood is of interest in clinical medicine and medicolegal situations. The tabular presentation of drug blood concentrations on pp. 757 to 759 is intended as a source of information and as a guide to the available literature. It should be recognized that the figures given are often based on a few cases and are subject to change as more information accumulates. Furthermore, the significance of blood concentrations depends on numerous factors, and the table should be consulted with full recognition of the role of modifying influences.

*IMPORTANCE OF
DRUG SERUM
CONCENTRATIONS*

The determination of drug serum concentrations is not important when the pharmacological effects of the drug can be easily monitored. For example, in the use of coumarin anticoagulants or antihypertensive drugs, the effects of the drugs provide a good indication for adequacy of serum levels and dosage. On the other hand, there are drugs that are used prophylactically, such as phenytoin, quinidine, and others, which provide therapeutic problems in the absence of knowledge of their serum concentrations. The determination of phenytoin in the serum is useful also for revealing noncompliance with the physician's instructions.

The relationship between serum concentration and its pharmacological effect is complicated by numerous factors such as (1) tolerance, (2) drug interactions, (3) the underlying disease, (4) protein binding, and (5) active metabolites.

The role of tolerance, drug interactions, and underlying disease in modifying the relationship between serum concentration and drug effect is easily understood. The importance of protein binding and the role of active metabolites are not always appreciated.

The role of protein binding is illustrated by the following problem.

Much of this information has been compiled and kindly provided by Dr. Charles L. Winek, Chief Toxicologist, County of Allegheny, and Professor of Toxicology, Duquesne University.

PROBLEM A. The therapeutic concentration of phenytoin is 20 mg/L. It is about 95% bound to serum albumin. In the case of uremia, hypoalbuminemia, or the presence of other drugs that displace phenytoin from its binding site, the bound fraction could go down to 90%. What will be the effect on the free drug fraction and the potential toxicity of phenytoin? If the total phenytoin concentration in the serum is reported to be 20 mg/L, the free fraction will be 2 mg, which is twice as much as it would be with normal albumin binding and could be toxic.[5]

The complicating effect of active metabolites is demonstrated in the case of propranolol. This drug is metabolized to 4-hydroxy-propranolol, which is an active β blocker. If one knows the serum concentration of propranolol, it still may not be possible to state the intensity of β blockade. Other complicating factors may result from the application of radioimmunoassays. In a few instances the biological activity— usually of an endogenous compound—and the concentration as measured by radioimmunoassay do not correlate well.

DEFINITION OF BLOOD CONCENTRATIONS

therapeutic blood concentration The concentration of drug in blood, serum, or plasma after therapeutically effective dosage in humans. The values in the table are generally those reported with oral administration of the drug.

toxic blood concentration The concentration of drug in blood, serum, or plasma associated with serious toxic symptoms in humans.

lethal blood concentration The concentration of drug in blood, serum, or plasma that has been reported to cause death or is so far above therapeutic or toxic concentrations that it might cause death in humans.

•   •   •

The following table gives the therapeutic, toxic, and lethal blood concentrations of a large number of drugs.

Drug and chemical blood concentrations*

Compound	Therapeutic or "normal" concentration	Toxic concentration	Lethal concentration
Acetaminophen (Tylenol)	10-20 mg/L	400 mg/L	1500 mg/L
Acetazolamide (Diamox)	10-15 mg/L	—	—
Acetohexamide (Dymelor)	21-56 mg/L		—
Acetone		200-300 mg/L	550 mg/L
Aluminum	0.13 mg/L	—	
Ammonia	500-1700 mg/L		—
Aminophylline (Theophylline)	10-20 mg/L		—
Amitriptyline (Elavil)	50-200 μg/L	400 μg/L	10-20 mg/L
Amphetamine	20-30 μg/L	—	2 mg/L
Arsenic	0.0-20 μg/L	1.0 mg/L	15 mg/L
Barbiturates			
Short-acting	1 mg/L	7 mg/L	10 mg/L
Intermediate-acting	1-5 mg/L	10-30 mg/L	30 mg/L
Phenobarbital	~10 mg/L	40-60 mg/L	80-150 mg/L
Barbital	~10 mg/L	60-80 mg/L	100 mg/L
Benzene	—	Any measurable	0.94 mg/L
Beryllium	Tissue levels generally used (lung and lymph)		
Boron (boric acid)	0.8 mg/L	40 mg/L	50 mg/L
Bromide	50 mg/L	0.5-1.5 g/L	2 g/L
Brompheniramine (Dimetane)	8-15 μg/L	—	—
Cadmium	0.1-0.2 μg/L	50 μg/L	—
Caffeine	—	—	>100 mg/L
Carbamazepine (Tegretol)	2 mg/L	8-10 mg/L	—
Carbon monoxide	1% saturation of Hb	15-35% saturation of Hb	50% saturation of Hb
Carbon tetrachloride	—	20-50 mg/L	—
Carisoprodol (Rela, Soma)	10-40 mg/L	—	—
Chloral hydrate (Noctec)	10 mg/L	100 mg/L	250 mg/L
Chloroform	—	70-250 mg/L	390 mg/L
Chlordiazepoxide (Librium)	1.0-3.0 mg/L	5.5 mg/L	20 mg/L
Chlorpheniramine	—	20-30 mg/L	—
Chlorpromazine (Thorazine)	0.5 mg/L	1-2 mg/L	3-12 mg/L
Chlorpropamide (Diabinese)	30-140 mg/L	—	—
Chlorprothixine (Taractan)	0.04-0.3 mg/L	—	—
Codeine	25 μg/L		—
Copper	1-1.5 mg/L	5.4 mg/L	
Cyanide	0.15 mg/L	—	>5 mg/L
DDT	13 μg/L	—	—
Desipramine (Norpramin)	0.59-1.4 mg/L	—	10-20 mg/L
Dextropropoxyphene (Darvon)	50-200 μg/L	5-10 mg/L	57 mg/L†
Diazepam (Valium)	0.5-2.5 mg/L	5-20 mg/L	>50 mg/L

From Winek, C.L.: Tabulation of therapeutic, toxic and lethal concentrations of drugs and chemicals in blood, Clin. Chem. **22:**832, 1976.
*Some common brand names that may be more familiar than the generic name, alternative forms (e.g., aminophylline/theophylline), and the like are given parenthetically.
†McBay reports much lower values.

Continued.

Drug and chemical blood concentrations—cont'd

Compound	Therapeutic or "normal" concentration	Toxic concentration	Lethal concentration
Dieldren	1.5 μg/L	—	—
Digitoxin	20-35 μg/L	—	320 μg/L
Digoxin	0.6-1.3 μg/L	2-9 μg/L	—
Dinitro-o-cresol	—	30-40 μg/L	75 mg/L
Diphenhydramine (Benadryl)	5 mg/L	10 mg/L	—
Divinyl oxide	—	—	700 mg/L
Doxepin (Sinequan)	—	—	>10 mg/L
Ethanol	—	1.5 g/L	>3.5 g/L
Ethchlorvynol (Placidyl)	5 mg/L	20 mg/L	150 mg/L
Ethinamate (Valmid)	5-10 mg/L	—	—
Ethosuximide (Zarontin)	25-75 mg/L	—	—
Ethyl chloride	—	—	400 mg/L
Ethyl ether	0.9-1.0 g/L	—	1.4-1.89 g/L
Ethylene glycol	—	1.5 g/L	2-4 g/L
Fluoride	0.5 mg/L	—	2 mg/L
Glutethimide (Doriden)	0.2 mg/L	10-80 mg/L	30-100 mg/L
Gold (sodium aurothiomalate)	3-6 mg/L	—	—
Halothane (Fluothane)	—	—	200 mg/L
Hydrogen sulfide	—	—	0.92 mg/L
Hydromorphone (Dilaudid)	—	—	0.1-0.3 mg/L
Imipramine (Tofranil)	0.05-0.16 mg/L	0.7 mg/L	2 mg/L
Iron	500 mg/L (erythrocytes)	6 mg/L (serum)	—
Isopropanol	—	3.4 g/L	—
Lead	0.05-1.3 mg/L	1.3 mg/L	—
Lidocaine	2 mg/L	6 mg/L	—
Lithium	4.2-8.3 mg/L	13.9 mg/L	13.9-34.7 mg/L
LSD (lysergic acid diethylamide)	—	1-4 μg/L	—
Magnesium	0.8-1.3 mmol/L	—	0.5 mmol/L
Manganese	0.15 mg/L	4.6 mg/L	—
Meperidine (Demerol)	600-650 μg/L	5 mg/L	30 mg/L
Meprobamate	10 mg/L	100 mg/L	200 mg/L
Mercury	60-120 μg/L	—	—
Methadone	480-860 μg/L	2 mg/L	>4 mg/L
Methamphetamine	—	5 mg/L	40 mg/L
Methanol	—	200 mg/L	>890 mg/L
Methapyrilene	2 μg/L	30-50 mg/L	>50 mg/L
Methaqualone (Quaalude)	5 mg/L	10-30 mg/L	>30 mg/L
Methsuximide (Celontin)	2.5-7.5 mg/L	—	—
Methylene chloride	—	—	>280 mg/L
Methylenedioxyamphetamine (MDA)	—	—	4-10 mg/L
Methyprylon (Noludar)	10 mg/L	30-60 mg/L	100 mg/L
Morphine	0.1 mg/L	—	0.05-4 mg/L
Nickel	0.41 mg/L	—	—

	Drug and chemical blood concentrations—cont'd		
Compound	Therapeutic or "normal" concentration	Toxic concentration	Lethal concentration
Nicotine	—	10 mg/L	5-52 mg/L
Nitrofurantoin (Furadantin)	1.8 mg/L	—	—
Nortriptyline (Aventyl)	1.2-1.6 μg/L	5 mg/L	13 mg/L
Orphenadrine	—	2 mg/L	4-8 mg/L
Oxalate	2 mg/L	—	10 mg/L
Papaverine	1 mg/L	—	—
Paraldehyde	50 mg/L	200-400 mg/L	500 mg/L
Paramethoxyamphetamine (PMA)	—	—	2-4 mg/L
Pentazocine (Talwin)	0.14-0.16 mg/L	2-5 mg/L	10-20 mg/L
Perphenazine (Trilafon)	—	1 mg/L	—
Phencyclidine	—	>0.5 mg/L	1.0 mg/L
Phenmetrazine	—	—	4 mg/L
Phensuximide (Milontin)	10-19 mg/L	—	—
Phenylbutazone (Butazolidin)	100 mg/L	—	—
Phenytoin (Dilantin)	5-22 mg/L	50 mg/L	100 mg/L
Phosphorus	Concentration in tissues usually used	—	—
Primidone (Mysoline)	10 mg/L	50-80 mg/L	100 mg/L
Probenecid (Benemid)	100-200 mg/L	—	—
Procainamide	6 mg/L	10 mg/L	—
Prochlorperazine (Compazine)	—	1 mg/L	—
Promazine (Sparine)	—	1 mg/L	—
Propoxyphene	50-200 μg/L	5-2 mg/L	57 mg/L
Propranolol (Inderal)	0.025-0.2 mg/L	—	8-12 mg/L
Propylhexedrine (Benzedrex)	—	—	2-3 mg/L
Quinidine	3-6 mg/L	10 mg/L	30-50 mg/L
Quinine	—	—	12 mg/L
Salicylate (acetylsalicylic acid)	20-100 mg/L	150-300 mg/L	500 mg/L
Strychnine	—	2 mg/L	9-12 mg/L
Sulfadiazine	80-150 mg/L	—	—
Sulfadimethoxine (Madribon)	80-100 mg/L	—	—
Sulfaguanidine	30-50 mg/L	—	—
Sulfanilamide	100-150 mg/L	—	—
Sulfisoxazole (Gantrisin)	90-100 mg/L	—	—
Theophylline	20-100 mg/L	—	—
Thioridazine (Mellaril)	1-1.5 mg/L	10 mg/L	20-80 mg/L
Tin	0.12 mg/L	—	—
Tolbutamide (Orinase)	53-96 mg/L	—	—
Toluene	—	—	10 mg/L
Tribromoethanol	—	—	90 mg/L
Trichloroethane	—	—	0.01-1 g/L
Trimethobenzamide (Tigan)	1.0-2.0 mg/L	—	—
Warfarin	1.0-10 mg/L	—	—
Zinc	0.68-1.36 mg/L	—	—
Zoxazolamine (Flexin)	3-13 mg/L	—	—

REFERENCES

1. Beller, G.A., Smith, T.W., Abelmann, W.H., Haber, E., and Hood, W.B.: Digitalis intoxication: a prospective clinical study with serum level correlations, N. Engl. J. Med. **284:**989, 1971.

2. Koch-Weser, J.: Serum drug concentrations as therapeutic guides, N. Engl. J. Med. **287:**227, 1972.

3. Koch-Weser, J., and Klein, S.W.: Procainamide dosage schedules, plasma concentrations and clinical effects, JAMA **215:**1454, 1971.

4. McBay, A.J.: Toxicological findings in fatal poisonings, Clin. Chem. **19:**361, 1973.

5. Reidenberg, M.M.: Protein binding of diphenylhydantoin and desmethylimipramine in plasma from patients with poor renal function, N. Engl. J. Med. **285:**264, 1971.

6. Thomson, P.D., Rowland, M., and Melmon, K.L.: Influence of heart failure, liver disease, and renal failure on the disposition of lidocaine in man, Am. Heart J. **82:**417, 1971.

7. Winek, C.L.: Tabulation of therapeutic, toxic and lethal concentrations of drugs and chemicals in blood, Clin. Chem. **22:**832, 1976.

Comparison of selected effects
of commonly abused drugs

Some selected effects of commonly abused drugs are summarized in the table shown on pp. 762 to 763. This table is intended for quick reference only. Greater detail on the subject is available in Chapter 31 dealing with contemporary drug abuse.

Drug category	Physical dependence	Characteristics of intoxication
Opiates (see p. 321 for classification)	Marked	Analgesia with or without depressed sensorium; pinpoint pupils (tolerance does not develop to this action); patient may be alert and appear normal; respiratory depression with overdose
Barbiturates	Marked	Patient may appear normal with usual dose, but narrow margin between doses needed to prevent withdrawal symptoms and toxic dose is often exceeded and patient appears "drunk," with drowsiness, ataxia, slurred speech, and nystagmus on lateral gaze; pupil size and reaction normal; respiratory depression with overdose
Nonbarbiturate sedatives Glutethimide (Doriden)	Marked	Pupils dilated and reactive to light; coma and respiratory depression prolonged; sudden apnea and laryngeal spasm common
Antianxiety agents* ("minor tranquilizers")	Marked	Progressive depression of sensorium as with barbiturates; pupil size and reaction normal; respiratory depression with overdose
Ethanol	Marked	Depressed sensorium, acute or chronic brain syndrome, odor on breath, pupil size and reaction normal
Amphetamines	Mild to absent	Agitation with paranoid thought disturbance in high doses; acute organic brain syndrome after prolonged use; pupils dilated and reactive; tachycardia, elevated blood pressure, with possibility of hypertensive crisis and CVA; possibility of convulsive seizures
Cocaine	Absent	Paranoid thought disturbance in high doses, with dangerous delusions of persecution and omnipotence; tachycardia; respiratory depression with overdose
Marijuana	Absent	Milder preparations: drowsy, euphoric state with frequent inappropriate laughter and disturbance in perception of time or space (occasional acute psychotic reaction reported); stronger preparations such as hashish: frequent hallucinations or psychotic reaction; pupils normal, conjunctivas injected (marijuana preparations frequently adulterated with LSD, tryptamines, or heroin)
Psychotomimetics LSD, STP, tryptamines, mescaline, morning glory seeds	Absent	Unpredictable disturbance in ego function, manifest by extreme lability of affect and chaotic disruption of thought, with danger of uncontrolled behavioral disturbance; pupils dilated and reactive to light
Phencyclidine	Unknown	Disinhibition, agitation, confusion, chaotic thought disturbance, unpredictable behavior, hypertension, miosis, respiratory collapse, cardiovascular collapse, death
Anticholinergic agents	Absent	Nonpsychotropic effects such as tachycardia, decreased salivary secretion, urinary retention, and dilated, nonreactive pupils plus depressed sensorium, confusion, disorientation, hallucinations, and delusional thinking
Inhalants†	Unknown	Depressed sensorium, hallucinations, acute brain syndrome; odor on breath; patient often with glassy-eyed appearance

Modified from Dimijian, G.G.: Drug Ther. 1:7, 1971.
*Meprobamate (Equanil), chlordiazepoxide (Librium), diazepam (Valium), ethchlorvynol (Placidyl), and ethinamate (Valmid).
†The term *inhalant* is used to designate a variety of gases and highly volatile organic liquids, including the aromatic glues, paint thinners, gasoline, some anesthetic agents, and amylnitrite. The term excludes liquids sprayed into the nasopharynx (droplet transport required) and substances that must be ignited before administration (such as marijuana).

Characteristics of withdrawal	"Flashback" symptoms	Masking of symptoms of illness or injury during intoxication
Rhinorrhea, lacrimation, and dilated, reactive pupils, followed by gastrointestinal disturbances, low back pain, and waves of gooseflesh; convulsions not a feature unless heroin samples were adulterated with barbiturates	Not reported	An important feature of opiate intoxication, due to analgesic action, with or without depressed sensorium
Agitation, tremulousness, insomnia, gastrointestinal disturbances, hyperpyrexia, blepharoclonus (clonic blink reflex), acute brain syndrome, major convulsive seizures	Not reported	Only in presence of depressed sensorium or after onset of acute brain syndrome
Similar to barbiturate withdrawal syndrome, with agitation, gastrointestinal disturbances, hyperpyrexia, and major convulsive seizures	Not reported	Same as in barbiturate intoxication
Similar to barbiturate withdrawal syndrome, with danger of major convulsive seizures	Not reported	Same as in barbiturate intoxication
Similar to barbiturate withdrawal syndrome, but with less likelihood of convulsive seizures	Not reported	Same as in barbiturate intoxication
Lethargy, somnolence, dysphoria, and possibility of suicidal depression; brain syndrome may persist for many weeks	Infrequently reported	Drug-induced euphoria or acute brain syndrome may interfere with awareness of symptoms of illness or may remove incentive to report symptoms of illness
Similar to amphetamine withdrawal	Not reported	Same as in amphetamine intoxication
No specific withdrawal symptoms	Infrequently reported	Uncommon with milder preparations; stronger preparations may interfere in same manner as psychotomimetic agents
No specific withdrawal symptoms; symptomatology may persist for indefinite period after discontinuation of drug	Commonly reported as late as 1 year after last dose	Affective response or psychotic thought disturbance may remove awareness of, or incentive to report, symptoms of illness
No specific withdrawal symptoms	Occasionally reported	Same as in LSD intoxication
No specific withdrawal symptoms; mydriasis may persist for several days	Not reported	Pain may not be reported as a result of depression of sensorium, acute brain syndrome, or acute psychotic reaction
No specific withdrawal symptoms	Infrequently reported	Same as in anticholinergic intoxication

Half-lives of drugs in normal subjects

Drug	Half-life (hours)						Major route of elimination
	<1.0 ± 0.5	2 ± 0.5	4 ± 1.5	12 ± 6	24 ± 6	>30	
Acetaminophen		X					Hepatic
Acetazolamide			X				Renal
Acetylsalicylic acid	X						Renal (hepatic)
Allopurinol							Renal
Amantadine				X			Renal
Amikacin		X					Renal
Amiloride			X				Renal
p-Aminosalicylic acid	X						Renal (hepatic)
Amobarbital					X		Hepatic
Amoxicillin	X						Renal
Amphetamine				X			Hepatic (renal)
Amphotericin B					X		Nonrenal
Ampicillin	X						Renal (hepatic)
Antipyrine				X			Hepatic
Atropine					X		Renal (hepatic)
Aurothiomalate sodium						X	Renal
Barbital						X	Renal
Bupivacaine		X					Hepatic
Calcitonin	X						—
Carbamazepine						X	Hepatic
Carbenicillin	X						Renal (hepatic)
Cefazolin		X					Renal
Cephalexin	X						Renal
Cephalothin	X						Renal (hepatic)
Chloramphenicol		X					Hepatic (renal)
Chlordiazepoxide				X			Hepatic
Chlorpromazine					X		Hepatic
Chlorpropamide						X	Hepatic (renal)
Chlortetracycline			X				Renal (hepatic)

Modified from Bennett W.M., et al.: Ann. Intern. Med. **86**:754, 1977; and Pagliaro, L.A., and Benet, L.Z.: J. Pharmacokinet. Biopharm. 3:353, 1975.

Drug	Half-life (hours)						Major route of elimination
	<1.0 ± 0.5	2 ± 0.5	4 ± 1.5	12 ± 6	24 ± 6	>30	
Clindamycin		X					Hepatic (renal)
Cloxacillin	X						Hepatic (renal)
Colchicine	X						Renal (hepatic)
Colistimethate			X				Renal
Cortisone	X						Hepatic
Cyclophosphamide			X				Hepatic (renal)
Cycloserine				X			Renal
Cytarabine		X					Nonrenal
Dapsone					X		Renal
Desipramine					X		Hepatic
Diazepam						X	Hepatic (renal)
Diazoxide					X		Renal
Dicloxacillin	X						Renal (hepatic)
Dicumarol					X		Nonrenal
Digitoxin						X	Hepatic (renal)
Digoxin						X	Renal (nonrenal)
Diphenoxylate		X					Hepatic
Doxycycline				X			Renal (hepatic)
Ephedrine			X				Renal (hepatic)
Ethambutol			X				Renal
Ethosuximide						X	Hepatic (renal)
Furosemide	X						Renal
Gentamicin		X					Renal
Glutethimide				X			Hepatic
Griseofulvin				X			—
Guanethidine						X	Renal (nonrenal)
Haloperidol					X		Renal (hepatic)
Heparin		X					Nonrenal
Hydralazine			X				Hepatic (renal)
Hydrocortisone	X						Hepatic
Indomethacin		X					Hepatic (renal)
Insulin	X						Nonrenal
Isoniazid		X					Hepatic (renal)
Kanamycin		X					Renal
Lidocaine		X					Hepatic (renal)
Lincomycin			X				Hepatic (renal)
Lithium					X		Renal
Meperidine			X				Hepatic (renal)
Meprobamate				X			Hepatic (renal)
6-Mercaptopurine	X						Hepatic
Methacycline				X			Hepatic (renal)
Methadone				X			Hepatic (renal <21%)
Methaqualone				X			Hepatic
Methicillin	X						Renal (hepatic)
Methimazole				X			Renal
Methyltestosterone			X				Hepatic
Minocycline				X			Hepatic

Continued.

Drug	Half-life (hours)						Major route of elimination
	<1.0 ± 0.5	2 ± 0.5	4 ± 1.5	12 ± 6	24 ± 6	>30	
Minoxidil			X				Nonrenal
Morphine		X					Hepatic
Nafcillin	X						Hepatic (renal)
Nalidixic acid	X						Renal (hepatic)
Nitrofurantoin	X						Renal
Nitroglycerin	X						Hepatic
Nortriptyline					X		Hepatic
Oxacillin	X						Renal (hepatic)
Oxyphenbutazone						X	Hepatic
Oxytetracycline				X			Renal (hepatic)
Penicillin G	X						Renal
Pentazocine			X				Hepatic
Pentobarbital						X	Hepatic
Phenacetin	X						Hepatic
Phenobarbital						X	Hepatic (renal)
Phenylbutazone						X	Hepatic
Phenytoin					X		Hepatic (renal)
Pralidoxime	X						Hepatic (renal)
Prednisolone		X					Hepatic
Probenecid				X			Nonrenal (renal)
Procainamide		X					Renal (hepatic)
Propoxyphene			X				Hepatic (renal >23%)
Propranolol			X				Hepatic
Propylthiouracil	X						Renal
Pseudoephedrine			X				Renal
Quinidine			X				Nonrenal (renal 12% to 36%)
Reserpine							Nonrenal
Rifampicin			X				Hepatic
Salicylic acid			X				Renal (hepatic)
Spectinomycin		X					Renal
Streptomycin		X					Renal
Sulfadiazine				X			Renal
Sulfamethoxazole				X			Renal
Sulfamethoxypyridazine					X		Renal
Sulfinpyrazone			X				Hepatic
Sulfisoxazole			X				Renal
Testosterone		X					Hepatic
Tetracycline				X			Renal (hepatic)
Theophylline			X				Hepatic
Thiothixene						X	Hepatic
l-Thyroxine						X	Hepatic
Tobramycin		X					Renal
Tolbutamide				X			Hepatic
l-Triiodothyronine					X		Hepatic
Trimethoprim				X			Renal
Vancomycin			X				Renal
Warfarin						X	Nonrenal

Index